One Health Integration

One Health Integration

Global Perspectives on Animal Health and Sustainable Agriculture

Edited by

Pratik Subhash Gaikwad
Vivek Harishankar Shukla
Pintu Choudhary

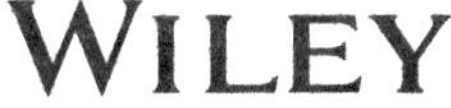

This edition first published 2026

Registered Offices
John Wiley & Sons, Inc., 111 River Street, Hoboken, NJ 07030, USA
John Wiley & Sons Ltd, New Era House, 8 Oldlands Way, Bognor Regis, West Sussex, PO22 9NQ, UK

For details of our global editorial offices, customer services, and more information about Wiley products visit us at www.wiley.com.

The manufacturer's authorized representative according to the EU General Product Safety Regulation is Wiley-VCH GmbH, Boschstr. 12, 69469 Weinheim, Germany, e-mail: Product_Safety@wiley.com.

Wiley also publishes its books in a variety of electronic formats and by print-on-demand. Some content that appears in standard print versions of this book may not be available in other formats.

Library of Congress Cataloging-in-Publication Data has been applied for:

Hardback: 9781394295951
ePDF: 9781394295975
epub: 9781394295968
obook: 9781394295982

Cover Design: Wiley
Cover Image: © Rifat Creations/stock.adobe.com, © Komola/stock.adobe.com, © Creative Worlds/stock.adobe.com, © Pinak/stock.adobe.com, © djvstock/stock.adobe.com, © Kateryna Kovarzh/stock.adobe.com, © Ramcreative/stock.adobe.com, © Salamatik/stock.adobe.com

STIX Two Text 9.5/12.5 by Lumina Datamatics

SKY10132471_112625

Contents

List of Contributors *xiii*
Preface *xvii*
About the Companion Website *xix*

1 Global Overview of Veterinary Sciences *1*
Khalida Shaikh, Drishti Dange, Zainab Ali Abbas Magar, and Pratik Subhash Gaikwad
1.1 Introduction *2*
1.1.1 Definition and Scope of Veterinary Sciences *2*
1.1.2 Historical Evolution of Veterinary Medicine *2*
1.1.3 Current Trends and Innovations *2*
1.2 Role of Veterinary Sciences in Public Health *3*
1.2.1 Veterinary Contributions to Public Health *3*
1.2.2 Disease Prevention and Control *4*
1.2.3 Zoonotic Diseases *5*
1.3 Veterinary Sciences and Food Security *6*
1.3.1 Livestock Health and Productivity *7*
1.3.2 Safe Food Practices *7*
1.4 Environmental Sustainability *8*
1.4.1 Sustainable Agricultural Practices *8*
1.4.2 Impact of Veterinary Practices on Ecosystems *9*
1.4.3 Role in Biodiversity Conservation *10*
1.5 Contemporary Challenges in Veterinary *10*
1.5.1 Emerging Infectious Diseases *11*
1.5.2 Antimicrobial Resistance *11*
1.5.3 Climate Change and Animal Health *12*
1.6 One Health *13*
1.6.1 Concept and Principles *13*
1.6.2 One Health Framework *14*
1.6.3 Applications of One Health in Veterinary Sciences *15*
1.7 Global Initiatives and Frameworks *16*
1.7.1 World Organisation for Animal Health (WOAH) *16*
1.7.2 Food and Agriculture Organization *18*
1.7.3 Global Collaborations *19*
1.8 Future Directions *19*
1.8.1 Research Opportunities for Innovations *20*
1.8.2 Educational Strategies *20*

1.8.3 Policy Development *21*
1.9 Conclusion *22*
References *22*

2 One Health Approach Worldwide and Challenges in Collaboration *33*
I Made Dwi Mertha Adnyana, Ni Luh Gede Sudaryati, Dwinka Syafira Eljatin, Ronald Pratama Adiwinoto and Zito Viegas da Cruz
2.1 Introduction to the One Health Approach *34*
2.2 Case Studies on Successful Health Collaborations *35*
2.2.1 Rabies Control Worldwide *35*
2.2.2 Avian Influenza Response Worldwide *37*
2.2.3 Zoonotic Disease Control Worldwide *39*
2.2.4 Antimicrobial Resistance Worldwide *40*
2.3 One Health Event in Recent Global Health Events *41*
2.3.1 The Role of One's Health in Handling the COVID-19 Pandemic *41*
2.3.2 Health in Facing the Threat of Antimicrobial Resistance *43*
2.3.3 One Health in Mitigating the Impacts of Climate Change on Health *45*
2.3.4 One Health and Zoonotic Disease Control *46*
2.3.5 One Health in Addressing the Global Health Crisis of Neglected Tropical Diseases *47*
2.3.6 Comparative Summary of Case Studies on Successful One Health Collaboration *48*
2.4 Technology and Innovation in the One Health Field *48*
2.4.1 Digital Surveillance Systems *48*
2.4.2 Genomic Sequencing *50*
2.4.3 Technological Innovations and Their Applications in the One Health Field *51*
2.5 Overcoming Challenges in Cross-disciplinary Cooperation *51*
2.5.1 Institutional Barriers *51*
2.5.2 Cultural and Disciplinary Differences *53*
2.5.3 Resource Constraints *54*
2.5.4 Data Sharing and Privacy Issues *54*
2.6 Conclusion *55*
Abbreviations *55*
References *56*

3 Connection of Human, Animal, and Environmental Health: A One Health Perspective *63*
Budi Utomo
3.1 Introduction *63*
3.2 Interdependence of Human, Animal, and Environmental Well-being *64*
3.2.1 Animals as Vectors of Disease in Human *66*
3.2.2 Animals as Sentinels of Human Health *67*
3.2.3 Animals in Biomedical Research *67*
3.3 Addressing Zoonotic Diseases Through a Holistic Approach *68*
3.4 AMR: A One Health Perspective *70*
3.4.1 AMR Overview *70*
3.4.2 Lack of New Antibiotics Development *71*
3.4.3 Strategies to Combat AMR *72*
3.4.4 Impact of AMR on Animal Health *73*
3.4.5 Environmental Factors *73*
3.5 Global Implications of Environmental Health on Public Health *75*

3.6 Conclusion *76*
References *77*

4 Integrating One Health into Global Veterinary Education *81*
Delower Hossain, Ridwan Olamilekan Adesola, Easrat Jahan Esha, Nasir Uddin, Oluwaseun Adeolu Ogundijo, Olamilekan Gabriel Banwo, Adetolase Azizat Bakre, Amitush Dutta, Mir Mohammad Ali, AHM Musleh Uddin and Sabiha Zarin Tasnim Bristi
4.1 Introduction *82*
4.2 Current State of Veterinary Education *84*
4.2.1 Traditional Veterinary Curricula *84*
4.2.2 Gaps and Limitations in Current VE Models *85*
4.2.3 Overview of Existing One Health Programs *86*
4.3 Transformative Strategies for Veterinary Education *87*
4.3.1 Rethinking Curriculum Design *87*
4.3.2 Core Competencies in One Health *88*
4.3.3 Incorporating Public Health and Environmental Science *89*
4.3.4 Innovative Pedagogical Methods *91*
4.3.5 Leveraging Technology for One Health Education *93*
4.3.6 Assessment and Evaluation Techniques *94*
4.4 Institutional One Health Model: A Global Perspective *95*
4.4.1 Utrecht University, the Netherlands *95*
4.4.2 University of California, Davis, United States *95*
4.4.3 University of Minnesota, United States *97*
4.4.4 Royal Veterinary College, UK *97*
4.4.5 University of Tokyo, Japan *97*
4.4.6 University of Veterinary and Animal Sciences, Pakistan *98*
4.4.7 One Health Institute, Chattogram Veterinary and Animal Sciences University, Bangladesh *98*
4.4.8 Kerala Veterinary and Animal Sciences University, India *99*
4.4.9 University of Nairobi, Kenya *99*
4.4.10 University of Pretoria, South Africa *99*
4.4.11 University of Ibadan, Ibadan, Nigeria *100*
4.4.12 Queensland Alliance for One Health Sciences, University of Queensland, Australia *100*
4.4.13 Lessons Learned and Key Takeaways *100*
4.5 Fostering Interdisciplinary Learning Environments *100*
4.5.1 Building Collaborative Partnerships *100*
4.5.2 Creating Interdisciplinary Courses and Modules *103*
4.5.3 Utilizing Problem-based Learning *104*
4.5.4 Incorporating Fieldwork and Practical Experiences *104*
4.5.5 Promoting Cross-disciplinary Research Projects *105*
4.5.6 Enhancing Communication and Leadership Skills *106*
4.6 Building Institutional Capacity *106*
4.6.1 Faculty Training and Development *106*
4.6.2 Infrastructure and Resource Allocation *107*
4.6.3 Policy and Institutional Support *108*
4.6.4 Funding and Sustainability *108*
4.7 Research and Innovation in One Health *108*
4.7.1 Promoting Interdisciplinary Research *108*
4.7.2 Innovative Research Methodologies *109*

4.7.3 Case Studies of Impactful One Health Research 109
4.8 Global Perspectives on One Health Education 110
4.8.1 Regional Case Studies: Africa, Asia, Europe, and the Americas 110
4.8.2 Adapting One Health Education to Local Contexts 111
4.8.3 International Collaboration and Exchange Programs 111
4.9 Policy and Advocacy 112
4.9.1 Role of Veterinary Associations and Organizations 112
4.9.2 Roles of Development Partners and Organizations 114
4.9.3 Influencing Policy at the National and International Levels 115
4.9.4 Advocacy Strategies for One Health Integration 116
4.10 Future Directions in One Health Education 116
4.11 Conclusion 117
Abbreviations 118
Author Contributions 119
Conflicts of Interest 119
Acknowledgments 119
Dedication 119
References 119

5 Advanced Veterinary Sciences for Sustainable Agriculture and Global Food Security 135
Abdullah Ahmed Butt and Zahra Ahmed
5.1 Introduction 136
5.1.1 Impacts of Animal Diseases on Food Production and Global Food Security 136
5.2 Technological Innovations in Veterinary Medicine and Agriculture 138
5.2.1 Advancements in Diagnostics and Disease Surveillance 139
5.2.2 Emerging Technologies for Disease Prevention and Control 140
5.3 One Health Approach: Integrating Veterinary and Human Health 141
5.3.1 One Health: Relevance to Agriculture and Food Security 141
5.4 Nutrition and Feed Management for Livestock Health 142
5.4.1 Importance of Balanced Nutrition for Animal Health and Productivity 143
5.4.2 Innovations in Feed Formulation and Delivery Systems 143
5.4.3 Sustainable Feed Production Practices 144
5.5 Disease Control and Biosecurity Measures 145
5.5.1 Strategies for Preventing and Managing Infectious Disease in Livestock 145
5.5.2 Biosecurity Protocols for Farms and Food Production Facilities 146
5.5.3 Role of Vaccination in Disease Control and Eradication 147
5.6 Climate Change and Veterinary Challenges 148
5.6.1 Impact of Climate Change on Animal Health and Agriculture 148
5.6.2 Adaptation Strategies for Livestock Farming in Changing Environmental Conditions 149
5.6.3 Mitigation Measures to Reduce the Environmental Footprint of Animal Agriculture 150
5.7 Veterinary Extension and Capacity Building 151
5.7.1 Importance of Education and Training in Veterinary Sciences for Sustainable Agriculture 151
5.7.2 Extension Services to Disseminate Best Practices and Innovations 152
5.7.3 Capacity Building Initiatives for Veterinary Professionals in Developing Countries 153
5.8 Challenges and Future Directions 155
5.8.1 Identifying Challenges in Veterinary Medicine and Agriculture 155
5.8.2 Opportunities for Future Research and Collaboration 156
5.8.3 Exemplary Projects Showcasing the Application of Advanced Veterinary Sciences 157

5.8.4 Lessons Learned and Recommendations for Future Interventions *158*
5.9 Conclusion *159*
References *160*

6 Global Zoonotic Diseases and Public Health: A One Health Perspective *165*
Delower Hossain, Shamsaldeen Ibrahim Saeed, Daniel Jesuwenu Ajose, Chidozie Freedom Egbu, Ridwan Olamilekan Adesola, Oluwaseun Adeolu Ogundijo, Olamilekan Gabriel Banwo, Fernando Ulloa, and Sabiha Zarin Tasnim Bristi
6.1 Introduction *166*
6.2 Emerging Trends in Global Zoonotic Diseases *167*
6.2.1 Distribution of Zoonotic Diseases Globally *167*
6.2.2 Factors Driving the Emergence and Spread of Zoonotic Diseases *168*
6.2.3 Epidemiology of Emerging and Re-emerging Zoonotic Diseases (December 2019–January 2025) *171*
6.2.4 Challenges in Predicting and Controlling Zoonoses *176*
6.2.5 Economic and Societal Effects of Zoonotic Disease Outbreaks *176*
6.3 One Health Strategies for Disease Surveillance and Prevention *177*
6.3.1 Principles of the One Health Approach *177*
6.3.2 Interconnectivity of the One Health Component Parts *177*
6.3.3 Multidisciplinary Approaches to Disease Surveillance and Prevention *178*
6.3.4 Integrated Surveillance Systems for Rapid Diagnosis and Swift Action of Zoonoses *180*
6.4 Collaborative Approaches in Pandemic Preparedness *181*
6.4.1 Understanding the Risk of Zoonotic Disease Pandemics *181*
6.4.2 International Frameworks for Pandemic Preparedness and Response *181*
6.4.3 Importance of Multisectoral Collaboration in Pandemic Response *182*
6.4.4 Role of Interdisciplinary Collaboration in Pandemic Preparedness *182*
6.4.5 Vaccine Development and Distribution *183*
6.4.6 Public Awareness and Community Engagement Initiatives *183*
6.5 Social and Ecological Dimensions of Zoonotic Diseases *184*
6.5.1 Impact of Socio-economic Factors on Zoonotic Disease Transmission *184*
6.5.2 Role of Environmental Factors in Zoonotic Disease Emergence and Spread *185*
6.5.3 Role of Cultural Practices and Behavior Changes in Zoonotic Disease Emergence and Spread *186*
6.5.4 Importance of Sustainable Land Use and Wildlife Conservation in Disease Prevention *187*
6.6 Case Studies and Examples of Global Zoonoses Control and OH Integration *188*
6.6.1 Successful One Health Interventions *188*
6.6.2 Lessons Learned from Previous Zoonotic Outbreaks *189*
6.7 Challenges and Opportunities *191*
6.7.1 Barriers to Implementing One Health *191*
6.7.2 Strategies for Overcoming Challenges *192*
6.8 Conclusion *193*
Abbreviations *194*
Author Contributions *194*
Conflicts of Interest *194*
References *194*

7 Advancing Veterinary Medicine for Biodiversity Conservation and Global Wildlife Health *209*
Sonam Bhatt, Anil Kumar, Arzoo Nisha, Ashish Tripathi, R. S. K. Mandal, Rohit Jaiswal and Bhavna
7.1 Intersection of Veterinary Medicine and Wildlife Conservation *210*
7.1.1 Health Assessment, Disease Monitoring, Surveillance, and Control *210*

7.1.2 Captive Propagation and Reintroduction/Wildlife Rehabilitation and Release *211*
7.1.3 Identification of Critical Health Factors with Impact on Wildlife Population Dynamics *211*
7.1.4 Integrated Approaches to Protect Ecosystem *211*
7.1.5 Wildlife Management *212*
7.1.6 Conflict Resolution *212*
7.1.7 Legal and Ethical Considerations *212*
7.1.8 Research and Innovation *213*
7.1.9 Public Education and Advocacy *214*
7.2 Addressing Health Challenges in Diverse Ecosystems *214*
7.2.1 Veterinarians in Wildlife Conservation *214*
7.2.2 Addressing Intensive Livestock Farming *215*
7.2.3 Ecological Medicine *216*
7.2.4 Integrating Ecosystem Health in Veterinary Curriculum *217*
7.3 One Health Initiatives for Biodiversity Protection *217*
7.3.1 Threats to Biodiversity Addressed by One Health *218*
7.3.2 Role of Veterinarians in One Health for Biodiversity *218*
7.3.3 Holistic One Health Strategies for Advancing Global Health *220*
7.4 Conclusion *222*
References *222*

8 Emerging Global Technologies in Veterinary Sciences *227*
Benedict Terkula Iber, Pranshul Sethi, Ramandeep Saini, Nainci Dhiman, and Ayush Madan
8.1 Introduction *228*
8.1.1 Overview of Veterinary Sciences *228*
8.1.2 Conventional vs. Advanced Methods in Veterinary Sciences *229*
8.1.3 Importance of Technological Advancements in Veterinary Medicine *230*
8.2 Diagnostic Technologies *230*
8.2.1 Imaging Techniques in Veterinary Diagnostics *231*
8.2.2 Molecular Diagnostics in Veterinary Medicine *233*
8.2.3 Point-of-care Testing Devices for Rapid Diagnosis *235*
8.3 Treatment and Therapeutic Technologies *236*
8.3.1 Advanced Surgical Techniques in Veterinary Medicine *237*
8.3.2 Emerging Therapies in Veterinary Oncology *238*
8.3.3 Rehabilitation and Physiotherapy for Animals *238*
8.3.4 Gene Therapy and Regenerative Medicine for Animals *239*
8.3.5 Nanotechnology Applications for Drug Delivery in Animals *239*
8.3.6 Immunotherapy and Vaccines: Advancements in Preventative Medicine *239*
8.4 Digital Health and Telemedicine *239*
8.4.1 Teleconsultation Services for Remote Diagnosis *240*
8.4.2 Wearable Health Monitoring Devices for Pets *240*
8.4.3 Remote Surgery Guidance: Advancements in Teleoperation *241*
8.4.4 Mobile Applications for Animal Healthcare *242*
8.5 Impact of Technology on Animal Welfare and Management *243*
8.5.1 Precision Livestock Farming *243*
8.5.2 Use of VR in Animal Training *247*
8.6 Technological Innovations in Animal Nutrition *247*
8.6.1 Precision Feeding System for Livestock *247*
8.6.2 Nutrigenomics in Animal Nutrition Research *248*

8.6.3 Smart Feeders and Automated Diet Management *250*
8.7 Future Perspectives *250*
8.8 Conclusion *251*
References *251*

9 Global Policy Frameworks and Future Directions for Veterinary Sciences *257*
Bernabé Vidal, Lorenzo Verger, Linda Ternova, and Gustavo J. Nagy
9.1 Introduction *258*
9.2 International Policies Shaping Veterinary Sciences *258*
9.2.1 Origins and Early Drivers of International Collaboration for Animal Disease Control *258*
9.2.2 Incorporation of Veterinary Sciences into the Global Public Health Sphere *259*
9.2.3 New Fields of Action, New Policies: Animal Welfare and Wildlife Health *260*
9.2.4 Development of Holistic Health Concepts *261*
9.2.5 Current International Policies on OH and Planetary Health *261*
9.3 Collaborative Frameworks for Global Health Initiatives *263*
9.3.1 Introduction to Collaborative Frameworks: Origins and Core Concepts *263*
9.3.2 Global Health Stakeholders, Evolving Relationships, and Interdisciplinarity *264*
9.3.3 Key Principles, Strategies, and Successful Initiatives for Effective Development *266*
9.3.4 Current Situation, Barriers, and Problems *267*
9.4 Anticipated Future Trends and Policy Considerations *268*
9.4.1 Veterinary Sciences, Policies, and Public Health Challenges and Trends *268*
9.4.2 Climate Change, Environmental Shifts, Increased Endemic Areas, and the Emergence of Zoonotic Vector-borne Diseases *270*
9.4.3 Science and Policy in Action: Future Trends and Challenges in Decision-making in Animal Health and Epidemiology *271*
9.4.4 The United Nations SDGs Framework for Addressing Future Global Challenges in Veterinary Science and Policies *271*
9.4.5 Planetary Health: A Bibliometric Review of Current and Expected Trends and Policy Implications *272*
9.5 Summary of Chapter *275*
9.5.1 International Policies Shaping Veterinary Sciences *275*
9.5.2 Collaborative Frameworks for Global Health Initiatives (GHIs) *275*
9.5.3 Future Trends and Policy Considerations *275*
9.5.4 Bibliometric Research Findings (2017–2024) *275*
9.6 Conclusion *276*
References *276*

10 Challenges, Opportunities, and Future Directions in One Health Collaboration *283*
Ahmed Abdulkadir Hassan-Kadle, Zainab Ali Abbas Magar, Aamir Muse Osman and Pratik Subhash Gaikwad
10.1 Introduction *284*
10.2 Current Landscape of One Health Collaboration *284*
10.3 Challenges in One Health Collaboration *284*
10.3.1 Lack of Integrated One Health Approach *285*
10.3.2 Sectionalism and Fragmented Governance *286*
10.3.3 Resource Constraints *287*
10.3.4 Communication Barriers *287*
10.3.5 Conflicting Agendas *288*

10.3.6 Leadership and Continuity Challenges *288*
10.3.7 Cultural and Behavioral Differences *289*
10.3.8 Knowledge and Data Sharing Obstacles *289*
10.4 Opportunities in One Health Collaboration *290*
10.4.1 Strengthening Surveillance and Response *291*
10.4.2 Ensuring Sustainable Food Systems *291*
10.4.3 Promoting Environmental Sustainability *292*
10.4.4 Facilitating Research and Development *292*
10.4.5 Building Public Trust and Advocacy *293*
10.5 Future Directions in One Health Collaboration *293*
10.5.1 One Health Governance *294*
10.5.2 Multisectoral Communication and Coordination *295*
10.5.3 Building Sustainable One Health Systems *295*
10.5.4 Interdisciplinary Research *295*
10.5.5 Public–Private Partnerships in One Health *296*
10.5.6 Investing in One Health Education *296*
10.5.7 Ethical Considerations in Implementing One Health Practices *297*
10.5.8 Leveraging New Technologies and Tools *297*
10.5.9 Untapped Opportunities for Global Collaborations *298*
10.5.10 Envisioning a Sustainable and Healthier Future *299*
10.6 Conclusion *299*
References *300*

11 Interactive Learning and Practical Applications of One Health *307*
Vivek Harishankar Shukla, Pintu Choudhary and Pratik Subhash Gaikwad
11.1 Introduction *308*
11.2 One Health: A Holistic Approach to Learning and Interconnectivity *308*
11.2.1 Importance of Interdisciplinary Education *309*
11.3 Innovative Teaching Methodologies *310*
11.3.1 Problem-based Learning *312*
11.3.2 Simulations *312*
11.3.3 Field-based Experiences *312*
11.4 Case Studies in One Health *313*
11.4.1 Real-world Applications *313*
11.4.2 Success Stories and Lessons Learned *313*
11.5 Challenges in One Health Education *316*
11.5.1 Curriculum Integration *317*
11.5.2 Resource Limitations *317*
11.5.3 Interdisciplinary Collaboration *317*
11.6 Opportunities for Enhancing One Health Learning *318*
11.7 Conclusion *318*
References *318*

Multiple-choice Questions (MCQs) on One Health *323*
Vivek Harishankar Shukla and Pratik Subhash Gaikwad
Introduction *323*

Index *325*

List of Contributors

Ridwan Olamilekan Adesola
Department of Veterinary Medicine
University of Ibadan
Ibadan
Nigeria

Ronald Pratama Adiwinoto
Department of Public Health
Hang Tuah University
Surabaya city
Indonesia

I Made Dwi Mertha Adnyana
Department of Medical Professions
Universitas Jambi
Jambi City
Indonesia

Indonesian Society of Epidemiologists Daerah Khusus Ibukota
Jakarta
Indonesia

Royal Society of Tropical Medicine and Hygiene
London
United Kingdom

Zahra Ahmed
Department of Pharmacology
King Edward Medical University
Lahore
Pakistan

Daniel Jesuwenu Ajose
Department of Microbiology
North-West University
Mmabatho
South Africa

Mir Mohammad Ali
Department of Aquaculture
Sher-e-Bangla Agricultural University (SAU)
Dhaka
Bangladesh

Adetolase Azizat Bakre
Department of Veterinary Medicine
University of Ibadan
Ibadan
Nigeria

Olamilekan Gabriel Banwo
Department of Veterinary Medicine
University of Ibadan
Ibadan
Nigeria

Sonam Bhatt
Department of Veterinary Medicine
BASU
Patna, Bihar
India

Bhavna
Department of Veterinary Gynaecology and Obstetrics
BASU
Patna, Bihar
India

Sabiha Zarin Tasnim Bristi
Department of Veterinary Medicine and Animal Sciences (DIVAS)
Università degli Studi di Milano (UNIMI)
Lodi
Italy

Abdullah Ahmed Butt
Department of Food Science and Technology
Government College University
Faisalabad
Pakistan

Pintu Choudhary
Department of Food Technology
College of Agricultural Engineering and Technology
Dr Rajendra Prasad Central Agricultural University
Samastipur, Bihar
India

Zito Viegas da Cruz
Department of Epidemiological Surveillance
Serviçu Municipal da Saúde de Bobonaro
Maliana City
Timor-Leste

Drishti Dange
School of Biotechnology and Bioinformatics
D Y Patil Deemed to be University
Navi Mumbai, Maharashtra
India

Nainci Dhiman
Chandigarh College of Technology
Chandigarh Group of Colleges
Greater Mohali, Punjab
India

Amitush Dutta
Department of Animal Nutrition
Sylhet Agricultural University
Sylhet
Bangladesh

Chidozie Freedom Egbu
Department of Agriculture and Animal Health
University of South Africa
Roodepoort
South Africa

Department of Agricultural Science Education
Alvan Ikoku Federal University of Education
Owerri, Imo State
Nigeria

Dwinka Syafira Eljatin
Indonesian Society of Epidemiologists
Jakarta
Indonesia

Department of Medical
Institut Teknologi Sepuluh Nopember
Surabaya City
Indonesia

Easrat Jahan Esha
Fleming Fund Country Grant to Bangladesh
DAI Global
Dhaka
Bangladesh

Pratik Subhash Gaikwad
School of Biotechnology and Bioinformatics
D Y Patil Deemed to be University
Navi Mumbai, Maharashtra
India

Ahmed Abdulkadir Hassan-Kadle
Somali One Health Centre
Abrar University
Mogadishu
Somalia

Delower Hossain
Department of Medicine and Public Health
Sher-e-Bangla Agricultural University (SAU)
Dhaka
Bangladesh

Department of Veterinary Medicine and Animal Sciences (DIVAS)
Università degli Studi di Milano (UNIMI)
Lodi
Italy

Benedict Terkula Iber
Department of Fisheries and Aquaculture
Joseph Sarwuan Tarka University (Formerly, Federal University of Agriculture Makurdi)
Makurdi, Benue State
Nigeria

Institute of Tropical Aquaculture and Fisheries (AKUATROP)
Universiti Malaysia Terengganu
Kuala Nerus, Terengganu
Malaysia

Rohit Jaiswal
Department of Livestock Products Technology
BASU
Patna, Bihar
India

Anil Kumar
Department of Veterinary Medicine
BASU
Patna, Bihar
India

Ayush Madan
Department of Biotechnology
People's University
Bhopal, Madhya Pradesh
India

Institute of Tropical Aquaculture and Fisheries (AKUATROP)
Universiti Malaysia Terengganu
Kuala Nerus, Terengganu
Malaysia

Zainab Ali Abbas Magar
School of Biotechnology and Bioinformatics
D Y Patil Deemed to be University
Navi Mumbai, Maharashtra
India

R. S. K. Mandal
Department of Veterinary Medicine
BASU
Patna, Bihar
India

Gustavo J. Nagy
Graduate Programme in Environmental Sciences and Institute of Ecology and Environmental Sciences (IECA)
University of the Republic (FC-UdelaR)
Montevideo
Uruguay

Arzoo Nisha
Department of Veterinary Medicine
BASU
Patna, Bihar
India

Oluwaseun Adeolu Ogundijo
Department of Veterinary Public Health and Preventive Medicine
University of Ibadan
Ibadan
Nigeria

Aamir Muse Osman
Somali One Health Centre
Abrar University
Mogadishu
Somalia

Ministry of Livestock, Forestry, and Range
Federal Government of Somalia
Mogadishu
Somalia

Shamsaldeen Ibrahim Saeed
Nanotechnology in Veterinary Medicine Research Group
Universiti Malaysia Kelantan (UMK)
Pengkalan Chepa
Malaysia

Department of Microbiology
University of Nyala
Nyala
Sudan

Ramandeep Saini
Chandigarh College of Technology
Chandigarh Group of Colleges
Greater Mohali, Punjab
India

Pranshul Sethi
College of Pharmacy
Shri Venkateshwara University
Gajraula, Uttar Pradesh
India

Chitkara College of Pharmacy
Chitkara University
Rajpura, Punjab
India

Khalida Shaikh
School of Biotechnology and Bioinformatics
D Y Patil Deemed to be University
Navi Mumbai, Maharashtra
India

Vivek Harishankar Shukla
Department of Livestock Products Technology
Mumbai Veterinary College Parel
Mumbai, Maharashtra
India

Maharashtra Animal and Fishery Sciences University
Nagpur, Maharashtra
India

Ni Luh Gede Sudaryati
Department of Biology
Universitas Hindu Indonesia
Denpasar City
Indonesia

Linda Ternova
Faculty of Medicine Carl Gustav Carus
TUD Dresden University of Technology
Dresden
Germany

Ashish Tripathi
Department of Veterinary Medicine
BASU
Patna, Bihar
India

AHM Musleh Uddin
Department of Surgery and Theriogenology
Sylhet Agricultural University
Sylhet
Bangladesh

School of Animal and Veterinary Science
University of Adelaide
Roseworthy
Australia

Nasir Uddin
Centre for Integrative Conservation
Chinese Academy of Sciences
Xishuangbanna
People's Republic of China

Fernando Ulloa
Escuela de Graduados, Facultad de Ciencias Veterinarias
Universidad Austral de Chile
Valdivia
Chile

Budi Utomo
Department of Public Health & Preventive Medicine
Airlangga University
Surabaya
Indonesia

Lorenzo Verger
Department of Public Health
University of the Republic (FVET-UdelaR)
Montevideo
Uruguay

Zoonosis Division
Ministry of Public Health (MSP)
Montevideo
Uruguay

Bernabé Vidal
Graduate Programme in Environmental Sciences
University of the Republic (FC-UdelaR)
Montevideo
Uruguay

Preface

The health of humans, animals, and the environment is intricately connected, and this connection is becoming increasingly critical in light of global challenges such as emerging diseases, climate change, and antimicrobial resistance. *One Health Integration: Global Perspectives on Animal Health and Sustainable Agriculture* addresses these pressing issues through a multidisciplinary approach, offering an in-depth exploration of how veterinary sciences, environmental management, and human health intersect within the One Health framework.

Chapter 1 lays the groundwork by introducing the fundamentals of veterinary science, underscoring its crucial role in advancing both animal and public health. It establishes a foundation for understanding how veterinarians contribute to disease prevention and animal welfare, as well as to broader public health outcomes. Chapter 2 explores the concept of One Health, tracing its development and elucidating its core principles. It highlights the necessity of integrated policies and collaborative efforts to tackle complex health challenges that transcend species and national boundaries.

Chapter 3 investigates the nexus between animal health and global food systems, detailing how veterinary interventions enhance food safety, boost livestock productivity, and diminish the risk of zoonotic disease transmission. Chapter 4 showcases real-world case studies that exemplify the practical application of the One Health approach across various regions. These examples highlight successful strategies in zoonotic disease surveillance, wildlife conservation, and pandemic preparedness, illustrating the importance of cross-sector collaboration in achieving health benefits.

Chapter 5 addresses the pressing issue of antimicrobial resistance, investigating how this global threat is driven by interconnected practices in human medicine, veterinary applications, and environmental exposure. It emphasizes the need for coordinated stewardship efforts across all sectors. Chapter 6 focuses on technological advancements that support One Health goals, featuring innovations such as genomic tools, biosensors, and remote diagnostics that are revolutionizing disease monitoring and control in both veterinary and public health sectors.

Recognizing the significance of capacity-building, Chapter 7 focuses on education and training reforms within veterinary and allied health curricula. It highlights successful educational programs that promote interdisciplinary learning and prepare future professionals for collaborative practice. Chapter 8 discusses institutional frameworks and policy integration, stressing the essential role of governments, international organizations, academic institutions, and NGOs in implementing One Health through effective governance and communication.

Chapter 9 examines sustainable agriculture through the lens of veterinary science, focusing on how veterinarians contribute to climate-smart livestock management, animal welfare, and minimizing environmental impact. It explores how veterinary practices align with sustainable development goals, particularly in relation to food security and climate change mitigation. Chapter 10 synthesizes the key themes from the earlier chapters and envisions the future of the One Health approach. It advocates for enhanced leadership, increased investment in research, and stronger global partnerships to address the complex challenges at the intersection of human, animal, and environmental health.

Chapter 11 emphasizes the significance of experiential learning- and field-based education in deepening the understanding of One Health principles. It demonstrates how real-world exposure to health challenges and interdisciplinary collaboration can enrich learning and foster effective solutions to global health problems.

This book is intended for a diverse audience, including veterinary professionals, students, researchers, educators, and policymakers. It combines theoretical frameworks, real-world applications, and educational insights to promote integrated thinking and encourage collaboration. The content of the book is designed to be valuable for academic, research, and policy development while fostering collective action. Through this work, we aspire to strengthen the collective commitment to preserving the balance between humans, animals, and the environment, ultimately contributing to a more sustainable and healthier world.

Dr. Pratik Subhash Gaikwad
Assistant Professor,
School of Biotechnology and Bioinformatics,
D Y Patil Deemed to be University,
Navi Mumbai, Maharashtra – 400614, India.

About the Companion Website

This book is accompanied by a companion website:

https://www.wiley.com/go/pratikgaikwad/onehealth

This website includes:

Multiple-choice Questions (MCQs) on One Health

- **Introduction**
- **Section I:** One Health Approach
- **Section II:** Zoonotic Diseases
- **Section III:** Public Health
- **Section IV:** Epidemiology
- **Section V:** Climate Change, Environmental Health, and Urbanization
- **Section-wise Answer Key**

1

Global Overview of Veterinary Sciences

*Khalida Shaikh, Drishti Dange, Zainab Ali Abbas Magar, and Pratik Subhash Gaikwad**

School of Biotechnology and Bioinformatics, D Y Patil Deemed to be University, Navi Mumbai, Maharashtra, India

*Corresponding author: pratik.gaikwad@dypatil.edu

TABLE OF CONTENTS

1.1 Introduction
  1.1.1 Definition and Scope of Veterinary Sciences
  1.1.2 Historical Evolution of Veterinary Medicine
  1.1.3 Current Trends and Innovations
1.2 Role of Veterinary Sciences in Public Health
  1.2.1 Veterinary Contributions to Public Health
  1.2.2 Disease Prevention and Control
  1.2.3 Zoonotic Diseases
1.3 Veterinary Sciences and Food Security
  1.3.1 Livestock Health and Productivity
  1.3.2 Safe Food Practices
1.4 Environmental Sustainability
  1.4.1 Sustainable Agricultural Practices
  1.4.2 Impact of Veterinary Practices on Ecosystems
  1.4.3 Role in Biodiversity Conservation
1.5 Contemporary Challenges in Veterinary
  1.5.1 Emerging Infectious Diseases
  1.5.2 Antimicrobial Resistance
  1.5.3 Climate Change and Animal Health
1.6 One Health
  1.6.1 Concept and Principles
  1.6.2 One Health Framework
  1.6.3 Applications of One Health in Veterinary Sciences
1.7 Global Initiatives and Frameworks
  1.7.1 World Organisation for Animal Health (WOAH)
  1.7.2 Food and Agriculture Organization
  1.7.3 Global Collaborations
1.8 Future Directions
  1.8.1 Research Opportunities for Innovations
  1.8.2 Educational Strategies
  1.8.3 Policy Development
1.9 Conclusion
  References

One Health Integration: Global Perspectives on Animal Health and Sustainable Agriculture. First Edition.
Edited by Pratik Subhash Gaikwad, Vivek Harishankar Shukla and Pintu Choudhary.

Companion Website: https://www.wiley.com/go/pratikgaikwad/onehealth

1.1 Introduction

Veterinary science is vital for animal health, public health, and food security. Veterinarians diagnose, treat, and prevent diseases in animals, with a focus on sustainable practices and disease management in response to growing demand for animal products and zoonotic disease concerns. This chapter explores the global development of veterinary science, highlighting professionals, innovations, and international frameworks. It emphasizes the "One Health" approach, connecting animal, human, and environmental health and examines how technologies like precision medicine, genomics, and AI are transforming veterinary practice, crucial for public health and sustainability.

1.1.1 Definition and Scope of Veterinary Sciences

Veterinary sciences focus on the health, welfare, and medical treatment of animals, from pets to livestock and wildlife [1]. It integrates disciplines such as biology, medicine, and agriculture to diagnose conditions, develop treatments, and prevent diseases across species [2]. This interdisciplinary approach allows veterinarians to address health issues from routine care to advanced procedures [3]. Veterinary science plays a critical role in public health, food safety, and zoonotic disease control [4, 5], embodying the "One Health" concept, which links human, animal, and environmental health [6, 7]. Veterinarians monitor cross-species diseases, ensure the safety of animal-derived food, and contribute to epidemiological research [4, 5]. The field also emphasizes animal welfare [8], supports sustainable farming practices [9], and contributes to conservation efforts [10]. Additionally, veterinary science is crucial for comparative medicine, using animal models to enhance human healthcare [9]. Through its broad scope, veterinary science ensures the well-being of both animals and humans, while advancing medical knowledge and promoting global food security and ecosystem sustainability [9, 11].

1.1.2 Historical Evolution of Veterinary Medicine

The historical evolution of veterinary medicine showcases the deep and evolving relationship between humans and animals. Veterinary practice began in early societies where animals were integral for labor, companionship, and sustenance.

In ancient Egypt, treatments for cattle, dogs, and other domesticated animals were documented in hieroglyphs, demonstrating early knowledge of animal care [12]. Ancient Indian texts like the Sushruta Samhita described procedures for treating horses and elephants, vital for transport and warfare [13]. A major milestone occurred in 1762 with the founding of the first veterinary school in Lyon, France, marking the shift to scientific animal care [14].

In the nineteenth century, veterinary medicine progressed significantly alongside human medicine, marked by breakthroughs such as Louis Pasteur's identification of microorganisms and the creation of vaccines for anthrax and rabies [15]. The twentieth century brought innovations like antibiotics, improved surgical methods, and diagnostic technologies, including X-rays and MRIs. Specializations in fields like ophthalmology and cardiology emerged [13]. By the twenty-first century, molecular biology and genetics revolutionized diagnostics and treatments [13]. The evolution of veterinary medicine highlights the ongoing commitment to animal welfare, benefiting both animal and human health [15].

1.1.3 Current Trends and Innovations

In recent decades, veterinary sciences have undergone a significant transformation, integrating advanced technologies and innovative approaches across multiple domains. Telemedicine has emerged as an essential part of veterinary care, enabling remote consultations and monitoring. This became particularly important during the COVID-19 pandemic, improving accessibility and reducing costs [16, 17]. Genetic advancements, such as gene therapy and CRISPR, have expanded the field, offering potential treatments for genetic disorders and improving livestock traits [18].

AI and machine learning are transforming diagnostics by facilitating early disease detection, forecasting outbreaks, and improving surgical accuracy [19, 20]. Regenerative medicine, including stem cell therapy, provides new solutions for chronic conditions like joint diseases and spinal injuries [18]. A stronger focus on animal welfare has led to innovations in pain management, behavioral therapies, and environmental enrichment, improving the overall well-being of animals [18]. Furthermore, veterinary sciences play a vital role in public health through the One Health approach, addressing zoonotic diseases and contributing to global health security [9, 18].

As the field continues to evolve, it must tackle challenges such as climate change, habitat destruction, and emerging diseases, requiring interdisciplinary collaboration [9]. This progress reflects a growing respect for animals and the interconnectedness of all life, positioning veterinary science to enhance animal care, public health, and sustainability.

1.2 Role of Veterinary Sciences in Public Health

Veterinary science holds a pivotal place in public health by tackling major health concerns that affect both humans and animals. Veterinarians are responsible for managing zoonotic diseases, such as rabies, avian influenza, and bovine tuberculosis, that spread from animals to humans. Through their specialized knowledge, veterinarians help detect and prevent the spread of these illnesses, playing a vital role in protecting global health [21, 22]. Their responsibilities also involve adhering to international disease surveillance systems like the International Health Regulations (IHR), ensuring timely response to emerging threats [23]. This integration of veterinary expertise with public health efforts underscores the need for collaborative strategies in disease control and prevention.

Veterinarians also safeguard food safety and security by ensuring that livestock products like meat, milk, and eggs are free from contamination. Through regular health checks, inspections, and regulatory compliance, they uphold public trust in the food supply [24, 25]. In biomedical research, veterinarians use animal models to develop vaccines and treatments that benefit both species, supporting the One Health approach, which links human, animal, and environmental well-being [21, 22].

Additionally, veterinary professionals contribute to environmental health by managing wildlife, controlling vectors like mosquitoes and ticks, and preserving biodiversity [18]. Their efforts help maintain balanced ecosystems, which in turn support human health [26]. In times of crisis, such as natural disasters or disease outbreaks, veterinarians are key responders, helping manage animal welfare and prevent disease transmission, thereby strengthening community resilience [18, 23].

Urban expansion and growing rates of pet ownership are contributing to emerging challenges in the control of zoonotic diseases. This underscores the vital role of integrating veterinary services into public health frameworks, particularly in resource-constrained regions [27].

1.2.1 Veterinary Contributions to Public Health

Veterinary contributions to public health span diverse domains, significantly influencing both animal and human well-being. Veterinarians act as critical guardians of public health, working to prevent, detect, and respond to health threats emerging at the interface of animal and human populations [28, 29].

A major area of impact is food safety. Veterinarians are integral to maintaining the quality and safety of animal-derived food products [30]. They oversee every stage of the production chain from farm to table by implementing rigorous inspection systems, monitoring livestock health, inspecting processing facilities, and certifying the safety of meat, dairy, and egg products [30]. These efforts are essential in preventing the entry of contaminated food into the supply chain, thus reducing the global burden of foodborne diseases. Veterinary science also plays a vital role in combating zoonotic diseases those transmitted between animals and humans. Veterinarians monitor disease patterns in both domestic and wild animals, helping identify potential reservoirs and transmission routes [31]. Early detection through this surveillance allows for rapid intervention, preventing outbreaks from escalating into larger public health crises.

In research, veterinarians contribute to the development of vaccines, diagnostics, and therapies benefiting both humans and animals [32]. Breakthroughs in human medicine, such as insulin therapy for diabetes originally developed through canine research [33] and advancements in cancer and infectious disease treatments, often stem from veterinary studies. Veterinarians also contribute to environmental health by monitoring wildlife populations and assessing ecological risks [34]. Their work helps detect environmental degradation and pollutant exposure in animals, which often parallels risks to human health [35]. In addition to their technical roles, veterinarians engage in public health education, informing farmers, pet owners, and the public about disease prevention, animal care, and the significance of the human–animal bond [36]. They raise awareness about zoonotic diseases and promote safe practices for interacting with animals of all kinds.

Veterinarians play a vital role in public health education. They educate animal owners, farmers, and the general public about proper animal care, disease prevention, and the importance of the human–animal bond in promoting overall well-being [36]. This educational role extends to raising awareness about zoonotic diseases and teaching people how to interact safely with animals, whether they are pets, livestock, or wildlife.

1.2.2 Disease Prevention and Control

Disease prevention and control form a cornerstone of veterinary public health efforts, encompassing a wide array of strategies and interventions aimed at maintaining the health of animal populations and, by extension, safeguarding human health [30].

At the heart of disease prevention in veterinary medicine is the implementation of comprehensive vaccination programs. Veterinarians develop and administer vaccines to protect animals against a wide range of infectious diseases, many of which have zoonotic potential [32]. These vaccination efforts not only protect individual animals but also contribute to herd immunity, reducing the overall disease burden in animal populations and minimizing the risk of transmission to humans.

The evolution of such preventive strategies has been shaped by key milestones in the history of veterinary medicine (Figure 1.1). Beyond vaccination, veterinarians emphasize the importance of good animal husbandry practices in disease prevention. This involves educating farmers and animal owners about proper nutrition, sanitation, and animal [37]. By promoting optimal living conditions and care for animals, veterinarians help create environments that are less conducive to disease emergence and spread. This includes guidance on proper waste management, vector control, and biosecurity measures to prevent the introduction and spread of pathogens in animal populations [38].

In the event of disease outbreaks, veterinarians play a crucial role in controlling the spread. They employ strategies like quarantine, treatment protocols, and, when necessary, culling to prevent the disease from spreading to other animals or humans, especially in zoonotic cases [39]. Veterinarians are also instrumental in disease surveillance, conducting regular health checks and analyzing data to identify emerging health patterns and diseases [40]. This proactive approach allows for early intervention and containment before a potential public health crisis develops.

Biosecurity measures have gained importance in recent years, and veterinarians work with farms, animal facilities, and pet owners to implement protocols that control pathogen introduction. These measures include controlling access to facilities, introducing new animals safely, and ensuring proper cleaning and disinfection [38]. In addition, veterinarians play an important role in policymaking, offering expert advice on animal health regulations, import/export policies, and guidelines for controlling outbreaks [41]. Their involvement at the policy level ensures a comprehensive and effective approach to disease prevention.

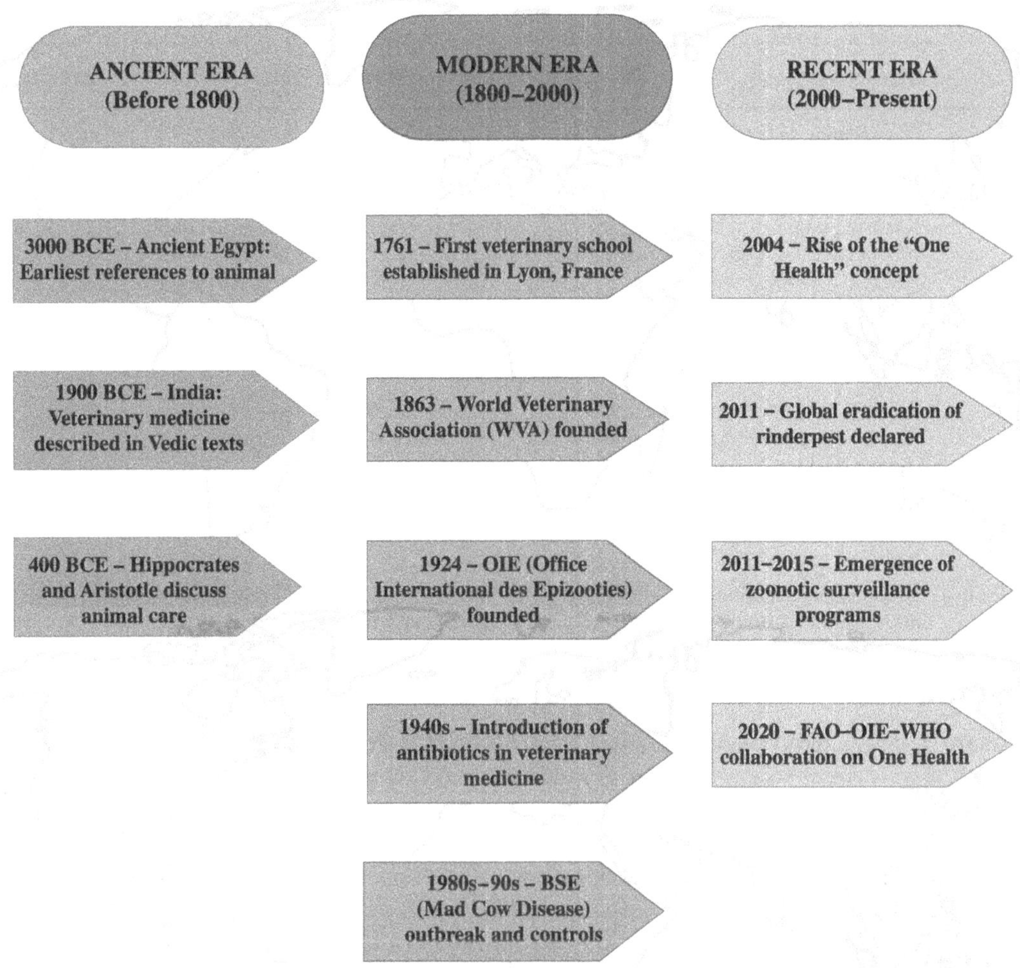

Figure 1.1 Historical timeline of veterinary medicine.

Lastly, the "One Health" approach, which recognizes the interconnectedness of human, animal, and environmental health, is increasingly embraced by veterinarians. By collaborating with human health professionals and environmental scientists, veterinarians contribute to a more holistic and effective strategy for disease prevention and control across these domains.

1.2.3 Zoonotic Diseases

Zoonotic diseases those transmissible between animals and humans account for a large share of all infectious diseases and pose major global public health risks [42]. Veterinary science is central to understanding, preventing, and managing these threats to both human and animal populations.

Veterinarians study the ecology, reservoirs, and transmission cycles of zoonotic pathogens, working to identify the environmental and biological factors that facilitate their spread to humans [43, 44]. These diseases are caused by a diverse range of pathogens viruses, bacteria, parasites, and fungi each requiring specific diagnostic and control strategies [45, 46]. The emergence of diseases like COVID-19 underscores the need for robust animal

Table 1.1 Veterinary contributions to public health.

Role	Description	Relevant WOAH programs	References
Zoonotic Disease Management	Surveillance, diagnosis, and control of diseases like rabies, avian influenza, and brucellosis.	WOAH guidelines on zoonotic disease management and One Health initiatives.	[51]
Food Safety	Ensuring safe meat, dairy, and egg products through veterinary inspections and HACCP principles.	WOAH standards on food production safety and collaborations with Codex Alimentarius.	[52]
Public Health Education	Promoting responsible pet ownership, vaccination campaigns, and hygiene practices to reduce zoonotic risks.	WOAH public awareness initiatives and veterinary education campaigns.	[53]
Disease Outbreak Management	Rapid response to emerging diseases in livestock to prevent outbreaks and protect human health.	WOAH emergency management procedures for livestock disease control.	[54]
Vector-Borne Disease Control	Managing vector populations (e.g., ticks, mosquitoes) to reduce diseases like Rift Valley fever and Lyme disease.	WOAH guidance on vector-borne disease prevention and control.	[55]
Animal Vaccination Programs	Designing vaccination schedules to prevent animal diseases and reduce zoonotic transmission risks.	WOAH Vaccine Banks for fast deployment during disease outbreaks.	[56]

surveillance systems to detect and contain future pandemics early [47]. Prevention is a cornerstone of veterinary efforts, including widespread vaccination programs like those for rabies, which have significantly reduced global cases. Veterinarians also develop new vaccines for emerging diseases and promote hygiene, biosecurity, and public education to minimize transmission risks [48].

During outbreaks, veterinarians help implement critical control measures quarantining, treatment, and sometimes culling to curb disease spread [39]. They collaborate closely with public health officials, embodying the One Health approach that links human, animal, and environmental health. Veterinary research advances our understanding of zoonotic transmission, identifies risk factors, and supports the development of treatments and prevention strategies [49]. Additionally, veterinarians combat antimicrobial resistance (AMR) by advocating for responsible antibiotic use and exploring alternative disease management practices [50].

Overall, veterinary sciences are vital in the ongoing fight against zoonotic diseases, contributing significantly to global health security through research, surveillance, prevention, and collaborative response efforts. To provide a concise overview of these diverse roles, Table 1.1 summarizes the major areas of veterinary involvement and their associated public health impacts.

1.3 Veterinary Sciences and Food Security

The intersection of veterinary sciences and food security is critical, particularly as the global population grows and climate change pressures food systems [26]. Veterinary professionals are pivotal in maintaining livestock health, which directly impacts the quality, safety, and quantity of food available for human consumption [57]. Their responsibilities go beyond treating illnesses they develop preventive health strategies, manage disease outbreaks, and provide expert guidance on husbandry practices to enhance productivity and sustainability [58].

By controlling zoonotic diseases at their animal sources, veterinarians help prevent human infections and food supply disruptions, protecting public health and maintaining consumer confidence [59]. They also uphold food safety by enforcing rigorous standards for meat, dairy, and eggs, ensuring these products are free from contaminants and safe for consumption [59]. Veterinary research into genetics and breeding has improved livestock traits like disease resistance, productivity, and environmental adaptability, helping meet the growing demand for protein in a sustainable way [60].

Environmental sustainability is another key area where veterinary sciences contribute. Veterinarians are innovating in efficient production systems that utilize alternative feeds, reduce greenhouse gas emissions, and manage animal waste effectively [61]. In aquaculture, they help maintain the health of aquatic species and ensure sustainable practices in fish farming and harvesting [62]. Veterinary involvement in global trade is vital as well. Their expertise in preventing and controlling transboundary animal diseases helps secure international markets and food availability [63, 64]. Amid climate change, veterinarians are developing heat-tolerant livestock breeds, vaccines for new diseases, and adaptive strategies to preserve animal health in evolving environments [65].

Veterinary sciences form the backbone of a secure, safe, and sustainable food system. Through disease control, food safety, genetic innovation, and environmental stewardship, veterinarians are essential in safeguarding food security for current and future generations.

1.3.1 Livestock Health and Productivity

Livestock health and productivity are crucial for global food security and agricultural economies. Veterinarians play a key role in safeguarding animal health and improving production efficiency through disease prevention, treatment, and modern management practices that help herds and flocks thrive worldwide [66].

Prevention is central to veterinary care. Veterinarians create customized vaccination programs to protect animals from local and emerging diseases, ensuring timely and effective immunity [67]. Parasite control is another vital area, involving a mix of treatments, pasture management, and selective breeding to combat internal and external parasites [68]. Biosecurity is critical in disease prevention. Veterinarians work with farm managers to implement strict protocols to limit pathogen entry and spread, including visitor control, quarantine of new animals, and facility designs that minimize cross-contamination. These practices support animal health, growth, reproduction, and overall productivity.

Nutrition is another domain where veterinarians contribute significantly. They collaborate with nutritionists to develop species-specific, stage-appropriate diets, using tools like computer modeling to optimize feed plans [1]. These strategies enhance productivity and the quality of meat, milk, and eggs [69]. Vets also monitor and adjust diets based on conditions and goals. Veterinary science has advanced reproductive health through technologies like artificial insemination, improving breeding efficiency and genetic progress. Embryo transfer accelerates elite genetics multiplication [70]. Vets partner with geneticists to apply genomic selection and tools promoting traits such as disease resistance and feed efficiency, improving livestock sustainability [71].

Animal welfare is another priority. Veterinarians uphold welfare standards, ensuring better product quality and consumer trust [72]. They assist in developing traceability and quality assurance programs that support food safety and facilitate international trade. Looking ahead, veterinary science leads sustainable livestock efforts exploring genome editing, incorporating indigenous knowledge, and managing resources efficiently [73]. As the sector faces climate change and emerging diseases, veterinarians are advancing adaptive strategies, including heat-tolerant breeds, new vaccines, and precision farming technologies to optimize animal health [74].

Veterinary professionals' evolving role integrates data-driven tools to enhance health, welfare, and productivity while reducing environmental impact. Their expertise ensures sustainable development, supports agricultural economies, and reinforces global food security.

1.3.2 Safe Food Practices

Veterinary sciences are vital for food security, ensuring safety throughout the food production chain from farm to fork. On farms, veterinarians maintain livestock health by developing tailored health plans, including vaccinations, parasite control, and biosecurity to prevent disease spread [75]. They also oversee medication use in food-producing animals, ensuring compliance with guidelines to prevent harmful residues in meat, milk, and eggs [76].

Veterinarians advise on nutrition and animal welfare, both of which enhance product safety. Proper nutrition keeps animals healthy, while good welfare reduces stress and disease risk, improving the safety and quality of animal products [77]. Disease surveillance is another key responsibility vets monitor animal health, interpret test results, and respond quickly to outbreaks, enabling early detection of pathogens and reducing public health risks [78]. In slaughterhouses and processing plants, veterinary inspectors ensure only safe animal products enter the food chain. They conduct antemortem inspections to detect illness and postmortem examinations of carcasses to identify diseases, parasites, or abnormalities [79]. Vets also enforce hygiene standards and sanitation protocols, preventing contamination during processing. They supervise Hazard Analysis and Critical Control Points (HACCP) systems to control food safety risks [80, 81].

Veterinary public health professionals influence food safety regulations at both national and global levels. They research foodborne pathogens, AMR, and contamination detection methods, guiding evidence-based food safety policies [57, 82]. The "One Health" approach linking human, animal, and environmental health positions veterinarians as leaders in addressing AMR and promoting responsible antibiotic use [83]. Veterinarians also control zoonotic diseases at their animal sources, preventing them from entering the food supply. Since many emerging infectious diseases originate in animals, vets are central to protecting public health [84]. They contribute to sustainability by researching alternative feeds, waste management strategies, and methods to reduce greenhouse gas emissions [85]. As climate change alters disease patterns, veterinary sciences will be key in adapting food systems.

In conclusion, veterinary sciences are essential to food security through livestock health, disease control, and food safety. Their expertise supports resilient, sustainable food systems that ensure a safe and adequate food supply for the growing global population.

1.4 Environmental Sustainability

Environmental sustainability in veterinary medicine focuses on reducing the ecological impact of animal care while supporting ecosystem health. This includes resource conservation, waste reduction, and eco-friendly technologies in clinics. Veterinarians adopt practices like energy-efficient tools, water-saving systems, and safe medical waste disposal. The field also addresses the environmental footprint of animal agriculture and pet ownership by promoting sustainable pet food, responsible breeding, and shelter adoptions [86]. These efforts reflect a growing commitment within veterinary science to support both animal and environmental well-being, contributing to a more sustainable future.

1.4.1 Sustainable Agricultural Practices

Veterinary medicine plays a vital role in promoting sustainable farming, especially in livestock management. Beyond treating sick animals, veterinarians help balance animal welfare, farm profitability, and environmental protection [87]. A major shift in veterinary practices is the move toward disease prevention. This proactive approach reduces antibiotic use, combats AMR, and limits harmful residues in soil and water.

Veterinarians prevent illnesses primarily through enhanced biosecurity keeping farms clean and controlling animal exposure to people, equipment, and other animals. This creates a protective barrier to reduce disease entry [88]. Tailored vaccination programs based on regional risks also boost herd immunity and reduce the need for medications [89]. Vets further support animal welfare by advising on better housing, handling, and transport. Reduced stress improves immune function, allowing animals to resist diseases naturally.

Nutrition is another critical area. Vets collaborate with nutritionists to design species-specific diets that improve digestion and nutrient absorption, boosting animal health and reducing environmental waste [90]. In breeding, veterinarians assist in selecting animals with traits for disease resistance and adaptability, producing livestock that needs fewer resources supporting both productivity and sustainability [91]. In aquaculture, veterinary professionals enhance sustainability by maintaining fish health without excessive antibiotic use. They help design farms that promote water quality and minimize environmental pollution [92]. Vets are also at the forefront of precision farming using sensors and data analytics to monitor animal health in real time, enabling early interventions and efficient resource use.

Education is a key part of veterinary involvement in sustainable agriculture. Vets train farmers and workers on best practices for animal health, welfare, and eco-friendly management, spreading sustainable knowledge across the farming community [93].

Veterinary medicine supports sustainable farming by preventing disease, improving animal welfare and nutrition, guiding responsible breeding, advancing aquaculture, and integrating technology. As agriculture faces increasing challenges from climate change and food insecurity, veterinarians are central to building resilient, ethical, and environmentally sound farming systems.

1.4.2 Impact of Veterinary Practices on Ecosystems

The relationship between veterinary practices and ecosystems is complex, involving both beneficial contributions and potential environmental challenges. At its core, veterinary medicine aims to enhance animal health and welfare, but the tools used especially pharmaceuticals can sometimes lead to unintended ecological consequences.

One of the primary concerns is the use of veterinary pharmaceuticals in both livestock and companion animals. Livestock in intensive farming systems often receive antibiotics, antiparasitic, and growth-promoting agents. Pets, too, are commonly treated with various drugs throughout their lives. These substances often enter the environment through animal waste, runoff, or improper disposal. Once in soil or water, they can affect microbial communities, aquatic organisms, and the food chain [94].

In aquatic ecosystems, for instance, certain antibiotics and anti-inflammatory drugs have been shown to impair reproduction, behavior, and organ function in fish and other wildlife. The environmental presence of antibiotics also drives the development of AMR. Low-level exposure promotes the survival of resistant bacteria, which can spread through water, wildlife, and even air, posing significant risks to animal and human health [95].

Veterinary waste, including syringes, gloves, packaging, and surgical materials, adds another environmental burden. Plastics in veterinary waste can persist in the environment for decades, harming wildlife through ingestion or entanglement. Sharps and other biohazardous materials, if improperly managed, can also spread pathogens or injure animals [96]. In response, the veterinary profession is increasingly implementing eco-conscious practices. Clinics are adopting waste management protocols, promoting safe disposal of pharmaceuticals, recycling where possible, and using biodegradable materials [97]. Treatment approaches are also evolving. Veterinarians now favor targeted, evidence-based therapies over broad-spectrum preventive drug use, reducing the environmental load of pharmaceuticals. There's growing interest in alternative treatments, including herbal remedies and bacteriophage therapy, which may carry fewer environmental risks [98].

Veterinarians also play an essential role in managing the health of ecosystems through zoonotic disease control, wildlife conservation, and sustainable farming. By monitoring diseases that spread between animals and humans, veterinarians help prevent outbreaks that could disrupt ecosystems and endanger public health. Wildlife vets work to protect endangered species, rehabilitate injured animals, and support rewilding programs. They often conduct research to assess ecosystem health, using wildlife as indicators of environmental quality.

In agriculture, veterinarians encourage sustainable livestock practices that benefit both animals and the environment [99]. This includes advocating for improved housing, nutrition, and welfare. For example, pasture-based systems not only improve animal well-being but also enhance soil health, promote biodiversity, and reduce reliance on pharmaceuticals compared to intensive feedlots. Veterinarians are also helping educate pet owners about sustainability. This includes advising on eco-friendly pet food choices, reducing pet overpopulation through responsible breeding and adoption, and promoting the safe disposal of pet waste and medications [86].

The "One Health" approach has become a guiding principle in modern veterinary science. It emphasizes the interconnectedness of human, animal, and environmental health. This holistic perspective is increasingly integrated into veterinary training and research, promoting practices that safeguard ecological well-being while maintaining high standards of animal care. Veterinary schools now include environmental science and sustainability in their curricula, preparing graduates to consider ecological impacts in their work. Researchers are developing new tools and methods such as precision livestock farming and green veterinary pharmaceuticals that aim to reduce the footprint of veterinary care.

Veterinary practices can affect ecosystems, and the profession is evolving to reduce its environmental impact. Veterinarians are actively contributing to ecological sustainability through waste reduction, responsible medication use, disease surveillance, and education. By embracing the One Health model and adopting sustainable innovations, veterinary medicine can support both animal health and environmental stewardship. The future of veterinary practice depends on collaboration across disciplines bringing together veterinarians, ecologists, policymakers, and the public to build a more sustainable and resilient world.

1.4.3 Role in Biodiversity Conservation

Veterinary medicine plays a vital role in global biodiversity conservation, particularly through the work of wildlife veterinarians. These professionals address the challenges of endangered species, working in remote areas to care for at-risk animals, monitor populations, and develop protection strategies [100].

Veterinarians contribute significantly to captive breeding programs, ensuring the physical and genetic health of endangered species. They oversee reproductive health, artificial insemination, and genetic diversity to avoid inbreeding [101]. Additionally, they assist in reintroducing animals to the wild by conducting health checks, vaccinations, and monitoring postrelease survival [102]. In wildlife rehabilitation, vets treat injured or displaced animals, providing critical care following natural disasters or human impact. This work also offers valuable insights into the health of wild populations and environmental stressors [103].

Veterinary research helps develop solutions for wildlife diseases that threaten biodiversity, such as white-nose syndrome in bats and chytrid fungus in amphibians [104]. Vets in zoos also contribute to conservation by ensuring the health of captive animals, which supports broader conservation efforts [105]. Furthermore, vets address human–wildlife conflicts by collaborating with ecologists and communities to minimize negative interactions [106]. The veterinary profession is essential in One Health initiatives, linking human, animal, and environmental health. Vets track diseases that spread between wildlife, domestic animals, and humans, supporting both public health and conservation [107]. They also play a key role in wildlife crime forensics, helping to protect endangered species from poaching and illegal trade [108, 109]. Through education and public outreach, vets raise awareness of biodiversity, advocating for the interconnectedness of all life [110].

Veterinary medicine is crucial for biodiversity conservation. Vets contribute through direct care, ecological research, breeding programs, wildlife crime forensics, and innovative technologies, all of which help protect Earth's biodiversity.

1.5 Contemporary Challenges in Veterinary

Contemporary challenges in veterinary medicine are diverse and complex, reflecting the rapidly changing landscape of animal health and welfare. Veterinarians today face the dual task of embracing new medical technologies while combating emerging infectious diseases, AMR, and the impact of climate change on animal health.

Increased global trade and travel have contributed to the spread of diseases, making disease control and prevention even more crucial [111].

In companion animal practice, rising expectations for advanced care have added pressure, while economic constraints and ethical considerations further complicate decision-making. The need for a One Health approach, which recognizes the interconnectedness of human, animal, and environmental health, requires veterinarians to address not only individual animal welfare but also broader public health and ecological concerns [112]. Moreover, challenges such as burnout, lack of diversity, and shifting societal expectations demand that veterinarians balance quality care with accessibility and affordability. As the profession evolves, veterinarians must remain adaptable, committed to lifelong learning, and prepared to tackle these complex issues to ensure the well-being of both animals and humans in a rapidly changing world.

1.5.1 Emerging Infectious Diseases

Emerging infectious diseases present a significant challenge for veterinary medicine, with their rapid spread and the complex interactions between pathogens, hosts, and the environment [113]. Diseases like avian influenza (H5N1, H7N9), West Nile virus, and African swine fever show how these threats can cross species barriers, causing economic and zoonotic impacts [114–116]. Globalization has accelerated their spread, as seen with COVID-19, highlighting the interconnectedness of human, animal, and environmental health [117].

Veterinarians play a critical role in combating these emerging threats through early detection, surveillance, and control. They must stay informed about new pathogens and use advanced diagnostic tools like Polymerase Chain Reaction (PCR) assays and next-generation sequencing for rapid pathogen identification [118, 119]. Prevention and treatment require innovation, including biosecurity protocols, vaccination programs, quarantine procedures, and, when necessary, culling [120]. The zoonotic potential of many emerging diseases underscores the importance of the One Health approach, which recognizes the links between human, animal, and environmental health [121]. Veterinarians must collaborate with human health professionals, environmental scientists, and policymakers to predict, prevent, and respond to outbreaks [122]. Additionally, global cooperation and coordinated efforts are essential for controlling disease spread, with veterinarians contributing to global surveillance networks [59].

Addressing emerging infectious diseases requires scientific expertise, technological innovation, and collaboration. Veterinarians must continue to adapt and innovate to safeguard animal health, public health, and ecosystems.

1.5.2 Antimicrobial Resistance

AMR is a major global health threat, arising when microorganisms become resistant to antimicrobial drugs, undermining the effectiveness of treatments in both veterinary and human medicine [123]. The overuse and misuse of antibiotics, particularly in animal farming for growth promotion and disease prevention, have driven this crisis. Antibiotics are also often misused in pet care, contributing to resistance [83, 124]. AMR poses risks to both animal and human health. Resistant bacteria can enter the food chain through animal products like meat, dairy, and eggs, and spread to humans through direct contact with animals. This leads to infections that are difficult to treat with standard antibiotics.

Veterinarians play a key role in combating AMR by ensuring judicious antibiotic use. They are responsible for selecting the right drug, dose, and duration to maintain long-term efficacy [125]. Diagnostic testing also helps reduce unnecessary antibiotic use. In addition, veterinarians are exploring nonantibiotic alternatives, such as probiotics, bacteriophages, and immunomodulatory agents, and emphasizing preventive strategies like improved hygiene, vaccination, and biosecurity to reduce reliance on antimicrobials [126].

Education is vital in the fight against AMR. Veterinarians educate farmers, pet owners, and animal handlers on the risks of AMR and the importance of completing prescribed antibiotic courses [127]. Furthermore,

Table 1.2 Antimicrobial resistance in veterinary practices.

Resistant pathogen	Affected animal species	Commonly used antimicrobials	WOAH guidelines/interventions	References
Escherichia coli (ESBL-producing)	Cattle, swine, poultry	Cephalosporins, fluoroquinolones	WOAH advocates for prudent use of antimicrobials and surveillance programs.	[130]
Staphylococcus aureus (MRSA)	Cattle (mastitis cases)	Beta-lactams, macrolides	WOAH emphasizes infection control measures and monitoring to prevent resistance.	[131]
Salmonella spp. (MDR)	Poultry, swine	Tetracyclines, beta-lactams	WOAH recommends biosecurity practices and alternative treatments.	[132]
Klebsiella pneumoniae (MDR)	Cattle, swine	Carbapenems, cephalosporins	WOAH urges strict hygiene and infection control practices to reduce MDR pathogens.	[133]
Campylobacter jejuni	Poultry	Fluoroquinolones, macrolides	WOAH promotes improved sanitation, biosecurity, and reduced antibiotic dependency.	[134]
Pseudomonas aeruginosa (MDR)	Dogs, Cats	Beta-lactams, aminoglycosides	WOAH recommends infection surveillance and tailors antibiotic treatments.	[135]

veterinarians contribute to AMR surveillance by collecting and reporting resistance data, supporting policy development, and guiding research into new treatments and resistance mitigation strategies [128].

Tackling AMR effectively also necessitates a One Health approach, integrating veterinary, human, and environmental health sectors [129]. This multidisciplinary collaboration enhances the effectiveness of AMR response strategies through shared knowledge, coordinated actions, and joint policy development. Table 1.2 illustrates the impact of AMR in veterinary practices.

AMR is a complex and urgent challenge for veterinary medicine. It demands a multifaceted approach that combines judicious antibiotic use, exploration of alternative treatments, extensive education, and rigorous monitoring. As stewards of animal health and key players in public health, veterinarians bear a significant responsibility in addressing this global threat. Their efforts in combating AMR not only protect animal health but also play a crucial role in safeguarding human health and maintaining the efficacy of these vital medicines for future generations. The ongoing battle against AMR underscores the need for continued research, innovation, and collaboration across all health sectors to preserve the effectiveness of antimicrobial drugs and ensure the health of both animals and humans in the face of this growing threat.

1.5.3 Climate Change and Animal Health

Climate change is a significant global challenge that affects both humans and animals [136]. Rising temperatures are altering ecosystems and impacting animal health in various ways. Warmer climates allow disease-carrying insects like ticks and mosquitoes to spread into new regions, exposing animals to diseases they haven't encountered before. Diseases once limited to tropical areas are now emerging in cooler regions like Europe and North America. Figure 1.2 illustrates how climate change affects animal health through changes in disease patterns, thermal stress, and food security issues.

Extreme weather events, such as floods, droughts, hurricanes, and wildfires, are becoming more frequent due to climate change, threatening animal health by depriving them of food, water, and shelter, and causing separation from their owners [137]. These events weaken animals' immune systems, making them more susceptible to disease. Heatwaves, in particular, impact farm animals like cows and chickens, leading to heat stress, reduced food intake, lower production, fertility issues, and increased vulnerability to illness [138]. This harms animal health and threatens food supply and farmers' livelihoods.

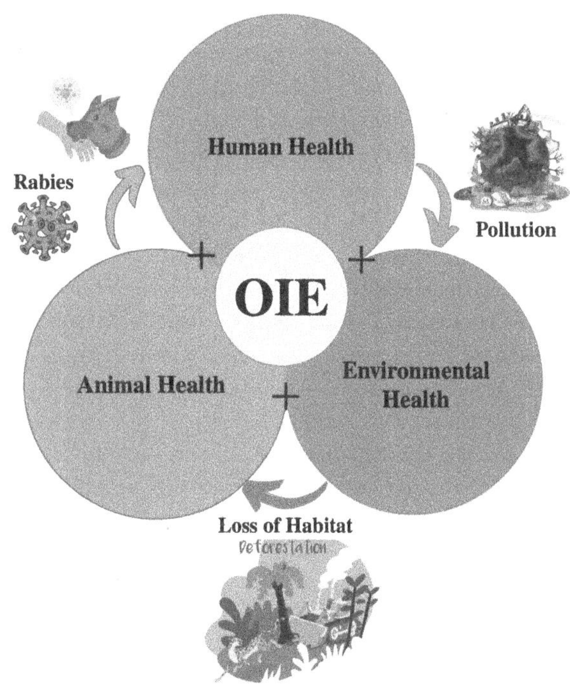

Figure 1.2 One health framework visualization.

Veterinarians are adapting to these challenges by developing heat-tolerant animals and improving animal housing to keep them cool. As diseases spread, they are revising vaccination and parasite control strategies, staying informed about emerging diseases [56]. Veterinarians are also promoting sustainable farming practices to reduce greenhouse gas emissions from livestock, improving animal diets to decrease methane production, and exploring environmentally friendly farming methods like insect farming and algae-based feeds [139, 140]. In wildlife conservation, veterinarians monitor and protect species affected by climate change [141].

Overall, climate change presents numerous challenges for animal health, requiring veterinarians to adapt, innovate, and collaborate to address both direct and indirect effects. Their work goes beyond treating animals; they play a crucial role in climate change mitigation and promoting sustainability.

1.6 One Health

One Health is an integrated, unifying approach that aims to sustainably balance and optimize the health of people, animals, and ecosystems. It recognizes the interconnection between humans, animals, plants, and their shared environment. This approach is especially relevant in understanding and addressing complex health challenges such as emerging infectious diseases, AMR, food safety, and climate change, which lie at the interface of human, animal, and environmental health [141].

1.6.1 Concept and Principles

The One Health approach is a holistic, multidisciplinary framework emphasizing the interdependence of human, animal, and environmental health. It promotes collaboration among experts in medicine, veterinary science, public health, environmental science, and agriculture to tackle challenges like zoonotic diseases, AMR, foodborne illnesses, and ecological degradation [142]. By addressing root causes such as deforestation, unsustainable agriculture, habitat destruction, and antibiotic misuse One Health enables preventive, sustainable solutions. It focuses on early intervention, cross-sectoral strategies, and shared expertise to enhance disease control, protect biodiversity, improve food safety, and increase resilience against emerging health threats. This collaborative model strengthens health systems and supports the well-being of humans, animals, and ecosystems.

The concept represents a transformative shift in global health. Rather than isolating human, animal, and environmental health, One Health recognizes their deep interconnection and promotes integrated approaches for better outcomes [143]. Though ancient knowledge recognized these links, the modern One Health framework gained momentum in the late twentieth and early twenty-first centuries amid rising concerns about emerging infectious diseases and environmental impacts on health.

Core principles include interconnectedness and interdisciplinary collaboration among medicine, veterinary science, ecology, social sciences, and public policy [144]. One Health promotes a holistic view of health, emphasizing prevention, inclusivity, and equity, particularly for marginalized populations. It also values traditional and indigenous knowledge systems [145]. With its transboundary focus, One Health addresses global issues like climate change and urbanization that require international cooperation. It aligns with sustainable development goals, recognizing that long-term health depends on healthy ecosystems and responsible resource use. These principles are reflected in joint surveillance systems for zoonoses, monitoring of ecological shifts, and studies of human–animal interactions [146]. Although challenges exist such as breaking down disciplinary silos and navigating political complexities the approach offers a comprehensive and efficient path toward health security and sustainability [147].

1.6.2 One Health Framework

The One Health framework provides a structured model to implement the approach's principles across human, animal, and environmental domains [148]. It promotes intersectoral collaboration and effective governance, as shown in Figure 1.3. At its core is governance, which establishes cross-sectoral committees or task forces including experts in public health, veterinary medicine, environmental science, and social sciences. These bodies set priorities, allocate resources, and ensure integration of One Health into policies at all levels. Good governance relies on clear communication, accountability, and conflict-resolution mechanisms.

Shared knowledge is another pillar, involving standardized data collection, joint analysis, and real-time information sharing. Centralized or interoperable platforms allow professionals from different fields to collaborate, interpret data, and address complex health issues more effectively [149]. Workforce development is essential for multidisciplinary success. Training programs foster collaboration skills, systems thinking, and continuous learning. Curricula across medical, veterinary, and environmental sciences now increasingly reflect One Health principles, preparing professionals for evolving challenges [150].

Surveillance and monitoring enable early detection and response to threats across sectors. Integrated systems combine human and animal disease surveillance, environmental monitoring, and technological tools like Geographic Information System (GIS) and big data analytics to build a comprehensive risk picture [151]. Research and innovation support interdisciplinary studies exploring the human–animal–environment interface. These efforts focus on new methods, risk assessment tools, and practical interventions. Importantly, this research must inform policies and real-world actions [152]. Communication and outreach engage policymakers, practitioners, and the public. Clear messaging about the interconnectedness of health helps build support for collaborative strategies. Tactics include public awareness campaigns and stakeholder forums.

Lastly, policy and legislation create the legal foundation for One Health implementation. This includes revising laws, developing supportive policies, and securing funding. Laws must be flexible to adapt to emerging global challenges and facilitate cooperation across sectors. Together, these framework elements create a roadmap for coordinated responses to health threats, reinforcing that addressing interconnected issues demands more than scientific expertise it requires effective governance, policy, and collaboration.

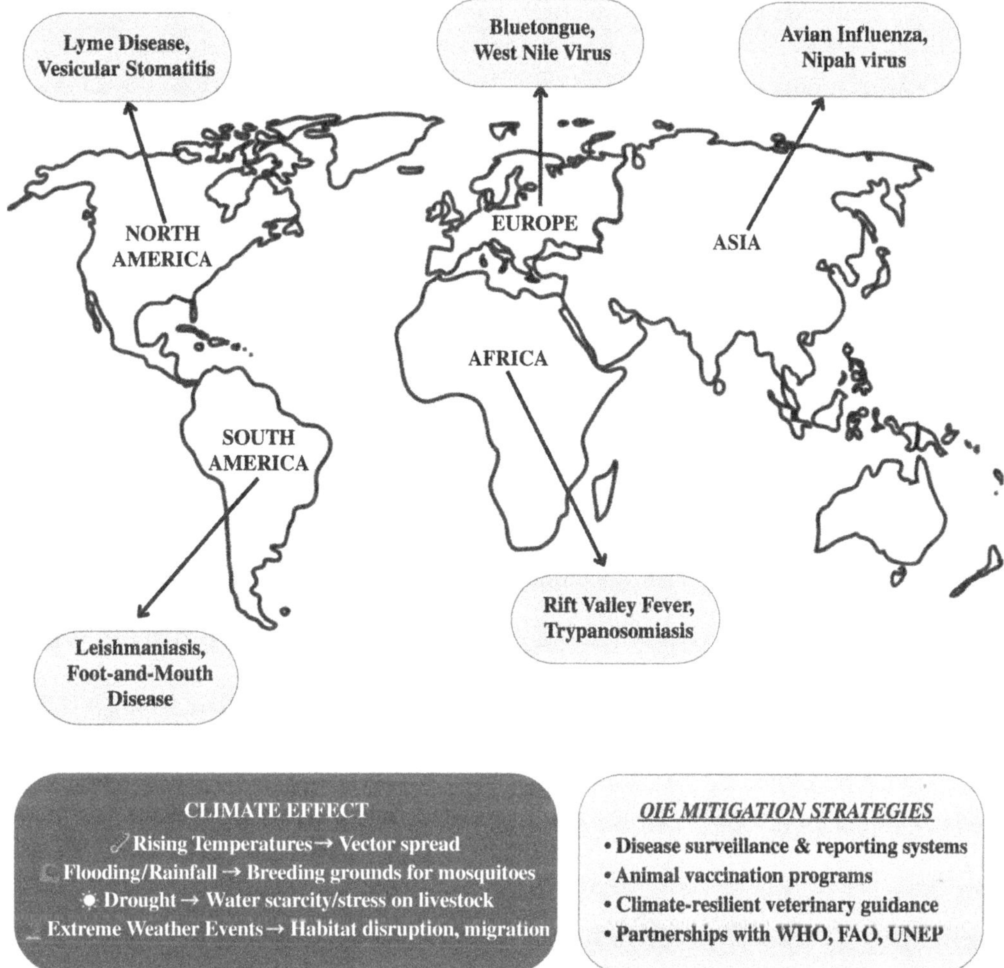

Figure 1.3 Impact of climate change on animal health.

1.6.3 Applications of One Health in Veterinary Sciences

Veterinary sciences play a pivotal role in One Health, reflecting the close ties between animal health, human well-being, and environmental balance. In zoonotic disease management, veterinarians collaborate with public health professionals to conduct joint surveillance and develop strategies for diseases like rabies, influenza, and coronaviruses. Research on wildlife reservoirs and interspecies disease transmission helps predict and mitigate pandemics [153].

Food safety and security also benefit from veterinary expertise. Veterinarians oversee the safety of food from farm to table, detect pathogens, and manage contamination risks. They help curb AMR by promoting prudent antibiotic use, developing alternatives, and monitoring resistance trends. Moreover, they support sustainable livestock practices that reduce environmental impact while maintaining productivity [154].

The One Health approach also sheds light on the relationship between environmental health and animal welfare. Veterinarians study how habitat loss, climate change, and pollution affect animal disease patterns. Animals often act as sentinels, signaling broader ecological problems. This insight supports early warnings for human and ecosystem health [155]. Veterinarians are central to combating AMR. They reduce antibiotic use by improving animal housing, nutrition, and disease prevention methods. By tracking resistance in animals, they contribute vital data to global AMR surveillance. Coordinated efforts between human and veterinary medicine are key to addressing AMR effectively [156].

In the realm of vector-borne diseases, veterinary scientists study disease ecology to inform integrated control strategies. As climate change shifts vector populations, veterinarians help monitor and forecast new disease risks. Comparative medicine using animal models to study shared diseases offers insights into disease mechanisms and therapies that benefit both humans and animals. This interdisciplinary research exemplifies One Health collaboration.

1.7 Global Initiatives and Frameworks

Global initiatives are crucial for tackling challenges in health, food security, and sustainability. The World Organisation for Animal Health (WOAH) leads efforts to prevent and control animal diseases, supporting both animal welfare and public health. The Food and Agriculture Organization (FAO) works to enhance food security and promote sustainable agriculture worldwide. Together, these organizations develop international policies, support disease surveillance, and improve farming practices. Their collaborative frameworks ensure a coordinated global response to emerging threats, aiming to build resilient food systems and safeguard both human and animal health in a changing world.

These organizations, through coordinated global collaborations, develop and implement frameworks that facilitate the sharing of knowledge, resources, and expertise. Together, they contribute to a unified approach aimed at safeguarding global health, ensuring food security, and fostering environmental sustainability, thereby addressing the interconnected challenges of today's world [157].

Table 1.3 summarizes major programs, frameworks, and partnerships that have been launched or supported by global organizations to tackle pressing challenges in animal and public health, including zoonoses, AMR, and capacity building.

1.7.1 World Organisation for Animal Health (WOAH)

The WOAH plays a central role in promoting global animal health and welfare, serving as a key pillar of the One Health approach. Founded in 1924, the OIE has grown into a pivotal intergovernmental organization working with its 182 member countries to tackle complex challenges at the intersection of animal health, human well-being, and environmental integrity [163].

At the heart of the OIE's mission is its commitment to developing and maintaining international standards for animal health and zoonoses. These standards, detailed in the *Terrestrial and Aquatic Animal Health Codes and Manuals*, are regularly updated and serve as the global benchmark for disease surveillance, control, animal welfare, and the safe trade of animals and animal products [164]. These standards are foundational to global trade, providing the scientific basis for World Trade Organization (WTO) members to resolve disputes over animal-related products. This role underscores the OIE's function in harmonizing animal health protection with safe trade, ensuring food security and economic stability [165].

The OIE operates the World Animal Health Information System (WAHIS), a global platform for collecting, analyzing, and sharing real-time data on animal diseases and zoonoses. WAHIS acts as an early warning system, alerting the international community to disease outbreaks and potential zoonotic threats. It supports timely decision-making and is accessible to both member countries and the public, enhancing global awareness and coordination [166].

As a center of scientific expertise, the OIE unites global experts to provide evidence-based recommendations for disease control, including zoonoses. Its scientific commissions and working groups address emerging diseases,

Table 1.3 Key global initiatives in veterinary sciences.

Organization	Mandate	Notable veterinary-related projects	Contribution to one health framework	References
World Organisation for Animal Health (WOAH)	Improve animal health worldwide and ensure safe international trade of animal products.	Development of global disease reporting systems and veterinary capacity-building.	Collaborates with WHO and FAO to control zoonotic outbreaks.	[158]
Food and Agriculture Organization (FAO)	Improve livestock health and promote sustainable food production practices.	Emergency Prevention System (EMPRES) for transboundary disease prevention.	Focuses on livestock health as part of sustainable food systems and zoonotic risk control.	[159]
World Health Organization (WHO)	Coordinate global health efforts, including zoonotic disease control.	Supports veterinary collaboration in disease surveillance and early warning systems.	Facilitates integrated responses to zoonotic diseases like avian influenza and COVID-19.	[82]
Centers for Disease Control and Prevention (CDC)	Focus on public health protection, including veterinary-related disease control.	Developed the One Health Zoonotic Disease Prioritization Tool to manage zoonotic risks.	Promotes research and education to manage zoonotic transmission routes.	[160]
European Food Safety Authority (EFSA)	Ensure food safety by improving animal health practices.	Provides risk assessments on antimicrobial resistance and zoonotic pathogens.	Supports EU-wide strategies to reduce antimicrobial use in veterinary practices.	[161]
International Livestock Research Institute (ILRI)	Enhance animal health and welfare in developing nations.	Focuses on livestock vaccines, disease prevention strategies, and sustainable farming practices.	Links animal health to poverty reduction and improved public health outcomes.	[162]

AMR, and other critical issues, contributing to global policy through research-driven insights. This scientific leadership extends to facilitating research partnerships and promoting innovation in animal health and welfare [158, 167].

To strengthen veterinary infrastructure worldwide, the OIE implements the Performance of Veterinary Services (PVS) Pathway, a framework for evaluating and improving national veterinary systems. The program helps countries build capacity, upgrade legislation, and improve disease detection and prevention systems. Through tailored support, the OIE fosters resilient veterinary services essential for protecting animal and public health [168, 169].

The OIE's role in the *Tripartite Alliance* alongside the World Health Organization (WHO) and the FAO embodies the One Health approach. This collaboration addresses key areas such as AMR, zoonotic diseases, and food safety. Through coordinated research and shared strategies, the alliance offers integrated solutions to complex health threats across human, animal, and environmental domains [158]. Beyond health standards, the OIE also leads efforts in animal welfare, recognizing the link between welfare, animal productivity, and public health. It develops global welfare guidelines and promotes training, workshops, and educational outreach to enhance veterinary and policy expertise across member countries. This capacity building helps countries respond more effectively to evolving challenges.

In response to emerging global concerns like climate change, the OIE has expanded its scope to consider environmental factors affecting animal health. The organization now addresses how ecological changes influence disease transmission and animal populations. This evolving focus underscores its commitment to a holistic One Health vision that integrates environmental sustainability [65].

As global health challenges become more complex and interconnected, the OIE's leadership in One Health through surveillance, policy, science, and collaboration remains indispensable. In parallel, the FAO has emerged as a key player in tackling urgent health threats like AMR, highlighting the need for unified global efforts to safeguard health, food security, and sustainability [170].

1.7.2 Food and Agriculture Organization

The FAO of the United Nations stands as a cornerstone in the global fight against hunger and malnutrition. More than just a food aid agency, the FAO plays a vital role in the One Health approach, acknowledging the deep connections between human health, animal welfare, and environmental sustainability [171].

At the heart of the FAO's mission is its focus on ensuring food safety and quality throughout the entire food chain from farm to fork. This comprehensive strategy involves setting and implementing food safety standards to protect public health and support international trade. By promoting good agricultural practices, supporting the establishment of food safety management systems, and encouraging multisectoral collaboration, the FAO contributes to building safer and more resilient global food systems [172]. In the One Health context, the FAO's work in animal health and production is especially significant. Recognizing the link between livestock production, human well-being, and environmental health, the FAO promotes sustainable practices that balance productivity with animal welfare and ecological responsibility. This includes encouraging genetic diversity, ethical animal husbandry, and innovative farming methods that reduce environmental impact while maintaining food production efficiency.

The FAO has also emerged as a global leader in addressing AMR, a growing threat to both human and animal health [173]. Through a broad array of interventions, the FAO promotes responsible antimicrobial use in agriculture. This includes educating farmers and veterinarians, advocating for policy reform, supporting the development of vaccines and alternatives to antibiotics, and helping countries implement systems to monitor antimicrobial usage. These efforts aim to preserve antimicrobial efficacy for future generations.

The Emergency Prevention System (EMPRES) is one of the FAO's flagship initiatives for combating transboundary threats to animal and plant health. By integrating advanced surveillance with rapid response mechanisms, EMPRES allows early detection and swift management of outbreaks. This program exemplifies the One Health approach, acknowledging that pests and diseases affecting animals and plants can have significant consequences for human health and global food security [174].

A cornerstone of the FAO's strategy is its commitment to capacity building in member countries. Understanding that sustainable development must be locally driven, the FAO provides technical assistance and training to enhance national capabilities. Whether it's formulating food safety laws or training professionals in disease control, the organization empowers countries to manage their food systems more effectively and sustainably [175].

The FAO's work is also distinguished by its emphasis on collaboration and knowledge exchange. Acting as a global platform, the organization brings together governments, researchers, NGOs, and industry leaders to share insights and drive innovation in food and agriculture. These collaborations extend through partnerships with other UN bodies and international stakeholders, facilitating the transfer of best practices and research findings across borders.

Looking ahead, the FAO's leadership in the One Health domain is becoming increasingly vital. Climate change is transforming agricultural ecosystems, population growth is intensifying pressure on food systems, and new health threats are arising at the intersections of humans, animals, and the environment. These dynamics demand integrated solutions, and the FAO with its broad scope and expertise is uniquely positioned to develop sustainable food systems that support human, animal, and environmental health [176].

Ultimately, the FAO's efforts encapsulate the essence of the One Health philosophy that the health of people, animals, and ecosystems is interconnected. By addressing these shared challenges through coordinated, evidence-based strategies, the FAO contributes not only to eradicating hunger but also to creating a healthier, more harmonious world for all.

1.7.3 Global Collaborations

Global collaborations in the One Health domain mark a transformative shift in how the international community addresses complex health issues. These initiatives go beyond traditional disciplinary and national boundaries, fostering coordinated efforts to tackle challenges at the human–animal–environment interface [177].

The Tripartite Alliance comprising the WHO, WOAH, and FAO is the foundation of global One Health efforts. Since its formation in 2010, this alliance has demonstrated the power of interagency collaboration in addressing shared health threats. Its work spans zoonoses, AMR, and food safety, creating unified strategies and guidelines that inform both national and global policies. Through combined resources and expertise, the Tripartite has improved disease surveillance, bolstered response capabilities, and championed integrated solutions to global health concerns [175].

The One Health Global Leaders Group on Antimicrobial Resistance, established in 2020, addresses the critical issue of AMR through high-level advocacy. Comprising leaders from governments, industry, and civil society, the group takes a multisectoral approach to counter AMR's drivers in human, animal, and environmental health [178]. By promoting policy reform, encouraging innovation, and raising awareness, the group plays a vital role in safeguarding antimicrobial effectiveness for future generations.

The Global Health Security Agenda (GHSA), launched in 2014, emphasizes health security on a global scale. While broader in scope than One Health, many GHSA initiatives align with its principles. With over 70 partners, GHSA fosters global cooperation, enhances national disease response systems, and strengthens capacities for preventing and managing infectious threats [179]. Its collaborative model enables the exchange of expertise and reinforces resilience in health systems worldwide. The United Nations Environment Programme (UNEP) officially joined the Tripartite Alliance in 2021, expanding it into a Quadripartite partnership. This move highlights the critical role of environmental health in the One Health framework [180]. UNEP brings vital expertise in ecosystem preservation and pollution control, enhancing efforts to address emerging risks such as habitat loss and environmental contamination that influence disease dynamics.

The World Bank's One Health Operational Framework provides a practical guide for integrating One Health principles into development planning, especially in low- and middle-income countries. By offering structured guidance for project design, implementation, and evaluation, this framework supports the mainstreaming of One Health into national strategies, bridging policy and action for lasting impact. The One Health European Joint Programme (OH EJP) exemplifies the benefits of regional cooperation. Bringing together 44 partners from 22 countries, the OH EJP fosters research and innovation relevant to policymakers and public health authorities [181]. By aligning research with real-world needs, the program ensures scientific findings translate into effective health interventions. Additionally, it nurtures a new generation of One Health professionals through training and collaboration, strengthening the field's long-term capacity.

Though diverse in scope and structure, these collaborations share a unified vision: a holistic approach to health that transcends sectoral silos. They reflect the growing awareness that contemporary health threats, ranging from pandemics to climate-induced disease emergence, require collective, cross-sectoral responses [182]. As these partnerships expand, their influence on shaping global health strategies will continue to grow. Beyond addressing immediate threats, they are laying the foundation for resilient health systems prepared for future challenges. Together, these global collaborations are bringing the One Health vision closer to reality: a healthier, more sustainable future where human, animal, and environmental health are protected in unison.

1.8 Future Directions

Education is continually evolving, shaped by emerging technologies, changing societal demands, and a growing emphasis on innovation. To build more inclusive and adaptable systems, we must integrate research, teaching strategies, and policy development to meet the diverse needs of today's learners. Research offers vital insights into improving teaching methods, student engagement, and curriculum design. Technological advancements and data-driven tools allow for personalized learning, while innovative strategies promote collaboration and critical thinking. Simultaneously, education policy must adapt to support these changes and respond to emerging challenges.

A holistic focus on research, teaching innovation, and policy reform is essential for creating environments that foster creativity, resilience, and lifelong learning. By prioritizing this intersection, we can shape a more effective and future-ready education system.

1.8.1 Research Opportunities for Innovations

The future of One Health research holds great promise for transformative innovations that can reshape our approach to global health challenges. Several key areas stand out for their potential impact.

Advanced surveillance systems are at the forefront. Integrating technologies like artificial intelligence and machine learning into health monitoring could revolutionize our ability to detect and respond to threats [183]. Imagine a global sensor network that collects data on environmental conditions, animal health, and human well-being analyzed in real time by intelligent algorithms. Such systems could identify early warning signs of disease outbreaks, enabling rapid action before issues escalate [184]. The microbiome the vast community of microorganisms living in humans, animals, and the environment is another promising area. Research into these microbial ecosystems may unlock new ways to prevent and treat diseases. For example, manipulating the gut microbiome could strengthen immune systems or help control antibiotic-resistant infections. Applications might range from sustainable agriculture to ecosystem restoration and disease management [185].

Climate change is a pressing global issue, and One Health research is well-positioned to study its health impacts. Shifting climate patterns influence the spread of vector-borne diseases, disrupt food systems, and affect the health of both people and animals. One Health studies can guide adaptive strategies like climate-resilient agriculture or disease control programs for vulnerable populations [186]. The field of genomics offers exciting opportunities as well. Studying the genetic basis of disease susceptibility across species could lead to more targeted treatments. Future health strategies may combine personal genetic data with environmental and animal health factors to deliver more precise, ecosystem-informed healthcare.

Zoonotic diseases, which transfer from animals to humans, remain a major global concern. Developing predictive models for outbreaks could help prevent future pandemics. These models would integrate diverse data sources from wildlife patterns to human behavior and climate conditions using machine learning to identify emerging threats [187]. Sustainable agriculture also falls within One Health's scope. As populations grow, there's increasing pressure to boost food production without compromising the environment. One Health research can guide innovations that reduce antibiotic use, cut greenhouse gas emissions, and promote biodiversity all while maintaining food security [188].

Finally, understanding the economic value of One Health interventions is crucial. New economic models could reveal how integrated health strategies yield long-term savings by preventing disease and preserving ecosystems. In all these areas, it's essential to maintain a holistic view recognizing that improvements in one area can benefit the entire system. By fostering cross-sector collaboration, embracing innovation, and prioritizing the health of people, animals, and the environment, One Health research can help build a healthier, more resilient world [189].

1.8.2 Educational Strategies

The future success of the One Health approach depends on our ability to educate and inspire the next generation of professionals, policymakers, and the public. Innovative educational strategies are essential to build a strong foundation in One Health principles and their real-world applications.

A central strategy is the development of interdisciplinary curricula that break traditional academic boundaries. Imagine veterinary, medical, environmental, and social science students working together on complex health challenges. These programs would promote systems thinking and collaborative problem-solving, helping learners understand the connections between human, animal, and environmental health [190]. To cultivate leadership, global health leadership programs must go beyond academic training. Scenario-based learning can prepare future leaders to respond to crises, make decisions under uncertainty, and communicate across cultures and disciplines [177]. These immersive experiences will build the confidence and skills needed to lead in diverse, complex environments.

The digital era offers tremendous potential for expanding access to One Health education. E-learning platforms, MOOCs, and virtual simulations can reach global audiences regardless of location or resources. A veterinary student in rural India, for instance, could use VR to simulate outbreak responses with peers worldwide, all under expert guidance [191]. Community-based education is vital for successful One Health implementation. Participatory research involving local residents in monitoring animal health or environmental changes empowers communities while enriching scientific understanding. This grassroots involvement builds trust and fosters lasting commitment to One Health values [192].

Professional exchange programs can deepen expertise and broaden perspectives. By working on wildlife conservation in Africa or urban health in Asia, participants gain diverse, hands-on experiences and build global networks. These relationships and insights are invaluable in addressing transboundary health issues [193]. For working professionals, continuing education remains crucial. Online workshops, webinars, and short courses offer flexible ways to stay updated with the latest research and practices. These programs support professionals in applying One Health principles in fields like clinical care, public health, and policy. Equally important are public awareness campaigns that communicate the essence of One Health to broader audiences. Engaging content through museums, media, or storytelling can highlight how daily choices affect the health of people, animals, and the environment. These creative approaches inspire societal understanding and support for One Health goals [194].

Ultimately, One Health education must go beyond information-sharing to foster a mindset. We must nurture curiosity, empathy, and global citizenship in learners of all ages. By empowering individuals with knowledge and passion, we can cultivate a generation of One Health champions ready to build a healthier, more sustainable future for all.

1.8.3 Policy Development

Developing effective policy frameworks is essential for translating One Health principles into action. As we look to the future, several policy directions can help operationalize this holistic approach.

At the forefront is the creation of integrated health policies that bridge human, animal, and environmental health sectors. For example, national health strategies could include joint disease surveillance, cross-sectoral research, and shared resources. These integrated policies would better reflect the interconnected nature of health and lead to more comprehensive outcomes [195]. The introduction of One Health Impact Assessments (OHIAs) offers a proactive policy tool. Similar to environmental impact assessments, OHIAs would ensure that proposed initiatives such as urban development or agricultural reforms are evaluated for their broader health effects. This would institutionalize a One Health perspective in policymaking and improve long-term outcomes [196].

On a global scale, strengthening international governance is key. This could involve enhancing the roles of WHO, FAO, and WOAH to promote One Health, or establishing a dedicated global body to coordinate cross-border collaboration, standard-setting, and information sharing. Such governance is essential for addressing transboundary health threats [197]. Sustainable funding mechanisms are another critical pillar. Dedicated grants, public–private partnerships, and allocations from national budgets can support research, training, and implementation of One Health programs. Without reliable funding, many innovative approaches remain theoretical [177].

Robust legal frameworks are needed to regulate zoonotic disease control, antimicrobial use, and environmental protection. For instance, antibiotic use in livestock might be more tightly regulated to combat AMR, while wildlife trade laws can reduce zoonotic risks and protect biodiversity. Intersectoral collaboration policies help overcome bureaucratic fragmentation. These might mandate joint task forces, shared budgets, and routine coordination between departments of health, agriculture, and environment. Institutionalizing collaboration ensures One Health becomes embedded in governance structures [198].

In international development, aligning aid and projects with One Health principles enhances sustainability. For example, agricultural programs could promote ecosystem health alongside food production, helping to prevent disease emergence and environmental degradation. As data sharing becomes increasingly vital, policies must support rapid, secure exchange of information across sectors and borders. Clear protocols will ensure data are available during crises while protecting privacy and national interests.

Urban planning policies should consider One Health impacts in an increasingly urbanized world. These might promote green spaces to reduce heat and support biodiversity, while limiting disease risks from dense human–animal interactions [199]. Lastly, climate change adaptation policies must embrace a One Health lens. Strategies might address shifting disease patterns, food insecurity, and biodiversity loss due to environmental stress, ensuring resilience across species and systems [200].

Moving forward, effective One Health policy requires ongoing collaboration, flexibility, and innovation. By embedding a systems-thinking approach in policy frameworks, governments can anticipate and mitigate future threats building a healthier, more resilient world for all.

1.9 Conclusion

This chapter underscores the pivotal role of veterinary sciences within the One Health framework, highlighting their contributions to animal health, disease prevention, and food security while addressing significant challenges such as emerging infectious diseases and AMR. Despite advancements in technology and interdisciplinary collaboration, limitations persist in the form of resource constraints and the need for robust surveillance systems. Future research should focus on leveraging innovative technologies for real-time disease detection, fostering interdisciplinary education, and developing integrated policies that enhance collaboration across sectors. By addressing these gaps, the One Health approach can further advance global health outcomes and promote sustainability for humans, animals, and the environment.

References

1 Yeates, J. *Veterinary Science: A Very Short Introduction*. Vol. 554. Oxford: Oxford University Press; 2018. https://doi.org/10.1093/actrade/9780198790969.001.0001.

2 Hobson-West, P. and Jutel, A. Animals, veterinarians and the sociology of diagnosis. *Soc. Health Illn.* 2020; 42(2): 393–406. https://doi.org/10.1111/1467-9566.13017.

3 Battaglia, A.M. and Steele, A.M. *Small Animal Emergency and Critical Care for Veterinary Technicians-E-Book*. 4th ed. St. Louis, MO: Elsevier Health Sciences; 2020.

4 King, L.J. Veterinary medicine and public health at CDC. *Morb. Mortal Wkly. Rep.* 2006; 55: 7–9.

5 Van Knapen, F. Veterinary public health: past, present, and future. *Vet. Q.* 2000; 22(2): 61–62. https://doi.org/10.1080/01652176.2000.9695026.

6 Ferguson, D.C. Veterinary sciences—a forum for one medicine, one health. *Vet. Sci.* 2014; 1(1): 1–2. https://doi.org/10.3390/vetsci1010001.

7 Potter, P. "One medicine" for animal and human health. *Emerg. Infect. Dis.* 2004; 10(12): 2269. https://doi.org/10.3201/eid1012.AC1012.

8 Dawkins, M.S. A user's guide to animal welfare science. *Trends Ecol. Evol.* 2006; 21(2): 77–82. https://doi.org/10.1016/j.tree.2005.10.017.

9 Christopher, M.M. A new decade of veterinary research: societal relevance, global collaboration, and translational medicine. *Front. Vet. Sci.* 2015; 2: 1–4. https://doi.org/10.3389/fvets.2015.00001.

10 Engdawork, A., Belayhun, T., and Aseged, T. The role of reproductive technologies and cryopreservation of genetic materials in the conservation of animal genetic resources: a review. *Ecol. Genet. Genom.* 2024; 31: 100250. https://doi.org/10.1016/j.egg.2024.100250.

11 Rollin, B.E. Integrating science and well-being. *Vet. Clin. North Am. Small Anim.* 2020; 50(4): 899–904. https://doi.org/10.1016/j.cvsm.2020.03.009.

12 Binois, A. Excavating the history of ancient veterinary practices. *Vet. Rec.* 2015; 176(22): 564–569. https://doi.org/10.1136/vr.h991.

13 Jones, S.D. and Koolmees, P.A. Veterinary medicine and animal health, 2000–2020. In: *A Concise History of Veterinary Medicine. New Approaches to the History of Science and Medicine*, 329–368. Cambridge: Cambridge University Press; 2022. https://doi.org/10.1017/9781108354929.009.

14 Stephens, G. Animal health and veterinary sciences. In: *Using the Agricultural, Environmental, and Food Literature*, 74–127. New York: Marcel Decker, CRC Press; 2002. https://doi.org/10.1201/9780203909119.

15 Woods, A. Animals in the history of human and veterinary medicine. In: *The Routledge Companion to Animal-Human History*, 147–170. London: Routledge; 2018. https://doi.org/10.4324/9780429468933.

16 Devi, S., Singh, R.D., Ghasura, R.S., et al. Telemedicine: a new rise of hope to animal health care sector—a review. *Agric. Rev.* 2015; 36(2): 153–158. https://doi.org/10.5958/0976-0741.2015.00018.5.

17 Abu-Seida, A.M., Abdulkarim, A., and Hassan, M.H. Veterinary telemedicine: a new era for animal welfare. *Open Vet. J.* 2024; 14(4): 952. https://doi.org/10.5455/OVJ.2024.v14.i4.2.

18 Mohanty, I. Role of a veterinarian in present society and One Health approach. *J. Livest. Sci.* 2014; 5: 18–22.

19 Min, P.K., Mito, K., and Kim, T.H. The evolving landscape of artificial intelligence applications in animal health. *Indian J. Anim. Res.* 2024; 58(10): 1793–1798. https://doi.org/10.18805/IJAR.BF-1742.

20 Hamadani, A., Ganai, N.A., Hamadani, H., et al. Applications and impact of artificial intelligence in veterinary sciences. In: *A Biologist's Guide to Artificial Intelligence*, 139–150. London, UK: Academic Press; 2024. https://doi.org/10.1016/B978-0-443-24001-0.00009-9.

21 Khan, M., Junaid, M., Kousar, U., et al. Veterinary interventions and public health implications: zoonotic disease perspective. *J. Asian Dev. Stud.* 2023; 12(4): 870–878. https://doi.org/10.62345/jads.2023.12.4.68.

22 Cersosimo, G. The role and responsibility of the veterinary profession in the One Health approach. *Salute Soc.* 2024; XXIII(3): 117–130.

23 Primrose, S.B. Zoonotic diseases. In: *Microbiology of Infectious Disease: Integrating Genomics with Natural History*, 233–238. Oxford: Oxford Academic; 2022. https://doi.org/10.1093/oso/9780192863843.003.0030.

24 Xue, Y. Preventing zoonotic diseases: an investigation into veterinary medicine's role in public health. *J. Clin. Med. Res.* 2024; 5(1): 41–43. https://doi.org/10.32629/jcmr.v5i1.1781.

25 Berdah, D., Noûs, C. Veterinary expertise, public health and animal contagion: the control of bovine tuberculosis in France and UK, 1860–1960. In: *Animals and Epidemics. Interspecies Entanglements in Historical Perspective.* Bohlau Verlag Koln; 2023.

26 Brugère-Picoux, J., Leroy, E., Angot, J.L., et al. Santé humaine et santé animale. *Bull. Acad. Natl. Med.* 2022; 206(1): 138–145. https://doi.org/10.1016/j.banm.2021.11.008.

27 Basit, A., Yasin, U., Hashmi, H.A., et al. Pets diseases and public health: zoonosis, transmission and treatment: a review. *Indus J. Biosci. Res.* 2024; 2(02): 1059–1071. https://doi.org/10.70749/ijbr.v2i02.327.

28 Das, U. Veterinary public health: the planetary path to one health. In: *Global Applications of One Health Practice and Care* (ed. S. Yasobant and D. Saxena), 113–124. Harshey, PA: IGI Global; 2019. https://doi.org/10.4018/978-1-5225-6304-4.ch005.

29 Saleem, M.I., Mahfooz, A., Zaka, F., et al. Public health awareness of zoonosis through veterinary profession. In: *Zoonosis*, 594–611. Faisalabad, Pakistan: Unique Scientific Publishers; 2023. https://doi.org/10.47278/book.zoon/2023.044.

30 Verma, S., Malik, Y.S., Singh, G., et al. *Core Competencies of a Veterinary Graduate*. Singapore: Springer; 2024.

31 Vicente, J., Vercauteren, K.C., and Gortázar, C. *Diseases at the Wildlife-Livestock Interface*. Cham: Springer International Publishing; 2021.

32 Carpenter, A., Waltenburg, M.A., Hall, A., et al. Vaccine preventable zoonotic diseases: challenges and opportunities for public health progress. *Vaccines* 2022; 10(7): 993. https://doi.org/10.3390/vaccines10070993.

33 Gerstein, H.C., Rutty, C.J. Insulin therapy: the discovery that shaped a century. *Can. J. Diabetes* 2021; 45(8): 798–803. https://doi.org/10.1016/j.jcjd.2021.03.002.

34 Masurkar, S. Exploring the impact of environmental factors on animal health: a veterinary perspective. *Rev. Electron. Vet.* 2024; 25(1): 120–138.

35 Bean, T.G. and Rattner, B.A. Environmental contaminants of health-care origin: exposure and potential effects in wildlife. In: *Health Care and Environmental Contamination* (ed. D. Brunk), 87–122. Amsterdam: Elsevier; 2018. https://doi.org/10.1016/B978-0-444-63857-1.00006-1.

36 Maréchal, L., Barcelos, A.M., Cole, J., et al. Human–animal welfare: the interconnectedness of human well-being and animal welfare. In: *Introduction to Human-Animal Interaction* (ed. P. McCardle), 65–78. London: London: Routledge; 2024.

37 Van Herten, J. and Meijboom, F.L.B. Veterinary responsibilities within the one health framework. *Food Ethics* 2019; 3: 109–123.

38 Robertson, I.D. Disease control, prevention and on-farm biosecurity: the role of veterinary epidemiology. *Engineering* 2020; 6(1): 20–25. https://doi.org/10.1016/j.eng.2019.10.004.

39 Thrusfield, M. *Veterinary Epidemiology*. 4th ed. Oxford: John Wiley and Sons; 2018.

40 Kumar, H.C., Hiremath, J., Yogisharadhya, R., et al. Animal disease surveillance: its importance and present status in India. *Indian J. Med. Res.* 2021; 153(3): 299–310. https://doi.org/10.4103/ijmr.IJMR_740_21.

41 Bishop, K.A. and Huwa, J.J. *Introduction to Government Plant and Animal Disease Monitoring and Prevention Programs in the United States*. Institute for Defense Analyses: Alexandria, VA; 2020. IDA Document NS D-14345, 34p.

42 Rahman, M.T., Sobur, M.A., Islam, M.S., et al. Zoonotic diseases: etiology, impact, and control. *Microorganisms* 2020; 8(9): 1405. https://doi.org/10.3390/microorganisms8091405.

43 Usmani, M.W., Rizvi, F., Shakir, M.Z., et al. Factors influencing the emergence and re-emergence of zoonotic infectious diseases in livestock and human populations. *Zoonosis* 2023; 1: 316–326. https://doi.org/10.47278/book.zoon/2023.023.

44 Salkeld, D., Hopkins, S., and Hayman, D. *Emerging Zoonotic and Wildlife Pathogens: Disease Ecology, Epidemiology, and Conservation*. Oxford: Oxford University Press; 2023. https://doi.org/10.1093/oso/9780198825920.001.0001.

45 Recht, J., Schuenemann, V.J., Sánchez-Villagra, M.R. Host diversity and origin of zoonoses: the ancient and the new. *Animals* 2020; 10(9): 1672. https://doi.org/10.3390/ani10091672.

46 Michel, A.L., Van Heerden, H., Prasse, D., et al. Pathogen detection and disease diagnosis in wildlife: challenges and opportunities. *Rev. Sci. Tech.* 2021; 40(1): 105–118.

47 Haider, N., Rothman-Ostrow, P., Osman, A.Y., et al. COVID-19—zoonosis or emerging infectious disease? *Front. Public Health* 2020; 8: 596944. https://doi.org/10.3389/fpubh.2020.596944.

48 Agrawal, I. and Varga, C. Assessing and comparing disease prevention knowledge, attitudes, and practices among veterinarians in Illinois, United States of America. *Prev. Vet. Med.* 2024; 228: 106223. https://doi.org/10.1016/j.prevetmed.2024.106223.

49 Warimwe, G.M., Francis, M.J., Bowden, T.A., et al. Using cross-species vaccination approaches to counter emerging infectious diseases. *Nat. Rev. Immunol.* 2021; 21(12): 815–822.

50 Frey, E. The role of companion animal veterinarians in One Health efforts to combat antimicrobial resistance. *J. Am. Vet. Med. Assoc.* 2018; 253(11): 1396–1404. https://doi.org/10.2460/javma.253.11.1396.

51 Pimentel, L.C. and Taylor, E.V. Surveillance for zoonotic diseases. In: *Concepts and Methods in Infectious Disease Surveillance* (ed. L.M. Lee), 92–106. Hoboken: Wiley Blackwell; 2014. https://doi.org/10.1002/9781118928646.ch10.

52 Shekel, V.F., Kurtyak, B.M., Padovsky, A.I., and Dembitska, I.S. Veterinary aspects of protection peoples' health and role VET departments in the sanitary food safety according to requirements OIE. *Sci Messin. LNU Vet. Med. Biotechnol. Vet. Sci.* 2018; 20: 357–361. https://doi.org/10.15421/nvlvet8371.

53 Saleem, M.I., Mahfooz, A., Khan, M.S., et al. Role of veterinary students in propagation of awareness regarding the public health education of zoonotic diseases. In: *Zoonosis*, 627–642. Faisalabad, Pakistan: Unique Scientific Publishers; 2023. https://doi.org/10.47278/book.zoon/2023.046.

54 Thakur, S.D. Early warning systems, disease management, and biosecurity in disasters. In: *Management of Animals in Disasters*, 25–37. Singapore: Springer Nature Singapore; 2022. https://doi.org/10.1007/978-981-16-9392-2_3.

55 Wilson, A.L., Courtenay, O., Kelly-Hope, L.A., et al. The importance of vector control for the control and elimination of vector-borne diseases. *PLoS Negl. Trop Dis.* 2020; 14: e0007831. https://doi.org/10.1371/journal.pntd.0007831.

56 Thomas, S., Abraham, A., Rodríguez-Mallon, A., et al. Challenges in veterinary vaccine development. In: *Vaccine Design: Methods and Protocols, Volume 2. Vaccines for Veterinary Diseases*, 3–34. New York: Humana press; 2022. https://doi.org/10.1371/journal.pntd.0007831.

57 Hernandez, E., Llonch, P., and Turner, P.V. Applied animal ethics in industrial food animal production: exploring the role of the veterinarian. *Animals* 2022; 12: 678. https://doi.org/10.3390/ani12060678.

58 Ferri, M. and Lloyd-Evans, M. The contribution of veterinary public health to the management of the COVID-19 pandemic from a One Health perspective. *One Health* 2021; 12: 100230. https://doi.org/10.1016/j.onehlt.2021.100230.

59 Sharan, M., Vijay, D., Yadav, J.P., et al. Surveillance and response strategies for zoonotic diseases: a comprehensive review. *Sci. One Health* 2023; 2: 100050. https://doi.org/10.1016/j.soh.2023.100050.

60 Van Marle-Köster, E. and Visser, C. Genomics for the advancement of livestock production: a South African perspective. *S. Afr. J. Anim. Sci.* 2018; 48: 808–817. https://doi.org/10.4314/sajas.v48i5.2.

61 Marcombes, L. Veterinary sustainability. *Med. Writ.* 2022; 31: 30–35.

62 Ibrahim, M., Ahmad, F., Yaqub, B., et al. Current trends of antimicrobials used in food animals and aquaculture. In: *Antibiotics and Antimicrobial Resistance Genes in the Environment*, 39–69. Amsterdam: Elsevier; 2020. https://doi.org/10.1016/B978-0-12-818882-8.00004-8.

63 Perry, B.D., Robinson, T.P., and Grace, D.C. Animal health and sustainable global livestock systems. *Animal* 2018; 12: 1699–1708. https://doi.org/10.1017/S1751731118000630.

64 Lewis, C.E. and Roth, J. Challenges in having vaccines available to control transboundary diseases of livestock. *Curr. Issues Mol. Biol.* 2021; 42: 1–40. https://doi.org/10.21775/cimb.042.001.

65 Magiri, R., Muzandu, K., Gitau, G., et al. Impact of climate change on animal health, emerging and re-emerging diseases in Africa. In: *African Handbook of Climate Change Adaptation*, 1–18. Cham, Switzerland: Springer; 2020. https://doi.org/10.1007/978-3-030-42091-8_19-1.

66 Trujillo, S.L. Enhancing the welfare of working equids: an imperative in development and humanitarian scenarios. PhD dissertation; Portugal: Universidade Fernando Pessoa Porto; 2020.

67 Leyland, T. A path to prosperity: new directions for African livestock. *Gates Open Res.* 2019; 3: 148.
68 Whittemore, C.T. *Animal Farming: The Story Behind the Livestock Industry*. Netherlands: Brill; 2023.
69 Lean, I.J., Van Saun, R., and DeGaris, P.J. Energy and protein nutrition management of transition dairy cows. *Vet. Clin. Food Anim. Pract.* 2018; 34: 1–21.
70 Mikkola, M. Utilization of sexed semen in dairy cattle. *J. Anim. Sci.* 2018; 96(Suppl 3): 51–52.
71 Mrode, R., Ojango, J.M.K., Okeyo, A.M., and Mwacharo, J.M. Genomic selection and use of molecular tools in breeding programs for indigenous and crossbred cattle in developing countries: current status and future prospects. *Front. Genet.* 2019; 9: 694. https://doi.org/10.3389/fgene.2018.00694.
72 Jerlström, J., Berg, C., Karlsson, A., et al. A formal model for assessing the economic impact of animal welfare improvements at bovine and porcine slaughter. *Animal Welfare*. 2022; 31(3): 361–371. https://doi.org/10.7120/09627286.31.4.004.
73 Rexroad, C., Vallet, J., Matukumalli, L.K., et al. Genome to phenome: improving animal health, production, and well-being—a new USDA blueprint for animal genome research 2018–2027. *Front. Genet.* 2019; 10: 327. https://doi.org/10.3389/fgene.2019.00327.
74 Britt, J.H., Cushman, R.A., Dechow, C.D., et al. Invited review: learning from the future—a vision for dairy farms and cows in 2067. *J. Dairy Sci.* 2018; 101(5): 3722–3741. https://doi.org/10.3168/jds.2017-14025.
75 Kumbhar, U.T. Veterinary interventions in livestock agriculture: enhancing productivity and welfare. *Rev. Electron. Vet.* 2024; 25(1): 160–180.
76 Anadón, A., Martínez-Larrañaga, M.R., Ares, I., and Martínez, M.A. Regulatory aspects for the drugs and chemicals used in food-producing animals in the European Union. In: *Veterinary Toxicology*, 103–131. Academic Press; 2018. https://doi.org/10.1016/B978-0-12-811410-0.00007-6.
77 Tobin, G. and Schuhmacher, A. Nutrition, feeding, and animal welfare. In: *The UFAW Handbook on the Care and Management of Laboratory and Other Research Animals*, 191–219. Boca Raton, FL, USA: CRC Press; 2024. https://doi.org/10.1002/9781119555278.ch13.
78 Buller, H., Adam, K., Bard, A., et al. Veterinary diagnostic practice and the use of rapid tests in antimicrobial stewardship on UK livestock farms. *Front. Vet. Sci.* 2020; 7: 569545. https://doi.org/10.3389/fvets.2020.569545.
79 Bayantassova, S.M., Nurgaliyev, B.E., Muhanbetkalieva, G.S., and Dzhumagulova, S.K. Veterinary-sanitary inspection of poultry, fish, beekeeping, and plant products. Almanah Publishing house; 2022.
80 Surono, S. Development of competency standards for good hygienic practices facilitators to enhance food safety assurance. *Asian J. Eng. Soc. Health* 2024; 3(5): 893–912. https://doi.org/10.46799/ajesh.v3i5.300.
81 Motarjemi, Y. and Warren, B.R. Hazard analysis and critical control point system (HACCP). In: *Food Safety Management*, 799–818. San Diego, CA: Academic Press; 2023. https://doi.org/10.1016/B978-0-12-820013-1.00017-6.
82 Erkyihun, G.A. and Alemayehu, M.B. One Health approach for the control of zoonotic diseases. *Zoonoses* 2022; 2(1): 963.
83 Caneschi, A., Bardhi, A., Barbarossa, A., and Zaghini, A. The use of antibiotics and antimicrobial resistance in veterinary medicine, a complex phenomenon: a narrative review. *Antibiotics* 2023; 12(3): 487. https://doi.org/10.3390/antibiotics12030487.
84 Patil, S.V. Zoonotic disease surveillance and control: safeguarding both animal and human populations. *Rev. Electron. Vet.* 2024; 25(1): 452–463.
85 Garcia, S.N., Osburn, B.I., and Jay-Russell, M.T. One Health for food safety, food security, and sustainable food production. *Front. Sustain. Food Syst.* 2020; 4: 1. https://doi.org/10.3389/fsufs.2020.00001.
86 Koytcheva, M.K., Sauerwein, L.K., Webb, T.L., et al. A systematic review of environmental sustainability in veterinary practice. *Top. Companion Anim. Med.* 2021; 44: 100550. https://doi.org/10.1016/j.tcam.2021.100550.
87 Rees, G.M., Reyher, K.K., Barrett, D.C., and Buller, H. "It's cheaper than a dead cow": understanding veterinary medicine use on dairy farms. *J Rural Stud.* 2021; 86: 587–598. https://doi.org/10.1016/j.jrurstud.2021.07.020.
88 Lau, T.C.W. Prophylactic fictions: immunity and biosecurity. PhD dissertation. University of Pennsylvania; 2018.

89 Day, M.J., Crawford, C., Marcondes, M., and Squires, R.A. Recommendations on vaccination for Latin American small animal practitioners: a report of the WSAVA vaccination guidelines group. *J. Small Anim. Pract.* 2020; 61(6): E1–E35. https://doi.org/10.1111/jsap.13125.

90 Pawar, J. Nutritional strategies for enhancing animal health and performance: a veterinary approach. *Rev. Electron. Vet.* 2024; 25(1): 139–159.

91 Pal, A. and Chakravarty, A.K. *Genetics and Breeding for Disease Resistance of Livestock*. Cambridge, MA, USA: Academic Press; 2019.

92 Araujo, G.S., Silva, J.W.A., Cotas, J., and Pereira, L. Fish farming techniques: current situation and trends. *J. Mar. Sci. Eng.* 2022; 10(11): 1598. https://doi.org/10.3390/jmse10111598.

93 Shaikh, T.A., Rasool, T., and Lone, F.R. Towards leveraging the role of machine learning and artificial intelligence in precision agriculture and smart farming. *Comput. Electron. Agric.* 2022; 198: 107119. https://doi.org/10.1016/j.compag.2022.107119.

94 Tian, M., He, X., Feng, Y., et al. Pollution by antibiotics and antimicrobial resistance in livestock and poultry manure in China, and countermeasures. *Antibiotics* 2021; 10(5): 539. https://doi.org/10.3390/antibiotics10050539.

95 Serwecińska, L. Antimicrobials and antibiotic-resistant bacteria: a risk to the environment and to public health. *Water* 2020; 12(12): 3313. https://doi.org/10.3390/antibiotics10050539.

96 Iepsen, S.E.L., Martini, L., Iepsen, G.L., et al. Management of waste in veterinary hospitals: challenges, risks and opportunities. *Cad. Pedagógico.* 2024; 21(4): e3872–e3872. https://doi.org/10.54033/cadpedv21n4-137.

97 Schiavone, S.C.M., Smith, S.M., Mazariegos, I., et al. Environmental sustainability in veterinary medicine: an opportunity for teaching hospitals. *J. Vet. Med. Educ.* 2022; 49(2): 260–266. https://doi.org/10.3138/jvme-2020-0125.

98 Zhu, F. A review on the application of herbal medicines in the disease control of aquatic animals. *Aquaculture* 2020; 526: 735422. https://doi.org/10.1016/j.aquaculture.2020.735422.

99 Willette, M., Rosenhagen, N., Buhl, G., et al. Interrupted lives: welfare considerations in wildlife rehabilitation. *Animals* 2023; 13(11): 1836. https://doi.org/10.3390/ani13111836.

100 Gray, J. Challenges of compassionate conservation. *J. Appl. Anim. Welf Sci.* 2018; 21(suppl 1): 34–42. https://doi.org/10.1080/10888705.2018.1513840.

101 Blackett, T., Marsh, S., Groves, G., et al. Core fundamental standard of practice for captive wild animals. *Wild Welfare* 2020. https://wildwelfare.org/wp-content/uploads/Core-Fundamental-Standard-of-Practice-for-Captive-Wild-Animals-Oct2020.pdf (accessed on 11 November 2010).

102 Mullineaux, E. and Pawson, C. Trends in admissions and outcomes at a British wildlife rehabilitation centre over a ten-year period (2012–2022). *Animals* 2023; 14(1): 86. https://doi.org/10.3390/ani14010086.

103 Cerda, J.R. and Webb, T.L. Wildlife conservation and preserving biodiversity: impactful opportunities for veterinarians? *J. Am. Vet. Med. Assoc.* 2023; 261(7): 1077–1085. https://doi.org/10.2460/javma.23.02.0094.

104 Verant, M. and Bernard, R.F. White-nose syndrome in bats: conservation, management, and context-dependent decision making. In: *Wildlife Disease and Health in Conservation*, 273–291. Johns Hopkins University; 2023.

105 Miranda, R., Escribano, N., Casas, M., et al. The role of zoos and aquariums in a changing world. *Annu. Rev. Anim. Biosci.* 2023; 11(1): 287–306. https://doi.org/10.1146/annurev-animal-050622-104306.

106 König, H.J., Kiffner, C., Kramer-Schadt, S., et al. Human–wildlife coexistence in a changing world. *Conserv. Biol.* 2020; 34(4): 786–794.

107 Thorat, G. One Health approach: integrating veterinary medicine into public health and environmental conservation. *Rev. Electron. Vet.* 2024; 25(1): 181–193.

108 Parry, N.M.A. and Stoll, A. The rise of veterinary forensics. *Forensic Sci. Int.* 2020; 306: 110069. https://doi.org/10.1016/j.forsciint.2019.110069.

109 Martinez, B., Reaser, J.K., Dehgan, A., et al. Technology innovation: advancing capacities for the early detection of and rapid response to invasive species. *Biol Invasions* 2020; 22(1): 75–100. https://doi.org/10.1007/s10530-019-02146-y.

110 Moore, R.M. Parallels between biodiversity and human diversity: a mandate to improve ecological and organizational health and vitality. *J. Zoo Wildl. Med.* 2023; 53(4): 633–643. https://doi.org/10.1638/2022-0081.

111 Stephens, T. (ed.) *One Welfare in Practice: The Role of the Veterinarian.* CRC Press; 2021.

112 Panel, O.H.H.L.E., Hayman, D.T., Adisasmito, W.B., et al. Developing one health surveillance systems. *One Health* 2023; 17: 100617. https://doi.org/10.1016/j.onehlt.2023.100617.

113 Bloom, D.E. and Cadarette, D. Infectious disease threats in the twenty-first century: strengthening the global response. *Front. Immunol.* 2019; 10: 549. https://doi.org/10.3389/fimmu.2019.00549.

114 Subbarao, K. The critical interspecies transmission barrier at the animal–human interface. *Trop. Med. Infect. Dis.* 2019; 4(2): 72. https://doi.org/10.3390/tropicalmed4020072.

115 Naveed, A., Eertink, L.G., Wang, D., and Li, F. Lessons learned from West Nile Virus infection: vaccinations in equines and their implications for One Health approaches. *Viruses* 2024; 16(5): 781. https://doi.org/10.3390/v16050781.

116 Guberti, V., Khomenko, S., Masiulis, M., and Kerba, S. *African Swine Fever in Wild Boar: Ecology and Biosecurity.* FAO; 2022.

117 De Sadeleer, N. and Godfroid, J. The story behind COVID-19: animal diseases at the crossroads of wildlife, livestock and human health. *Eur. J. Risk Regul.* 2020; 11(2): 210–227. https://doi.org/10.1017/err.2020.45.

118 Neujahr, A.C., Loy, D.S., Loy, J.D., et al. Rapid detection of high consequence and emerging viral pathogens in pigs. *Front. Vet. Sci.* 2024; 11: 1341783. https://doi.org/10.3389/fvets.2024.1341783.

119 Das, B., Ellis, M., and Sahoo, M. Veterinary diagnostics: growth, trends, and impact. In: *Evolving Landscape of Molecular Diagnostics*, 227–242. Amsterdam: Elsevier; 2024. https://doi.org/10.1016/B978-0-323-99316-6.00007-X.

120 Galles, B. A literature review of the psychosocial impacts on livestock producers and veterinary responders involved with depopulation during and after an animal health emergency. *Capstone Experience* 2023. https://digitalcommons.unmc.edu/coph_slce/263.

121 Singh, S., Sharma, P., Pal, N., et al. Holistic one health surveillance framework: synergizing environmental, animal, and human determinants for enhanced infectious disease management. *ACS Infect. Dis.* 2024; 10(3): 808–826. https://doi.org/10.1021/acsinfecdis.3c00625.

122 Ogunseitan, O.A. One health and the environment: from conceptual framework to implementation science. *Environ. Sci. Policy Sustain. Dev.* 2022; 64(2): 11–21. https://doi.org/10.1080/00139157.2022.2021792.

123 Ahmed, S.K., Hussein, S., Qurbani, K., et al. Antimicrobial resistance: impacts, challenges, and future prospects. *J. Med. Surg. Public Health* 2024; 2: 100081. https://doi.org/10.1016/j.glmedi.2024.100081.

124 Ifedinezi, O.V., Nnaji, N.D., Anumudu, C.K., et al. Environmental antimicrobial resistance: implications for food safety and public health. *Antibiotics* 2024; 13(11): 1087. https://doi.org/10.3390/antibiotics13111087.

125 Adebisi, Y.A. Balancing the risks and benefits of antibiotic use in a globalized world: the ethics of antimicrobial resistance. *Global Health* 2023; 19(1): 27. https://doi.org/10.1186/s12992-023-00930-z.

126 Singha, B., Singh, V., and Soni, V. Alternative therapeutics to control antimicrobial resistance: a general perspective. *Front. Drug Discov.* 2024; 4: 1385460. https://doi.org/10.3389/fddsv.2024.1385460.

127 Fuller, W., Kapona, O., Aboderin, A.O., et al. Education and awareness on antimicrobial resistance in the WHO African region: a systematic review. *Antibiotics* 2023; 12(11): 1613. https://doi.org/10.3390/antibiotics12111613.

128 Chindelevitch, L., Jauneikaite, E., Wheeler, N.E., et al. Applying data technologies to combat AMR: current status, challenges, and opportunities on the way forward. *arXiv preprint arXiv:2208.04683.* 2022. https://doi.org/10.48550/arXiv.2208.04683.

129 Samajdar, S.S., Chatterjee, N., Sarkar, S., et al. Antimicrobial resistance in human health: a comprehensive review of One Health approach. *Bengal Phys. J.* 2024; 11(1): 18–23. https://doi.org/10.5005/jp-journals-10070-8039.

130 Malik, H., Singh, R., Kaur, S., et al. One Health assessment of poultry and cattle farms as reservoirs for ESBL-producing *Escherichia coli. bioRxiv* 2024. https://doi.org/10.1101/2024.09.22.614308.

131 Monistero, V. Characterization of staphylococci and streptococci isolated from bovine mastitis: genotypes, virulence profiles and antimicrobial resistance patterns of *Staphylococcus aureus* strains and *Streptococcus uberis* strains. Tutor: P. Moroni; Coordinatore: F. Ceciliani. Università degli Studi di Milano; 2022 May 19. 34. ciclo, Anno Accademico 2021. https://hdl.handle.net/2434/927922.

132 Lamichhane, B., Mawad, A.M.M., Saleh, M., et al. Salmonellosis: an overview of epidemiology, pathogenesis, and innovative approaches to mitigate the antimicrobial resistant infections. *Antibiotics* 2024; 13(1): 76. https://doi.org/10.3390/antibiotics13010076.

133 Sebola, D.C. A study of the transmission pathways of organisms associated with nosocomial infections at a veterinary academic hospital. PhD dissertation. South Africa: University of Pretoria; 2023.

134 Bukari, Z., Emmanuel, T., Woodward, J., et al. The global challenge of *Campylobacter*: antimicrobial resistance and emerging intervention strategies. *Trop. Med. Infect. Dis.* 2025; 10(1): 25. https://doi.org/10.3390/tropicalmed10010025.

135 Scott, A.C. Phenotypic and molecular characterisation of pseudomonas aeruginosa infections from companion animals and potential reservoirs of antibacterial resistance in humans. PhD dissertation. The University of Liverpool; 2018.

136 Romm, J. *Climate Change: What Everyone Needs to Know*. Oxford, UK: Oxford University Press; 2022.

137 Sergio, F., Blas, J., and Hiraldo, F. Animal responses to natural disturbance and climate extremes: a review. *Global Planet. Change* 2018; 161: 28–40. https://doi.org/10.1016/j.gloplacha.2017.10.009.

138 Stephen, C. and Duncan, C. (eds.) *Climate Change and Animal Health*. Boca Raton, FL, USA: CRC Press; 2022.

139 Wijerathna-Yapa, A. and Pathirana, R. Sustainable agro-food systems for addressing climate change and food security. *Agriculture* 2022; 12(10): 1554. https://doi.org/10.3390/agriculture12101554.

140 Samberger, C. Algae as nature-based solutions for climate change adaptation. In: *Algae as a Natural Solution for Challenges in Water-Food-Energy Nexus: Toward Carbon Neutrality*, 871–890. Singapore: Springer Nature Singapore; 2024. https://doi.org/10.1007/978-981-97-2371-3_32.

141 Hernandez, E., Fawcett, A., Brouwer, E., et al. Speaking up: veterinary ethical responsibilities and animal welfare issues in everyday practice. *Animals* 2018; 8(1): 15. https://doi.org/10.3390/ani8010015.

142 Rai, B.D., Tessema, G.A., Fritschi, L., et al. The application of the One Health approach in the management of five major zoonotic diseases using the World Bank domains: a scoping review. *One Health* 2024; 18: 100695. https://doi.org/10.1016/j.onehlt.2024.100695.

143 Rüegg, S.R., Nielsen, L.R., Buttigieg, S.C., et al. A systems approach to evaluate One Health initiatives. *Front. Vet. Sci.* 2018; 5: 23. https://doi.org/10.3389/fvets.2018.00023.

144 El-Ansary, H. One Health: perspectives on the interconnectedness of human, animal, and environmental health. In: *Routledge Handbook of Climate Change and Health System Sustainability*, 273–284. London: Routledge; 2024.

145 Abunna, F., Mamo, G., and Megersa, B. One Health–a holistic solution for sustainable management of globalization-driven public health challenges. *Ethiop. Vet. J.* 2022; 26(2): 107–131. https://doi.org/10.4314/evj.v26i2.7.

146 ENETWILD-consortium, Zanet, S., Vada, R., et al. Literature review on worldwide surveillance systems targeting transboundary zoonotic and emerging diseases within the holistic One-Health perspective. *EFSA Support. Publ.* 2022; 19(12): 7767E. https://doi.org/10.2903/sp.efsa.2022.EN-7767.

147 Destoumieux-Garzón, D., Mavingui, P., Boetsch, G., et al. The one health concept: 10 years old and a long road ahead. *Front. Vet. Sci.* 2018; 5: 14. https://doi.org/10.3389/fvets.2018.00014.

148 Pinillos, R.G. (ed.) *One Welfare: A Framework to Improve Animal Welfare and Human Well-Being*. Wallingford, UK: CAB International; 2018. https://doi.org/10.1079/9781786393845.0000.

149 Smits, P. and Champagne, F. Governance of health research funding institutions: an integrated conceptual framework and actionable functions of governance. *Health Res. Policy Syst.* 2020; 18: 1–19. https://doi.org/10.1186/s12961-020-0525-z.

150 Errecaborde, K.M., Wuebbolt Macy, K., Pekol, A., et al. Factors that enable effective one health collaborations—a scoping review of the literature. *PLOS ONE* 2019; 14(12): e0224660. https://doi.org/10.1371/journal.pone.0224660.

151 Langran, G. *Time in Geographic Information Systems*. London: Taylor & Francis; 1992.
152 Bordier, M., Uea-Anuwong, T., Binot, A., et al. Characteristics of One Health surveillance systems: a systematic literature review. *Prev. Vet. Med.* 2020; 181: 104560. https://doi.org/10.1016/j.prevetmed.2018.10.005.
153 Mumford, E.L., Martinez, D.J., Tyance-Hassell, K., et al. Evolution and expansion of the One Health approach to promote sustainable and resilient health and well-being: a call to action. *Front. Public Health* 2023; 10: 1056459. https://doi.org/10.3389/fpubh.2022.1056459.
154 Horvat, O. and Kovačević, Z. Human and veterinary medicine collaboration: synergistic approach to address antimicrobial resistance through the lens of planetary Health. *Antibiotics* 2025; 14(1): 38. https://doi.org/10.3390/antibiotics14010038.
155 Schneider, M.C., Munoz-Zanzi, C., Min, K.D., and Aldighieri, S. One Health from concept to application in the global world. In: *Oxford Research Encyclopedia of Global Public Health*. Oxford, UK: Oxford University Press; 2019. https://doi.org/10.1093/acrefore/9780190632366.013.29.
156 McEwen, S.A. and Collignon, P.J. Antimicrobial resistance: a one health perspective. In: *Antimicrobials Resistance in Bacteria of Livestock and Companion Animals*, 521–547. Washington, DC: American Society for Microbiology Press; 2018. https://doi.org/10.1128/9781555819804.ch25.
157 Bhatia, R. *National Framework for One Health*. New Delhi: Food and Agriculture Organization; 2021.
158 De La Rocque, S., Errecaborde, K.M.M., Belot, G., et al. One Health systems strengthening in countries: tripartite tools and approaches at the human-animal-environment interface. *BMJ Global Health* 2023; 8(1): e011236. https://doi.org/10.1136/bmjgh-2022-011236.
159 Welte, V.R. and Terán, M.V. Emergency prevention system (EMPRES) for transboundary animal and plant pests and diseases: the EMPRES-livestock: an FAO initiative. *Ann. N. Y. Acad. Sci.* 2004; 1026(1): 19–31. https://doi.org/10.1196/annals.1307.003.
160 Anderson, D. A disaster veterinary contingency plan utilizing the one health model and the World Organization for Animal Health Guidelines. Master's thesis. Middle Tennessee State University; 2023.
161 Chatzopoulou, S., Eriksson, N.L., Eriksson, D., et al. Improving risk assessment in the European food safety authority: lessons from the European Medicines Agency. *Front. Plant Sci.* 2020; 11: 349. https://doi.org/10.3389/fpls.2020.00349.
162 Donadeu, M., Nwankpa, N., Abela-Ridder, B., et al. Strategies to increase adoption of animal vaccines by smallholder farmers with focus on neglected diseases and marginalized populations. *PLoS Negl. Trop. Dis.* 2019; 13(2): e0006989. https://doi.org/10.1371/journal.pntd.0006989.
163 Behravesh, C.B. One Health: people, animals, and the environment. *Emerg. Infect. Dis.* 2016; 22(4): 766.
164 Escobar, L.S., Jara, W.H., Nizam, Q.N.H., and Plavšić, B. The perspective of the world organisation for animal health. In: *Advances in Agricultural Animal Welfare*, 169–182. Oxford, UK: Woodhead Publishing; 2018. https://doi.org/10.1016/B978-0-08-101215-4.00009-2.
165 Wang, J. OIE international standards on aquatic animals. In: *Aquatic Emergency Preparedness and Response Systems for Effective Management of Transboundary Disease Outbreaks in Southeast Asia: Proceedings of ASEAN Regional Technical Consultation*. Tigbauan, Iloilo, Philippines: Aquaculture Department, Southeast Asian Fisheries Development Center, 80. 2018.
166 Caceres, P., Awada, L., Weber-Vintzel, L., et al. The World Animal Health Information System as a tool to support decision-making and research in animal health. *Rev. Sci. Tech.* 2023; 42: 242–251. https://dx.doi.org/10.20506/rst.42.3367.
167 Belot, G., Caya, F., Errecaborde, K.M., et al. IHR-PVS National Bridging Workshops, a tool to operationalize the collaboration between human and animal health while advancing sector-specific goals in countries. *PLOS ONE* 2021; 16(6): e0245312. https://doi.org/10.1371/journal.pone.0245312.
168 Pinto Ferreira, J., Gochez, D., Jeannin, M., et al. From OIE standards to responsible and prudent use of antimicrobials: supporting stewardship for the use of antimicrobial agents in animals. *JAC Antimicrob. Resis.* 2022; 4(2): dlac017. https://doi.org/10.1093/jacamr/dlac017.

169 Palić, D. and Scarfe, A.D. Biosecurity in aquaculture: practical veterinary approaches for aquatic animal disease prevention, control, and potential eradication. In: *Biosecurity in Animal Production and Veterinary Medicine: From Principles to Practice*, 497–523. Wallingford, UK: CABI; 2019. https://doi.org/10.1079/9781789245684.0497.

170 World Organisation for Animal Health Sub-Region (W.I.S.A.). *OIE Virtual Workshop for Veterinary Education Establishments (VEEs) and Veterinary Statutory Bodies (VSBs) in South Asia and Iran*; South Asia and Iran 19–20 April, 2022.

171 Ali, W., Ali, M., Ahmad, M., et al. Application of modern techniques in animal production sector for human and animal welfare. *Turk. J. Agric. Food Sci. Technol.* 2020; 8(2): 457–463. https://doi.org/10.24925/turjaf.v8i2.457-463.3159.

172 Boliko, M.C. FAO and the situation of food security and nutrition in the world. *J. Nutr. Sci. Vitaminol.* 2019; 65: S4–S8. https://doi.org/10.3177/jnsv.65.S4.

173 White, A. and Hughes, J.M. Critical importance of a One Health approach to antimicrobial resistance. *EcoHealth* 2019; 16: 404–409. https://doi.org/10.1007/s10393-019-01415-5.

174 Tounkara, K., Couacy-Hymann, E., and Diall, O. Transboundary animal diseases (TADs) surveillance and control (including national veterinary services, regional approach, regional and international organisations, GF-TAD). In: *Transboundary Animal Diseases in Sahelian Africa and Connected Regions*, 53–68. Cham: Springer; 2019. https://doi.org/10.1007/978-3-030-25385-1_4.

175 Sinclair, J.R. Importance of a One Health approach in advancing global health security and the Sustainable Development Goals. *Rev. Sci. Tech.* 2019; 38(1): 145–154. https://doi.org/10.20506/rst.38.1.2949.

176 Zhang, T., Nickerson, R., Zhang, W., et al. The impacts of animal agriculture on One Health—bacterial zoonosis, antimicrobial resistance, and beyond. *One Health* 2024; 18: 100748. https://doi.org/10.1016/j.onehlt.2024.100748.

177 Mackenzie, J.S. and Jeggo, M. The one health approach—why is it so important? *Trop. Med. Infect. Dis.* 2019; 4(2): 88. https://doi.org/10.3390/tropicalmed4020088.

178 Collignon, P.J. and McEwen, S.A. One health—its importance in helping to better control antimicrobial resistance. *Trop. Med. Infect. Dis.* 2019; 4(1): 22. https://doi.org/10.3390/tropicalmed4010022.

179 Armstrong-Mensah, E.A. and Ndiaye, S.M. Global health security agenda implementation: a case for community engagement. *Health Security* 2018; 16(4): 217–223. https://doi.org/10.1089/hs.2017.0097.

180 Curry-Lindahl, K. United Nations Environment Programme. In: *Earthcare: Global Protection of Natural Areas*, 740–753. London: Routledge; 2019.

181 Brown, H.L., Passey, J.L., Getino, M., et al. The One Health European Joint Programme (OHEJP), 2018–2022: an exemplary one health initiative. *J. Med. Microbiol.* 2020; 69(8): 1037. https://doi.org/10.1099/jmm.0.001228.

182 Cowan, E.S., Dill, L.J., and Sutton, S. Collective healing: a framework for building transformative collaborations in public health. *Health Promot. Pract.* 2022; 23(3): 356–360. https://doi.org/10.1177/15248399211032607.

183 Rajpurkar, P., Chen, E., Banerjee, O., et al. AI in health and medicine. *Nat. Med.* 2022; 28(1): 31–38. https://doi.org/10.1038/s41591-021-01614-0.

184 Javaid, M., Haleem, A., Rab, S., et al. Sensors for daily life: a review. *Sens. Int.* 2021; 2: 100121. https://doi.org/10.1016/j.sintl.2021.100121.

185 Gilbert, J.A., Blaser, M.J., Caporaso, J.G., et al. Current understanding of the human microbiome. *Nat. Med.* 2018; 24(4): 392–400. https://doi.org/10.1038/nm.4517.

186 Srivastav, A.L., Dhyani, R., Ranjan, M., et al. Climate-resilient strategies for sustainable management of water resources and agriculture. *Environ. Sci. Pollut. Res.* 2021; 28(31): 41576–41595. https://doi.org/10.1007/s11356-021-14332-4.

187 Becker, D.J., Albery, G.F., Sjodin, A.R., et al. Optimising predictive models to prioritise viral discovery in zoonotic reservoirs. *Lancet Microbe* 2022; 3(8): e625–e637. https://www.thelancet.com/journals/lanmic/article/PIIS2666-5247(22)00028-3/fulltext.

188 Harwood, R.R. A history of sustainable agriculture. In: *Sustainable Agricultural Systems*, 3–19. Boca Raton: CRC Press; 2020.

189 Scholthof, K.B.G. The greening of one health: plants, pathogens, and the environment. *Annu. Rev. Phytopathol.* 2024; 62: 401–421. https://doi.org/10.1146/annurev-phyto-121423-042102.

190 Bresalier, M., Cassidy, A., and Woods, A. One health in history. In: *One Health: The Theory and Practice of Integrated Health Approaches* (ed. J. Zinsstag, E. Schelling, M. Whittaker. et al.), 1–14. Wallingford UK: CABI; 2021.

191 Jung, Y. and Lee, J. Learning engagement and persistence in massive open online courses (MOOCs). *Comput. Educ.* 2018; 122: 9–22. https://doi.org/10.1016/j.compedu.2018.02.013.

192 Haldane, V., Chuah, F.L., Srivastava, A., et al. Community participation in health services development, implementation, and evaluation: a systematic review of empowerment, health, community, and process outcomes. *PLOS ONE* 2019; 14(5): e0216112. https://doi.org/10.1371/journal.pone.0216112.

193 González-Carriedo, R., Anderson, A.A., King, K.M., et al. Developing critical consciousness for culturally responsive teaching: an international teacher exchange program. *Teach. Dev.* 2024; 28(5): 740–758. https://doi.org/10.1080/13664530.2024.2353591.

194 Aguirre, A.A., Longcore, T., Barbieri, M., et al. The one health approach to toxoplasmosis: epidemiology, control, and prevention strategies. *EcoHealth.* 2019; 16(2): 378–390. https://doi.org/10.1007/s10393-019-01405-7.

195 Zinsstag, J., Schelling, E., Crump, L., et al. (eds.) *One Health: The Theory and Practice of Integrated Health Approaches*. Wallingford UK: CABI; 2021.

196 Buse, K., Mays, N., Colombini, M., et al. *Making Health Policy*, 3rd ed. New York: McGraw Hill; 2023.

197 Zurn, M. *A Theory of Global Governance: Authority, Legitimacy, and Contestation.* Oxford: Oxford University Press; 2018.

198 Najafi, M., Mosadeghrad, A.M., and Arab, M. Mechanisms of intersectoral collaboration in the health system: a scoping review. *Iran J. Public Health* 2023; 52(11): 2299. https://doi.org/10.18502/ijph.v52i11.14030.

199 World Health Organization. *Global Action Plan on Physical Activity 2018–2030: More Active People for a Healthier World.* Geneva: World Health Organization; 2019.

200 Zinsstag, J., Crump, L., Schelling, E., et al. Climate change and One Health. *FEMS Microbiol. Lett.* 2018; 365(11): fny085. https://doi.org/10.1093/femsle/fny085.

2

One Health Approach Worldwide and Challenges in Collaboration

I Made Dwi Mertha Adnyana[1,2,3]*, *Ni Luh Gede Sudaryati*[4], *Dwinka Syafira Eljatin*[2,5], *Ronald Pratama Adiwinoto*[6] *and Zito Viegas da Cruz*[7]

[1] *Department of Medical Professions, Faculty of Medicine and Health Science, Universitas Jambi, Telanaipura, Jambi City, Indonesia*
[2] *Associate Epidemiologist, Indonesian Society of Epidemiologists, Daerah Khusus Ibukota Jakarta, Indonesia*
[3] *Royal Society of Tropical Medicine and Hygiene, London, United Kingdom*
[4] *Department of Biology, Faculty of Information Technology and Science, Universitas Hindu Indonesia, Denpasar city, Indonesia*
[5] *Department of Medical, Faculty of Medicine and Health, Institut Teknologi Sepuluh Nopember Jl. Raya ITS, Surabaya City, Indonesia*
[6] *Department of Public Health, Faculty of Medicine, Hang Tuah University, Komplek Barat RSAL Dr. Ramelan, Surabaya City, Indonesia*
[7] *Department of Epidemiological Surveillance, Serviçu Municipal da Saúde de Bobonaro, Maliana City, Timor-Leste*

*Corresponding author: i.madedwimertha@unja.ac.id

TABLE OF CONTENTS

2.1 Introduction to the One Health Approach
2.2 Case Studies on Successful Health Collaborations
 2.2.1 Rabies Control Worldwide
 2.2.2 Avian Influenza Response Worldwide
 2.2.3 Zoonotic Disease Control Worldwide
 2.2.4 Antimicrobial Resistance Worldwide
2.3 One Health Event in Recent Global Health Events
 2.3.1 The Role of One's Health in Handling the COVID-19 Pandemic
 2.3.2 Health in Facing the Threat of Antimicrobial Resistance
 2.3.3 One Health in Mitigating the Impacts of Climate Change on Health
 2.3.4 One Health and Zoonotic Disease Control
 2.3.5 One Health in Addressing the Global Health Crisis of Neglected Tropical Diseases
 2.3.6 Comparative Summary of Case Studies on Successful One Health Collaborations
2.4 Technology and Innovation in the One Health Field
 2.4.1 Digital Surveillance Systems
 2.4.2 Genomic Sequencing
 2.4.3 Technological Innovations and Their Applications in the One Health Field
2.5 Overcoming Challenges in Cross-disciplinary Cooperation
 2.5.1 Institutional Barriers
 2.5.2 Cultural and Disciplinary Differences
 2.5.3 Resource Constraints
 2.5.4 Data Sharing and Privacy Issues
2.6 Conclusion
 Abbreviations
 References

One Health Integration: Global Perspectives on Animal Health and Sustainable Agriculture. First Edition.
Edited by Pratik Subhash Gaikwad, Vivek Harishankar Shukla and Pintu Choudhary.

Companion Website: https://www.wiley.com/go/pratikgaikwad/onehealth

2.1 Introduction to the One Health Approach

The One Health approach establishes a comprehensive framework for addressing complex global health challenges through multisectoral collaboration across local, national, and international levels, with the objective of optimizing health outcomes for humans, animals, plants, and their shared environments (Figure 2.1). This concept emphasizes collaboration across multiple sectors and disciplines at the local, national, and international levels. The One Health strategy integrates various fields and promotes a comprehensive understanding of health interconnections [1].

The origins of the One Health approach can be traced back to the nineteenth century, when researchers began identifying connections between diseases affecting humans and animals. In 1855, Rudolf Virchow, a German doctor widely regarded as the founder of modern pathology, introduced the term "zoonosis" to describe illnesses that can spread from animals to humans [2]. The contemporary One Health framework emerged in the early 2000s, crystallizing in 2004 when the Wildlife Conservation Society's *One World, One Health* symposium established

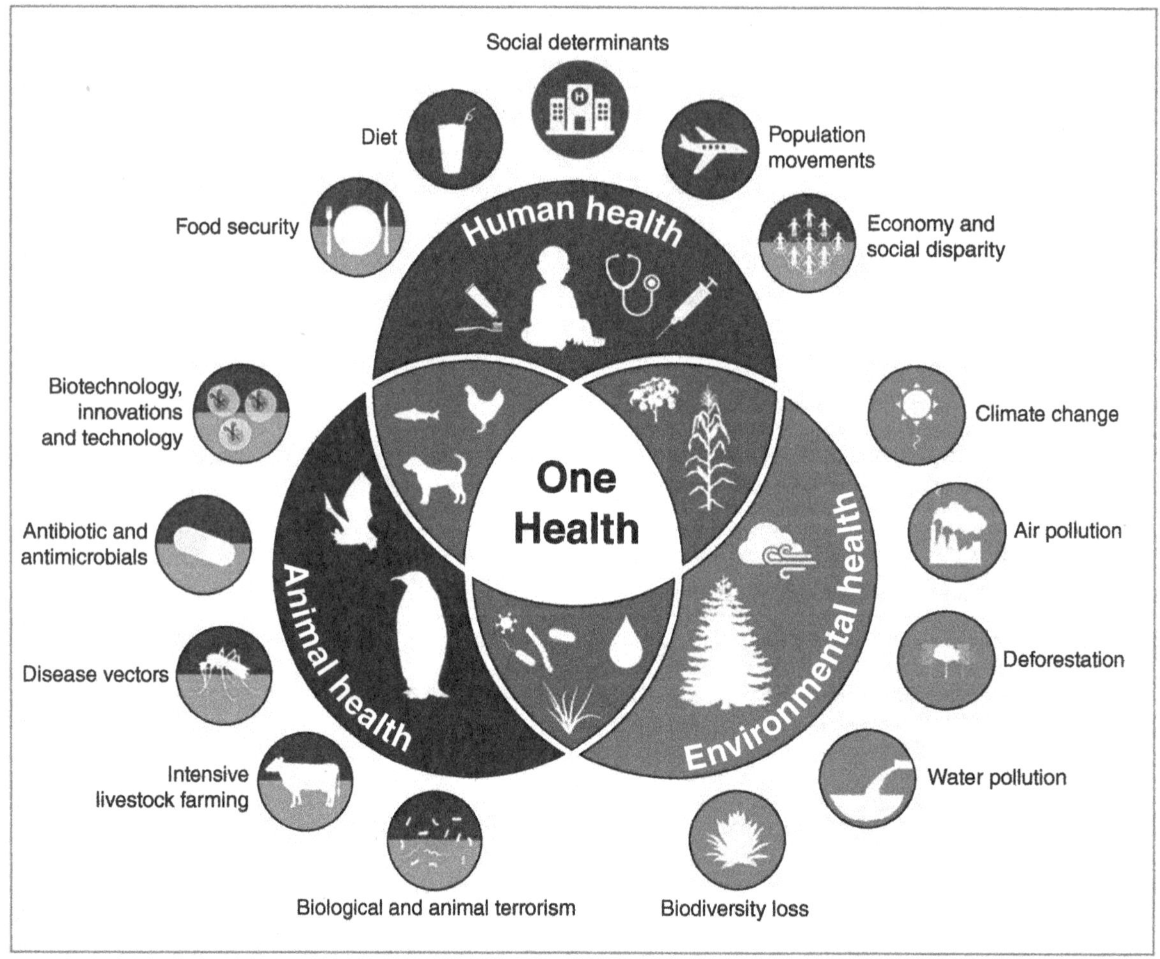

Figure 2.1 The "One Health" concept, which describes the interconnected relationships among human, animal, and environmental health.

the Manhattan Principles, which comprises 12 recommendations designed to foster preventative approaches to epizootic diseases while preserving ecosystem integrity through holistic, interdisciplinary methodologies [3].

Factors such as climate change, population expansion, urban development, and alterations in land use have increased the likelihood of zoonotic and other infectious diseases [4]. The COVID-19 pandemic epitomizes the necessity of a One Health approach, demonstrating how a virus with presumed animal origins transmitted to humans through complex human–animal–environment interactions can rapidly escalate into a global crisis, requiring coordinated multidisciplinary solutions [5]. A One Health strategy is based on various principles and frameworks. A key tenet is the interconnectedness of human, animal, and environmental well-being. Additional principles include cross-disciplinary cooperation, fairness, and justice in global health [6]. The established One Health framework emphasizes integrated surveillance systems, cross-sectoral data sharing for disease emergence prevention, and collaborative capacity building that leverages advanced technologies for early detection and response to health threats affecting the human–animal–environment interface [4].

The tripartite collaboration between the World Health Organization (WHO), Food and Agriculture Organization (FAO), and World Organization for Animal Health (WOAH) provides a structured framework for addressing health risks at the human–animal–ecosystem nexus and establishing governance mechanisms for coordinated global responses [7]. In addition, the systems thinking in the One Health framework developed by Laing et al. [8] provides a systematic approach for analyzing complex health issues. The framework incorporates six key aspects: social and ecological context, knowledge and understanding, stakeholders and networks, practices and behavior patterns, values and beliefs, and outcomes and impacts of the program. Global health initiatives have proliferated exponentially, with the Global Health Security Agenda (GHSA), a collaborative network spanning more than 70 nations, exemplifying international efforts to increase the worldwide capacity for prevention, detection, and response to infectious disease threats through the implementation of One Health principles at fundamental biological levels [9].

The One Health Workforce-Next Generation (OHW-NG) program is a targeted capacity-building initiative aimed at developing sustainable health workforces across Africa and Southeast Asia through evidence-based curriculum development, specialized training, and collaborative research networks. In Europe, the One Health European Joint Programme (OHEJP) is a significant collaborative effort uniting 44 partners across 22 EU member states. The African One Health Platform facilitates transnational cooperation through capacity enhancement, knowledge exchange mechanisms for disease management, improved surveillance systems, standardized reporting protocols, and policy advocacy that support One Health implementation across the continent [1].

Despite the growing momentum for the One Health approach, implementation faces persistent challenges, including disciplinary silos, institutional barriers, a lack of standardized evaluation frameworks, and funding limitations that impede the full realization of its potential [10]. On this basis, we present key points that can be adopted by various groups worldwide regarding the adoption of the One Health approach, along with the identification of challenges in the current, past, and future collaboration to improve global preparedness against health threats and contribute to the achievement of sustainable development goals (SDGs).

2.2 Case Studies on Successful Health Collaborations

2.2.1 Rabies Control Worldwide

Rabies is a deadly zoonotic disease that has long been a global health threat. This disease is caused by a virus of the genus Lyssavirus and is transmitted through bites or scratches from infected animals, especially dogs [1, 9]. Rabies causes approximately 59 000 human fatalities annually, with 95% of the mortality concentrated in Asian and African countries, underscoring the disproportionate burden on regions with limited healthcare infrastructure [11]. The global initiative to combat rabies aims to eliminate human fatalities caused by dog-transmitted rabies by 2030, in line with the objectives established by the WHO, FAO, and WOAH [7]. Given the intricate relationships among humans, animals, and ecosystems in the transmission and management of rabies, a One Health approach is crucial for eradicating this disease [11]. Key strategies for rabies control include decreasing the incidence of rabies in canine populations, enhancing public knowledge about rabies prevention and treatment, improving accessibility to affordable and efficient postexposure prophylaxis (PEP), and enhancing rabies monitoring and incident reporting mechanisms [12].

The evolution of rabies control methodologies represents a paradigm shift from the ineffective and inhumane mass culling of stray dogs in the early twentieth century to evidence-based preventative approaches initiated by Louis Pasteur's groundbreaking 1885 development of the first human rabies vaccine, a pivotal advancement that fundamentally transformed prevention strategies [13, 14]. In the mid-twentieth century, mass dog vaccination programs were implemented in several countries, mainly Europe and North America, and were quite effective. In Asia and Africa, where resources are limited, rabies control faces greater challenges than it does in other regions. However, successful pilot programs in Sri Lanka and the Philippines have demonstrated that eliminating rabies is a viable approach [15].

Effective rabies control requires close collaboration among multiple stakeholders. Collaborative strategies involve coordination between the human health, animal health, and environmental sectors, as well as active participation from communities and nongovernmental organizations [16]. Comprehensive rabies control frameworks necessitate multifaceted collaborative strategies: (i) cross-sectoral governance teams comprising representatives from Ministries of Health, Agriculture, Animal Health institutes, research organizations, and civil society to develop evidence-based policies and coordinate implementation; (ii) integrated surveillance systems that synthesize human and animal rabies reporting for comprehensive epidemiological assessment and rapid outbreak response; (iii) joint capacity-building programs for human and animal health professionals in diagnosis, prevention, and control methodologies; and (iv) community engagement through public awareness campaigns coupled with interdisciplinary research examining transmission dynamics and intervention efficacy [17].

A framework illustrating a collaborative approach to controlling rabies worldwide is presented in Figure 2.2. In this section, we highlight several successful strategies for controlling rabies worldwide, focusing on large-scale dog vaccination programs aimed at addressing the disease at its source. According to the WHO, the immunization of at least 70% of the canine population is necessary to disrupt the rabies transmission cycle [18]. Mass dog

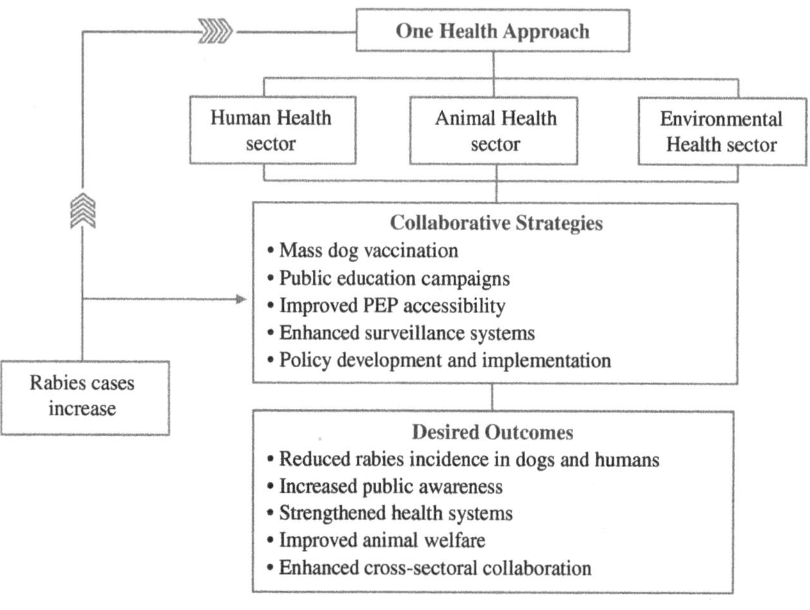

Figure 2.2 Health rabies control framework.

vaccination campaigns have demonstrated remarkable efficacy in eliminating canine-mediated rabies across diverse geographical and socioeconomic contexts, including Latin American countries [11] and Tanzania [13, 19]. Implementation strategies necessarily encompass comprehensive dog population mapping, sophisticated vaccine cold-chain logistics, vaccination workforce training, and innovative delivery mechanisms, such as mobile vaccination teams and community volunteer networks, which have proven particularly effective in achieving adequate coverage in rural and remote areas [20]. Another approach is to raise public awareness of rabies and its prevention. Public education campaigns aim to change people's behavior regarding responsible dog keeping, the importance of dog vaccination, and actions to be taken after an animal bite by providing education in schools, using social media, and celebrating World Rabies Day every September 2.828 to increase global awareness [21]. Research in the Philippines has revealed that intensive educational campaigns involving schools and communities have significantly contributed to the success of rabies elimination programs [22].

Although preventive canine vaccination remains the optimal intervention, accessible and affordable PEP is an essential component of comprehensive rabies elimination programs. Research from India has demonstrated that the implementation of cost-effective intradermal PEP protocols substantially expanded treatment access and contributed to measurable reductions in rabies mortality [18, 21]. The integration of these three initiatives into one health framework has shown promising results for rabies control in various countries [23].

The implementation of integrated rabies control strategies has resulted in significant positive impacts on public and animal health in many parts of the world, such as the Philippines, where the "Rabies-Free Philippines by 2020" program, launched in 2007, achieved significant success. Through an integrated approach involving mass dog vaccination, public education, and increased access to PEP, the Philippines reduced human rabies-related deaths by 82% from 2008 to 2018. Several provinces have declared themselves rabies free, indicating the effectiveness of community-based approaches and cross-sector collaboration [22]. A transformative demonstration program in Tanzania's Serengeti region established a proof-of-concept for rabies elimination in resource-constrained rural African settings, where achieving greater than 70% canine vaccination coverage produced substantial reductions in both human and animal rabies incidence while simultaneously highlighting the value of community engagement and digital technology integration, specifically smartphone applications for enhanced surveillance and monitoring operations [21].

Sri Lanka's comprehensive national rabies program exemplifies a sustained long-term commitment to disease elimination, documenting a remarkable reduction in human rabies mortality from 377 cases in 1973 to 25 cases in 2018 through the strategic implementation of free canine vaccination, systematic stray dog sterilization, expanded PEP access, and innovative public–private partnerships that enhanced both program coverage and sustainability [24]. Mexico successfully eliminated dog-borne rabies through a long-term control program that began in 1990. Key strategies include annual mass dog vaccination, active surveillance, and intensive public education. The country achieved dog-borne rabies-free status in 2019, reinforcing the importance of long-term political commitment and consistency in program implementation [25].

Thailand has made significant progress in rabies control through its "Thailand Rabies Free by 2020" program. The country is implementing a One Health approach that involves close collaboration between the ministries of health and agriculture and the local government. Key strategies include free dog vaccination, the sterilization of stray dogs, and intensive public education campaigns [26]. Consequently, the number of deaths from rabies decreased from hundreds of cases per year in the 1980s to only a few in the 2010s. The three flagship programs mass vaccination, public awareness education, and increased access to PEP can contribute to reducing the incidence of rabies in the future.

2.2.2 Avian Influenza Response Worldwide

Avian influenza (AI), commonly known as bird flu, is a contagious illness triggered by type A influenza viruses that can affect various types of poultry, including domestic and wild birds [27]. AI viruses are categorized into two groups on the basis of their severity in poultry: highly pathogenic AI (HPAI) and less pathogenic AI (LPAI) [28].

HPAI viruses, predominantly H5 and H7 subtypes, cause severe, often fatal disease in poultry populations and present significant zoonotic potential for human transmission, whereas LPAI viruses maintain a natural reservoir status in global wild waterfowl populations, particularly Anseriformes and Charadriiformes [29].

Migratory waterfowl movement patterns serve as the primary mechanism for transcontinental and transboundary AI virus dissemination, whereas domestic poultry outbreaks are concentrated in regions characterized by intensive production systems, particularly Southeast Asia, the Middle East, and Africa, with transmission amplified through inadequate biosecurity measures, live bird trading networks, and environmental factors, including climate and land-use changes that alter the interface dynamics of wild-domestic birds [30, 31]. Figure 2.3 illustrates the progress and future trajectories of AI worldwide. While AI outbreaks have historical documentation

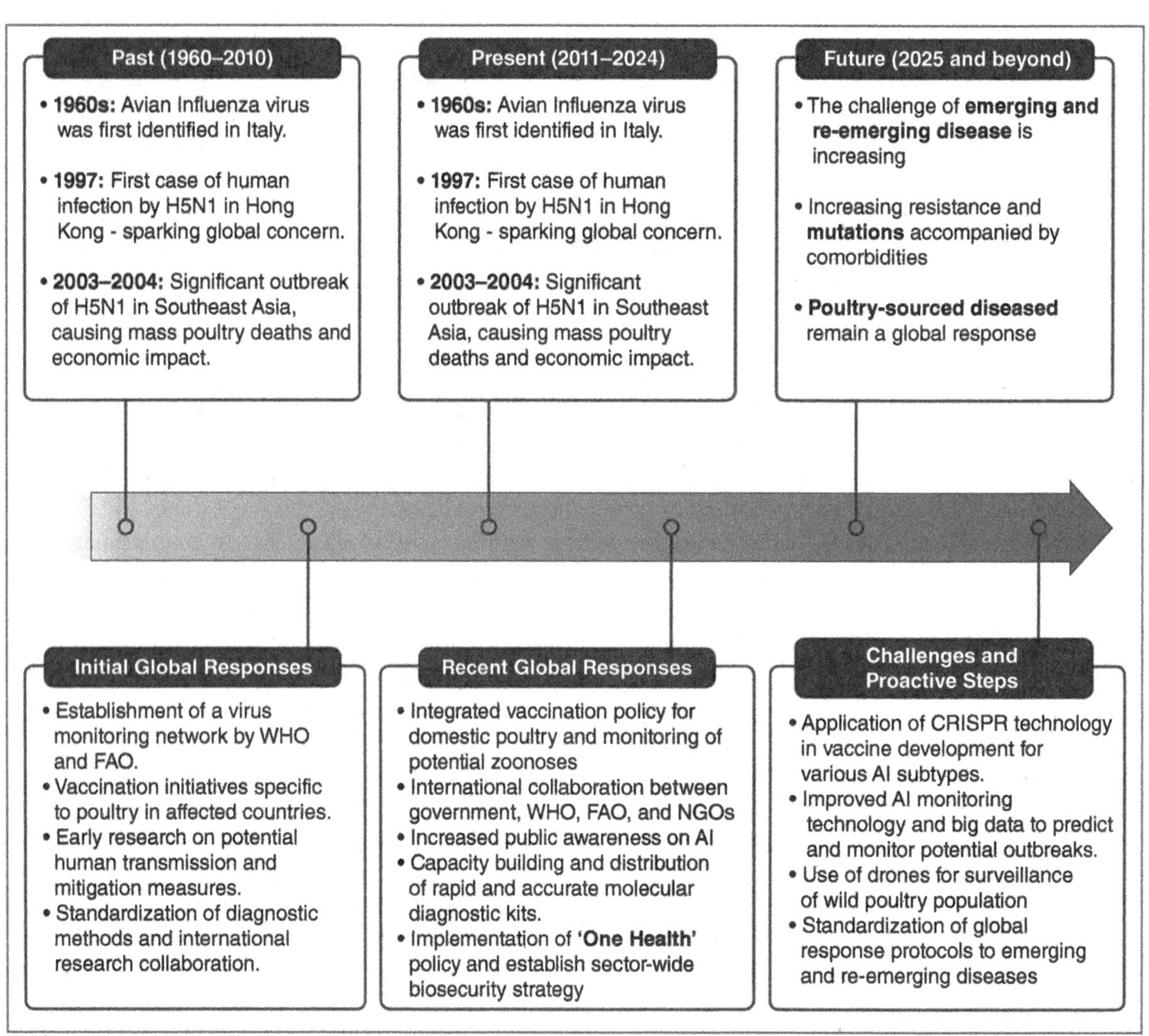

Figure 2.3 A comprehensive timeline illustrating the evolution of AI (H5N1) and global responses from 1960 to 2025. *Remarks*: The diagram is structured into three main temporal sections: past (1960–2010), present (2011–2024), and future (2025 and beyond). The upper timeline tracks significant historical events, including the initial identification of the AI virus in Italy during the 1960s, the first human H5N1 infection in Hong Kong in 1997, and a substantial outbreak in Southeast Asia from 2003 to 2004. The lower section of the diagram outlines the corresponding global responses and initiatives during this period.

dating to the early twentieth century, contemporary epidemiological patterns reveal marked increases in frequency, geographic distribution, and economic impact, exemplified by the watershed 1996 HPAI H5N1 emergence in Southeast Asia, which subsequently expanded globally, causing substantial poultry industry losses and public health threats through zoonotic transmission, followed by significant outbreaks, including H7N9 in China (2013–present) with hundreds of human infections, intercontinental H5N8 spread (2014–2015), and ongoing global H5N1 clade 2.3.4.4.4 dissemination affecting wild and domestic avian populations across multiple continents since 2020 [27, 31–33].

The global response to AI challenges has evolved toward comprehensive One Health approaches integrating animal, human, and environmental health through multifaceted intervention strategies: (i) development of integrated surveillance systems synthesizing animal health, public health, and wild bird monitoring data via real-time information technology platforms facilitating analysis and exchange between countries and international organizations; (ii) substantial laboratory capacity enhancement through infrastructure investment and personnel training for rapid, accurate viral diagnostics; (iii) establishment of international reference laboratory networks supporting viral characterization and vaccine development; (iv) implementation of stringent biosecurity standards throughout poultry production chains, including compartmentalization and zoning systems; (v) strategic vaccination programs tailored to local epidemiological contexts; (vi) development of rapid response protocols for outbreak management; (vii) community engagement and education targeting stakeholders throughout the poultry value chain; and (viii) strengthened international cooperation mechanisms exemplified by the WOAH-FAO Network of Expertise on Animal Influenza (OFFLU) and the Global Initiative on Sharing All Influenza Data (GISAID) [25, 34, 35].

2.2.3 Zoonotic Disease Control Worldwide

Diseases that can spread between animals and humans, either directly or indirectly, are known as zoonotic diseases. These zoonoses have emerged as major global issues because of their extensive effects on public health, economic systems, and food security [36]. More than 60% of human infectious diseases originate from animal reservoirs, with approximately 75% of newly emerging infectious diseases in the past two decades exhibiting zoonotic transmission patterns, exemplified by the globally consequential outbreaks of influenza, rabies, Ebola, and the COVID-19 pandemic [37]. The distribution and prevalence of zoonotic diseases vary globally and are influenced by various factors, such as bioclimatic, ecological, and agricultural practices and socioeconomic conditions [38]. Developing countries, especially those in tropical and subtropical regions, often face a greater burden of zoonotic diseases owing to a combination of environmental risk factors and limited resources for disease control [39].

Contemporary epidemiological research has demonstrated that anthropogenic environmental changes, particularly climate alteration and deforestation, function as primary drivers of zoonotic disease emergence and transmission across global ecosystems [40]. Rocklöv and Dubrow [41] established causal linkages between climate parameters (temperature and precipitation patterns) and deforestation processes with the expanded geographical ranges of arthropod vectors, including mosquitoes and ticks, thereby introducing transmission potential to previously nonendemic regions. Furthermore, deforestation has intensified human–wildlife interactions, creating new pathways for zoonotic pathogen transmission [42]. An illustration of this is the correlation between deforestation in the Amazon and increased malaria incidence [43].

Adnyana et al. [44] corroborated these findings, noting that ongoing bioclimatological shifts could increase the incidence of mosquito-borne diseases, posing a threat to public health. Additionally, the expansion of agricultural and livestock practices, coupled with increased human–wildlife contact, has fostered conditions conducive to the emergence and dissemination of novel zoonotic pathogens. The multifactorial etiology and complex transmission dynamics of zoonotic diseases necessitate comprehensive interdisciplinary management strategies that transcend traditional disciplinary boundaries [44, 45]. The One Health approach has gained empirical validation as an effective framework that integrates human, animal, and environmental health dimensions through cross-sectoral collaboration while addressing sustainability imperatives, as conceptualized by Zinsstag et al. [11].

The operationalization of One Health principles in zoonotic disease control encompasses multiple integrated components: (i) harmonized surveillance systems that synthesize human and animal health data to facilitate rapid outbreak detection and coordinated response mechanisms; (ii) transdisciplinary research initiatives investigating transmission dynamics, ecological determinants, and intervention efficacy; (iii) specialized education programs that incorporate One Health paradigms within veterinary and medical curricula; and (iv) policy frameworks designed to address interconnected health domains simultaneously across human–animal–environment interfaces [11].

The application of the One Health approach has yielded positive outcomes in the management of zoonotic diseases worldwide. Research conducted in Tanzania has illustrated the efficacy of a comprehensive surveillance system for identifying and addressing rabies outbreaks. This initiative, which combines human and animal health data, led to a substantial decrease in rabies cases among both humans and animals [46]. This achievement highlights the importance of intersectoral cooperation in managing diseases that spread between animals and humans. In Southeast Asian countries, the implementation of comprehensive One Health strategies for AI control has demonstrably reduced human infection risk through multifaceted interventions, including targeted poultry vaccination campaigns, enhanced biosecurity protocols throughout production chains, and community engagement programs, demonstrating the effectiveness of integrated approaches for addressing complex zoonotic transmission systems [18, 47].

European antimicrobial resistance (AMR) research has provided compelling evidence supporting One Health interventions, with Dutch investigators demonstrating that coordinated reductions in veterinary antimicrobial usage coupled with human antimicrobial stewardship programs produced concurrent decreases in resistant bacterial populations across both the human and animal sectors, empirically validating the interconnected nature of resistance ecology across species boundaries [48]. In North America, the Canadian government established the Canadian Integrated Program for Antimicrobial Resistance Surveillance (CIPARS), which employs a health strategy to track AMR in the food supply chain.

The program has successfully identified AMR trends and informed policies for the wider use of antibiotics in the agricultural and human health sectors. The implementation of an integrated One Health approach to leishmaniasis control in Brazil has led to successful ecological intervention design, the synchronization of vector surveillance methodologies, canine reservoir management strategies, and human treatment protocols to achieve measurable reductions in both human and animal disease incidence, providing evidence that coordinated cross-sectoral interventions effectively address complex transmission cycles involving multiple host species [49, 50]. This evidence suggests that a One Health approach is effective in addressing the complexity of zoonotic diseases across multiple global contexts. Successful implementation relies on multisectoral collaboration, data integration, and tailoring interventions to local needs.

Various countries have implemented regulations in line with the One Health principle, such as the European One Health Action Plan against AMR in the European Union, the National Center for Emerging and Zoonotic Infectious Diseases in the United States, the National Standing Committee on Zoonoses in India, and the Kenya One Health Strategy 2019–2023 [51]. Although the One Health approach encounters obstacles such as departmental isolation, limited resources, and difficulties in coordination, several effective strategies have been employed with encouraging outcomes. These include collaborative monitoring, combined vaccination efforts, community awareness programs, skill enhancement initiatives, and the development of comprehensive policies that integrate multiple sectors [52].

2.2.4 Antimicrobial Resistance Worldwide

The global health community is increasingly concerned with the increase in AMR cases worldwide. AMR represents an escalating tripartite threat to the human, animal, and environmental health sectors globally and is defined by the WHO as the ability of microorganisms to survive therapeutic concentrations of previously effective antimicrobial compounds. Although AMR naturally emerges through microbial genetic adaptation, improper overuse of antimicrobial agents has greatly accelerated this process. The WHO has identified AMR as one of the ten most significant threats to global health. Current epidemiological data attribute approximately 1.27 million direct fatalities to antibiotic-resistant bacterial infections in 2019, with projections indicating a potential escalation to 10 million annual deaths by 2050 if intervention measures remain inadequate, compounded by estimated annual economic losses approaching US$100 trillion through impacts on healthcare systems, agricultural productivity, and global economic development [8, 53].

The global AMR distribution exhibits pronounced geographical heterogeneity, with a disproportionate burden concentrated in low- and middle-income countries (LMICs), driven by multifactorial determinants, including inappropriate antimicrobial prescribing and consumption patterns across the human and veterinary sectors; inadequate water, sanitation, and hygiene infrastructure; fragile healthcare delivery systems; insufficient regulatory frameworks governing antimicrobial access and usage; increased globalization facilitating transboundary pathogen movement; and environmental alterations influencing microbial ecology and resistance transmission pathways [54]. Contemporary AMR epidemiology reveals evolutionary trends, including increasing resistance to carbapenems and colistin antibiotics of last resort [55], the proliferation of multidrug-resistant organisms such as methicillin-resistant *Staphylococcus aureus* (MRSA) and extended-spectrum beta-lactamase (ESBL)-producing *Enterobacteriaceae* [6], increasing AMR among zoonotic pathogens with transmission potential across species barriers [56], and the detection of resistance determinants in environmental matrices, including surface water and soil, indicating the establishment of complex resistance reservoirs beyond clinical settings [49].

The global AMR response encompasses diverse intervention strategies across the One Health spectrum: the implementation of antimicrobial stewardship programs within healthcare institutions to optimize prescribing practices [55]; the development of novel vaccines to reduce infection-driven antimicrobial demand [57]; the enhancement of biosecurity protocols in agricultural systems; the exploration of antibiotic alternatives in livestock production [58]; the advancement of rapid diagnostic technologies for pathogen identification and susceptibility determination [59]; the establishment of integrated surveillance networks, including the WHO's Global Antimicrobial Resistance and Use Surveillance System; the formation of reference laboratory consortia for standardized resistance monitoring; the deployment of genomics-based surveillance platforms [60]; and the implementation of early warning systems to detect emerging resistance patterns [61].

2.3 One Health Event in Recent Global Health Events

2.3.1 The Role of One's Health in Handling the COVID-19 Pandemic

The SARS-CoV-2 virus, which originated in Wuhan, China, in late 2019 triggered an unparalleled global health emergency known as the COVID-19 pandemic [62]. This crisis has affected virtually every facet of human existence worldwide, with the virus rapidly spreading across nations, infecting hundreds of millions, and claiming millions of lives. In addition to its immediate health implications, the pandemic has significantly disrupted the global economic, social, and political landscape [5, 63]. The unprecedented scale and multidimensional impacts of the COVID-19 pandemic exposed fundamental vulnerabilities in global health security architecture, catalyzing renewed recognition of the One Health framework as an essential paradigm for addressing complex health challenges at the human, animal, and environmental interfaces [64].

The COVID-19 pandemic epitomizes the multifaceted dimensions of One Health, encompassing zoonotic viral emergence at wildlife–human interfaces, accelerated global transmission through interconnected travel networks, and cascading impacts across food systems and agricultural value chains, necessitating coordinated interventions through transdisciplinary collaboration among medical professionals, veterinarians, virologists, and environmental scientists investigating viral origins, developing vaccines, and establishing comprehensive surveillance systems [44]. Many countries have adopted health strategies for pandemic preparedness and response at the policy level. International organizations, such as the World Organization for Animal Health (WOAH), have increased their collaboration to support health implementation at the global level [8].

While One Health approach has proven valuable in dealing with the COVID-19 pandemic, its implementation faces challenges such as the lack of a coordinated governance framework, gaps in capacity and resources between developing and developed countries, and weaknesses in the global surveillance system [65]. Two notable examples of One Health success during the COVID-19 response emerged at the global and national levels: unprecedented scientific collaboration across disciplinary boundaries facilitated rapid vaccine development through accelerated research timelines while maintaining rigorous safety standards [2]; concurrently, Vietnam and New Zealand implemented comprehensive One Health strategies integrating human health measures with environmental interventions and animal surveillance to effectively contain viral transmission within their borders [66].

The experience of dealing with the COVID-19 pandemic has provided valuable lessons for future health collaborations (Figure 2.4). These include the importance of integrated early warning systems, "whole of government" and "whole of society" approaches, investment in One Health research and development, strengthening of global health systems, and effective communication and community engagement [67]. The One Health approach is becoming increasingly important in the face of global health threats. Climate change, deforestation, urbanization, and increased human–animal interactions are likely to increase the risk of emerging zoonotic diseases. Therefore, strengthening the global health framework should be a priority on the international health agenda [4].

A fundamental lesson emerging from the pandemic response centers on the imperative for integrated surveillance systems that synthesize data across human, animal, and environmental health sectors, enabling earlier detection of emerging threats, identification of spillover events, and implementation of targeted preventive measures before pathogens establish sustained human-to-human transmission [68]. The pandemic has highlighted the importance of interdisciplinary approaches to research and development. Collaboration among virologists, epidemiologists, ecologists, and social scientists has proven invaluable for understanding the dynamics of the spread of COVID-19 and developing effective mitigation strategies [45]. The weaknesses in global health systems and inequalities in access to healthcare revealed during the pandemic emphasize the need for a more inclusive and equitable health approach [69]. Investments in strengthening the health system, especially in LMICs, should be a priority on the global health agenda [70].

The pandemic accelerated technological integration within One Health frameworks, demonstrating how big data analytics, artificial intelligence, and Internet of Things applications can transform disease surveillance, predictive modeling, and response capabilities; create digital ecosystems that enhance early warning systems; facilitate real-time data sharing across sectors; and enable precision interventions during outbreaks [71]. The COVID-19 pandemic highlighted the importance of effective risk communication and community involvement. A comprehensive One Health strategy should encompass efficient communication methods to enhance the public's understanding of the interrelationships among humans, animals, and environmental well-being [65]. To improve global readiness for future pandemics, enhancing global governance mechanisms for health, including aligning policies and standards across nations, is crucial [72].

Despite demonstrated efficacy during the COVID-19 pandemic, the One Health approach faces persistent implementation challenges, including methodological difficulties in quantifying intervention impacts, knowledge gaps regarding zoonotic emergence mechanisms, and entrenched institutional silos that impede intersectoral coordination, necessitating strategic investment priorities to strengthen global implementation capacity through the development of specialized educational curricula, integrated surveillance infrastructure, and regulatory frameworks that incentivize cross-sectoral collaboration [53]. By capitalizing on the insights gained from the COVID-19 crisis and persistently reinforcing the One Health strategy, we can increase our capacity to foresee, avert, and address future health challenges. Through worldwide cooperation and collective dedication to the health of our planet, we can forge a more secure and enduring world for future generations.

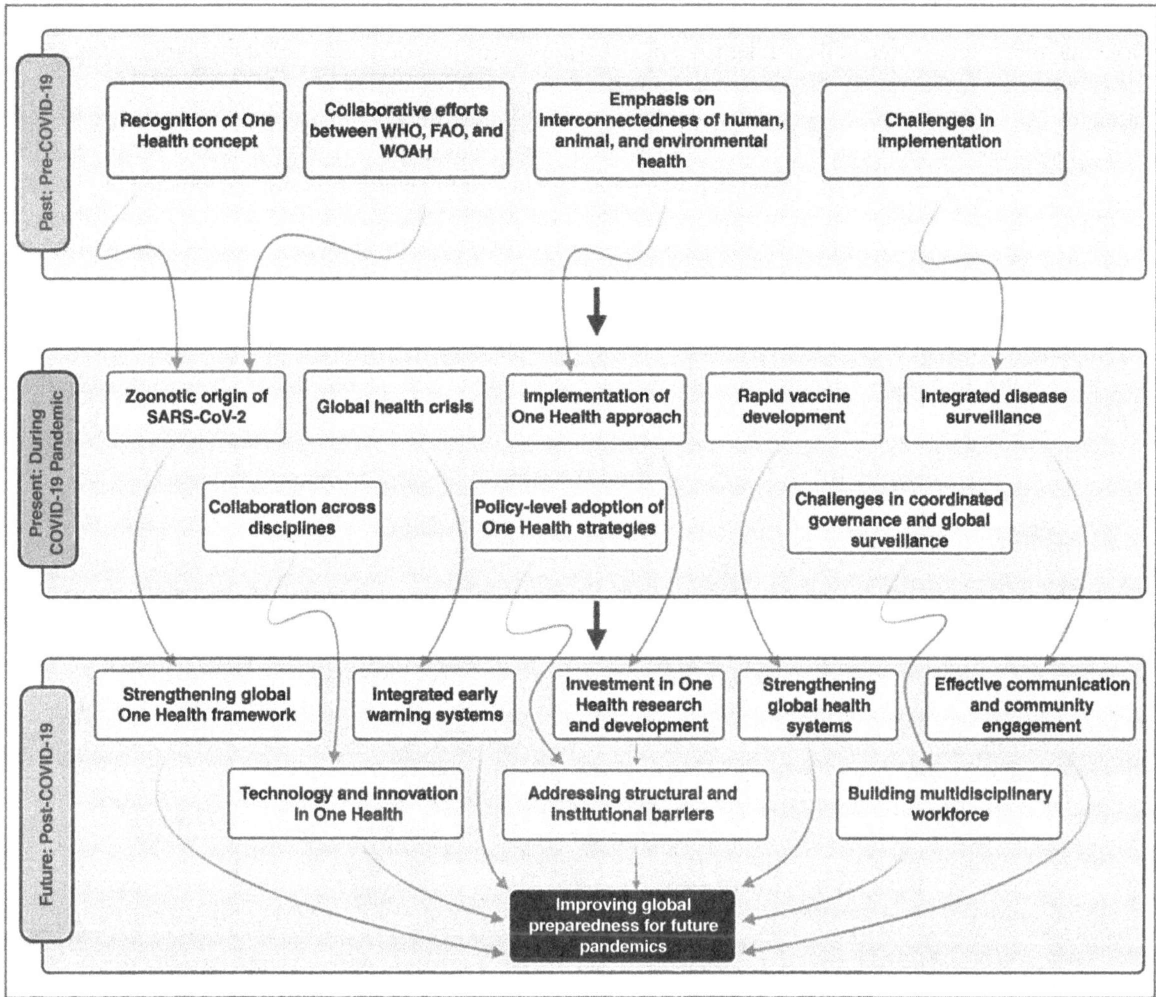

Figure 2.4 Evolution of the One Health approach in three phases: pre-COVID-19, during the COVID-19 pandemic, and post-COVID-19. *Remarks*: The first phase involved the recognition of the One Health concept and interagency collaboration. The second phase describes the response to the pandemic, including the zoonotic origin of SARS-CoV-2, the global health crisis, and rapid vaccine development. The third phase focuses on the future, emphasizing the strengthening of the global health framework, the integration of early warning systems, and investment in research. All these phases lead to the ultimate goal of improving global preparedness for future pandemics through multidisciplinary approaches, technological innovation, and addressing structural and institutional barriers.

2.3.2 Health in Facing the Threat of Antimicrobial Resistance

AMR represents one of the most formidable public health challenges of the twenty-first century, with the WHO projecting 10 million annual deaths by 2050 without effective intervention, underscoring the necessity of implementing holistic One Health strategies that address the complex interrelationships between human, animal, and environmental determinants of resistance emergence and transmission [50]. AMR transmission is intricately connected to human, animal, and environmental factors. In human populations, the inappropriate use of antibiotics and inadequate infection control measures contribute to the development and dissemination of resistant bacteria. The agricultural sector functions as a significant reservoir and amplifier of AMR through the widespread application of antimicrobials for growth promotion and prophylaxis in healthy animals, whereas environmental matrices, including soil, water, and sediment, serve as both repositories and conduits for resistant bacteria and mobile genetic elements carrying resistance determinants [73].

Antimicrobial-resistant organisms traverse complex transmission networks involving multiple pathways, including foodborne dissemination through the consumption of contaminated animal products, direct zoonotic transfer through occupational exposure, nosocomial spread within healthcare facilities, and environmental dissemination through contaminated wastewater, agricultural runoff and wildlife vectors. This necessitates a systems-based understanding of effective intervention design. The One Health approach to combat AMR involves various interconnected strategies. These include establishing comprehensive surveillance networks [8], implementing programs for responsible antimicrobial use, enhancing measures to prevent and control infections [18], promoting scientific innovation and investigation [74], expanding educational initiatives and public awareness [75], and upgrading sanitation infrastructure and water access [76]. Figure 2.5 illustrates the conceptual framework for applying the One Health paradigm in the context of AMR.

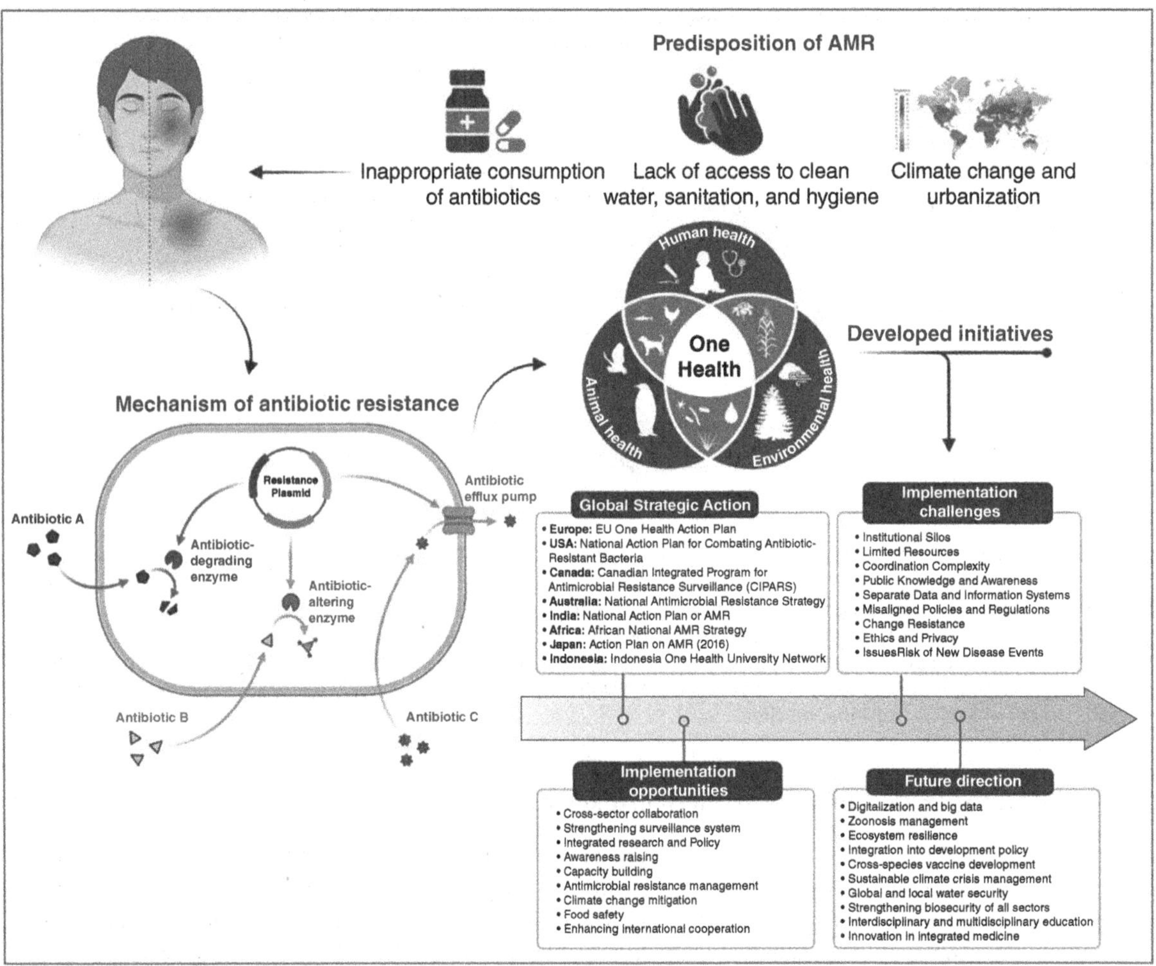

Figure 2.5 Antimicrobial resistance (AMR) issues and future directions for the implementation of the "One Health" approach.

The global governance architecture addressing AMR has evolved substantially, with the 2015 WHO Global Action Plan on AMR establishing One Health as the foundational framework for national action plans, reinforced through tripartite collaboration between the WHO, FAO, and WOAH, complemented by specialized initiatives including the Global Antibiotic Research and Development Partnership and the Fleming Fund, and strategically coordinated through United Nations Interagency mechanisms promoting synchronized action across sectors.

Empirical evaluations of One Health implementation for AMR control have demonstrated promising outcomes, with Munkholm et al. [77] documenting strengthened surveillance systems and more comprehensive control programs in countries adopting integrated approaches, whereas economic analyses by Gilbert et al. [31] revealed significant cost efficiencies compared with siloed sectoral interventions. However, methodological challenges in quantifying the direct impacts on resistance prevalence persist because of complex ecological interactions and extended timeframes required for measurable shifts in resistance epidemiology.

The prospects and challenges of the One Health concept for AMR eradication include several important aspects. Strengthening cross-sectoral collaboration requires improvement [10]. Capacity building in AMR surveillance, antimicrobial stewardship, and research in LMICs is a top priority [78]. Emerging technologies, including whole-genome sequencing, metagenomic surveillance, big data analytics, and artificial intelligence, offer transformative potential for understanding resistance transmission dynamics, predicting emergence patterns, and designing precise interventions. However, successful implementation necessitates adaptation to local socioeconomic, cultural, and ecological conditions through participatory approaches that engage communities as active partners rather than passive recipients [79]. Expanding the focus of health to address the socioeconomic factors underlying inappropriate antibiotic use and the spread of AMR is also important [80]. The development of standardized metrics and indicators to measure the effectiveness of the One Health approach in addressing AMR is critical for program evaluation and improvement [81].

2.3.3 One Health in Mitigating the Impacts of Climate Change on Health

Global climate change poses a significant threat with widespread consequences for environmental, human, and animal health. The Food and Agriculture Organization (FAO) reported that global surface temperatures have risen by 1.1 °C since preindustrial times and are expected to meet or surpass 1.5 °C in the near future without substantial reduction efforts [82]. These temperature elevations lead to severe climate shifts that negatively impact health, resulting in infectious diseases, poor nutrition, mental health issues and fatalities from natural calamities.

The One Health approach provides an integrated framework for addressing climate–health challenges through coordinated mitigation and adaptation strategies that recognize the intricate interconnections between ecological disruption and disease emergence in human and animal populations. The effects of climate change on human health include heightened risks of vector-borne illnesses, such as malaria and dengue [83]; waterborne diseases, such as cholera and diarrhea [84]; and cardiovascular and respiratory conditions caused by extreme heat [85]. Climate change affects the geographic distribution and population dynamics of many animal species, increases the risk of zoonotic diseases, and affects livestock productivity and feed availability [86].

The environmental effects include ecosystem degradation, biodiversity loss, and changes in biogeochemical cycles. Increased ocean temperatures and acidification lead to coral reef bleaching and the disruption of marine ecosystems, whereas climate change alters plant growth patterns and accelerates desertification [87]. The One Health approach to climate change mitigation establishes a comprehensive intervention framework that integrates environmental protection with animal and human health promotion through five key components: integrated surveillance networks monitoring climate-sensitive diseases across species boundaries, interdisciplinary research examining climate–health relationships at multiple scales, cross-sectoral capacity building developing specialized expertise, integrated policy mechanisms transcending traditional governance silos, and community education initiatives empowering local climate resilience [38, 41, 88].

The implementation of One Health interventions in climate-vulnerable regions has demonstrated measurable impacts, exemplified by Bangladesh's integrated program synthesizing water resource management with sustainable agriculture and public health initiatives to successfully reduce the incidence of waterborne disease while increasing food security in coastal communities facing sea-level rise and saltwater intrusion. In sub-Saharan Africa, a One Health approach to savannah ecosystem management has helped reduce human–wildlife conflicts and improve the health of pastoral communities while conserving biodiversity. Other successful programs and policies that apply the One Health approach to mitigate the health impacts of climate change include the "EcoHealth" program in Southeast Asia, the Global Zoonotic Disease Surveillance Network (GZDN), FAO's "Climate-Smart Agriculture" initiative, and the "Planetary Health" Project in coastal cities [89].

To strengthen the One Health approach to climate change mitigation, several policy recommendations can be considered, including (i) increasing investment in interdisciplinary research linking climate change, ecosystem health, and human–animal health; (ii) developing national and international policy frameworks that explicitly integrate the One Health approach into climate change mitigation and adaptation strategies; (iii) strengthening collaboration between the health, agriculture, environment, and urban planning sectors in the development and implementation of climate-related policies; (iv) enhancing the capacity of health and veterinary systems to address climate-related health threats through training, infrastructure, and appropriate technologies; (v) encouraging community participation and local wisdom in the development of the One Health strategy for climate change mitigation; and (vi) integrating education on One Health and climate change into school and college curricula [90].

The One Health paradigm establishes a holistic framework acknowledging the interdependence of environmental, animal, and human systems in addressing the multifaceted challenges of climate change, enhancing intervention efficacy through cross-sectoral collaboration, while recognizing that successful implementation requires robust political commitment, resource mobilization, and fundamental shifts in how societies conceptualize health and sustainability. This methodology underscores the importance of cross-sectoral and interdisciplinary cooperation in achieving optimal health outcomes for all living entities and ecosystems. Through the use of integrated monitoring systems, cross-disciplinary research, skill development, cohesive policies, and initiatives focused on educating and empowering communities, the One Health approach can facilitate the more effective and efficient identification and management of health threats associated with climate change.

2.3.4 One Health and Zoonotic Disease Control

The One Health framework provides a methodological foundation for addressing zoonotic disease pathogens transmissible between animals and humans through the recognition of complex bidirectional transmission dynamics occurring at human–animal interfaces within shared ecological contexts. The importance of a health approach to zoonotic control stems from its capacity to address the intricate interactions among humans, animals, and ecosystems that contribute to the emergence and proliferation of zoonotic diseases [91]. By combining various fields, including human and veterinary medicine, disease biology, ecology, and social sciences, this approach allows for a more comprehensive and efficient method of identifying, preventing, and controlling zoonotic outbreaks.

Major zoonotic diseases exhibit distinct epidemiological patterns determined by pathogen characteristics, host range dynamics, and environmental conditions. Globally significant examples include zoonotic influenza viruses, rabies lyssavirus, West Nile virus, and emerging threats such as Ebola, all of which share common risk factors, including direct contact with infected animal reservoirs, consumption of contaminated animal products, and ecological disruptions facilitating vector proliferation or novel host interactions [92]. Research has shown that rapid urban expansion, deforestation, and climate change increase the risk of zoonotic transmission.

The operationalization of One Health principles for zoonotic outbreak management requires synchronized collaborative mechanisms linking human health, animal health, and environmental sectors through integrated surveillance systems; early warning capabilities; and coordinated response protocols exemplified in AI control through concurrent poultry surveillance, rapid laboratory diagnostics, and farm-level biosecurity implementation, complemented by public education on hygienic practices and animal handling safety [69]. Through synchronized interventions, including canine vaccination campaigns, community education initiatives, and enhanced PEP accessibility, Thailand's implementation of comprehensive One Health rabies control programs has significantly reduced human mortality [93]. West Africa's 2014–2016 Ebola response demonstrated how integrated wildlife surveillance, human contact tracing, and community engagement effectively contained viral spread, providing empirical evidence for the efficacy and cost-effectiveness of One Health approaches relative to conventional sectoral interventions [94].

The policy implications and recommendations for strengthening health systems via a One Health approach include several key aspects. First, a legal and policy framework that supports cross-sector collaboration, including the establishment of a national coordination mechanism for One Health, is needed. Second, investment in human resource capacity building in epidemiology, veterinary medicine, and environmental science is essential for building a competent workforce via a One Health approach. Third, strengthening integrated surveillance systems and laboratories that can detect zoonotic threats early should be prioritized. In addition, integrating health into health education curricula and professional training can help build long-term understanding and capacity. Increased community engagement and risk communication are also important to ensure public support for the One Health initiative. Finally, international cooperation and information sharing regarding zoonotic threats must be strengthened to support a more effective global response to future pandemics [95].

2.3.5 One Health in Addressing the Global Health Crisis of Neglected Tropical Diseases

A group of infectious diseases known as neglected tropical diseases (NTDs) predominantly affects impoverished populations in tropical and subtropical regions. Despite their substantial effects on the health and quality of life of billions of individuals globally, these ailments are frequently disregarded in health initiatives [96]. NTDs include diverse pathogens, including soil-transmitted helminthiases, schistosomiasis, lymphatic filariasis, onchocerciasis, trachoma, and leishmaniasis, collectively affecting more than one billion people globally, with profound economic and social ramifications beyond direct morbidity and mortality through productivity reduction and impaired cognitive development in children, thereby perpetuating intergenerational poverty cycles [52].

NTD transmission dynamics are governed by complex, interconnected factors: anthropogenic environmental alterations, including climate change, urbanization, deforestation, and land-use conversion, modify vector behavior and reservoir ecology, expanding NTD geographical distribution; intensified human–animal–environment interfaces increase zoonotic transmission risk exemplified by malaria and leishmaniasis incidence patterns at settlement–wildlife boundaries; and socioeconomic determinants, including extreme poverty, inadequate water and sanitation infrastructure, and healthcare access limitations, further exacerbate disease burden with gender inequities, imposing additional barriers to prevention and treatment access for women and girls [97].

The One Health framework provides a comprehensive architecture for addressing NTD complexities through the transdisciplinary integration of public health, veterinary medicine, ecology, and social sciences, requiring coordinated implementation through cross-sectoral collaboration mechanisms that synchronize human–animal disease surveillance, ecologically informed vector management, and public health interventions targeting socioeconomic risk factors, exemplified by China's successful schistosomiasis control program combining human mass drug administration with animal vaccination, waste management protocols, and environmental modifications [95, 98].

Integrated NTD prevention and control strategies represent core One Health interventions: preventive chemotherapy through mass drug administration campaigns; innovative vector control technologies, including genetically modified mosquito- and Wolbachia-based approaches [99]; strengthened water, sanitation, and hygiene (WASH) infrastructure development [100]; community-centered health education programs promoting behavioral change; comprehensive zoonotic surveillance networks [2]; and strategic animal vaccination protocols reducing pathogen reservoir capacity. To improve the implementation of One Health in NTD management, several policy recommendations can be considered, such as strengthening legal and regulatory frameworks that support cross-sector collaboration and data sharing, increasing funding for One Health research, building multidisciplinary workforce capacity [101], integrating NTD management into broader health programs, strengthening integrated surveillance systems, and addressing the underlying social determinants of NTD health [102].

The One Health approach to NTD management offers transformative potential for reducing the global disease burden through sustainable, cost-effective interventions targeting root causes rather than symptoms, although success ultimately depends on political commitment, cross-sectoral coordination mechanisms, and sustained research investment while requiring fundamental paradigm shifts toward collaborative, innovative, and equitable approaches to global health challenges. By recognizing this complexity, stakeholders can develop more effective and sustainable strategies to address the burden of NTDs in the future. The integration of knowledge from multiple disciplines not only improves our understanding of disease dynamics but also paves the way for innovative interventions that address the root causes of NTDs. The successful implementation of One Health status in NTD management will require a paradigm shift in understanding and addressing global health challenges, with a focus on collaboration, innovation, and equity.

2.3.6 Comparative Summary of Case Studies on Successful One Health Collaboration

The case studies discussed earlier have shown the diversity of the application of the One Health approach to different infectious disease conditions and challenges. Table 2.1 presents a comparative summary of these case studies, highlighting the key stakeholders, implementation strategies, outcomes, challenges, and lessons learned from each collaboration. This synthesis illustrates how One Health principles have been operationalized across diverse settings to address health challenges at the human–animal–environment interface in the region. The comparative analysis revealed common patterns in successful One Health collaboration, including multisectoral coordination mechanisms, integrated surveillance systems, community engagement, and sustainable funding structures.

2.4 Technology and Innovation in the One Health Field

2.4.1 Digital Surveillance Systems

Technological advancements have fundamentally transformed cross-sectoral disease monitoring capabilities, enabling the unprecedented integration of surveillance data across human, animal, and environmental domains through digital platforms that increase the efficiency and effectiveness of One Health implementation [53]. Digital surveillance systems are a key component of modern health approaches that enable the collection, analysis, and dissemination of health data in real time and at an unprecedented scale. Information and communication technology (ICT) has transformed the manner in which we monitor, track, and respond to health threats. Technology-based surveillance systems enable the early detection of disease outbreaks, long-term monitoring of health trends, and faster and more effective response coordination [103].

Advanced artificial intelligence and machine learning algorithms analyze complex health datasets by identifying subtle patterns and anomalies undetectable through conventional analysis, facilitating precise outbreak prediction and early identification of emerging pathogens through the automated processing of heterogeneous data streams spanning clinical records, laboratory diagnostics, environmental parameters, and animal health indicators [104]. Geospatial technologies and digital mapping play important roles in modern disease surveillance systems. Geographic information systems (GIS) and web-based mapping technologies enable the visualization and analysis of the spatial distribution of diseases, environmental risk factors, and animal population dynamics in an area [105]. The digital surveillance technologies employed in the One Health approach extend beyond human

Table 2.1 Comparative summary of case studies on successful One Health collaboration.

Study	Key stakeholders	Implementation strategies	Outcomes	Challenges	Lessons learned	References
Rabies Control	WHO, FAO, WOAH, Ministries of Health, Veterinary Services, Local Communities	Mass dog vaccination (>70% coverage), public awareness campaigns, improved access to postexposure prophylaxis (PEP), integrated surveillance systems	82% reduction in human rabies deaths in Philippines (2008–2018), Significant reduction in Tanzania's Serengeti region, Thailand reduced cases from hundreds to few	Resource limitations in rural areas, coordination between sectors, cultural beliefs about dogs	Cross-sector collaboration is essential, community engagement improves success, sustainable funding mechanisms needed	[13, 19–21]
Avian Influenza Response	National governments, Poultry industry, FAO, WHO, WOAH, Wildlife authorities	Integrated surveillance systems, laboratory capacity building, biosecurity enhancement, strategic vaccination, rapid response protocols	Reduced human cases of H5N1, improved early detection systems, enhanced international cooperation	Viral evolution and adaptation, trade implications, resource disparities between countries	Real-time data sharing crucial, reference laboratory networks effective, compartmentalization protects healthy populations	[33]
COVID-19 Pandemic Management	WHO, National health systems, research institutions, pharmaceutical companies	Cross-disciplinary collaboration, extensive surveillance systems, vaccine development, national preparedness plans	Rapid vaccine development, effective management in countries using One Health approach (e.g. Vietnam, New Zealand)	Lack of coordinated governance, resource gaps between countries, weak global surveillance	Need for integrated early warning systems, importance of interdisciplinary approaches, necessity of equitable health systems	[66]
Antimicrobial Resistance	WHO, FAO, WOAH, Healthcare systems, pharmaceutical industry, agricultural sector	Surveillance networks, antimicrobial stewardship programs, infection prevention and control, Research and innovation	Stronger AMR surveillance systems in countries adopting One Health, cost savings compared to separate sectoral approaches	Sector coordination challenges, limited resources, differing stakeholder priorities	Cross-sectoral collaboration essential, Capacity building in LMICs critical, need for standardized metrics	[53, 77]
Neglected Tropical Diseases	WHO, National health systems, Research institutions, NGOs, Local communities	Interdisciplinary cooperation, joint monitoring, vector control, public health initiatives	Successful schistosomiasis control in China, improved management of leishmaniasis in Brazil	Environmental changes affecting disease vectors, socioeconomic barriers, gender disparities	Holistic frameworks effectively addressing socioeconomic determinants crucial, community engagement vital	[65]

health, encompassing the monitoring of animal well-being and environmental factors. Remote sensing devices and unmanned aerial vehicles have been used to track wildlife populations, observe habitat changes, and assess ecosystem health markers that may influence zoonotic disease dynamics [93].

Specific examples of digital tools and platforms used in One Health disease surveillance include ProMED, EMPRES-i, HealthMap, PREDICT, and EpiCore. These systems enable the rapid reporting of disease outbreaks, monitoring of global animal health threats, mapping of global disease trends, identification of new zoonotic disease threats, and rapid verification of disease outbreak reports [34]. The key benefits of digital surveillance systems in the One Health approach include the rapid identification of emerging health threats, the integration of data from multiple sources, improved accuracy of disease prediction and analysis, data collection from remote areas, and real-time data sharing among global stakeholders [106]. Implementation challenges for digital surveillance systems encompass critical governance considerations regarding data privacy and security, equity concerns in technological access that risk perpetuating global health disparities, technical barriers, including a lack of standardized data formats and interoperability frameworks, epistemological challenges in ensuring information accuracy and relevance across contexts, and sustainability constraints requiring continuous infrastructure investment and technological capacity development [107].

Addressing these obstacles and realizing the full potential of digital surveillance systems through a One Health approach requires coordinated action from diverse stakeholders. This involves establishing robust regulatory guidelines to safeguard data privacy, allocating resources to digital infrastructure and skill development in developing nations, and enhancing the consistency and compatibility of global data platforms. Furthermore, strengthening the connection between digital surveillance systems and public health decision-making is crucial. This can be achieved by enhancing data literacy among policymakers and healthcare professionals and creating analytical tools that can convert complex information into practical insights [53].

2.4.2 Genomic Sequencing

Genomic sequencing technologies have undergone revolutionary advancements since the initial Human Genome Project, with contemporary platforms, including Illumina NovaSeq and Oxford Nanopore Technologies MinION, enabling complete genome characterization within hours rather than months, dramatically expanding research capabilities and creating transformative applications across the One Health spectrum [81]. This technological advancement has created new opportunities for research and health applications via the One Health approach. Genomic data provide crucial insights into relationships among pathogens, hosts, and the environment. Genome sequencing enables the rapid detection and characterization of emerging pathogens, aiding in the outbreak response [108]. By comparing pathogen genomes with different hosts, scientists can trace transmission routes and identify factors that facilitate interspecies jumps. Genomic analyses have revealed resistance mechanisms and tracked the spread of resistance genes, including their potential to cause disease outbreaks [109]. Understanding the genomic structure of pathogens can accelerate the development of targeted interventions and increase global disease control efforts [38].

Genomic technologies have revolutionized zoonotic disease investigations through three primary applications: molecular epidemiology, which enables high-resolution reconstruction of transmission chains during outbreaks, facilitating precisely targeted control interventions; pathogen ecology research, which identifies viral reservoir hosts through genomic characterization across species boundaries; and predictive epidemiology, which employs wildlife virome analysis to identify novel pathogens with pandemic potential before human spillover occurs [108, 110]. Recent case studies have demonstrated the utility of genomic sequencing via the One Health approach, particularly in response to the COVID-19 pandemic. Genomic sequencing has played a key role in understanding the origin, transmission, and evolution of SARS-CoV-2. Phylogenetic analysis of viral genomes from different countries has helped track the global spread of the virus and identify variants of concern. Grubaugh et al. [111] used sequencing data to identify and track the spread of alpha variants (B.1.1.7) to inform public health policy.

In Asia, Li et al. [112] used genome sequencing to confirm human-to-human transmission during the early stages of the pandemic in Wuhan, China.

Genomic surveillance has proven indispensable for monitoring AI evolution, with studies in South Korea by Ahrberg et al. [113] employing whole-genome analysis to characterize highly pathogenic H5N8 virus reassortment patterns and migration dynamics, whereas European investigations by Lean et al. [33] identified specific mutations conferring enhanced pathogenicity and mammalian transmission potential in circulating H5N1 strains complemented by North American research using phylodynamic approaches to reconstruct West Nile virus spread and adaptation determinants across continental boundaries [114].

The 2014–2016 West African Ebola epidemic demonstrated the critical role of genomic sequencing in the outbreak response, with Dudas et al. [115] employing phylogenetic analysis to reconstruct viral transmission networks across national boundaries, quantify intervention effectiveness, and identify superspreader events. Deng et al. [116] subsequently established real-time genome sequencing protocols in the Democratic Republic of Congo, which directly informed contact tracing priorities and control measure implementation. The future of genomic sequencing via the One Health approach is promising, with several innovative directions. These include the development of portable sequencing technologies, such as the Oxford Nanopore MinION, for field-based genomic analysis and metagenomic sequencing for comprehensive microbial community analysis [117].

Future genomic applications in One Health will be transformed by several converging innovations: the integration of machine learning algorithms with genomic analysis to predict zoonotic potential and AMR evolution; the development of genomic early warning systems synthesizing sequence data with epidemiological and environmental parameters for preemptive intervention; and multiomics approaches combining genomics with transcriptomics, proteomics, and metabolomics to comprehensively characterize host–pathogen interactions across species boundaries [118]. These technological advances continue to create new opportunities for research and applications, promising a better understanding of zoonotic diseases and more effective strategies to address global health challenges. However, realizing the full potential of these technologies will require ongoing cross-disciplinary collaboration, investment in infrastructure, and the development of ethical and regulatory frameworks for responsible genomic data management and sharing.

2.4.3 Technological Innovations and Their Applications in the One Health Field

Technological advances are enabling factors for implementing the One Health approach and measuring program success in complex global health scenarios. Table 2.2 summarizes these technological innovations, detailing their specific applications in One Health, associated benefits and limitations, and examples of successful implementation worldwide. This overview demonstrates how emerging technologies have transformed our ability to detect, monitor, and respond to health threats at the human–animal–environment interface. While these technologies offer new capabilities for data collection, analysis, and sharing across sectors, their effective implementation requires addressing challenges related to equity in access, technical capacity, data standards and governance. Future progress in One Health will depend on how these technologies are harnessed and integrated into coordinated global health systems.

2.5 Overcoming Challenges in Cross-disciplinary Cooperation

2.5.1 Institutional Barriers

Interdisciplinary cooperation, particularly the One Health approach, has become crucial for addressing complex global challenges in animal health and sustainable agriculture. However, the implementation of this approach faces several institutional barriers. Structural impediments to One Health implementation include organizational

Table 2.2 Technological innovations and their applications in the One Health field.

Technology	Description	Applications in One Health	Benefits	Limitations	Implementation	Reference
Digital Surveillance Systems	ICT-based systems for data collection, analysis, and dissemination	Early outbreak detection, long-term health trend monitoring, response coordination	Real-time data collection, improved accuracy of predictions, enhanced global information sharing	Privacy concerns, unequal access to technology, data standardization issues	ProMED, EMPRES-i, HealthMap, PREDICT, EpiCore	[34, 35]
Artificial Intelligence and Machine Learning	Algorithms analyzing complex health datasets	Pattern detection in disease emergence, prediction of outbreaks, identification of zoonotic potential	Detection of trends missed by human analysis, faster processing of large datasets, more precise predictions	Requires quality training data, black box decision-making, technical expertise needed	AI-powered disease forecasting models, Automated syndromic surveillance	[25, 37]
Genomic Sequencing	Determination of complete DNA sequence of organisms	Pathogen characterization, transmission route tracing, AMR mechanism identification	Rapid detection of emerging pathogens, understanding of host relationships, tracking evolutionary changes	Cost, technical requirements, complex data interpretation	COVID-19 variant tracking, Avian influenza mutation monitoring, AMR gene identification	[58, 81, 116]
Geographic Information Systems	Spatial analysis and mapping technologies	Visualization of disease distribution, environmental risk factor analysis, animal population dynamics	Integration of multiple data layers, spatial relationship identification, targeted intervention planning	Data quality dependency, technical expertise needed, resource-intensive	Mapping of zoonotic disease hotspots, vector distribution monitoring, environmental change analysis	[62, 105]
Mobile Technologies	Smartphone applications and portable devices	Field-based diagnostics, disease reporting, community engagement	Increased accessibility in remote areas, real-time data transmission, reduced reporting delays	Connectivity issues, user adoption challenges, battery limitations	Mobile reporting for rabies cases, smartphone-based diagnostic tools, community health worker support apps	[20, 116]
Portable Sequencing Technologies	Field-deployable genomic analysis devices	On-site pathogen identification, AMR detection, environmental sampling	Rapid results without laboratory infrastructure, field applicability, lower sample transportation needs	Higher error rates than lab-based methods, limited throughput, training requirements	Oxford Nanopore MinION for field diagnostics, Portable PCR systems, and On-site AMR detection	[109]
Blockchain Technology	Secure distributed ledger systems	Data integrity verification, supply chain tracking, secure information sharing	Transparent data transactions, tamper-proof records, enhanced traceability	Energy consumption, scalability issues, interoperability challenges	WHO's COVID-19 vaccine tracing, veterinary drug supply monitoring, disease outbreak verification	[119]
Internet of Things (IoT)	Connected sensors and devices	Environmental monitoring, animal health tracking, automated surveillance	Continuous data collection, early warning capabilities, reduced human resource needs	Connectivity requirements, data management challenges, security concerns	Wildlife tracking systems, environmental parameter monitoring, automated farm biosecurity	[4, 37, 46, 104]

fragmentation across the health, agricultural, and environmental sectors; distinct professional cultures with divergent priorities and operational methodologies; resource allocation imbalances that limit cross-sectoral initiatives; and policy frameworks that reinforce traditional sectoral boundaries rather than incentivize collaborative approaches. Many countries struggle with poor coordination between health, agriculture, and environmental ministries, leading to inefficient resource use [69].

Effective integration mechanisms have emerged to overcome institutional silos, including multisectoral coordination platforms exemplified by the Netherlands' One Health Platform, which establishes formal governance structures facilitating regular dialog, joint priority-setting, and coordinated decision-making across diverse stakeholders. Interdisciplinary training programs, such as the USAID-funded Health Workforce-Next Generation program, have successfully prepared professionals for multidisciplinary teamwork [120]. Information and communication technologies, including data-sharing platforms such as the Global Early Warning System (GLEWS), enable real-time information exchange regarding transboundary disease threats.

Successful institutional collaboration demonstrates the potential for interdisciplinary cooperation. For example, the Vietnam One Health University Network (VOHUN) has built a national capacity for health education and research [121], whereas the Kenya Zoonotic Disease Unit (ZDU) has strengthened zoonotic disease surveillance and response. The Tripartite Zoonoses Guide (TZG) provides an operational framework for multisectoral collaboration in addressing zoonotic diseases. Despite measurable progress in establishing cross-sectoral mechanisms, persistent challenges constrain global One Health implementation, including disparate legal and regulatory frameworks across jurisdictions, pronounced resource and capacity disparities between developed and developing nations, and the inherent complexity of addressing interconnected environmental and health challenges that transcend traditional institutional boundaries [95]. Overcoming these institutional barriers requires long-term commitment from governments, international organizations, and civil society to continuously strengthen cross-disciplinary collaboration.

2.5.2 Cultural and Disciplinary Differences

Cultural diversity presents significant implementation challenges for One Health initiatives, with divergent worldviews, values, practice norms, and knowledge systems influencing how professionals from different backgrounds conceptualize and address animal health and sustainable agricultural issues across geographical contexts [70]. Overcoming these challenges requires the development of cultural sensitivity, effective cross-cultural communication skills, and engagement with local stakeholders. Cultural competency training and knowledge exchange can help bridge these gaps.

Epistemological boundaries between scientific disciplines constitute formidable barriers to integration, as each field operates within distinct conceptual frameworks, methodological approaches, and specialized terminology, creating potential misunderstandings that impede effective communication and collaboration across sectoral boundaries. To address this, a common language and conceptual framework must be developed, facilitated by cross-disciplinary workshops and discussion forums [122]. The establishment of balanced interdisciplinary teams ensures diverse decision-making perspectives. Education plays a crucial role in addressing these challenges. Integrating the One Health concept into educational programs can help prepare future practitioners for interdisciplinary research.

Balancing productivity and environmental conservation present additional challenges in sustainable agriculture. Conflicting priorities between agronomists and ecologists require a holistic approach to develop sustainable practices for the future. Despite the cultural and epistemological challenges, innovative One Health initiatives have emerged globally. Southeast Asian programs have successfully integrated indigenous knowledge systems with contemporary scientific approaches to zoonotic disease management, whereas Latin American cross-sectoral cooperation has generated novel intervention programs addressing AMR while simultaneously enhancing food security outcomes. With a strong global perspective and commitment to collaboration, these challenges can be transformed into opportunities for innovation and progress in animal health and sustainable agriculture.

2.5.3 Resource Constraints

Resource constraints pose significant challenges to the global implementation of the One Health approach, particularly in LMICs [64]. These constraints include financial limitations, inadequate infrastructure, technological gaps, and shortages of trained personnel. Financial constraints frequently result in systematic underinvestment in critical One Health infrastructure, including integrated zoonotic disease surveillance networks, cross-sectoral laboratory capacity, and interdisciplinary training programs, whereas physical infrastructure deficiencies, particularly pronounced in rural and remote regions, further compromise disease prevention and control efforts [120]. The scarcity of professionals trained in the One Health approach presents another significant hurdle [89].

Addressing resource limitations requires innovative financing mechanisms that integrate contributions across relevant ministries, thereby increasing the available resource pools while simultaneously incentivizing cross-sectoral collaboration and joint program implementation. Leveraging local resources and traditional knowledge, such as integrating traditional medical systems with modern approaches, can expand animal health services in remote areas. The use of appropriate technologies, such as mobile applications for disease reporting and online learning platforms, can increase efficiency at a relatively low cost. International support and strategic partnerships are vital for addressing resource limitations. Organizations such as the WHO, FAO, and WOAH can provide technical assistance, training, and financial support to these countries. Innovative financing approaches, such as blended financing, which combines public and private resources, can help bridge funding gaps [123].

Integrating One Health principles into agricultural systems offers multifaceted benefits, including increased productivity, improved biosecurity, and a reduced risk of zoonotic diseases. However, the implementation of environmentally sustainable practices frequently encounters barriers related to knowledge deficits, technological limitations, and insufficient economic incentives that must be systematically addressed through coordinated research and development programs focused on One Health-aligned agricultural innovations [124]. Local capacity building in terms of human resources and infrastructure should be prioritized in global health efforts to improve health outcomes. With a holistic and sustainable approach, the integration of animal health and sustainable agriculture can contribute significantly to global health, food security, and sustainable development.

2.5.4 Data Sharing and Privacy Issues

Cross-disciplinary collaboration has become increasingly vital in addressing complex health issues, particularly in the application of the One Health concept. Data sharing across sectors is crucial for this approach, as it can facilitate the early detection of zoonotic disease outbreaks, improve public health interventions, and foster innovation in biomedical research. Critical barriers to cross-disciplinary data exchange identified by the European Center for Disease Prevention and Control include insufficient technological infrastructure for secure data transfer, incompatible data formats and terminologies between sectors, and fundamental concerns regarding data privacy and security that restrict information flow [125]. Kelly et al. [34] noted that privacy concerns often stem from potential misuse of sensitive data, risk of breaches, and legal uncertainty regarding liability for shared data.

Comprehensive solutions to data-sharing challenges require multidimensional approaches that span the technical, legal, and ethical domains. Advanced cryptographic techniques and robust anonymization methods minimize the risk of privacy violations. Blockchain-based systems, exemplified by the WHO's COVID-19 vaccine tracing pilot, establish tamper-resistant data integrity. Harmonized regulatory frameworks across jurisdictions provide essential legal clarity for cross-border data exchanges. The development of comprehensive regulatory frameworks and the harmonization of privacy standards between countries are crucial. While the EU's General Data Protection Regulation (GDPR) has become a global model, Kuo et al. [119] highlighted the need for further customization to accommodate biomedical and public health research requirements. Standardized protocols and frameworks, such as findable, accessible, interoperable, and reusable (FAIR) data principles, provide important guidance for scientific data management and sharing. Wilkinson et al. [126] reported that applying FAIR principles to one health project can improve research efficiency and facilitate cross-sector collaboration.

The development of integrated, user-friendly data-sharing platforms is key to overcoming these barriers. The WHO's Global Health Security Connect (GHS Connect) initiative, launched in 2022, exemplifies efforts to facilitate the real-time exchange of global health security information. Equitable participation within One Health data ecosystem requires particular attention to capacity development in LMICs, ensuring not only access to shared information but also the technical infrastructure, human resource capacity, and governance frameworks necessary for meaningful contributions to global data repositories [127]. In conclusion, building a safe, ethical, and effective data-sharing ecosystem to improve human, animal, and environmental health holistically requires a combination of technological solutions, strong legal frameworks, and clear guidelines.

2.6 Conclusion

The One Health approach has proven to be a crucial paradigm for addressing the complexity of global health challenges involving interactions among humans, animals, and the environment. Case studies from various countries illustrate the effectiveness of cross-sector collaboration in improving disease surveillance, accelerating outbreak responses, and developing more holistic interventions. Innovative technologies, such as digital surveillance systems and genomic sequencing, have played an important role in strengthening health capabilities, enabling the early detection of health threats and more in-depth analysis of disease dynamics. However, One Health implementation still faces significant challenges, including institutional barriers, cultural and disciplinary differences, resource limitations, data sharing, and privacy concerns. Addressing these challenges requires a multifaceted approach that includes strengthening policy frameworks, increasing investments in infrastructure and capacity building, and promoting dialog and understanding across disciplines. Continued global collaboration and cross-sector innovation will be key to addressing future health challenges and achieving development goals.

Abbreviations

AI: Artificial Intelligence; AMR: Antimicrobial Resistance; CDC: Centers for Disease Control and Prevention; CIPARS: Canadian Integrated Program for Antimicrobial Resistance Surveillance; COVID-19: Coronavirus Disease 2019; DRC: Democratic Republic of Congo; EMPRES-i: Emergency Prevention System for Animal Health; ESBL: Extended-Spectrum Beta-Lactamase; EU: European Union; FAIR: Findable, Accessible, Interoperable, and Reusable; FAO: Food and Agriculture Organization; GDPR: General Data Protection Regulation; GHSA: Global Health Security Agenda; GHS Connect: Global Health Security Connect; GIS: Geographic Information Systems; GISAID: Global Initiative on Sharing All Influenza Data; GLEWS: Global Early Warning System; GZDN: Global Zoonotic Disease Surveillance Network; H5N1: Hemagglutinin Type 5 and Neuraminidase Type 1; H5N8: Hemagglutinin Type 5 and Neuraminidase Type 8; H7N9: Hemagglutinin Type 7 and Neuraminidase Type 9; HPAI: Highly Pathogenic Avian Influenza; ICT: Information and Communication Technology; IoT: Internet of Things; LMICs: Low- and Middle-Income Countries; LPAI: Less Pathogenic Avian Influenza; MRSA: Methicillin-Resistant Staphylococcus aureus; NTDs: Neglected Tropical Diseases; OFFLU: WOAH-FAO Network of Expertise on Animal Influenza; OHEJP: One Health European Joint Programme; OHW-NG: One Health Workforce-Next Generation; WOAH: World Organization for Animal Health (Office International des Epizooties); PCR: Polymerase Chain Reaction; PEP: Postexposure Prophylaxis; ProMED: Program for Monitoring Emerging Diseases; SARS-CoV-2: Severe Acute Respiratory Syndrome Coronavirus 2; SDGs: Sustainable Development Goals;

TZG: Tripartite Zoonoses Guide; USAID: United States Agency for International Development; VOHUN: Vietnam One Health University Network; WASH: Water, Sanitation, and Hygiene; WHO: World Health Organization; WOAH: World Organization for Animal Health; ZDU: Zoonotic Disease Unit.

References

1 Centers for Disease Control and Prevention. *One Health Basics*. 2022. https://www.cdc.gov/one-health/about/?CDC_AAref_Val=https://www.cdc.gov/onehealth/basics/index.html (accessed 17 October 2024).

2 Karesh, W.B., Dobson, A., Lloyd-Smith, J.O., et al. Ecology of zoonoses: natural and unnatural histories. *Lancet* 2012; 380: e1936–e1945. https://doi.org/10.1016/S0140-6736(12)61678-X.

3 Gibbs, E.P.J. The evolution of One Health: a decade of progress and challenges for the future. *Vet Rec.* 2014; 174: 85–91. https://doi.org/10.1136/vr.g143.

4 Mackenzie, J.S. and Jeggo, M. The One Health approach—why is it so important? *Trop. Med. Infect. Dis.* 2019; 4: 88. https://doi.org/10.3390/tropicalmed4020088.

5 Haider, N., Rothman-Ostrow, P., Osman, A.Y., et al. COVID-19—zoonosis or emerging infectious disease? *Front Public Health* 2020; 8: e596944. https://doi.org/10.3389/fpubh.2020.596944.

6 Lerner, H. and Berg, C. The concept of health in One Health and some practical implications for research and education: what is One Health? *Infect. Ecol. Epidemiol.* 2015; 5: 25300. https://doi.org/10.3402/iee.v5.25300.

7 Food and Agriculture Organization. *Global Early Warning and Response System for Major Animal Diseases Including Zoonoses (Glews)*. 2024. https://www.fao.org/agriculture/animal-production-and-health/en/ (accessed 13 July 2024).

8 Laing, G., Duffy, E., Anderson, N., et al. Advancing One Health: updated core competencies. *CABI One Health* 2023: ohcs20230002. https://doi.org/10.1079/cabionehealth.2023.0002.

9 Armstrong-Mensah, E.A. and Ndiaye, S.M. Global health security agenda implementation: a case for community engagement. *Health Secur.* 2018; 16: 217–223. https://doi.org/10.1089/hs.2017.0097

10 Zinsstag, J., Schelling, E., Crump, L., et al. *One Health: The Theory and Practice of Integrated Health Approaches*. 2nd ed. The Netherlands: CABI Digital Library; 2023, https://www.cabidigitallibrary.org/doi/book/10.1079/9781789242577.0000

11 Hampson, K., Coudeville, L., Lembo, T., et al. Estimating the global burden of endemic canine rabies. *PLoS Negl. Trop. Dis.* 2015; 9: e0003709. https://doi.org/10.1371/journal.pntd.0003709.

12 Freuling, C.M., Hampson, K., Selhorst, T., et al. The elimination of fox rabies from Europe: determinants of success and lessons for the future. *Philos. Trans. R Soc. B Biol. Sci.* 2013; 368: 20120142. https://doi.org/10.1098/rstb.2012.0142.

13 Cleaveland, S., Lankester, F., Townsend, S., et al. Rabies control and elimination: a test case for One Health. *Vet. Rec.* 2014; 175: 188–193. https://doi.org/10.1136/vr.g4996.

14 Lankester, F., Hampson, K., Lembo, T., et al. Implementing Pasteur's vision for rabies elimination. *Science* 2014; 345: 1562–1564. https://doi.org/10.1126/science.1256306.

15 Häsler, B., Bazeyo, W., Byrne, A.W., et al. Reflecting on One Health in action during the COVID-19 response. *Front. Vet. Sci.* 2020; 7: e578649. https://doi.org/10.3389/fvets.2020.578649.

16 Lankester, F., Davis, A., Kinung'hi, S., et al. An integrated health delivery platform, targeting soil-transmitted helminths (STH) and canine mediated human rabies, results in cost savings and increased breadth of treatment for STH in remote communities in Tanzania. *BMC Public Health* 2019; 19: 1398. https://doi.org/10.1186/s12889-019-7737-6.

17 Zinsstag, J., Schelling, E., Waltner-Toews, D., and Tanner, M. From "one medicine" to "One Health" and systemic approaches to health and well-being. *Prev. Vet. Med.* 2011; 101: 148–156. https://doi.org/10.1016/j.prevetmed.2010.07.003.

18 Gongal, G., Ofrin, R., de Balogh, K., et al. Operationalization of One Health and tripartite collaboration in the Asia-Pacific region. *WHO South East Asia J. Public Health* 2020; 9: 21. https://doi.org/10.4103/2224-3151.282991.

19 Sambo, M., Cleaveland, S., Ferguson, H., et al. The burden of rabies in Tanzania and its impact on local communities. *PLoS Negl. Trop. Dis.* 2013; 7: e2510. https://doi.org/10.1371/journal.pntd.0002510.

20 Gibson, A.D., Ohal, P., Shervell, K., et al. Vaccinate-assess-move method of mass canine rabies vaccination utilising mobile technology data collection in Ranchi, India. *BMC Infect. Dis.* 2015; 15: 589–589. https://doi.org/10.1186/s12879-015-1320-2.

21 Cleaveland, S., Thumbi, S.M., Sambo, M., et al. Proof of concept of mass dog vaccination for the control and elimination of canine rabies. *Rev. Sci. Tech. OIE* 2018; 37: 559–568. https://doi.org/10.20506/rst.37.2.2824.

22 Lapiz, S.M.D., Miranda, M.E.G., Garcia, R.G., et al. Implementation of an intersectoral program to eliminate human and canine rabies: the Bohol rabies prevention and elimination project. *PLoS Negl. Trop. Dis.* 2012; 6: e1891. https://doi.org/10.1371/journal.pntd.0001891.

23 Abela-Ridder, B., Knopf, L., Martin, S., et al. The beginning of the end of rabies? *Lancet Glob. Health* 2016; 4: e780–e781. https://doi.org/10.1016/S2214-109X(16)30245-5.

24 Kumarapeli, V. and Awerbuch-Friedlander, T. Human rabies focusing on dog ecology—a challenge to public health in Sri Lanka. *Acta Trop.* 2009; 112: 33–37. https://doi.org/10.1016/j.actatropica.2009.06.009.

25 Vasey, B., Nagendran, M., Campbell, B., et al. Reporting guideline for the early-stage clinical evaluation of decision support systems driven by artificial intelligence: decide-AI. *Nat. Med.* 2022; 28: 924–933. https://doi.org/10.1038/s41591-022-01772-9.

26 Erkyihun, G.A. and Alemayehu, M.B. One Health approach for the control of zoonotic diseases. *Zoonoses* 2022; 2: 0037–0037. https://doi.org/10.15212/ZOONOSES-2022-0037.

27 Lai, S., Qin, Y., Cowling, B.J., et al. Global epidemiology of avian influenza a h5n1 virus infection in humans, 1997–2015: a systematic review of individual case data. *Lancet Infect. Dis.* 2016; 16: e108–e118. https://doi.org/10.1016/S1473-3099(16)00153-5.

28 Alexander, D.J. A review of avian influenza in different bird species. *Vet. Microbiol.* 2000; 74: 3–13. https://doi.org/10.1016/S0378-1135(00)00160-7.

29 Capua, I. and Alexander, D.J. Avian influenza: recent developments. *Avian Pathol.* 2004; 33: 393–404. https://doi.org/10.1080/03079450410001724085.

30 The Global Consortium for H5N8 and Related Influenza Viruses. Role for migratory wild birds in the global spread of avian influenza H5N8. *Science* 2016; 354: 213–217. https://doi.org/10.1126/science.aaf8852.

31 Gilbert, M., Golding, N., Zhou, H., et al. Predicting the risk of avian influenza a h7n9 infection in live-poultry markets across Asia. *Nat. Commun.* 2014; 5: 4116–4116. https://doi.org/10.1038/ncomms5116.

32 Gao, R., Cao, B., Hu, Y., et al. Human infection with a novel avian-origin influenza a (H7N9) virus. *N. Engl. J. Med.* 2013; 368: 1888–1897. https://doi.org/10.1056/nejmoa1304459.

33 Lean, F.Z.X., Vitores, A.G., Reid, S.M., et al. Gross pathology of high pathogenicity avian influenza virus H5N1 2021–2022 epizootic in naturally infected birds in the United Kingdom. *One Health* 2022; 14: 100392. https://doi.org/10.1016/j.onehlt.2022.100392.

34 Kelly, T.R., Machalaba, C., Karesh, W.B., et al. Implementing One Health approaches to confront emerging and re-emerging zoonotic disease threats: lessons from predict. *One Health Outlook* 2020; 2: 1. https://doi.org/10.1186/s42522-019-0007-9.

35 Adnyana, I.M.D.M., Utomo, B., Eljatin, D.S., and Setyawan, M.F. Developing and establishing attribute-based surveillance system: a review. *Prev. Med. Res. Rev.* 2024; 1: 76–83. https://doi.org/10.4103/PMRR.PMRR_54_23.

36 Degeling, C., Gilbert, G.L., Tambyah, P., et al. One Health and zoonotic uncertainty in Singapore and Australia: examining different regimes of precaution in outbreak decision-making. *Public Health Ethics* 2020; 13: 69–81. https://doi.org/10.1093/phe/phz017.

37 Adnyana, I.M., Utomo, B., Eljatin, D.S., and Sudaryati, N.L.G. One Health approach and zoonotic diseases in Indonesia: urgency of implementation and challenges. *Narra J.* 2023; 3: e257. https://doi.org/10.52225/narra.v3i3.257.

38 Adnyana, I.M.D.M., Eljatin, D.S., Sudaryati, N.L.G., et al. CRISPR-cas9 genome editing technology for zoonotic disease control in Indonesia: a comprehensive review. *J. Med. Health Technol.* 2024; 1: 21–39. https://doi.org/10.12962/j30466865.v1i1.1172.

39 Bidaisee, S. and Macpherson, C.N.L. Zoonoses and One Health: a review of the literature. *J. Parasitol. Res.* 2014; 2014: 1–8. https://doi.org/10.1155/2014/874345.

40 Salam, I., Adnyana, I.M.D.M., Karimah, R., et al. *Epidemiologi Zoonosis*. 1st ed. Bandung: CV, Media Sains Indonesia; 2024.

41 Rocklöv, J. and Dubrow, R. Climate change: an enduring challenge for vector-borne disease prevention and control. *Nat. Immunol.* 2020; 21: 479–483. https://doi.org/10.1038/s41590-020-0648-y.

42 Bloomfield, L.S.P., McIntosh, T.L., and Lambin, E.F. Habitat fragmentation, livelihood behaviors, and contact between people and nonhuman primates in Africa. *Landsc. Ecol.* 2020; 35: 985–1000. https://doi.org/10.1007/s10980-020-00995-w.

43 Lebov, J., Grieger, K., Womack, D., et al. A framework for One Health research. *One Health* 2017; 3: 44–50. https://doi.org/10.1016/j.onehlt.2017.03.004.

44 Adnyana, I.M.D.M. and Utomo, B. Dengue elimination challenges in Bali: a One Health perspective. *Natl. J. Commun. Med.* 2023; 14: 544–546. https://doi.org/10.55489/njcm.140820233034.

45 Destoumieux-Garzón, D., Mavingui, P., Boetsch, G., et al. The One Health concept: 10 years old and a long road ahead. *Front. Vet. Sci.* 2018; 5: 14. https://doi.org/10.3389/fvets.2018.00014.

46 Mtui-Malamsha, N., Sallu, R., Mahiti, G.R., et al. Ecological and epidemiological findings associated with zoonotic rabies outbreaks and control in Moshi, Tanzania, 2017–2018. *Int. J. Environ. Res. Public Health* 2019; 16: 2816. https://doi.org/10.3390/ijerph16162816.

47 Sharan, M., Vijay, D., Yadav, J.P., et al. Surveillance and response strategies for zoonotic diseases: a comprehensive review. *Sci. One Health* 2023; 2: 100050. https://doi.org/10.1016/j.soh.2023.100050.

48 Dorado-García, A., Smid, J.H., van Pelt, W., et al. Molecular relatedness of ESBL/AMPC-producing *Escherichia coli* from humans, animals, food and the environment: a pooled analysis. *J. Antimicrob. Chemother.* 2018; 73: 339–347. https://doi.org/10.1093/jac/dkx397.

49 Larsson, D.G.J., Andremont, A., Bengtsson-Palme, J., et al. Critical knowledge gaps and research needs related to the environmental dimensions of antibiotic resistance. *Environ. Int.* 2018; 117: 132–138. https://doi.org/10.1016/j.envint.2018.04.041.

50 Laxminarayan, R., Van Boeckel, T., Frost, I., et al. The Lancet infectious diseases commission on antimicrobial resistance: 6 years later. *Lancet Infect. Dis.* 2020; 20: e51–e60. https://doi.org/10.1016/S1473-3099(20)30003-7.

51 Centers for Disease Control and Prevention. *Updated Guidelines for Evaluating Public Health Surveillance Systems: Recommendations from the Guidelines Working Group*. 2001. http://www.cdc.gov/mmwr/preview/mmwrhtml/rr5013a1.html (accessed 13 April 2024).

52 Adiwinoto, R.P., Adnyana, I.M.D.M., and Soedarsono, T.Y.P.G. From silos to systems: reimagining zoonotic neglected tropical disease management through the lens of One Health. *Svāsthya Trends Gen. Med. Public Health* 2024; 1: e61. https://doi.org/10.70347/svsthya.v1i3.61.

53 Aenishaenslin, C., Häsler, B., Ravel, A., et al. Evaluating the integration of One Health in surveillance systems for antimicrobial use and resistance: a conceptual framework. *Front. Vet. Sci.* 2021; 8: e611931. https://doi.org/10.3389/fvets.2021.611931.

54 Årdal, C., Balasegaram, M., Laxminarayan, R., et al. Antibiotic development economic, regulatory and societal challenges. *Nat. Rev. Microbiol.* 2020; 18: 267–274. https://doi.org/10.1038/s41579-019-0293-3.

55 Dyar, O.J., Huttner, B., Schouten, J., and Pulcini, C. What is antimicrobial stewardship? *Clin. Microbiol. Infect.* 2017; 23: 793–798. https://doi.org/10.1016/j.cmi.2017.08.026.

56 Rousham, E.K., Unicomb, L., and Islam, M.A. Human, animal and environmental contributors to antibiotic resistance in low-resource settings: integrating behavioural, epidemiological and One Health approaches. *Proc. R Soc. B Biol. Sci.* 2018; 285: e20180332. https://doi.org/10.1098/rspb.2018.0332.

57 Chanvatik, S., Donnua, S., Lekagul, A., et al. Antibiotic use in mandarin production (*citrus reticulata blanco*) in major mandarin-producing areas in Thailand: a survey assessment. *PLoS One* 2019; 14: e0225172. https://doi.org/10.1371/journal.pone.0225172.

58 Aarestrup, F.M. and Woolhouse, M.E.J. Using sewage for surveillance of antimicrobial resistance. *Science* 2020; 367: 630–632. https://doi.org/10.1126/science.aba3432.

59 Burnham, C.-A.D., Leeds, J., Nordmann, P., et al. Diagnosing antimicrobial resistance. *Nat. Rev. Microbiol.* 2017; 15: 697–703. https://doi.org/10.1038/nrmicro.2017.103.

60 Seffren, V., Lowther, S., Guerra, M., et al. Strengthening the global One Health workforce: veterinarians in CDC-supported field epidemiology training programs. *One Health* 2022; 14: e100382. https://doi.org/10.1016/j.onehlt.2022.100382.

61 Frost, I., Van Boeckel, T.P., Pires, J., et al. Global geographic trends in antimicrobial resistance: the role of international travel. *J. Travel Med.* 2019; 26: taz036. https://doi.org/10.1093/jtm/taz036.

62 Utomo, B., Chan, C.K., Mertaniasih, N.M., et al. Comparison epidemiology between tuberculosis and COVID-19 in East Java Province, Indonesia: an analysis of regional surveillance data in 2020. *Trop. Med. Infect. Dis.* 2022; 7: 83. https://doi.org/10.3390/tropicalmed7060083.

63 Verguet, S., Hailu, A., Eregata, G.T., et al. Toward universal health coverage in the post-COVID-19 era. *Nat. Med.* 2021; 27: 380–387. https://doi.org/10.1038/s41591-021-01268-y.

64 Amuasi, J.H., Lucas, T., Horton, R., and Winkler, A.S. Reconnecting for our future: the Lancet One Health Commission. *Lancet* 2020; 395: 1469–1471. https://doi.org/10.1016/S0140-6736(20)31027-8.

65 Essack, S.Y. Environment: the neglected component of the One Health triad. *Lancet Planet Health* 2018; 2: e239. https://doi.org/10.1016/S2542-5196(18)30124-4.

66 Baker, M.G., Wilson, N., and Anglemyer, A. Successful elimination of COVID-19 transmission in New Zealand. *N. Engl. J. Med.* 2020; 383: e56. https://doi.org/10.1056/NEJMc2025203.

67 Carlson, C.J., Chipperfield, J.D., Benito, B.M., et al. Species distribution models are inappropriate for COVID-19. *Nat. Ecol. Evol.* 2020; 4: 770–771. https://doi.org/10.1038/s41559-020-1212-8.

68 Morse, S.S., Mazet, J.A.K., Woolhouse, M., et al. Prediction and prevention of the next pandemic zoonosis. *Lancet* 2012; 380: e1965. https://doi.org/10.1016/S0140-6736(12)61684-5.

69 Yasobant, S., Bruchhausen, W., Saxena, D., and Falkenberg, T. One Health collaboration for a resilient health system in India: learnings from global initiatives. *One Health* 2019; 8: e100096. https://doi.org/10.1016/j.onehlt.2019.100096.

70 Bardosh, K.L., de Vries, D.H., Abramowitz, S., et al. Integrating the social sciences in epidemic preparedness and response: a strategic framework to strengthen capacities and improve global health security. *Global Health* 2020; 16: e120. https://doi.org/10.1186/s12992-020-00652-6.

71 Hendriksen, R.S., Munk, P., Njage, P., et al. Global monitoring of antimicrobial resistance based on metagenomics analyses of urban sewage. *Nat. Commun.* 2019; 10: e1124. https://doi.org/10.1038/s41467-019-08853-3.

72 Busso, M., Chauvin, J.P., and Herrera L.N. Rural-urban migration at high urbanization levels. *Reg. Sci. Urban Econ.* 2021; 91: e103658. https://doi.org/10.1016/j.regsciurbeco.2021.103658.

73 Bikbov, B., Purcell, C.A., Levey, A.S., et al. Global, regional, and national burden of chronic kidney disease, 1990–2017: a systematic analysis for the global burden of disease study 2017. *Lancet* 2020; 395: 709–733. https://doi.org/10.1016/S0140-6736(20)30045-3.

74 Bakken, S. Quantitative and qualitative methods advance the science of clinical workflow research. *J. Am. Med. Inform. Assoc.* 2023; 30: 795–796. https://doi.org/10.1093/jamia/ocad056.

75 Hockenhull, J., Turner, A.E., Reyher, K.K., et al. Antimicrobial use in food-producing animals: a rapid evidence assessment of stakeholder practices and beliefs. *Vet. Rec.* 2017; 181: e510. https://doi.org/10.1136/vr.104304.

76 Collignon, P., Beggs, J.J., Walsh, T.R., et al. Anthropological and socioeconomic factors contributing to global antimicrobial resistance: a univariate and multivariable analysis. *Lancet Planet Health* 2018; 2: e398–e405. https://doi.org/10.1016/S2542-5196(18)30186-4.

77 Munkholm, L., Rubin, O., Bækkeskov, E., and Humboldt-Dachroeden, S. Attention to the tripartite's One Health measures in national action plans on antimicrobial resistance. *J. Public Health Policy* 2021; 42: 236–248. https://doi.org/10.1057/s41271-021-00277-y.

78 Gozdzielewska, L., King, C., Flowers, P., et al. Scoping review of approaches for improving antimicrobial stewardship in livestock farmers and veterinarians. *Prev. Vet. Med.* 2020; 180: e105025. https://doi.org/10.1016/j.prevetmed.2020.105025.

79 Benton, D.J., Wrobel, A.G., Roustan, C., et al. The effect of the d614g substitution on the structure of the spike glycoprotein of SARS-CoV-2. *Proc. Natl. Acad. Sci. U. S. A.* 2021; 118: e2022586118. https://doi.org/10.1073/pnas.2022586118.

80 Chandler, C.I.R. Current accounts of antimicrobial resistance: stabilisation, individualisation and antibiotics as infrastructure. *Palgrave Commun.* 2019; 5: e53. https://doi.org/10.1057/s41599-019-0263-4.

81 Amarasinghe, S.L., Su, S., Dong, X., et al. Opportunities and challenges in long-read sequencing data analysis. *Genome Biol.* 2020; 21: e30. https://doi.org/10.1186/s13059-020-1935-5.

82 Machalaba, C., Romanelli, C., Stoett, P., et al. Climate change and health: transcending silos to find solutions. *Ann. Glob. Health* 2015; 81: e445. https://doi.org/10.1016/j.aogh.2015.08.002.

83 Bashir, A. How climate change is changing dengue fever. *BMJ* 2023; 382: 1690. https://doi.org/10.1136/bmj.p1690.

84 Ahmed, J., Wong, L.P., Chua, Y.P., et al. Quantitative microbial risk assessment of drinking water quality to predict the risk of waterborne diseases in primary-school children. *Int. J. Environ. Res. Public Health* 2020; 17: 2774. https://doi.org/10.3390/ijerph17082774.

85 Vardoulakis, S., Giagloglou, E., Steinle, S., et al. Indoor exposure to selected air pollutants in the home environment: a systematic review. *Int. J. Environ. Res. Public Health* 2020; 17: 8972. https://doi.org/10.3390/ijerph17238972.

86 Yuan, P., Tan, Y., Yang, L., et al. Assessing transmission risks and control strategy for monkeypox as an emerging zoonosis in a metropolitan area. *J. Med. Virol.* 2023; 95: e28137. https://doi.org/10.1002/jmv.28137.

87 Huttner, B., Saam, M., Moja, L., et al. How to improve antibiotic awareness campaigns: findings of a WHO global survey. *BMJ Glob Health* 2019; 4: e001239. https://doi.org/10.1136/bmjgh-2018-001239.

88 Bloom, D.E., Black, S., and Rappuoli, R. Emerging infectious diseases: a proactive approach. *Proc. Natl. Acad. Sci. U. S. A.* 2017; 114: 4055–4059. https://doi.org/10.1073/pnas.1701410114.

89 Bordier, M., Delavenne, C., Nguyen, D.T.T., et al. One Health surveillance: a matrix to evaluate multisectoral collaboration. *Front. Vet. Sci.* 2019; 6: e00109. https://doi.org/10.3389/fvets.2019.00109.

90 Adnyana, I.M.D.M., Mahendra, K.A., and Raza, S.M. The importance of green education in primary, secondary and higher education: a review. *J. Environ. Sustain. Educ.* 2023; 1: 42–49. https://doi.org/10.62672/joease.v1i2.14.

91 Bird, B.H. and Mazet, J.A.K. Detection of emerging zoonotic pathogens: an integrated One Health approach. *Annu. Rev. Anim. Biosci.* 2018; 6: 121–139. https://doi.org/10.1146/annurev-animal-030117-014628.

92 GhaderiShekhiAbadi, P., Irani, M., Noorisepehr, M., and Maleki, A. Magnetic biosensors for identification of SARS-CoV-2, influenza, HIV, and Ebola viruses: a review. *Nanotechnology* 2023; 34: 272001. https://doi.org/10.1088/1361-6528/acc8da.

93 Adisasmito, W.B., Almuhairi, S., Barton Behravesh, C., et al. One Health action for health security and equity. *Lancet* 2023; 401: 530–533. https://doi.org/10.1016/S0140-6736(23)00086-7.

94 Lokuge, K., Caleo, G., Greig, J., et al. Successful control of Ebola virus disease: analysis of service based data from rural Sierra Leone. *PLoS Negl. Trop. Dis.* 2016; 10: e0004498. https://doi.org/10.1371/journal.pntd.0004498.

95 Elnaiem, A., Mohamed-Ahmed, O., Zumla, A., et al. Global and regional governance of One Health and implications for global health security. *Lancet* 2023; 401: 688–704. https://doi.org/10.1016/S0140-6736(22)01597-5.

96 George, A.M., Ansumana, R., de Souza, D.K., et al. Climate change and the rising incidence of vector-borne diseases globally. *Int. J. Infect. Dis.* 2024; 139: 143–145. https://doi.org/10.1016/j.ijid.2023.12.004.

97 Bain, L.E. and Awah, P.K. Eco-epidemiology: challenges and opportunities for tomorrow's epidemiologists. *Pan. Afr. Med. J.* 2014; 17: 3–6. https://doi.org/10.11604/pamj.2014.17.317.4080.

98 Cui, F., Yue, Y., Zhang, Y., et al. Advancing biosensors with machine learning. *ACS Sens.* 2020; 5: 3346–3364. https://doi.org/10.1021/acssensors.0c01424.

99 Utarini, A., Indriani, C., Ahmad, R.A., et al. Efficacy of Wolbachia-infected mosquito deployments for the control of dengue. *N. Engl. J. Med.* 2021; 384: 2177–2186. https://doi.org/10.1056/NEJMoa2030243.

100 Olea-Popelka, F., Muwonge, A., Perera, A., et al. Zoonotic tuberculosis in human beings caused by *Mycobacterium bovis*—a call for action. *Lancet Infect. Dis.* 2017; 17: e21–e25. https://doi.org/10.1016/S1473-3099(16)30139-6.

101 Ferrinho, P. and Fronteira, I. Developing One Health systems: a central role for the One Health workforce. *Int. J. Environ. Res. Public Health* 2023; 20: 4704. https://doi.org/10.3390/ijerph20064704.

102 Müller, B., Dürr, S., Alonso, S., et al. Zoonotic *Mycobacterium bovis*–induced tuberculosis in humans. *Emerg. Infect. Dis.* 2013; 19: 899–908. https://doi.org/10.3201/eid1906.120543.

103 Choi, J., Cho, Y., Shim, E., and Woo, H. Web-based infectious disease surveillance systems and public health perspectives: a systematic review. *BMC Public Health* 2016; 16: 1238. https://doi.org/10.1186/s12889-016-3893-0.

104 Bansal, S., Chowell, G., Simonsen, L., et al. Big data for infectious disease surveillance and modeling. *J. Infect. Dis.* 2016; 214: S375–S379. https://doi.org/10.1093/infdis/jiw400.

105 Franch-Pardo, I., Napoletano, B.M., Rosete-Verges, F., and Billa, L. Spatial analysis and GIS in the study of COVID-19. A review. *Sci. Total Environ.* 2020; 739: 140033. https://doi.org/10.1016/j.scitotenv.2020.140033.

106 Salathé, M. Digital epidemiology: what is it, and where is it going? *Life Sci. Soc. Policy* 2018; 14: 1. https://doi.org/10.1186/s40504-017-0065-7.

107 Brookes, V.J., HernÁNdez-Jover, M., Black, P.F., and Ward, M.P. Preparedness for emerging infectious diseases: pathways from anticipation to action. *Epidemiol. Infect.* 2015; 143: 2043–2058. https://doi.org/10.1017/S095026881400315X.

108 Didelot, X., Gardy, J., and Colijn, C. Bayesian inference of infectious disease transmission from whole-genome sequence data. *Mol. Biol. Evol.* 2014; 31: 1869–1879. https://doi.org/10.1093/molbev/msu121.

109 Hendriksen, R.S., Bortolaia, V., Tate, H., et al. Using genomics to track global antimicrobial resistance. *Front. Public Health* 2019; 7: 00242. https://doi.org/10.3389/fpubh.2019.00242.

110 Kusumaningrum, T., Latinne, A., Martinez, S., et al. Knowledge, attitudes, and practices associated with zoonotic disease transmission risk in North Sulawesi, Indonesia. *One Health Outlook* 2022; 4: 11. https://doi.org/10.1186/s42522-022-00067-w.

111 Grubaugh, N.D., Ladner, J.T., Lemey, P., et al. Tracking virus outbreaks in the twenty-first century. *Nat. Microbiol.* 2018; 4: 10–19. https://doi.org/10.1038/s41564-018-0296-2.

112 Li, T., Yang, Y., Qi, H., et al. CRISPR/cas9 therapeutics: progress and prospects. *Sig. Transduct. Target Ther.* 2023; 8: 36. https://doi.org/10.1038/s41392-023-01309-7.

113 Ahrberg, C.D., Choi, J.W., Lee, J.M., et al. Plasmonic heating-based portable digital PCR system. *Lab Chip* 2020; 20: 3560–3568. https://doi.org/10.1039/D0LC00788A.

114 Hadfield, J., Brito, A.F., Swetnam, D.M., et al. Twenty years of West Nile virus spread and evolution in the Americas visualized by nextstrain. *PLOS Pathog.* 2019; 15: e1008042. https://doi.org/10.1371/journal.ppat.1008042.

115 Dudas, G., Carvalho, L.M., Bedford, T., et al. Virus genomes reveal factors that spread and sustained the Ebola epidemic. *Nature* 2017; 544: 309–315. https://doi.org/10.1038/nature22040.

116 Deng, X., Achari, A., Federman, S., et al. Metagenomic sequencing with spiked primer enrichment for viral diagnostics and genomic surveillance. *Nat. Microbiol.* 2020; 5: 443–454. https://doi.org/10.1038/s41564-019-0637-9.

117 Maestre-Carballa, L., Navarro-López, V., and Martinez-Garcia, M. City-scale monitoring of antibiotic resistance genes by digital PCR and metagenomics. *Environ. Microbiome* 2024; 19: 16. https://doi.org/10.1186/s40793-024-00557-6.

118 Gorai, B., Sahoo, A.K., Srivastava, A., et al. Concerted interactions between multiple gp41 trimers and the target cell lipidome may be required for HIV-1 entry. *J. Chem. Inf. Model.* 2021; 61: 444–454. https://doi.org/10.1021/acs.jcim.0c01291.

119 Rwego, I.B., Babalobi, O.O., Musotsi, P., et al. One Health capacity building in sub-Saharan Africa. *Infect. Ecol. Epidemiol.* 2016; 6: 34032. https://doi.org/10.3402/iee.v6.34032.

120 Nguyen, T.T., Mai, T.N., Dang-Xuan, S., et al. Emerging zoonotic diseases in Southeast Asia in the period 2011–2022: a systematic literature review. *Vet. Q.* 2024; 44: 1–15. https://doi.org/10.1080/01652176.2023.2300965.

121 Morón-Duarte, L.S., Ramirez Varela, A., Bassani, D.G., et al. Agreement of antenatal care indicators from self-reported questionnaire and the antenatal care card of women in the 2015 Pelotas birth cohort, Rio Grande do Sul, Brazil. *BMC Pregnancy Childb.* 2019; 19: e410. https://doi.org/10.1186/s12884-019-2573-3.

122 Cleaveland, S., Sharp, J., Abela-Ridder, B., et al. One Health contributions towards more effective and equitable approaches to health in low- and middle-income countries. *Philos. Trans. R Soc. B Biol. Sci.* 2017; 372: e20160168. https://doi.org/10.1098/rstb.2016.0168.

123 Shenoy, S., Rajan, A.K., Rashid, M., et al. Artificial intelligence in differentiating tropical infections: a step ahead. *PLoS Negl. Trop. Dis.* 2022; 16: e0010455. https://doi.org/10.1371/journal.pntd.0010455.

124 European Centre for Disease Prevention and Control. *EU-Level Collaboration on Sharing Data for Early Detection and Response to Public Health Threats.* 2021. https://www.ecdc.europa.eu/en/publications-data/eu-level-collaboration-sharing-data-early-detection-and-response-public-health (accessed 13 July 2024).

125 Kuo, T.T., Kim, H.E., and Ohno-Machado, L. Blockchain distributed ledger technologies for biomedical and health care applications. *J. Am. Med. Inform. Assoc.* 2017; 24: 1211–1220. https://doi.org/10.1093/jamia/ocx068.

126 Marmot, M. and Wilkinson, R.G. Health and the psychosocial environment at work. In: *Social Determinants of Health*, 97–130. 2nd ed. United Kingdom: Oxford University Press; 2005. https://doi.org/10.1093/acprof:oso/9780198565895.003.06.

127 Steele, S.G., Toribio, J.A., Booy, R., and Mor, S.M. What makes an effective One Health clinical practitioner? Opinions of Australian One Health experts. *One Health* 2019; 8: e100108. https://doi.org/10.1016/j.onehlt.2019.100108.

3

Connection of Human, Animal, and Environmental Health: A One Health Perspective

*Budi Utomo**

Department of Public Health and Preventive Medicine, Airlangga University, Surabaya, Indonesia

*Corresponding author: budiutomo@fk.unair.ac.id

TABLE OF CONTENTS

3.1 Introduction
3.2 Interdependence of Human, Animal, and Environmental Well-being
 3.2.1 Animals as Vectors of Disease in Human
 3.2.2 Animals as Sentinels of Human Health
 3.2.3 Animals in Biomedical Research
3.3 Addressing Zoonotic Diseases Through a Holistic Approach
3.4 AMR: A One Health Perspective
 3.4.1 AMR Overview
 3.4.2 Lack of New Antibiotics Development
 3.4.3 Strategies to Combat AMR
 3.4.4 Impact of AMR on Animal Health
 3.4.5 Environmental Factors
3.5 Global Implications of Environmental Health on Public Health
3.6 Conclusion
 References

3.1 Introduction

The modern world is facing intricate and interconnected health issues, including the emergence of infectious diseases, the increase in antimicrobial resistance (AMR), and the health effects of climate change. The One Health concept offers an integrated framework that recognizes the interconnectedness of human health with the health of animals and the environment. It encourages collaboration across various disciplines and sectors to create comprehensive and sustainable health solutions.

This chapter examines the complex relationships among humans, animals, and the environment in the context of global health. It highlights the role of animals as vectors of diseases, indicators of environmental health, and participants in medical research. Additionally, the chapter investigates how a holistic approach can effectively tackle outbreaks of zoonotic diseases and the escalating threat of AMR. Finally, it underscores the impact of global environmental changes on public health and the necessity of enhancing adaptive and resilient health systems.

One Health Integration: Global Perspectives on Animal Health and Sustainable Agriculture. First Edition.
Edited by Pratik Subhash Gaikwad, Vivek Harishankar Shukla and Pintu Choudhary.

Companion Website: https://www.wiley.com/go/pratikgaikwad/onehealth

3.2 Interdependence of Human, Animal, and Environmental Well-being

Humans, animals, and the environment form an interdependent system where the well-being of one element directly influences the others. Animals both domestic and wild play crucial roles in human survival, contributing to food security, economic development, and medical advancements. Meanwhile clean air, water, and fertile soil sustained by healthy ecosystems are essential for both human and animal well-being. These interconnections form the basis of the One Health paradigm, which recognizes that safeguarding human health necessitates the concurrent protection of animal and environmental health.

To better understand the One Health paradigm, it is helpful to visualize the complex interconnections between human, animal, and environmental health. Figure 3.1 presents a conceptual model illustrating these interdependencies. This diagram illustrates the interconnectedness of human, animal, and environmental health. It highlights the flow of influence between sectors through shared exposures, food webs, and environmental pathways, emphasizing the need for integrated health approaches.

The One Health approach, endorsed by leading international organizations such as the World Health Organization (WHO), Food and Agriculture Organization (FAO), and World Organization for Animal Health (WOAH), promotes coordinated, multisectoral strategies to tackle shared health threats. It aligns closely with global goals like the United Nations (UN) Sustainable Development Goals (SDGs), especially those addressing health, food security, poverty alleviation, and environmental sustainability [2].

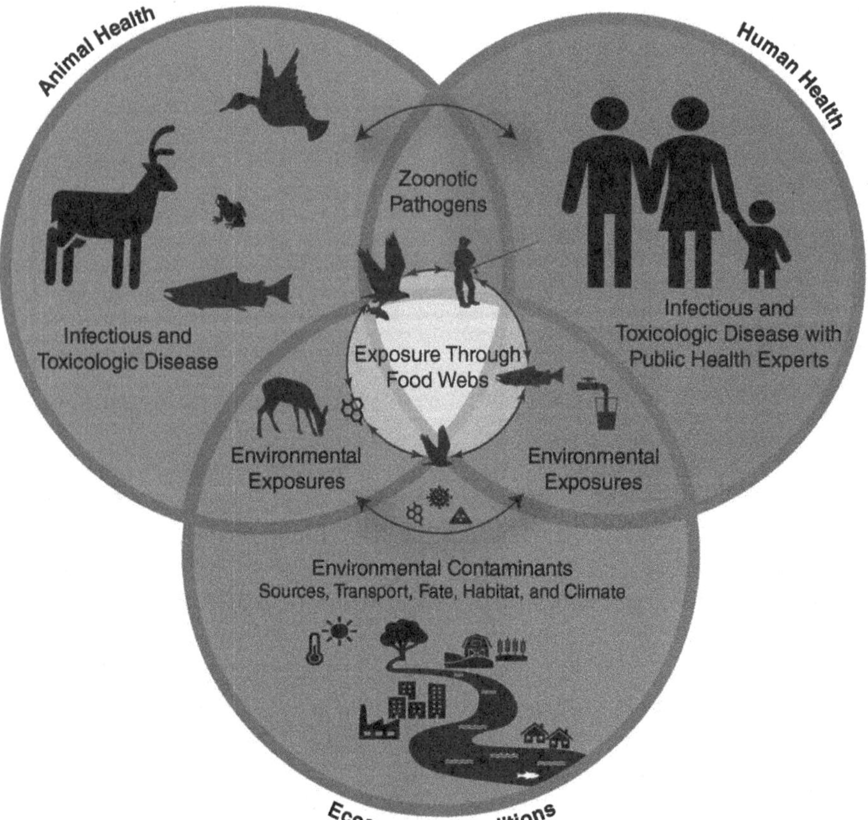

Figure 3.1 One Health conceptual model. *Source*: [1] /USGS/Public Domain.

Table 3.1 Factors contributing to the interdependence of human, animal, and environmental health.

Contributing factor	Impact on human health	Impact on animal health	Impact on environmental health	References
Zoonotic Disease Transmission	Increased risk of infectious diseases (e.g. Ebola, SARS, COVID-19)	Wildlife disease outbreaks; zoonotic pathogens complicating disease management	Disruption of ecosystems due to land use change or habitat intrusion	[3–6]
Antimicrobial Resistance (AMR)	Reduced effectiveness of treatments, prolonged illness	Treatment failures in veterinary medicine; spread of resistant pathogens	Contamination of water and soil with antibiotic residues; resistance in environmental microbes	[7–9]
Climate Change	Heat-related illnesses; expansion of vector-borne diseases (e.g. malaria, dengue)	Heat stress in livestock; habitat loss and reduced productivity	Biodiversity loss; ecosystem degradation; water scarcity	[10–12]
Intensive Agriculture and Livestock	Foodborne illnesses (e.g. *Salmonella, E. coli*); exposure to antibiotics and pesticides	Increased disease transmission due to overcrowding; animal welfare concerns	Land degradation; greenhouse gas emissions; agrochemical runoff pollution	[13–15]
Water, Sanitation, and Hygiene (WASH)	Diarrheal diseases (e.g. cholera, dysentery); skin and eye infections	Livestock diseases from contaminated water sources	Degraded aquatic ecosystems; pathogen proliferation	[16, 17]
Pollution (Air, Water, Soil)	Respiratory diseases, cancers, neurodevelopmental disorders	Bioaccumulation of toxins; reproductive and immune disorders	Soil degradation; eutrophication; loss of biodiversity	[18–20]
Deforestation and Habitat Loss	Increased human–wildlife contact leading to zoonotic spillover	Habitat loss; increased species extinction risk; stress-induced diseases	Disruption of ecological balance; soil erosion; carbon emissions	[21, 22]
Global Trade and Travel	Rapid spread of infectious diseases across borders	Transboundary animal diseases; spread of invasive species and pests	Unintentional transfer of pests and pathogens affecting biodiversity	[23, 24]

Originally, the One Health initiative was spearheaded by three organizations: FAO, WHO, and WOAH, collectively referred to as the “Tripartite” [2]. The addition of the United Nations Environment Programme (UNEP) expanded this alliance into the “Quadripartite,” signifying a more comprehensive approach that incorporates environmental factors into the One Health framework. This global strategy operates at various levels (local, national, and international) and promoting collaboration across sectors to achieve sustainable development and improve health outcomes for all (Table 3.1).

Within this context, animal health is not merely an ethical obligation but a strategic imperative for sustainable development. Maintaining healthy animal populations contributes significantly to food security, supports biomedical research, and underpins economic progress. In alignment with the United Nations SDGs, ensuring animal welfare and promoting responsible production systems are increasingly recognized as critical for advancing global health and economic resilience. This focus encompasses the entire agrifood system from production to consumption and involves a diverse array of stakeholders. By prioritizing animal welfare within this continuum, we invest in a healthier world for all [25].

In many resource-limited settings, livestock represent a critical livelihood asset, rendering animal health inextricably linked to human well-being. It is estimated that approximately 20% of global livestock production is lost each year due to animal diseases, thereby exacerbating poverty and undermining food security [25].

This burden is compounded by the fact that over 60% of human infectious diseases are zoonotic in origin, with approximately 75% of emerging infectious diseases arising from animals [26, 27]. Such figures highlight the inadequacy of siloed interventions and the necessity for integrated surveillance and control strategies that address human, animal, and environmental dimensions concurrently.

The core of the One Health strategy lies in the interdependencies among sectors and targeted interventions for crisis prevention and resilience. It extends to broader public health determinants, including nutrition, sanitation, pollution, and climate change. For example, poor hygiene and sanitation cause 1.5 million child deaths annually from diarrheal diseases, particularly in the Global South [28]. These statistics emphasize the urgent need for health systems that incorporate environmental and socio-economic realities. These interconnected risks are further magnified by the burden of zoonotic diseases, which highlight the importance of animal health as an integral component of public health efforts.

Humans share their environments with a wide variety of species in areas that are abundant with communicable diseases. While animals can act as vectors for human diseases, they also offer crucial roles in treatment and biomedical research. Living animals are essential for understanding human diseases and developing treatments. Thus, the health of animals and the environment directly impacts human health, necessitating a holistic approach to health initiatives [29].

Given the complexity of these interrelationships, it is essential to examine the specific roles animals play within the One Health framework. The following section discusses three interrelated aspects of the relationship between animals and human health: animals as vectors of disease in humans, animals as sentinels of human health, and animals in biomedical research.

3.2.1 Animals as Vectors of Disease in Human

Zoonotic diseases account for about 75% of emerging infectious diseases, many of which originate from wild animals acting as asymptomatic reservoirs [30]. These pathogens can spill over to humans, especially in contexts where human–animal interactions increase due to activities such as bushmeat handling, exotic animal trade, and habitat destruction. Wild animals, in particular, represent a poorly understood yet significant source of zoonotic threats to public health.

Despite increasing awareness of the health risks linked to interactions between humans, animals, and the environment, scientists have largely treated human and animal health as separate disciplines, while historians have overlooked this critical connection [31]. This gap in combining insights from different fields highlights the necessity of rethinking how we perceive and address zoonotic threats.

Animals, particularly wildlife and livestock, serve as primary vectors for a range of zoonotic diseases, playing a pivotal role in the transmission of pathogens that impact human health. The relationship between humans and animals is increasingly complex, influenced by activities such as habitat destruction, the wildlife trade, and agricultural practices, which escalate the risk of disease spillover. For instance, deforestation and urban expansion bring humans into closer proximity with wildlife, facilitating the transmission of diseases like Ebola and Lyme disease.

Additionally, the consumption and handling of bushmeat and live animals can introduce new pathogens to human populations, as seen in the case of HIV and SARS. Moreover, climate change further exacerbates these risks by altering animal migration patterns and extending the geographic range of certain diseases. According to the WHO [32], vector-borne diseases, transmitted by animals such as mosquitoes, account for over 700 000 deaths annually, underscoring the urgent need for a holistic approach to managing these risks.

To effectively manage the threat posed by zoonotic diseases, it is essential to recognize the interconnectedness of human, animal, and environmental health, advocating for a holistic approach that incorporates disease surveillance, habitat protection, and sustainable agricultural practices. Addressing these risks requires coordinated global efforts that not only focus on the immediate health threats but also tackle the underlying socio-environmental drivers that contribute to the emergence of new zoonotic diseases.

3.2.2 Animals as Sentinels of Human Health

The discovery of COVID-19 in various animals has underscored the deep connections between human, animal, and environmental health, highlighting the importance of animal disease surveillance for protecting human well-being [33]. The concept of animals as sentinels involves using them as early warning systems for potential health threats to humans.

For example, changes in animal behavior, health, or mortality rates can signal environmental hazards such as pollution, toxic substances, or the presence of infectious diseases. Animals like canaries were historically used in coal mines to detect dangerous gases, and today, wildlife and domestic animals continue to serve as critical indicators of environmental and public health risks.

Recent research has showcased a variety of species acting as effective sentinels. Other than bird, domestic cats could serve as potential sentinels for various parasitic, bacterial, and viral zoonoses, including SARS-CoV-2, *Toxoplasma gondii*, and *Trichinella* spp. This suggests their usefulness in monitoring the risks of zoonotic disease exposure to humans [34]. Also, study conducted in Southern Brazil utilized dogs as environmental sentinels to identify and monitor areas at risk for leptospirosis in humans, underscoring the importance of incorporating animal surveillance into public health strategies [35].

These proactive approaches not only help to prevent outbreaks but also provide valuable insights into the health of ecosystems, which are intrinsically linked to human well-being. Furthermore, the use of animals as sentinels aligns with the One Health framework, which emphasizes the interconnectedness of human, animal, and environmental health. By integrating data from animal surveillance into public health strategies, we can develop more effective and timely responses to health threats, ultimately safeguarding both human and animal populations. Strengthening animal disease surveillance programs and fostering interdisciplinary collaboration are essential steps in leveraging animals as sentinels to protect global health.

3.2.3 Animals in Biomedical Research

Animal research, while ethically complex, is essential in biomedical science. It enables scientists to study disease processes and develop new treatments that benefit both humans and animals [36]. Several factors underscore the importance of animals in this field:

- Studying animals is crucial for understanding human health due to their biological similarities to us some species, like mice, share over 98% of our DNA.
- Animals can develop many of the same health conditions, such as cancer and diabetes, allowing researchers to investigate disease processes and test treatments in controlled environments.
- The shorter lifespans also enable scientists to study them across entire lifecycles and multiple generations, which is vital for understanding disease progression. Thus, animal research is a key component in advancing human health.

In particular, various diseases have been extensively studied using specific animal models, providing critical insights into human health. Table 3.2 summarizes major health conditions investigated through animal research.

Despite ongoing controversies, animal research is vital for drug testing, safety assessments, and identifying side effects. Researchers, including those at Stanford, prioritize animal welfare and view their work as a privilege in advancing medical knowledge [41].

Beyond traditional medicine, animals have significantly advanced medical science and technology, leading to preventative measures and treatments for various diseases. While animal research gained prominence in the twentieth century, its roots extend back to ancient times. The outdated belief that animals lack sentience, as proposed by Descartes, is no longer a valid justification for their use in research [36].

Table 3.2 Health conditions studied using animal models.

Disease	Animal model	Research purpose	References
Cancer	Mice, rats, dogs	Tumor biology, drug efficacy testing	[37]
Diabetes	Mice, rats	Metabolic studies, insulin therapy research	[38]
Neurodegenerative Diseases	Fly	Alzheimer's, Parkinson's studies (drug discoveries)	[39]
Cardiovascular Diseases	Dogs, rats, rabbits	Heart disease mechanisms, treatment evaluation	[40]

Nonhuman primates, due to their close resemblance to humans, are a significant group in biomedical research, contributing greatly to advancements in human health and disease control. However, the ethical concerns surrounding animal research, including the use of marsupials, persist. Although anesthetics have been developed to reduce animal suffering, a strong movement opposes all animal research, regardless of potential human health benefits [42].

Animal research, while ethically contentious, remains an indispensable pillar of biomedical science, enabling the exploration of disease mechanisms and the development of novel therapies that benefit both humans and animals [36]. The rationale for employing animals in research is rooted in their biological parallels to humans – mice, for example, share over 98% of their DNA with humans. Many species naturally develop conditions such as cancer and diabetes, rendering them invaluable models for studying disease progression and evaluating therapeutic interventions under controlled conditions. Moreover, the shorter life cycles of many animals facilitate the observation of effects across generations, providing critical insights into long-term disease dynamics and inheritance patterns.

Despite persistent ethical debates, animal research continues to play a pivotal role in drug development, toxicological screening, and safety assessments. Institutions such as Stanford University underscore a steadfast commitment to animal welfare, recognizing that the pursuit of medical knowledge must be balanced with ethical responsibility [41]. While modern research emphasizes humane treatment, controversy endures, particularly concerning the use of higher-order species, including nonhuman primates and marsupials. Although the introduction of anesthetics and analgesics has mitigated suffering, opposition persists, driven by concerns over animal sentience and rights [42].

3.3 Addressing Zoonotic Diseases Through a Holistic Approach

The "One Health" concept acknowledges the interconnectedness of human health, animal health, and the environment, emphasizing the need for cross-sector collaboration to improve public health, food security, and trade. As globalization deepens these interconnections, One Health offers a holistic framework to tackle complex health issues.

This approach highlights the connections between human and animal well-being and healthy ecosystems, promoting interdisciplinary collaboration for the best health outcomes. This article examines One Health's core principles, historical roots, and transformative potential of One Health in addressing global health issues.

Initially focused on zoonoses diseases that transfer between animals and humans One Health has broadened to address socio-economic, environmental, and public health challenges [43]. This expanded focus includes maintaining healthy ecosystems, ensuring food security, alleviating poverty, and promoting fair trade practices [44]. One Health now also encompasses noncommunicable diseases like cancer and heart disease [45].

Consequently, One Health serves as a foundational framework for various international development initiatives, including the SDGs, the Sendai Framework for Disaster Risk Reduction, and global efforts for universal health security and combating antibiotic resistance [46, 47]. The COVID-19 pandemic has further underscored the necessity of a One Health approach.

Additionally, societal, economic, and demographic changes are reshaping lifestyles and dietary patterns, increasing pressure on food production resources. The One Health approach acknowledges the impact of these factors on noncommunicable diseases like heart disease and cancer [45].

The One Health concept recognizes the profound interconnectedness of human, animal, and environmental health, advocating for cross-sectoral collaboration to address shared public health challenges. Initially focused on zoonosis diseases transmitted between animals and humans, the framework has expanded to encompass environmental sustainability, food systems, and socio-economic factors, reflecting its holistic approach to global health [43].

Zoonotic diseases, which account for over 60% of human infectious diseases, underscore the urgent need for integrated surveillance, early detection, and coordinated response systems. The rising frequency of zoonotic outbreaks driven by climate change, deforestation, wildlife trade, and intensified agricultural practices demonstrates that human and animal health cannot be effectively managed in isolation [44] (Figure 3.2).

In response to these complexities, the One Health approach has become a strategic cornerstone for numerous global initiatives, including the SDGs, the Sendai Framework for Disaster Risk Reduction, and international efforts to combat AMR [46, 47]. The COVID-19 pandemic has further exposed systemic vulnerabilities at the human–animal–environment interface, highlighting the critical need for preventive, collaborative, and interdisciplinary strategies.

Additionally, demographic shifts and evolving consumption patterns are placing unprecedented pressure on global food systems and natural resources. These stressors not only exacerbate zoonotic risks but also contribute to broader public health challenges, emphasizing the importance of preserving ecosystem integrity and promoting sustainable food production practices.

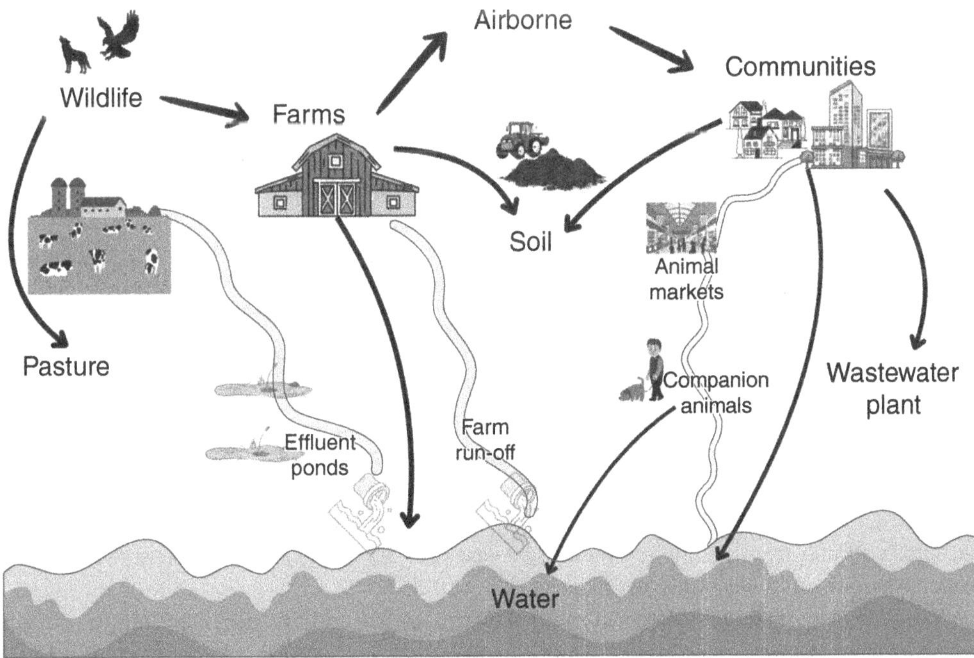

Figure 3.2 Transmission pathways of zoonotic diseases across human, animal, and environmental interfaces. *Source*: Adapted from [48].

3.4 AMR: A One Health Perspective

AMR has emerged as a formidable threat to health systems, food security, and sustainable development worldwide [39]. The widespread use – and frequent misuse – of antibiotics in human healthcare, veterinary practice, and agriculture has accelerated the evolution and dissemination of resistant microbes [7]. Because these sectors are interconnected, tackling AMR requires a One Health approach that recognizes the shared environments and pathways through which resistance can develop and spread.

The globalization of trade and travel, along with the intensification of food production, has enabled resistant organisms to cross borders with increasing ease [49]. Environmental factors, such as pharmaceutical waste and agricultural runoff, further contribute to the spread of resistance genes in soil and water ecosystems [50]. These overlapping drivers reinforce the need for coordinated, cross-disciplinary action rooted in One Health principles [17].

To fully grasp the scale and urgency of the challenge, it is essential to understand the current global burden of AMR, the trends in resistance development, and the consequences for both human and animal health.

The following sections will examine the global burden of AMR, the stagnation in antibiotic development, current strategies to address resistance, the impact on animal health, and the critical role of environmental factors in the spread of resistance.

3.4.1 AMR Overview

AMR is estimated to have caused 1.27 million deaths globally in 2019, with the highest burden falling on low- and middle-income countries [9]. The WHO has identified AMR as one of the top ten global public health threats, warning that without urgent action, common infections and minor injuries could once again become fatal [51].

AMR is an urgent global public health concern exacerbated by antibiotic misuse. This leads to severe illnesses, prolonged emergency room visits, and increased mortality. Overprescribing antibiotics, particularly in primary care where general practitioners account for 90% of prescriptions, often results from medicalizing self-limiting conditions and contributes to heightened side effects and readmission rates.

Multifaceted interventions, including antimicrobial stewardship programs, clinician audits, rapid point-of-care testing, delayed prescriptions, enhanced patient communication, and pragmatic primary care studies, are more effective than one-time efforts in reducing antibiotic misuse. Educating healthcare professionals and the public on proper antibiotic use is essential to raise awareness and prevent misuse.

Combating AMR requires collaboration among healthcare providers, policymakers, and researchers. By implementing evidence-based practices, we can slow the development of resistance and preserve antibiotic efficacy [44]. While antibacterial therapy was one of the twentieth century's greatest medical advancements, the rise of resistance threatens this progress. Addressing AMR from a One Health perspective recognizing the interconnectedness of humans, animals, and the environment is crucial for curbing the spread of resistant bacteria and promoting sustainability [17].

Infections caused by resistant bacteria can have outcomes twice as severe as those from susceptible strains due to delays in effective treatment, leading to increased morbidity, mortality, and healthcare costs [47]. The rise in infections occurs through two mechanisms: the emergence of new infections from resistant strains and the replacement of susceptible strains, exemplified by vancomycin-resistant *Enterococcus faecium* and *Acinetobacter* spp., which have become significant nosocomial pathogens [50].

AMR represents a pressing global public health crisis, fueled by the misuse and overuse of antibiotics, particularly in human healthcare. Inappropriate prescribing practices especially for self-limiting infections contribute to treatment failures, prolonged hospital stays, escalating healthcare costs, and increased mortality rates. In primary care settings, general practitioners account for approximately 90% of antibiotic prescriptions, highlighting the urgent need for targeted interventions [51].

Table 3.3 Mechanisms and drivers of AMR across sectors.

Sector	Mechanisms and drivers of AMR	Intersections with other sectors	References
Human Healthcare	Overprescription of antibiotics; misuse in outpatient settings; lack of diagnostics; poor infection control	Contributes to environmental contamination via hospital wastewater	[49, 52]
Animal Husbandry	Use of antibiotics for growth promotion and disease prevention; lack of veterinary oversight	AMR bacteria can spread to humans via food chain and environment	[50, 53]
Environment	Antibiotic residues from human and animal waste; pharmaceutical runoff; resistance genes in water and soil	Facilitates horizontal gene transfer among bacteria in soil and water system	[54]

Evidence indicates that multifaceted strategies, including antimicrobial stewardship programs, point-of-care diagnostics, delayed prescribing, clinician feedback, and enhanced patient–provider communication, are more effective than isolated measures in reducing antibiotic misuse. Public and professional education remains a cornerstone in raising awareness and fostering responsible antimicrobial use.

While antibiotic therapy marked a transformative milestone in twentieth-century medicine, the rapid spread of resistant pathogens now threatens to undo decades of progress [17]. Addressing AMR through a One Health approach which recognizes the interconnectedness of human, animal, and environmental health is critical for ensuring sustainable antimicrobial efficacy and safeguarding global health security [17].

Infections caused by resistant pathogens result in significantly worse outcomes compared to those caused by susceptible strains, largely due to delays in effective treatment [47]. Resistance can arise either through the emergence of novel resistant strains or the replacement of drug-susceptible strains with resistant ones. Notable examples include vancomycin-resistant *E. faecium* and multidrug-resistant *Acinetobacter* species, both of which have become formidable challenges in hospital settings [50]. Despite the escalating urgency of AMR, the development of new antibiotics has failed to keep pace with the emergence of resistant pathogens.

While human healthcare systems are a major contributor to AMR, the problem is not confined to clinical settings. AMR arises and spreads through a complex web of interactions involving animal agriculture and environmental contamination. Table 3.3 outlines the key mechanisms and drivers of AMR across various sectors, highlighting the interconnected factors contributing to its emergence and spread.

These interlinked mechanisms of AMR emergence demonstrate that no single intervention in isolation whether in human, animal, or environmental health can effectively curb resistance [8]. For example, antibiotic residues from agricultural runoff and pharmaceutical waste often contaminate soil and water systems, creating environmental reservoirs that facilitate the evolution and transmission of resistant genes [50]. Similarly, the prophylactic use of antimicrobials in livestock not only selects for resistant bacteria in animals but also enables the transmission of those organisms to humans via direct contact or through the food chain [49].

To effectively address these multifactorial drivers, integrated surveillance systems and coordinated policy frameworks are essential [17]. The next sections further explore how the lack of new antibiotic development, nosocomial infections, and inadequate WASH (water, sanitation, and hygiene) infrastructure compound the AMR crisis highlighting why cross-sectoral collaboration lies at the heart of sustainable AMR mitigation.

3.4.2 Lack of New Antibiotics Development

The rise of antibiotic-resistant bacteria presents an escalating risk to global health. While antibiotics have revolutionized medicine, the dwindling pipeline for new antibiotics limits our ability to treat common infections. The WHO has identified priority pathogens that pose significant threats due to their resistance patterns [55]. The slow development of new antibiotics is attributed to the high costs and risks associated with research and development, coupled with the lower profitability of antibiotics compared to drugs for chronic conditions [56].

Without new antibiotics, even minor infections could become life-threatening, jeopardizing simple surgeries and having a devastating impact, particularly in developing countries with limited healthcare access. Fortunately, initiatives are underway to incentivize antibiotic research and explore alternative therapies, such as phage therapy and antimicrobial peptides.

Infection control practices are vital for preventing the spread of germs and ensuring patient safety. Lapses in these practices can lead to Healthcare-Associated Infections (HAIs), placing a significant burden on healthcare resources [57]. Common issues include inadequate hand hygiene, improper PPE use, and poor clinical equipment sanitation. These lapses can occur in various settings, resulting in prolonged hospital stays, higher healthcare expenses, and the development of antibiotic-resistant bacteria [58].

Effective infection control measures include continuous education on hygiene practices, routine audits, and open communication among staff. Patient education on infection prevention is also crucial for creating a healthier environment. Additionally, deficiencies in WASH significantly impact public health, especially in developing countries, where poor hygiene contributes to diseases such as cholera and typhoid, disproportionately affects children, and leads to broader societal issues [59].

Investing in WASH programs can dramatically reduce infectious disease prevalence, improve health outcomes, and yield economic benefits by enhancing productivity and supporting SDG 6 for universal water and sanitation access [60].

The rise of antibiotic-resistant bacteria poses an escalating threat to global health. Although antibiotics have transformed modern medicine, the development of new antibiotics has significantly slowed. The WHO has listed priority pathogens that urgently require new treatments due to increasing resistance. However, pharmaceutical companies face major scientific, regulatory, and financial barriers: antibiotic research is costly, high-risk, and often less profitable than drugs for chronic diseases [56].

This stagnation endangers the effectiveness of existing antibiotics. Without new agents, routine infections may become life-threatening, and standard medical procedures such as surgeries or chemotherapy could carry unacceptable risk [47]. The impact is especially severe in low- and middle-income countries where healthcare systems are under-resourced and infection burdens are high. In response, global initiatives are promoting novel research models, financial incentives, and alternative therapies such as phage therapy, antimicrobial peptides, and host-directed strategies. Addressing this innovation gap is critical to preserving antimicrobial efficacy for future generations. Addressing this innovation gap is critical to preserving antimicrobial efficacy for future generations. Given the limited availability of new antibiotics, immediate and coordinated action is needed to mitigate resistance using the tools currently at our disposal [61].

3.4.3 Strategies to Combat AMR

Addressing the growing threat of AMR requires a global, multifaceted response, including:

- **Antibiotic Stewardship**: Raising awareness among healthcare professionals and the public about responsible antibiotic use is essential to slowing the rise of resistant bacteria [9].
- **Innovation in Treatment**: Investing in research and development of new antibiotics and alternative therapies to combat evolving resistance [61].
- **Infection Control Imperative**: Enforcing strong infection control measures in healthcare settings and communities to prevent the spread of resistant bacteria [57].

By raising awareness, promoting responsible antibiotic use, and investing in research, we can mitigate AMR's impact on human health.

Strategies to combat AMR must be comprehensive, interdisciplinary, and implemented across human, animal, and environmental sectors [17]. Key approaches include antimicrobial stewardship programs, strengthened surveillance systems, infection prevention and control (IPC) practices, and global policy coordination. These interventions aim not only to optimize antibiotic use but also to reduce transmission and emergence of resistant pathogens [53].

Combating AMR involves several key strategies:

- **Antibiotic Stewardship**: These initiatives focus on reducing unnecessary antibiotic use by educating clinicians and the public, ensuring that antibiotics remain effective for future generations [9].
- **Innovation in Treatment**: Developing new antibiotics and exploring alternative approaches, such as phage therapy or antimicrobial peptides, is critical to addressing the growing threat of resistance [61].
- **Infection Control**: Strict hygiene protocols in healthcare settings and improvements in WASH infrastructure, particularly in low-resource areas, are essential for preventing the spread of resistant pathogens [57].

A coordinated implementation of these approaches within a One Health framework is essential to mitigate AMR's far-reaching impact on human and planetary health.

3.4.4 Impact of AMR on Animal Health

AMR also significantly threatens animal health. Infected animals may face ineffective traditional antibiotic treatments, leading to prolonged illness and higher mortality rates [19]. The overuse of antibiotics in animals creates resistant bacteria, or "superbugs," which can spread within animal populations and potentially to humans through the food chain [49].

The economic implications of AMR in animals are severe. Ineffective antibiotics result in slower growth rates, reduced productivity, and higher mortality in livestock, leading to financial losses for farmers and higher food prices for consumers [9]. Furthermore, AMR threatens global food security, as healthy animals are essential for stable food production [62]. This underscores the interconnectedness of animal health, human health, and global food security.

AMR poses a growing threat not only to human health but also to animal health, which is often overlooked yet plays a vital role in the One Health framework. In veterinary contexts, infections caused by resistant bacteria can result in treatment failures, extended illness, and higher mortality rates among livestock and pets. The overuse and misuse of antibiotics in animals raised for food contribute to the development of resistant strains, which can spread within animal populations and eventually reach humans through direct contact or the food supply [49].

The implications of AMR go beyond animal welfare, impacting economic stability and food security. Ineffective treatments can lead to decreased productivity, higher veterinary expenses, and substantial financial losses for farmers and producers. This situation poses a threat to the stability of global food systems and can drive up food prices. Therefore, it is crucial to tackle AMR in animal populations in conjunction with efforts aimed at human and environmental health to protect both animal welfare and public health on a global scale [62].

3.4.5 Environmental Factors

Beyond the direct health impacts of climate change discussed previously, environmental factors also play a critical role in driving AMR and compounding public health challenges. AMR represents another major intersection where environmental, human, and animal health are tightly interconnected under the One Health framework.

AMR is influenced not only by antibiotic use in humans and animals but also by environmental factors. Key contributors include the following [63]:

- Many antibiotics are not fully metabolized and are excreted through urine and feces, entering the environment via wastewater treatment plants or through compost used in agriculture. This exposure to low antibiotic levels can promote the development of resistance in environmental bacteria.
- Bacteria can share genetic material through horizontal gene transfer, allowing resistant strains to impart their resistance genes to nonresistant bacteria, which may reside in places like wastewater treatment facilities and soil.

- Environmental pollutants, such as disinfectants and heavy metals, exert selective pressure similar to antibiotics, enabling bacteria with shared resistance traits to flourish.
- Climate change further compounds the issue, as rising temperatures can facilitate the transfer of resistance genes and enhance bacterial growth.

Addressing AMR effectively requires a One Health approach that acknowledges the environmental pathways of resistance and coordinates actions across sectors. Key strategies to mitigate this challenge include [9, 49, 64]:

- Upgrading wastewater treatment facilities to decrease the release of antibiotic residues into the environment.
- Promoting judicious antibiotic use in both human and veterinary medicine to limit the introduction of antibiotics into ecosystems.
- Encouraging sustainable agricultural practices, such as responsible manure management and exploring alternatives to antibiotics for livestock growth promotion.

Upgrading infrastructure, promoting antibiotic stewardship, and improving agricultural sustainability are critical interventions for limiting the emergence and spread of resistant pathogens across the human–animal–environment interface.

In parallel with AMR, climate change presents broader and multifaceted risks to public health. It threatens critical determinants such as clean air, safe drinking water, nutritious food, and stable shelter. Projections indicate that between 2030 and 2050, climate-related impacts could cause an additional 250 000 deaths annually due to malnutrition, malaria, diarrhea, and heat stress [65]. The economic burden is equally significant, with projected direct health costs reaching USD 2–4 billion per year by 2030 especially in regions with fragile health infrastructures [10].

To illustrate the breadth of health outcomes influenced by climate stressors, Figure 3.3 provides an overview of environmentally sensitive health risks.

As seen in Figure 3.3, climate change affects health both directly through rising temperatures, sea-level rise, and severe storms and indirectly by disrupting air quality, disease vector dynamics, water safety, food systems, and

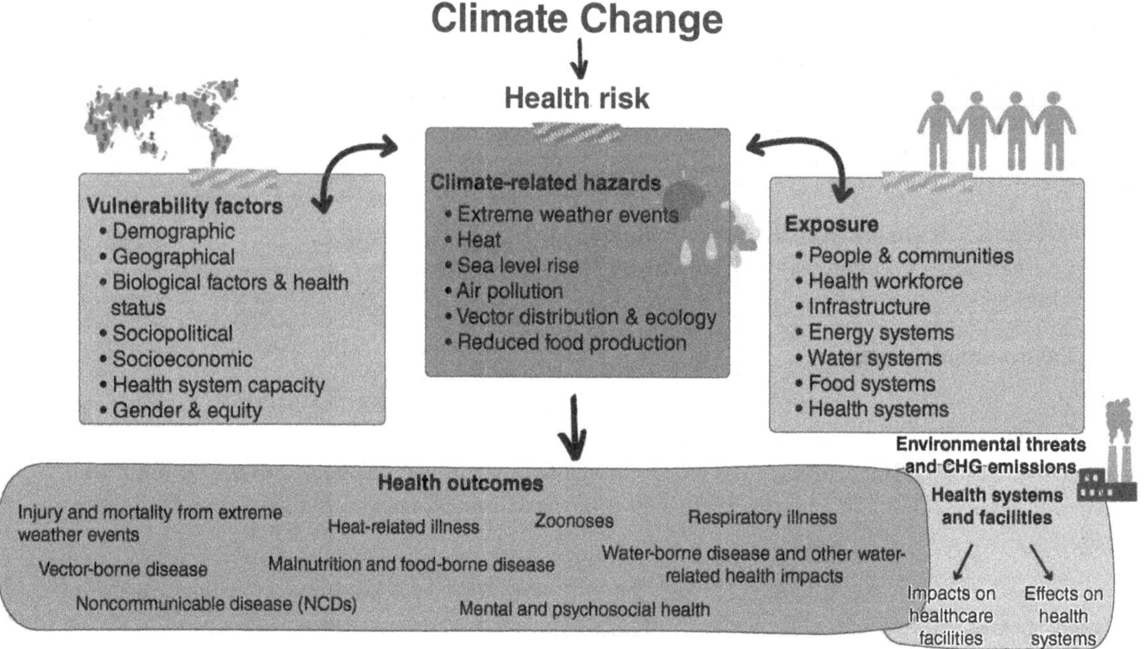

Figure 3.3 Overview of health risks sensitive to environmental changes. *Source*: Adapted from [10].

social stability. Vulnerable populations, including women, children, the elderly, and low-income communities, are disproportionately affected.

The degree of impact depends on various factors such as the level of environmental exposure, existing health conditions, and access to healthcare and infrastructure. Reducing these risks requires a well-coordinated public health response that strengthens resilience, improves preparedness, and ensures equity in adaptation measures.

In response, the WHO has proposed a threefold strategy to address climate-sensitive health risks. First, it encourages actions that reduce greenhouse gas emissions while improving health, including transitions to clean energy, sustainable transport, and healthier food systems. Second, the WHO supports building climate-resilient and environmentally sustainable health systems by integrating climate adaptation into universal health coverage and primary care. Last, it promotes proactive protection through enhanced disease surveillance, targeted adaptation strategies, and increased financial investment in health-related climate action.

Tackling environmental drivers of AMR alongside the health impacts of climate change requires a comprehensive, cross-sectoral One Health approach ensuring that interventions address root causes and build long-term health system resilience.

These environmental dynamics underscore the urgency of addressing AMR through an integrated framework that considers not only clinical and agricultural practices but also ecological conditions that enable resistance to spread. A deeper exploration of AMR within the One Health context is presented in the following section.

3.5 Global Implications of Environmental Health on Public Health

The intersection of environmental degradation and public health is no longer a localized issue it poses a profound and growing threat at a global scale. As climate change accelerates and AMR spreads through interconnected ecosystems, the health of populations worldwide becomes increasingly vulnerable. Understanding these global implications is crucial for formulating coordinated, cross-sectoral responses under the One Health framework.

Environmental health is a critical pillar in the One Health framework, with profound implications for global public health. Environmental degradation including air and water pollution, deforestation, inadequate waste management, and climate change directly and indirectly influences disease patterns, food and water safety, and population vulnerability. These impacts are disproportionately severe in low- and middle-income countries, where health systems are less equipped to cope with complex, overlapping environmental threats.

Pollution and climate change are key drivers of respiratory illnesses, cardiovascular disease, heat-related mortality, and the resurgence of vector-borne diseases such as malaria and dengue. Climate-induced changes in rainfall, temperature, and habitat alter the distribution and abundance of disease vectors, while rising sea levels and extreme weather events threaten the stability of water and food systems. In regions already struggling with undernutrition and poor infrastructure, these changes can push public health systems beyond capacity.

Environmental stressors also amplify risks at the human–animal–environment interface. For example, habitat loss and biodiversity reduction increase the frequency of human–wildlife interactions, elevating the risk of zoonotic spillover. Meanwhile, contaminated ecosystems can serve as reservoirs for antimicrobial-resistant pathogens, challenging infection control and threatening the effectiveness of modern medicine.

Globally, the economic and health burdens of environmental threats are substantial. The WHO estimates that nearly 24% of global deaths are linked to environmental factors [66]. Addressing these challenges requires multisectoral collaboration and investment in climate-resilient and environmentally sustainable health systems. Through One Health integration, public health policies can better anticipate environmental risks, strengthen global preparedness, and protect both human and animal populations across borders.

In recent years, global awareness has grown around the interconnection between environmental degradation and emerging health threats. Notably, the COVID-19 pandemic has highlighted the vulnerabilities in global systems and the consequences of neglecting ecological drivers of health crises. Land-use change, urban encroachment into natural habitats, and intensive agricultural practices have all increased the likelihood of zoonotic spillovers making the prevention of future pandemics a matter not only of medical preparedness but also of environmental governance.

Furthermore, AMR has become emblematic of environmental-public health entanglement. Environmental compartments such as soil, surface water, and wastewater serve as reservoirs and transmission pathways for resistant genes and pathogens. This environmental dimension of AMR, often overlooked in conventional health policy, underscores the need for holistic surveillance and intervention strategies that integrate environmental data with health outcomes. Environmental pollution from pharmaceuticals, especially antibiotics released through human and animal waste, further accelerates resistance in microbial populations, posing transboundary risks.

At the policy level, integrating environmental health indicators into national and international health assessments is increasingly recognized as essential. Initiatives like WHO's Health and Climate Change Country Profiles and UNEP's work on pollution and AMR provide frameworks for tracking environmental determinants of health [66]. The Global AMR Surveillance System (GLASS) has also begun including environmental sampling in certain regions, marking a shift toward more integrated, One Health-aligned monitoring [67].

To move from recognition to action, governments must prioritize upstream interventions by reducing industrial emissions, enforcing responsible pharmaceutical disposal, investing in green infrastructure, and improving urban planning. Simultaneously, international cooperation is vital. Environmental health threats do not respect borders, and effective mitigation demands harmonized global responses backed by sustained political commitment and funding.

Ultimately, environmental health is not a siloed concern but a global determinant of public health, economic stability, and equity. Ensuring a healthy planet is, fundamentally, ensuring a healthy population.

3.6 Conclusion

The interconnection between human, animal, and environmental health lies at the core of the One Health framework. As discussed in this chapter, the well-being of each domain is intricately linked animals act as vectors, sentinels, and subjects in biomedical research, while environmental conditions shape disease patterns and exposure risks across species. This interdependence demands a comprehensive and multisectoral approach to addressing global health challenges.

The analysis of zoonotic diseases underscores how emerging pathogens are not only threats to human populations but are often rooted in ecological disturbances, poor biosecurity, and intensified human–animal contact. Holistic strategies that include surveillance, education, ecosystem management, and equitable healthcare infrastructure are essential to preventing outbreaks and minimizing spillover risks. Moreover, animal health must be viewed not merely as a veterinary issue, but as a vital determinant of food security, economic stability, and public health resilience.

AMR exemplifies the profound interconnectedness of these domains. The overuse and misuse of antibiotics in human medicine and animal agriculture, combined with environmental contamination from pharmaceutical and agricultural waste, have accelerated the global spread of resistant pathogens. As outlined in this chapter, addressing AMR demands urgent, multisectoral collaboration: from curbing inappropriate antibiotic use in primary care to investing in new antimicrobials, enhancing WASH infrastructure, and mitigating environmental sources of resistance.

Environmental degradation, including pollution, biodiversity loss, and climate change, amplifies public health vulnerabilities. As shown in the final section, the global implications of environmental health reach far beyond ecological concerns they influence vector-borne diseases, respiratory illnesses, nutritional outcomes, and the broader social determinants of health. Therefore, integrating environmental stewardship into health planning is not optional, but essential for long-term sustainability.

However, this study has limitations. While it provides a broad overview of One Health principles, it does not delve deeply into specific case studies or regional variations in health challenges. Additionally, the discussion on AMR and environmental degradation could benefit from more detailed data on the economic and social impacts of these issues.

Future research should focus on developing practical, scalable One Health interventions, particularly in low-resource settings where health systems are most vulnerable. Further exploration of the economic and policy barriers to implementing One Health strategies is also needed. Additionally, studies should investigate the long-term effects of environmental changes on zoonotic disease dynamics and AMR spread, as well as the potential of emerging technologies, such as artificial intelligence and genomics, to enhance disease surveillance and response.

In conclusion, the One Health framework offers a vital pathway to addressing the interconnected health challenges of the twenty-first century. By fostering collaboration, integrating environmental stewardship, and prioritizing sustainable practices, we can build a healthier future for humans, animals, and the planet. This chapter serves as a call to action for researchers, policymakers, and practitioners to embrace the One Health vision and work collectively toward global health resilience.

References

1 U.S. Geological Survey (USGS). *One Health Conceptual Diagram*. 2024. https://www.usgs.gov/media/images/one-health-conceptual-diagram (accessed 29 April 2025).

2 FAO, OIE, WHO. *The Tripartite's Commitment Providing Multi-Sectoral, Collaborative Leadership in Addressing Health Challenges*. 2017. https://www.woah.org/app/uploads/2018/05/tripartite-2017.pdf (accessed 23 June 2024).

3 World Health Organization. *Environment and One Health*. https://www.who.int/europe/news-room/fact-sheets/item/environment-and-one-health (accessed 25 April 2025).

4 World Bank. *Safeguarding Animal, Human and Ecosystem Health: One Health at the World Bank*. https://www.worldbank.org/en/topic/agriculture/brief/safeguarding-animal-human-and-ecosystem-health-one-health-at-the-world bank (accessed 25 April 2025).

5 Food and Agriculture Organization. *One Health: Highlights and Challenges Shaping the Future*. https://www.fao.org/one-health/highlights/one-health--highlights-and-challenges-shaping-the-future/en (accessed 25 April 2025).

6 Thal, D.A. and Mettenleiter, T.C. One Health—key to adequate intervention measures against zoonotic risks. *Pathogens* 2023; 12(3): 415. https://doi.org/10.3390/pathogens12030415.

7 World Health Organization. *Global Action Plan on Antimicrobial Resistance*. Geneva: World Health Organization; 2015. https://iris.who.int/handle/10665/193736 (accessed 25 April 2025).

8 Larsson, D.G.J., Andremont, A., Bengtsson-Palme, J., et al. Critical knowledge gaps and research needs related to the environmental dimensions of antibiotic resistance. *Environ. Int.* 2018; 117: 132–138.

9 World Organization for Animal Health. *Antimicrobial Resistance*. https://www.woah.org/en/what-we-do/global-initiatives/antimicrobial-resistance/ (accessed 25 April 2025).

10 World Health Organization. *Climate Change and Health*. 2023. https://www.who.int/news-room/fact-sheets/detail/climate-change-and-health (accessed 25 April 2025).

11 FAO. *Animal Health and Climate Change*. 2020. https://openknowledge.fao.org/server/api/core/bitstreams/da3f8543-c638-4d98-9e23-d5a0db708ff3/content (accessed 26 April 2025).

12 World Meteorological Organization. *State of the Climate in Africa 2023*. Geneva: WMO; 2024.

13 Grace, D. Food safety in low and middle income countries. *Int. J. Environ. Res. Public Health* 2015; 12(9): 10490–10507. https://doi.org/10.3390/ijerph120910490.

14 World Health Organization. *Food Safety*. 2024. https://www.who.int/news-room/fact-sheets/detail/food-safety (accessed 25 April 2025).

15 FAO. *The State of the World's Land and Water Resources for Food and Agriculture–Systems at breaking point (SOLAW 2021) Synthesis report 2021*. Rome. https://doi.org/10.4060/cb7654en.

16 Gupta, J., Bai, X., Liverman, D.M., et al. A just world on a safe planet: a Lancet Planetary Health–Earth Commission report on earth-system boundaries, translations, and transformations. *Lancet Planet. Health* 2024; 8(10): e813–e873.

17 United Nations Environment Programme. *Bracing for Superbugs: Strengthening Environmental Action in the One Health Response to Antimicrobial Resistance*. Geneva: United Nations Environment Programme; 2023. https://doi.org/10.3389/fcimb.2022.873989.

18 World Health Organization. *Health Risks*. https://www.who.int/teams/environment-climate-change-and-health/air-quality-energy-and-health/sectoral-interventions/ambient-air-pollution/health-risks (accessed 25 April 2025).

19 Laborda, P., Sanz-García, F., Ochoa-Sánchez, L.E., et al. Wildlife and antibiotic resistance. *Front. Cell Infect. Microbiol.* 2022; 12: 873989.

20 WWF. *Living Planet Report 2022—Building a Nature-Positive Society* (ed. R.E.A. Almond, M. Grooten, D. Juffe Bignoli, and T. Petersen). Gland, Switzerland: WWF; 2022.

21 World Health Organization. *Connecting Global Priorities: Biodiversity and Human Health: A State of Knowledge Review*. 2015. https://www.who.int/publications/i/item/connecting-global-priorities-biodiversity-and-human-health (accessed 25 April 2025).

22 Brondízio, E.S., Settele, J., Díaz, S., and Ngo, H.T. (eds.) *The Global Assessment Report of the Intergovernmental Science-Policy Platform on Biodiversity and Ecosystem Services*. Bonn: IPBES; 2019.

23 United Nations. *Our Common Agenda—Report of the Secretary-General*. New York: United Nations; 2021.

24 Hulme, P.E. Unwelcome exchange: international trade as a direct and indirect driver of biological invasions worldwide. *One Earth* 2021; 4(5): 666–679.

25 Shaheen, M.N.F. The concept of One Health applied to the problem of zoonotic diseases. *Rev. Med. Virol.* 2022; 32: e2326. https://doi.org/10.1002/rmv.2326.

26 Meslin, F.X. Impact of zoonoses on human health. *Vet. Ital.* 2006; 42(4): 369–379.

27 Ruckert, A., Zinszer, K., Zarowsky, C., et al. What role for One Health in the COVID-19 pandemic? *Can. J. Public Health* 2020; 111(5): 641–644. https://doi.org/10.17269/s41997-020-00409-z.

28 Scotch, M., Odofin, L., and Rabinowitz, P. Linkages between animal and human health sentinel data. *BMC Vet. Res.* 2009; 5: 15. https://doi.org/10.1186/1746-6148-5-15.

29 Gebreyes, W.A., Dupouy-Camet, J., Newport, M.J., et al. The global One Health paradigm: challenges and opportunities for tackling infectious diseases at the human, animal, and environment interface in low-resource settings. *PLoS Negl. Trop. Dis.* 2014; 8: e3257. https://doi.org/10.1371/journal.pntd.0003257.

30 Alves, R.R.N. and da Silva Policarpo, I. Animals and human health: where do they meet? In: *Ethnozoology* (ed. R.R.N. Alves and U.P. Albuquerque), 233–259. London: Academic Press; 2018. https://doi.org/10.1016/B978-0-12-809913-1.00013-2.

31 WHO. *Vector-Borne Diseases*. 2024. https://www.who.int/news-room/fact-sheets/detail/vector-borne-diseases (accessed 25 April 2025).

32 Reif, J.S. Animal sentinels for environmental and public health. *Public Health Rep.* 2011; 126(Suppl 1): 50. https://doi.org/10.1177/00333549111260S108.

33 Selyemová, D., Antolová, D., Mangová, B., et al. Cats as a sentinel species for human infectious diseases–toxoplasmosis, trichinellosis, and COVID-19. *Curr. Res. Parasitol. Vector Borne Dis.* 2024; 6: 2–7. https://doi.org/10.1016/j.crpvbd.2024.100196.

34 Sohn-Hausner, N., Kmetiuk, L.B., da Silva, E.C., et al. One Health approach to leptospirosis: dogs as environmental sentinels for identification and monitoring of human risk areas in Southern Brazil. *Trop. Med. Infect. Dis.* 2023; 8: 9. https://doi.org/10.3390/tropicalmed8090435.

35 Domínguez-Oliva, A., Hernández-Ávalos, I., Martínez-Burnes, J., et al. The importance of animal models in biomedical research: current insights and applications. *Animals* 2023; 13(7): 1223. https://doi.org/10.3390/ani13071223.

36 Liu, C., Wu, P., Zhang, A., and Mao, X. Advances in rodent models for breast cancer formation, progression, and therapeutic testing. *Front. Oncol.* 2021; 11: 593337. https://doi.org/10.3389/fonc.2021.593337.

37 Singh, R., Gholipourmalekabadi, M., and Shafikhani, S.H. Animal models for type 1 and type 2 diabetes: advantages and limitations. *Front. Endocrinol.* 2024; 15: 1359685. https://doi.org/10.3389/fendo.2024.1359685.

38 Tello, J.A., Williams, H.E., Eppler, R.M., et al. Animal models of neurodegenerative disease: recent advances in fly highlight innovative approaches to drug discovery. *Front. Mol. Neurosci.* 2022; 15: 883358. https://doi.org/10.3389/fnmol.2022.883358.

39 Jia, T., Wang, C., Han, Z., et al. Experimental rodent models of cardiovascular diseases. *Front. Cardiovasc. Med.* 2020; 7: 588075. https://doi.org/10.3389/fcvm.2020.588075.

40 Stanford Medicine. *Why Animal Research*? https://med.stanford.edu/animalresearch/why-animal-research.html (accessed 29 April 2025).

41 National Academies of Sciences, Engineering, and Medicine. *Nonhuman Primate Models in Biomedical Research: State of the Science and Future Needs* (ed. O.C. Yost, A. Downey, and K.S. Ramos). Washington (DC): National Academies Press; 2023. https://doi.org/10.17226/26857.

42 Häsler, B., Cornelsen, L., Bennani, H., et al. A review of the metrics for One Health benefits. *Rev. Sci. Tech.* 2014; 33(2): 453–464. https://doi.org/10.20506/rst.33.2.2294.

43 World Health Organization (WHO). *WHO Traditional Medicine Strategy 2014–2023.* Geneva: World Health Organization (WHO); 2013.

44 Amuasi, J.H., Lucas, T., Horton, R., and Winkler, A.S. Reconnecting for our future: the Lancet One Health Commission. *Lancet (London, England)* 2020; 395(10235): 1469–1471.

45 Rupasinghe, N., Machalaba, C., Muthee, T., and Mazimba, A. *Stopping the Grand Pandemic: A Framework for Action-Addressing Antimicrobial Resistance Through World Bank Operations.* Washington DC: SIDALC Alliance of Agricultural Information Services; 2024.

46 Seifman, R. *SDGs: Why They Need to Include One Health. Impakter.* 2020. https://impakter.com/sdgs-why-include-one-health/ (accessed 11 April 2025).

47 O'Neill, J. *Tackling Drug-Resistant Infections Globally: Final Report and Recommendations. Government of the United Kingdom.* 2016. https://apo.org.au/node/63983 (accessed 25 April 2025).

48 Proboste, T., James, A., Charette-Castonguay, A., et al. Research and innovation opportunities to improve epidemiological knowledge and control of environmentally driven zoonoses. *Ann. Glob. Health* 2022; 88(1): 93. https://doi.org/10.5334/aogh.3770.

49 Van Boeckel, T.P., Pires, J., Silvester, R., et al. Global trends in antimicrobial resistance in animals in low- and middle-income countries. *Science* 2019; 365: eaaw1944. https://doi.org/10.1126/science.aaw1944.

50 Berendonk, T.U., Manaia, C.M., Merlin, C., et al. Tackling antibiotic resistance: the environmental framework. *Nat. Rev. Microbiol.* 2015; 13(5): 310–317. https://doi.org/10.1038/nrmicro3439.

51 Costelloe, C., Metcalfe, C., Lovering, A., et al. Effect of antibiotic prescribing in primary care on antimicrobial resistance in individual patients: systematic review and meta-analysis. *BMJ* 2010; 340: c2096. https://doi.org/10.1136/bmj.c2096.

52 Murray, C.J.L., Ikuta, K.S., Sharara, F., et al. Global burden of bacterial antimicrobial resistance in 2019: a systematic analysis. *Lancet* 2022; 399(10325): 629–655. https://doi.org/10.1016/S0140-6736(21)02724-0.

53 Tang, K.L., Caffrey, N.P., Nóbrega, D.B., et al. Restricting the use of antibiotics in food-producing animals and its associations with antibiotic resistance in food-producing animals and human beings: a systematic review and meta-analysis. *Lancet Planet Health* 2017; 1(8): e316–e327. https://doi.org/10.1016/S2542-5196(17)30141-9.

54 Karkman, A., Do, T.T., Walsh, F., et al. Antibiotic-resistance genes in waste water. *Trends Microbiol.* 2018; 26(3): 220–228. https://doi.org/10.1016/j.tim.2017.09.005.

55 World Health Organization. *WHO Bacterial Priority Pathogens List, 2024: Bacterial Pathogens of Public Health Importance to Guide Research, Development and Strategies to Prevent and Control Antimicrobial Resistance.* 2024. https://iris.who.int/bitstream/handle/10665/376776/9789240093461-eng.pdf?sequence=1 (accessed 21 May 2025).

56 Renwick, M.J., Brogan, D.M., and Mossialos, E. A systematic review and critical assessment of incentive strategies for discovery and development of novel antibiotics. *J. Antibiot. (Tokyo)* 2016; 69: 73–88. https://doi.org/10.1038/ja.2015.98.
57 World Health Organization. *Key Facts and Figures World Hand Hygiene Day*. https://www.who.int/campaigns/world-hand-hygiene-day/key-facts-and-figures (accessed 21 May 2025).
58 Centers for Disease Control and Prevention (CDC). *Antibiotic Resistance Threats in the United States, 2019*. Atlanta (GA): U.S. Department of Health and Human Services, CDC; 2019.
59 UNICEF, World Health Organization. *Progress on Household Drinking Water, Sanitation and Hygiene 2000–2022: Special Focus on Gender*. New York: UNICEF and WHO; 2023.
60 United Nations. *Sustainable Development Goal 6 Synthesis Report on Water and Sanitation*. New York: United Nations; 2018. FAO; 2021.
61 de Kraker, M.E.A., Stewardson, A.J., and Harbarth, S. Will 10 million people die a year due to antimicrobial resistance by 2050? *PLoS Med*. 2016; 13: e1002184. https://doi.org/10.1371/journal.pmed.1002184.
62 FAO (Food and Agriculture Organisation of the United Nations). *The FAO Action Plan on Antimicrobial Resistance 2021–2025: Supporting Innovation and Resilience in Food and Agriculture Sectors*. FAO; 2021. ISBN 978-92-5-134673-0.
63 Samreen, Ahmad, I., Malak, H.A., and Abulreesh, H.H. Environmental antimicrobial resistance and its drivers: a potential threat to public health. *J. Glob. Antimicrob. Resist*. 2021; 27: 101–11. https://doi.org/10.1016/j.jgar.2021.08.001.
64 Michael, I., Rizzo, L., McArdell, C.S., et al. Urban wastewater treatment plants as hotspots for the release of antibiotics in the environment: a review. *Water Res*. 2013; 47(3): 957–995. https://doi.org/10.1016/j.watres.2012.11.027.
65 Goh, D.L. *After COP29: What's Next for Climate and Health? APLN Commentary*. 2024. https://www.apln.network/analysis/commentaries/after-cop29-whats-next-for-climate-and-health (accessed 21 May 2025).
66 World Health Organization. *Preventing Disease through Healthy Environments: A Global Assessment of the Burden of Disease from Environmental Risks*. Geneva: WHO; 2016.
67 United Nations Environment Programme. *Environmental Dimensions of Antimicrobial Resistance: Summary for Policymakers*. Nairobi: UNEP; 2022.

4

Integrating One Health into Global Veterinary Education

Delower Hossain[1,2], Ridwan Olamilekan Adesola[3], Easrat Jahan Esha[4], Nasir Uddin[5], Oluwaseun Adeolu Ogundijo[6], Olamilekan Gabriel Banwo[3], Adetolase Azizat Bakre[3], Amitush Dutta[7], Mir Mohammad Ali[8], AHM Musleh Uddin[9,10] and Sabiha Zarin Tasnim Bristi[2]**

[1] *Department of Medicine and Public Health, Faculty of Animal Science and Veterinary Medicine, Sher-e-Bangla Agricultural University (SAU), Dhaka, Bangladesh*
[2] *Department of Veterinary Medicine and Animal Sciences (DIVAS), Università degli Studi di Milano (UNIMI), Lodi, Italy*
[3] *Department of Veterinary Medicine, Faculty of Veterinary Medicine, University of Ibadan, Ibadan, Nigeria*
[4] *Fleming Fund Country Grant to Bangladesh, DAI Global, Dhaka, Bangladesh*
[5] *Centre for Integrative Conservation, Xishuangbanna Tropical Botanical Garden, Chinese Academy of Sciences, Xishuangbanna, Yunnan, People's Republic of China*
[6] *Department of Veterinary Public Health and Preventive Medicine, University of Ibadan, Ibadan, Nigeria*
[7] *Department of Animal Nutrition, Faculty of Veterinary, Animal and Biomedical Sciences, Sylhet Agricultural University, Sylhet, Bangladesh*
[8] *Department of Aquaculture, Faculty of Fisheries and Marine Science, Sher-e-Bangla Agricultural University (SAU), Dhaka, Bangladesh*
[9] *Department of Surgery and Theriogenology, Faculty of Veterinary, Animal and Biomedical Sciences, Sylhet Agricultural University, Sylhet, Bangladesh*
[10] *School of Animal and Veterinary Science, University of Adelaide, Roseworthy Campus, Roseworthy, SA, Australia*

*Corresponding authors: delowervet@sau.edu.bd; delower.hossain@unimi.it; sabiha.bristi@unimi.it

TABLE OF CONTENTS

4.1 Introduction
4.2 Current State of Veterinary Education
4.2.1 Traditional Veterinary Curricula
4.2.2 Gaps and Limitations in Current VE Models
4.2.3 Overview of Existing One Health Programs
4.3 Transformative Strategies for Veterinary Education
4.3.1 Rethinking Curriculum Design
4.3.2 Core Competencies in One Health
4.3.2.1 Evolution of Thoughts in One Health
4.3.2.2 Background of the Competency Framework in One Health
4.3.3 Incorporating Public Health and Environmental Science
4.3.4 Innovative Pedagogical Methods
4.3.5 Leveraging Technology for One Health Education
4.3.6 Assessment and Evaluation Techniques
4.4 Institutional One Health Model: A Global Perspective
4.4.1 Utrecht University, the Netherlands
4.4.2 University of California, Davis, United States
4.4.3 University of Minnesota, United States
4.4.4 Royal Veterinary College, UK
4.4.5 University of Tokyo, Japan

One Health Integration: Global Perspectives on Animal Health and Sustainable Agriculture. First Edition.
Edited by Pratik Subhash Gaikwad, Vivek Harishankar Shukla and Pintu Choudhary.

Companion Website: https://www.wiley.com/go/pratikgaikwad/onehealth

4.4.6 University of Veterinary and Animal Sciences, Pakistan
4.4.7 One Health Institute, Chattogram Veterinary and Animal Sciences University, Bangladesh
4.4.8 Kerala Veterinary and Animal Sciences University, India
4.4.9 University of Nairobi, Kenya
4.4.10 University of Pretoria, South Africa
4.4.11 University of Ibadan, Ibadan, Nigeria
4.4.12 Queensland Alliance for One Health Sciences, University of Queensland, Australia
4.4.13 Lessons Learned and Key Takeaways
4.5 Fostering Interdisciplinary Learning Environments
4.5.1 Building Collaborative Partnerships
4.5.1.1 Partnerships with Medical Schools
4.5.1.2 Collaborations with Public Health Institutions
4.5.1.3 Collaboration with Environmental Science Institutions
4.5.2 Creating Interdisciplinary Courses and Modules
4.5.3 Utilizing Problem-based Learning
4.5.4 Incorporating Fieldwork and Practical Experiences
4.5.5 Promoting Cross-disciplinary Research Projects
4.5.6 Enhancing Communication and Leadership Skills
4.6 Building Institutional Capacity
4.6.1 Faculty Training and Development
4.6.2 Infrastructure and Resource Allocation
4.6.3 Policy and Institutional Support
4.6.4 Funding and Sustainability
4.7 Research and Innovation in One Health
4.7.1 Promoting Interdisciplinary Research
4.7.2 Innovative Research Methodologies
4.7.3 Case Studies of Impactful One Health Research
4.8 Global Perspectives on One Health Education
4.8.1 Regional Case Studies: Africa, Asia, Europe, and the Americas
4.8.2 Adapting One Health Education to Local Contexts
4.8.3 International Collaboration and Exchange Programs
4.9 Policy and Advocacy
4.9.1 Role of Veterinary Associations and Organizations
4.9.2 Roles of Development Partners and Organizations
4.9.3 Influencing Policy at the National and International Levels
4.9.4 Advocacy Strategies for One Health Integration
4.10 Future Directions in One Health Education
4.11 Conclusion
Abbreviations
Author Contributions
Conflicts of Interest
Acknowledgments
Dedication
References

4.1 Introduction

One Health (OH) is a concept that emphasizes the interconnections of human health with animal health (AH) and the environment. OH is a multidisciplinary approach that focuses on human–animal–environmental health and involves collaboration across various sectors to improve public health (PH) [1]. It focuses on the management of zoonotic diseases, antimicrobial resistance (AMR), and food safety. This concept encourages joint efforts across disciplines to achieve optimal health for people, animals, and the environment. It aims to mitigate risks and crises from contact between humans, animals, and diverse environments, promoting global interdisciplinary cooperation and communication [2]. Epidemic infectious diseases are causing significant burdens on PH and socioeconomic status. A new concept called OH should be used to respond better, integrating human, animal, and environmental health, whose interdependence requires the cooperation of experts from various disciplines and promotes cooperative governance for sharing information, joint response, and risk management. Infectious diseases can serve as a cross-country joint response and participation platform, addressing zoonotic, insect-borne, waterborne, and foodborne diseases (Figure 4.1) [3].

OH has gained importance in recent years because of changes in interactions among humans, animals, and the environment. Human populations are expanding, increasing contact with wild and domestic animals and providing more opportunities for diseases to spread between animals and humans. Climate and land use changes, such as deforestation and intensive farming practices, human–wildlife interactions, illegal wildlife trafficking, and bush meat consumption, also contribute to the spread of disease. The increased movement of people, animals, and animal products has led to the spread of zoonotic diseases, which affect millions of people and animals worldwide annually [3]. Like humans, animals are at risk of becoming sick from certain diseases and environmental hazards, serving as early warning signs of potential human illness [4].

OH issue encompasses zoonotic diseases, neglected tropical diseases, vector-borne diseases, AMR, food safety, environmental contamination, climate change, and other health threats shared by people, animals, and the

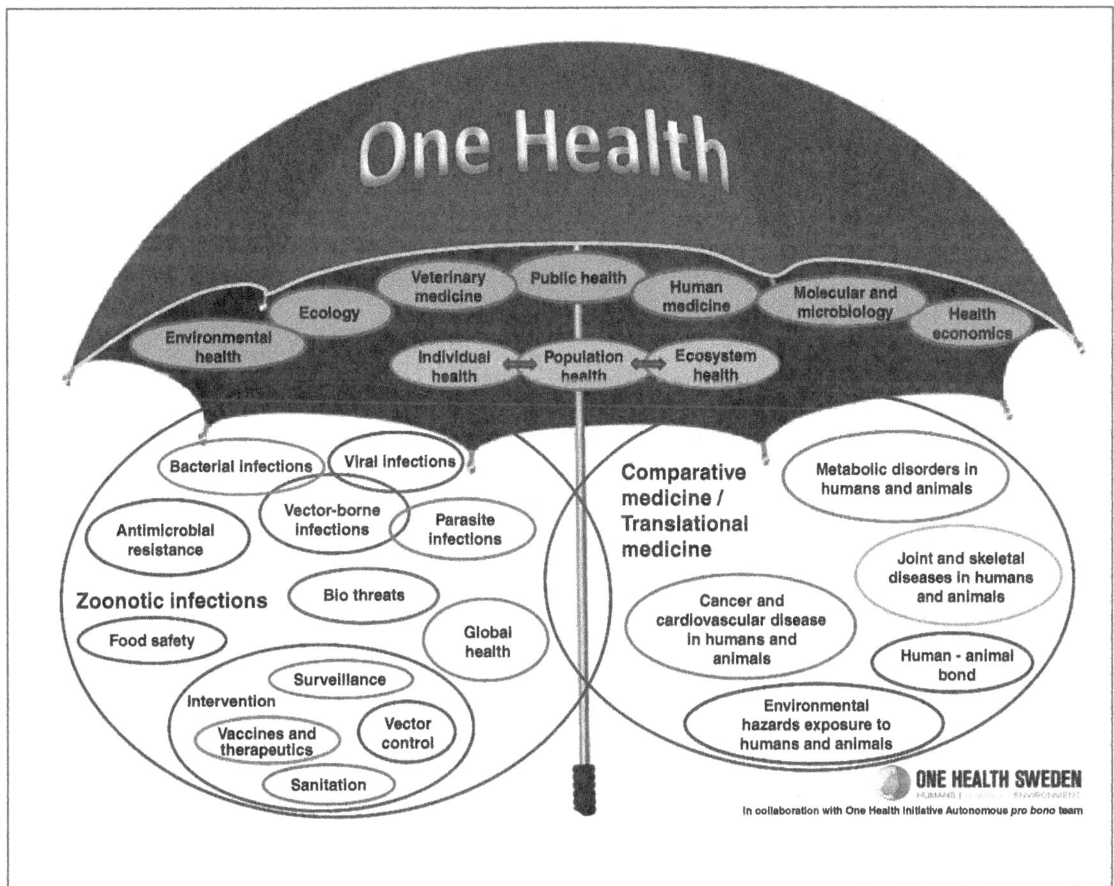

Figure 4.1 The "One Health Umbrella" illustrates the fundamental principles of the "One Health" concept [6]. *Remark*: The figure was drawn up by One Health Sweden and the One Health Initiative (OHI) and was republished with official permission [6]. Reproduced with permission of One Health Initiative.

environment [2]. These include antimicrobial-resistant germs that spread through communities, the food supply, healthcare facilities, and the environment. An OH approach can benefit chronic disease, mental health, injury, occupational health, and noncommunicable diseases through collaboration across disciplines and sectors [5].

Individual, population, and ecosystem health are three levels of OH, where animal and human health are two concepts used at the individual health level. The term "nonhuman animals" refers to all animal species except humans [4]. Separating humans from animals is a normative issue, especially in mental health. On the second level, population health is the term used in human medicine, veterinary medicine, and biology and refers to the overall health of a population, regardless of the species involved. Among several possible terms on the third level, the term "ecosystem health" is used.

4.2 Current State of Veterinary Education

The veterinary medical education (VME) program varies depending on the country and the university. The educational curricula in developed countries are more comprehensive than those in developing countries. In the United States, veterinary professionals focus more on pet animals, whereas in developing countries such as Bangladesh, India, and Pakistan, the focus remains on large animals, such as food animals.

4.2.1 Traditional Veterinary Curricula

There has been diversity in the curriculum of the VME program since the ancient period, and over the last 50 years, the curriculum has changed vigorously. A traditional veterinary curriculum is a comprehensive, structured educational program with four years or more of full-time theoretical study or equivalent. It also encompasses at least one year of hands-on clinical training for veterinary students, introducing them to real-world field scenarios. In this curriculum, students undertake preclinical studies for two to three years, covering fundamental, medical, and para-clinical sciences using diverse teaching approaches. Subsequently, they gain practical experience in clinical settings. This curriculum is designed to guide students through a progressive learning process, starting with studying normal animals and moving on to abnormal animals, clinical sciences, disease diagnosis, and treatment.

In different articles, Armistead and Pritchard discussed the changes needed in VME curricula in 1964, 1965, and 1970, with a focus on the integrated teaching of preclinical and clinical departments and clinical subjects [7–10]. At that time, the curricula were designed with two years of preclinical study, which was insufficient for vet students, and then turned into a three-year curriculum in Texas A&M and Tennessee with the help of Dean Armistead. For this purpose, both Armistead and Pritchard played significant roles. They agreed to reorient the curricula and teaching methods, as it was deemed insufficient for vet students to have only two years of preclinical courses [11, 12].

The number of veterinary schools and students increased (where) after the Health Manpower Training Act in 1971, allowing colleges to create new curricula and instructional methodologies. Although the University of Georgia adopted a competency-based curriculum for a selected number of students, many colleges later followed suit. In the 1980s, the curriculum was influenced by the explosion of knowledge, leading to debates on change. Iowa State implemented a semester system, Virginia-Maryland College of Veterinary Medicine used a block course body, and Mississippi State transitioned to problem-based learning (PBL) in 1993 to prepare vet students for the information age [13–17].

During the late 1980s and 1990s, the VME curriculum was impacted by the Paw National Veterinary Education Program grant [18]. After that, the preveterinary curriculum was changed to a flexible curriculum at the University of California, Davis (UC Davis) and Cornell University, while PBL and application-based exercises were introduced at the NC State and the University of Tennessee [19, 20]. Afterward, the Western University of Health

Sciences and other colleges accepted the PBL and application-based VME curriculum, which reflects the diversity of veterinary education (VE) [21].

4.2.2 Gaps and Limitations in Current VE Models

The gaps in VE models point to areas where current training fails to align with the needs and demands of integrated disease control practices covering humans, animals, and the environment. Some elaborate points on these gaps are as follows:

- **Emerging Scientific Disciplines**: Contemporary VE frequently falls behind in integrating advanced scientific disciplines such as molecular biology, genetics, and precision medicine. The significance of these domains is progressively growing due to the widespread adoption of modern diagnostic and therapeutic procedures in animal healthcare [22].
- **Overly Domestic Animal-based Learning**: Current veterinary practices emphasize domestic animals, especially in developing countries, which are very common. Therefore, the integration of other health issues, such as wildlife, human, and PH-related studies, is inevitable in VME systems [23].
- **Practical Clinical Skills**: Practical clinical training is insufficient. Several schools prioritize theoretical knowledge above practical application, resulting in students being inadequately prepared for surgical procedures, emergency treatment, and routine clinical assessments [24].
- **Cultural Competency and Communication**: Despite the importance of the OH idea for global health (GH), incorporating it into the veterinary curriculum has been sluggish. This strategy is crucial for tackling interrelated health problems beyond the human, animal, and environmental domains, particularly in the face of global challenges such as climate change and pandemics [25].

The limitations in VE models often stem from systemic and structural constraints within educational institutions and broader educational policy:

- **Resource Limitations**: A significant challenge faced by numerous veterinary schools is the lack of adequate funding, which limits their capacity to offer cutting-edge facilities, exposure to diverse live animal cases, and access to the newest training technology. This constraint can result in inequality in the caliber of education offered, specifically impacting hands-on skills development [21].
- **Geographical Limitations**: Veterinary colleges in isolated or countryside regions may encounter difficulties in obtaining seasoned faculty members and providing a wide range of clinical opportunities. Limiting students' exposure to a wide range of cases and advanced practice situations can potentially impede their preparedness for different professional environments [22].
- **Curricular Rigidity**: Sluggish curricular modifications in numerous veterinary schools can impede prompt upgrades that integrate novel knowledge and technologies. The inflexibility of these schools hinders their ability to adjust to swift advancements in veterinary research and practice, placing graduates at a disadvantage in the fiercely competitive job market [25].
- **Mental Health and Well-being**: Mental health and well-being are frequently overlooked in the veterinary curriculum despite the field experiencing high rates of burnout and mental health problems. Offering assistance and instruction in this field is essential for equipping students with the necessary skills to adequately handle the pressures and emotional difficulties associated with the job [26].

The existing VE model consists of several preveterinary and VE phases, with ongoing professional development essential to the overall approach. Continuing education (CE) is not dependent on time, location, or the preveterinary and veterinary curriculum. Instead, its purpose is to enhance clinical practice. The CE is the sole domain within the current virtual learning environment that constantly employs distant learning approaches, such as participating in seminars, workshops, conferences, and other formats [27].

The existing VE approach encompasses preveterinary methods. The world's inaugural veterinary school was established in Lyon, France in 1761. An extensive analysis of VME worldwide revealed the existence of 597 schools in 194 nations. Among these, 25% confer Doctor of Veterinary Medicine (DVM) degrees, whereas 5% confer Bachelor of Veterinary Science (BVSc) degrees. Furthermore, there are a total of 148 universities offering VME in 27 countries [28]. Various veterinary medical academic institutes provide degrees with 54 distinct titles and durations of VE, incorporating ongoing education as a fundamental component of their comprehensive approach. CE is not dependent on time, location, or the preveterinary or veterinary curriculum. Its focus is on enhancing clinical practice. The CE is the sole domain under the present Virtual Medical Education, which constantly employs distance learning techniques, such as participating in seminars, workshops, conferences, and other formats [28].

This has led to significant confusion due to the multiple nomenclatures for veterinary-related educational institutions worldwide. These veterinary medical academic institutes are designated departments, schools, institutions, academics, colleges/faculties, and even universities. In addition, these new universities also provide Bachelor of Science (BSc) programs in poultry science or dairy technology, which not only contribute to the existing uncertainty but also intensify competition in the labor market between BSc graduates and veterinary graduates. This issue is particularly problematic in the Indian subcontinent. In 1961, a US Agency for International Development (USAID) program resulted in the separation of the combined degree in veterinary science and animal husbandry (BSc Vet Sci and AH in Pakistan; BVSc in India) into two separate degrees: DVM and BSc in Animal Husbandry. In subsequent eras, India rectified these degrees, which were divided into two parts. More recently, in 2013, Pakistan also reverted to offering single and combined degrees. However, in Bangladesh, providing bifurcated degrees persists, leading to confusion in the job market and negatively impacting the quality of education and professional relationships among veterinarians. The dual degree course was initially established at Cornell University in 1871. It involves a four-year BSc in veterinary science and two additional years to obtain the DVM degree. The two-year DVM degree was subsequently transformed into a four-year standalone DVM degree. This modification was implemented by many Virtual Medical Artificial Intelligences to enhance the knowledge and expertise of veterinary students, namely, in the areas of disease diagnosis, treatment, and prevention [28]. The objective was also to address production-related concerns in livestock, wildlife, domesticated animals, and animals used in scientific settings [28].

However, there is a lack of consistency among Virtual Medical Artificial Intelligence programs, training facilities, and curricula, leading to graduates with diverse skills and expertise. According to a survey of 597 Veterinary Medical Associations of Interest (VMAIs), only 49 institutions have received accreditation from the American Veterinary Medical Association Council on Education (AVMA COE) on a global scale. Interestingly, no VMAIs from regions such as Africa and Asia are accredited. To ensure that VMAIs worldwide can produce graduates with superior knowledge and abilities to satisfy future demand, it is imperative to establish standardized core curricula, training, and lab facilities, as well as a uniform nomenclature for degrees and institutions [28, 29].

4.2.3 Overview of Existing One Health Programs

Various organizations currently run various kinds of health programs, all aiming to create interconnections among humans, animals, and the environment. Some of them are the Centers for Disease Control and Prevention (CDC)'s OH program, the World Health Organization (WHO) OH Initiative, the Food and Agriculture Organization (FAO) OH Approach, USAID OH Work, the World Organization for Animal Health (WOAH) OH Initiative, the Global OH Initiative, the PH England OH program, and regional OH networks. These programs focus on zoonotic diseases, AMR, emergency preparedness, food safety, sustainable agriculture, and disease management at the human–animal–environment interface. They also focus on research, education, and policy advocacy to address complex health challenges. The goal is to achieve better health outcomes globally by integrating health efforts across these domains. These organizations advocate and promote the OH approach through interdisciplinary collaboration with veterinary associations, human health organizations, environmental health agencies, and international organizations to address GH threats [29–31].

The 2022–2026 plan aims to increase and expand health system capacities in six key areas: OH, emerging and re-emerging zoonotic epidemics, endogenous diseases, food safety risks, AMR, and the environment. The plan promotes OH at the global, regional, and national levels, providing implementation guidance for countries, international partners, and nonstate actors. Its operational objectives include fostering multinational collaboration, learning, and knowledge exchange and promoting cooperation, shared responsibility, and inclusiveness. Coordination mechanisms for financing are being developed to support the plan's implementation, leveraging resources to address critical health threats and promote health for people, animals, plants, and the environment [4].

4.3 Transformative Strategies for Veterinary Education

Transformative strategies for VE are innovative approaches aimed at enhancing VE and practice. They focus on integrating new technologies, interdisciplinary learning, and hands-on experiences to prepare students for modern veterinary practice. By emphasizing the connections between human, animal, and environmental health through the OH model, these strategies aim to equip future veterinarians to address the evolving needs of AH, PH, and ecological sustainability.

4.3.1 Rethinking Curriculum Design

VE is an engaging and vibrant educational setting that provides accessible education that trains students to impact veterinary medicine and OH jointly. As the profession has advanced, an updated veterinary curriculum is needed to fulfil its aim.

Most traditional VE methods neglect broader aspects of human and environmental health, focusing only on AH. The traditional curriculum is designed to offer students fundamental knowledge and skills, according to Fanning et al. [32]. Basic sciences, such as anatomy, physiology, and pathology, are represented, along with professional courses and practical training complementing clinical skills. The key focal areas proposed by the Association of American Veterinary Medical Colleges (AAVMC) include those related to nutrition, husbandry, PH, pharmacology, toxicology, zoonotic and infectious diseases, and nutrition [33]. Students have engaged in practical experience through clinical rotations across several disciplines in the past two years. The current incomplete understanding of OH concepts within the existing veterinary curriculum limits the potential of students to appreciate the human–animal–environment interface, especially concerning emerging diseases and ecosystem health [34]. Second, there is little appreciation of wildlife health; hence, little is known about treating zoonotic diseases first isolated in animals [35]. This further indicates that little attention has been given to environmental factors. In addition, there is fragmented environmental education and a lack of training on the environmental impact of veterinary practices. Furthermore, the development of effective control measures is hampered since little attention has been given to AMR in environmental situations. On the other hand, these gaps in integrating the principles of OH, wildlife health, environmental consequences, and AMR make students inadequate to handle the complex interlinked problems they would encounter in their professional lives.

The application of the OH principle in veterinary curricula is supported because OH has shown great success in controlling health crises, including H1N1 influenza events, Ebola, rabies, monkeypox, and avian influenza (AI) [36–39]. These concrete examples illustrate how the coordination of environmental, animal, and human health leads to better disease surveillance, outbreak control, and improvements in PH. An integrated approach to VE would equip future veterinarians with a solid foundation to address the complex health problems of animals, humans, and the environment. These changes will nurture more comprehensive and integrated responses to new

GH threats. Through outreach in the community, students can discuss details of the resource limitations, cultural diversity, and diverse needs of the communities in which they will practice with their colleagues in medical and environmental science [40].

Additionally, OH education promotes critical thinking. The learning approach requires students to address health matters from different perspectives. Students must consider factors such as animal behavior, human habits, and the circumstances of the environment when trying to address zoonotic diseases or environmental health concerns [41]. Interprofessional learning environments foster students' communication and teamwork skills by allowing them to collaborate with peers from other disciplines within OH education projects. Therefore, OH concepts should be incorporated into any veterinary school curriculum because this will take a present student population and give them the essential competencies required to address contemporary veterinary care challenges, a good number of which are continuously on the rise.

4.3.2 Core Competencies in One Health

4.3.2.1 Evolution of Thoughts in One Health

The OH High-Level Expert Panel has endorsed OH as an integrated strategy that aims to maximize ecosystem, animal, and human health through cross-sector collaboration. This strategy is needed because it addresses global issues such as climate change, access to clean water, and sustainable development. It emphasizes how the health of people, animals, plants, and the environment is interconnected [42].

Traditionally, OH has been approached in two distinct schools of thought:

1. **Disease-centric Approach**: Historically, the emphasis has been on preventing and treating diseases that emerge at the interface of people, animals, plants, and ecosystems. Key priorities include combating antibiotic resistance, enhancing disease surveillance, strengthening biosecurity measures, and managing zoonotic diseases. This approach aims to minimize health risks and outbreaks through targeted interventions and collaborative efforts across sectors [42].
2. **System-level Approach**: A more recent evolution in OH thinking focuses on understanding the complex interactions among environmental, animal, plant, and human health at a systemic level. This perspective advocates the development of social–ecological systems that foster the well-being of all the components. It considers broader factors such as international capital flows, socioeconomic drivers, and environmental sustainability. Rather than solely focusing on disease prevention, this approach aims to cultivate resilient and sustainable systems that meet the needs of people, animals, and ecosystems over the long term [42].

This evolution in OH ideology reflects a shift from reactive disease management to proactive, holistic strategies that promote health and sustainability across interconnected systems. By integrating diverse perspectives and disciplines, OH continues evolving as a robust framework for comprehensively and sustainably addressing emerging GH challenges comprehensively and sustainably [43].

4.3.2.2 Background of the Competency Framework in One Health

OH, competency is the essential skill, knowledge, and attitudes that people should possess when training and addressing OH issues. Any group, project, policy, or organization that differs in approach and implementation but is constrained by a common objective or frequently follows operational principles defined by methods of systemic thinking, careful planning, and collaboration across disciplines is included in the wide range of OH initiatives [43]. The updated core OH capabilities represent the shift to system-based methods. This makes it possible for more competent professionals to adopt OH more broadly because they have the core abilities, know-how, and mindset needed for the program to be implemented successfully. Togami et al. [44] conducted a study that revealed gaps in the existing research, emphasized the difficulties in integrating OH competencies into educational programs, and offered suggestions for integrating these abilities into formal education curricula. The authors suggested that

OH education be incorporated into all disciplines (particularly underrepresented disciplines), emphasizing communication, coordination, collaboration, and practical and applied training. The resultant competencies proposed according to the study are categorized as health, knowledge, and local and global concerns concerning humans, animals, plants, and ecosystems (Table 4.1). This paradigm includes a slight movement to the second aspect of the OH concept, which is the broader assessment of the underlying causes of illness within a system, even while the primary emphasis is on competencies to respond to health risks. The existing OH competencies have been adapted to bolster this advancement in OH thinking and foster the evolution toward the second aspect (Figure 4.2). This was achieved by consulting with Network for Evaluation of One Health (NEOH) members, building on a history of publications, seminars, and conferences from the Network since 2014. The NEOH defines the characteristics of a single health project for evaluation to determine the instruments, frameworks, and indicators currently in use. In addition, they carried out a comprehensive analysis of the scientific literature and developed an assessment system [45]. Using this strategy, the underlying attitudes and beliefs of the community of practice were identified, leading to a consultation on principles that operate as the cornerstone of a long-term practitioner network. The authors and collaborators of the NEOH considered the competencies that an entry-level textbook for OH would need to cover to facilitate OH's successful adoption. Through a shared web platform, all writers received an initial set of suggested abilities on the basis of NEOH research, and the current literature, and feedback was requested from all.

After one of the writers integrated the remarks, a revised set of abilities was offered for a second iteration that was examined in 2021 with the current network of over 50 members. The finalized competencies were first presented at the OH conference in Oslo in November 2021 to obtain input from a larger audience. Table 4.2 and Figure 4.3 show nine fundamental competencies, which fall into three more significant categories: knowledge and awareness, values and attitudes, and skills. The present OH skills have been modified to support the advancement of OH thinking toward what is depicted in the second stream of Figure 4.2 and to further this breakthrough in OH. Building on a history of publications, seminars, and conferences from the Network since 2014, this was accomplished through consultation with NEOH members. To identify the tools, frameworks, and indicators currently in use, NEOH defines the features of a single health project for evaluation. They also created an assessment system and thoroughly examined scientific literature [45]. The community of practice's fundamental attitudes and beliefs were discovered through this technique, which resulted in consultation on the guiding principles for a long-term practitioner network.

4.3.3 Incorporating Public Health and Environmental Science

Given the interconnectedness of many of the most significant health and conservation issues of our time, professional groups such as ecologists, veterinarians, physicians, researchers, and conservation biologists must collaborate transdisciplinary [48]. Ecosystem health aims to bring a diverse range of academics and researchers together around a single, straightforward idea of health. Declining biodiversity and new diseases rank among the most complicated and broad ecological calamities that could affect our planet [49]. Collaboration is essential since health is the common thread that affects all life on the Earth [50].

Although Leopold, a conservationist, first proposed the idea of land health in the early 1940s, medical science advancements have increased since then [51]. The future is slowly drawing nearer for land health, just as Leopold foresaw [51]. To maintain the health of animals and people, veterinarians must advocate for conservation and environmental protection policies [52]. Numerous early research investigations, reports, medical essays, news pieces, journal papers, and magazine articles have linked the health of animals to that of humans [53, 54]. Chaddock [55] reported that viruses with various species hosts account for approximately 60% of the nearly 1500 diseases recognized to impact humans.

Humans are accidental or terminal hosts for a number of these new viral diseases that originated in animals or arthropods. For instance, although humans are not necessary for the formation and spread of the West Nile virus, they can become infected with it and experience life-threatening symptoms or even death.

Table 4.1 Recommended core competencies for One Health education.

Sr. No.	Health knowledge	Global and local issues in One Health	Professional characteristics
1	Proficiency in establishing and developing transdisciplinary OH sciences, encompassing PH, AH, environmental sciences, and contemporary agriculture.	To exhibit knowledge of the scientific, political, social, cultural, and historical facets of contemporary, complex health issues that lend themselves to the OH paradigm.	To exhibit knowledge of and proficiency with research and evaluation methodologies and apply scientific findings to practical settings in the context of policy and health program implementation.
2	Give an account of the genesis, development, and ecology of infectious disease agents affecting humans, animals, and plants that are significant to PH.	Explain the underlying biological theories, the range, and the intricacy of diseases that affect people, animals, plants, and the environment.	Describe the advantages and difficulties of using an integrative, interdisciplinary approach to studies of health issues at the interface between humans, animals, plants, and the environment.
3	Explain the principal pathways of toxin, pathogen, and resistance gene transmission, including exposures to animals, plants, and the environment; additionally, discuss vector-borne, waterborne, and airborne cycles.	Recognize how local and global variables influence the spread of disease inside and between nations and the effects of global change on health.	Convey scientific findings to the scientific community, non–health-related academics, the public, the media, and policymakers both orally and in writing.
4	Describe the epidemiologic concepts used to define issues pertaining to plants, animals, humans, and the environment. Recognize scientific concepts that affect the complex issues facing human, animal, plant, and environmental health today, such as biological complexity, genetic variety, and systems interconnections from individuals to ecosystems.	Recognize and comprehend the causes of disease and the environmental, animal, plant, and human determinants of health.	Clearly, exhibit scientific quantitative skills, including assessing experimental design, analyzing and interpreting scientific data, fostering discussions, and offering practical recommendations.
5	Recognize the common socioeconomic and cultural factors influencing health, such as resource security, education, cultural practices, home geography, poverty, and nutrition.	Examine and contrast the effects of illnesses and exposures on health and nonhealthy and the social, behavioral, political, and economic ramifications in various parts of the world.	Establish and oversee a competent transdisciplinary team that uses principles to carry out morally and scientifically good research that will influence policy.
6	Describe the application of therapeutic countermeasures, diagnostics, and bio-surveillance.	Identify key obstacles and chances for local and GH improvement through hands-on, applied training. Exhibit a fundamental comprehension of food safety both before and after production.	Create a strategy for incorporating new research discoveries into community programs, health policies, interventions, and public education in a financially viable, culturally appropriate, and sustainable way.
7	Describe the strategies utilized at the individual, group, and population levels to prevent illness and enhance the health of people, animals, plants, and the environment.	Recognize the roles and functions of the PH system and those of the federal, state, and municipal governments.	

Note: This table is modified from Togami et al. and Laing et al. [44, 46].

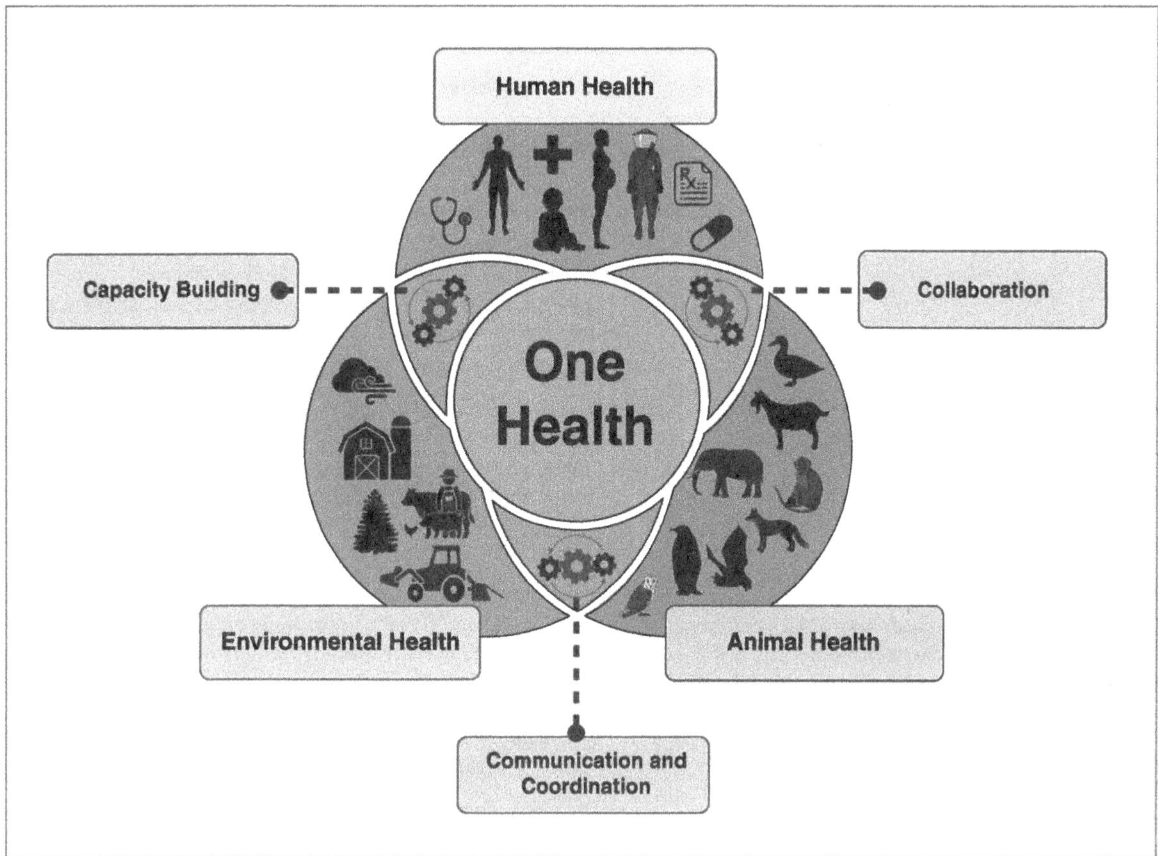

Figure 4.2 One Health concept encompasses two primary perspectives: (i) the interactions among humans, animals, plants, and the environment and (ii) the system that integrates all these components.

The need for a more thorough strategy to control emerging zoonotic diseases and the importance of veterinary care in society have been highlighted by the recent Ebola outbreak. Allela et al. [56] discovered measurable IgG antibodies against the Ebola virus in feral West African canines that had come into contact with the virus, mostly by eating infected dead animals and vomiting from people who had tested positive for the infection.

Understanding the connections among human, animal, and environmental health requires a multidisciplinary approach. Considering this GH paradigm, the veterinary profession must prepare [34]. Veterinarians can positively impact ecosystem health concerns where human, animal, and environmental health interact by completing biomedical training in comparative (trans-species) and population medicine (herd health) [57].

4.3.4 Innovative Pedagogical Methods

Beyond the veterinary sector, medical practitioners receive formal pedagogical education [58, 59]. Additionally, a study by Jason and Westberg [60] showed that most medical school faculty members were not prepared to be professional teachers. It has also been found that role models are essential for clinical teachers, so most clinical instructors in human medicine learn how to teach by observing other teachers in action [61]. As this process seems time-consuming and requires different types of testing and contemplation, efforts for faculty development and improved curricula have been added to medical teacher education [59, 62, 63]. However, clinical training

Table 4.2 Comparison of previously proposed competencies in One Health.

Rome synthesis major domains	Core competencies for One Health education
Management Capable of overseeing multidisciplinary groups; recognizes the duties and responsibilities of the group and its members; maintains team accountability	**Professional characteristics** • Recognizes the advantages and difficulties of a multidisciplinary approach. • Communicates with all audiences and stakeholders effectively. • Adopts morally and scientifically sound procedures. • Convert research into treatments, programs, and policies in a culturally appropriate and long-lasting way.
Communication and informatics Demonstrates diplomacy, negotiation skills, and conflict resolution abilities to foster cooperation	**Global and local issues in One Health** • Recognizes important difficulties and possibilities to enhance health globally and locally. • Comprehends the structure of stakeholders, both locally and globally; and is aware of the historical, cultural, political, economic, and scientific components of complex and emerging health problems
Values and ethics It has a great sense of self-awareness, values honesty, and is an integral proponent of change **Leadership** The ability to adapt to changing circumstances, comprehend both individual and group leadership styles, and understand the outside world (social, political, legal, and cultural) **Team and collaboration** Determines common values and objectives-builds trust-thinks strategically value the diversity of background, experience, culture, and discipline **Systems thinking** Understanding and adopting an OH strategy that recognizes an issue and its effects on the system, awareness of the big picture, and the interdependency of stakeholders.	**Health knowledge** • Knowledgeable in PH, AH, environmental sciences, and agriculture, among other transdisciplinary fields. • Familiarity with the genesis, ecology, and spread of infectious illnesses. grasps the fundamentals of epidemiology. • The capacity to recognize common cultural, social, and health-related factors. • Describes population-level, community-level, and individual-level interventions used to prevent disease.

Note: This table is modified from Togami et al., Laing et al., and Frankson et al. [44, 46, 47].

settings continue to face difficulties in obtaining pedagogical expertise for medical teachers as the fundamental pedagogical ideas in the teaching scripts seem missing [64]. Medical faculty members acquire pedagogical expertise when working with multilevel learners, which is a developmental approach they receive during their appointment. On the other hand, it has been proposed though not yet substantiated by empirical evidence, that academic physicians in the veterinary sector educate in a manner similar to how they are exposed throughout their education [65]. Observational learning also plays a vital role. According to Smith et al. [65], there is evidence that veterinary clinical educators can benefit from thinking aloud, role modeling, guided cognitive processes, breaking down specific experiences, providing opportunities for active practice, and providing feedback immediately.

It is interesting to note that gaps exist in the pedagogies and skill development of teacher educators for training student teachers. Professors anticipate these teacher educators to pick up knowledge on the job, but in the end, they rely on what they have learned as classroom instructors in college [66]. The need for faculty development

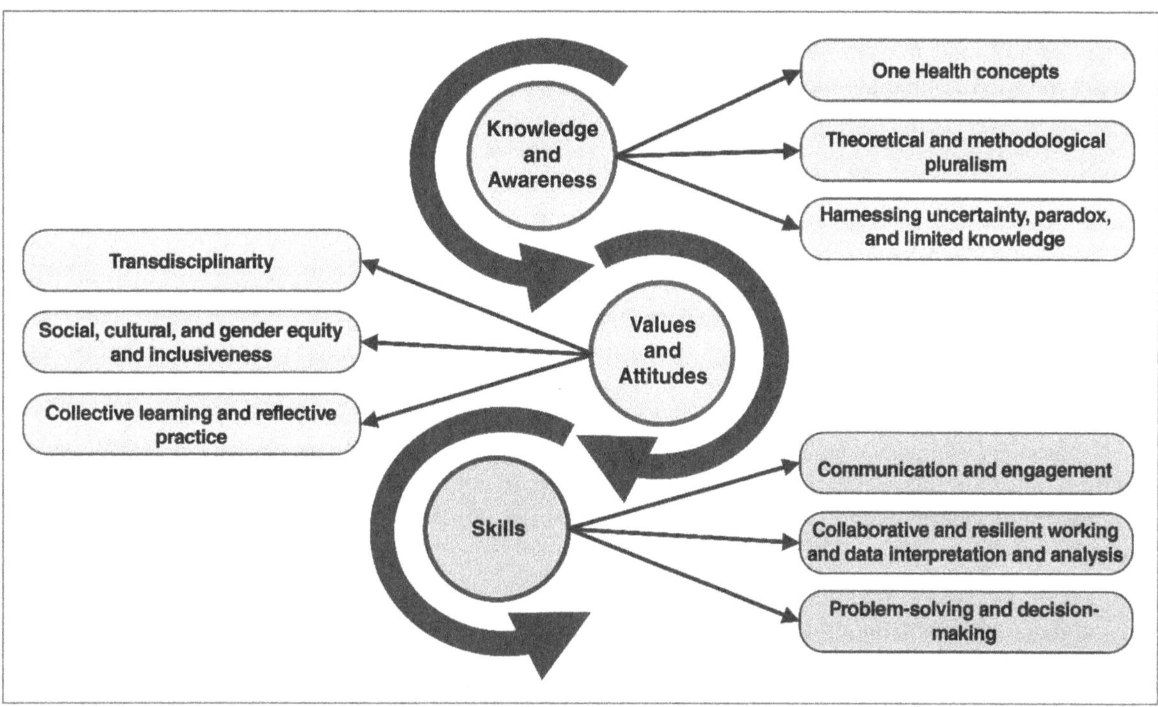

Figure 4.3 The nine updated NEOH One Health competences; include knowledge and awareness, values and attitudes, and skills. Adapted and modified from [46].

programs to improve teaching practices in higher education is a recurrent theme identified by researchers; however, there is disagreement over the best way to design these programs [67–69]. According to Wilkerson and Irby [59], teaching abilities are distinct from subject-matter competence, as they need to be comprised of professional, instructional, leadership, and organizational development. Another interesting strategy for teaching development is peer mentoring, particularly for more senior and experienced faculty members [68]. For example, nurse educators pick up teaching techniques from their mentors via on-the-job training [70]. This approach focuses on reflective, cooperative learning strategies among senior and junior faculty members. On the other hand, positive teacher development might not occur until educators are dissatisfied with their current teaching philosophies because teachers who experience low levels of teacher efficacy seem to believe that they are unable to instruct students in a way that can be beneficial to them [67]. According to Strand et al. [62], Steinert et al. [63], and Smith et al. [65], successful instructors and clinical teachers have similar characteristics. Harden and Crosby [71] stated that clinical instructors must assume tasks beyond the mentor or role model, including information suppliers, case facilitators, learner assessors, course designers, and resource producers. The key components of exceptional clinical teaching are noncognitive traits such as passion, social skills, and the capacity to assist, motivate, actively engage, and connect with students. Additionally, an ethnographic case study of veterinarians in clinical teaching revealed that a reflective approach to clinical teaching was useful for educators, as they built relationships with their students; these educators sought to provide a demanding but secure learning environment [72].

4.3.5 Leveraging Technology for One Health Education

The surge in zoonotic diseases underscores the critical need for competent OH professionals who understand and can manage complex relationships between animal, human, and environmental health [73]. Technological innovation can make this training more accessible and relevant for preparing these practitioners with the required competencies and tools to fight the increasing threat of zoonosis for improved health globally. Some of the challenges in OH education are indeed solved by online learning platforms, such as time zone variations and geographical distance [74]. As such, flexible curricula for learning, which allow students to study at any time and from any part of the world, can easily make OH education accessible through e-learning platforms. Only a few elements that can be housed within e-learning to make learning dynamic and engaging include virtual laboratories and videos. The learning process can also be made more fun with the integration of e-learning with gamification, virtual reality, and augmented reality technology.

Big data analytics enables trend, frequency, and pattern analyses of disease outbreaks since OH requires data. Using data analytics tools to synthesize and analyze data better prepares students for decision-making, initiating and supporting best practices against diseases that disrupt the ecosystem, and identifying patterns and correlations. Social media allows students to interact, exchange knowledge, and share educational resources. This can thus facilitate collaboration and information sharing and raise awareness to support PH activities [75].

Finally, through technology, coupled with empowering learners to fight challenges in the real world, OH education can be shifted toward greater efficiency, inclusion, and fun. In this context, we can use technology to improve the quality of OH education and prepare the next generation of OH professionals to safeguard health and the future of the planet.

4.3.6 Assessment and Evaluation Techniques

The only way to test the effectiveness of OH education is through the caliber of professionals it produces [1]. Therefore, we could use various models to assess and evaluate the quality of professionals and review the learning models to ensure that we release only the best and most competent professionals for managing OH issues worldwide. Assessment is thus an important and necessary concept in OH education. It enables educators to identify whether students have absorbed specific knowledge, skills, and behavior from the OH strategy and, therefore, to know if the set learning objectives for a particular interventionist program in a course are met [76]. According to the Mississippi Department of Education [77] and the CDC [78], this input informs improvements to the curriculum and instructional strategies. Evaluation takes the form of a planned process for collecting and analyzing data to arrive at an overall judgment regarding the effectiveness of an OH education program.

Summative assessment tools measure students' learning. It analyzes the skills and knowledge of students that they have learned by completing a unit or course. Modified essay questions, extended matching items, and multiple-choice questions are instructional strategies used in health education. These assessment strategies measure the application of information, understanding of basic ideas, and students' problem-solving abilities. In contrast, students self-evaluate their learning and performance through assignments, including written exams (MCQs, true/false, essays, MEQs, modified constructed answer questions), performance tests (checklists, global ratings, student logbooks), and reflective portfolios [79, 80].

OH calls for specialists from diverse disciplines to collaborate to ensure the health of humans, the environment, and animals. Therefore, group discussions, assignments, and presentations can be applicable in assessing a student's ability to work, team, and communicate as a group [81]. Teamwork skills are beneficial when working as a team to resolve PH problems through cooperation and communication. On the other hand, health is a priceless career. For this reason, practical examples in actual cases should be made part of the examination or assessment procedure to test students' critical thinking abilities, analyze complex issues by breaking them down, and offer, recommend, and devise the best possible solution. This will ensure that learners at the school are empowered with intellectual and practical competencies to succeed beyond school.

The integration of many assessment methodologies ensures that we will produce professionals who can understand, assess, and act on twenty-first-century PH concerns; they will be imbued with the requisite skills, knowledge, commitment, and abilities. These results help to assess the quality of the learning models and identify weaknesses.

4.4 Institutional One Health Model: A Global Perspective

To prepare grounded veterinarians in OH, it is necessary to incorporate conceptual and practical models of OH from the early stages of higher educational training. This integration can be achieved through strategic curriculum planning and the implementation of OH-focused required and elective courses at this institutional level [82, 83]. Universities' role in advancing OH through transdisciplinary research, education, and community engagement is of utmost importance [84].

Institutional OH models are essential in equipping the professional workforce with a vast knowledge of OH principles [85]. Several academic institutions have embraced the OH model and implemented it to address the unique challenges and priorities of their local and national contexts. This chapter, therefore, refers to several successful institutional models of OH worldwide. A comparative overview of the veterinary school and VE programs that incorporate One Health is presented in Table 4.3.

4.4.1 Utrecht University, the Netherlands

At Utrecht University in the Netherlands, advocacy for OH initiatives has been led through the One Health Centre of Excellence also called the Netherlands Centre for One Health (NCOH) which uses research and education to encourage interdisciplinary collaborations in tackling AMR, emerging and re-emerging infectious diseases, food safety, and environmental sustainability [86–88]. The interdisciplinary collaboration between veterinary, medical, and environmental science faculties and departments has produced translational research that informs policies and practices within different professions. Another way to engage institutions is through global Shared Socio-economic Pathways (SSPs), where the university collaborates with public and private partners to mitigate health risks and vulnerabilities [89]. The institution partners with the government, nongovernment agencies, and other research institutions to safeguard human, animal, and environmental health [90].

According to one of their joints OH postgraduate programs, a statement on their webpage reads,

> "*...Given the intimate relationship between animal and human health and the environment, the joint research programs of the Faculty of Veterinary Medicine, the Faculty of Science and UMC Utrecht constitute a unique center of excellence for OH. In collaboration with our public and private partners, we focus on the prevention of and fight against existing and emerging infectious diseases – both in humans and animals – including zoonoses and food safety pathogens, on the prevention and control of AMR, and on overcoming environmental risks...*" [91].

This further emphasized the commitment of the institution to propagating OH principles.

4.4.2 University of California, Davis, United States

UC Davis has an internationally recognized One Health Institute (OHI) for addressing GH issues. The OHI was established on the basis of the solid commitment of the UC Davis School of Veterinary Medicine to the OH approach, and it hosts the renowned Karen C. Drayer Wildlife Health Center. The Institute has led pioneering research, such as Predicting Infectious Disease Transmission (PREDICT) with USAID funds, to detect and reduce the risk of spillover of high threat zoonoses, leading to pandemics. More than 30 countries have benefited from the initiative in its endeavor to set up systems for the early detection of emerging infectious diseases. It also leads a number of collaborative efforts, including the One Health Workforce-Next Generation (OHW-NG) project, to train health professionals across Africa and Asia to address health risks using an OH approach [92]. Its innovative strategies range from climate change and food security to wildlife conservation, combining expertise in epidemiology, economics, and veterinary science. Several influential programs, including the California Raptor Center

Table 4.3 Comparative overview of veterinary education programs integrating One Health.

Universities	Location	Core components	Focus areas	Educational approaches
Utrecht University	The Netherlands	Netherlands Centre for One Health (NCOH); Shared Socio-economic Pathways (SSPs)	Antimicrobial resistance; Emerging and re-emerging infectious diseases; Food safety, and environmental sustainability	Postgraduate programs
University of California, Davis	USA	Karen C. Drayer Wildlife Health Center; One Health Workforce-Next Generation project; California Raptor Center and the Global Virome Project; Rx One Health Field Institute	Zoonoses; Climate change; Food security; Wildlife conservation; Emerging infectious diseases	Health professionals; undergraduate and postgraduate programs;
University of Minnesota	USA	One Health University Networks (OHUNs); the One Health Central and Eastern Africa (OHCEA) network; Southeast Asia One Health University Network (SEAOHUN)	Emerging infectious diseases	Research and training
Royal Veterinary College	UK	Network for Evaluation of One Health (NEOH)	Antimicrobial resistance; Emerging infectious diseases	Postgraduate programs
University of Tokyo	Japan	Southeast Asia One Health University Network (SEAOHUN)	Zoonoses; Environmental pollution; Disaster response; Governance; Education	Health professionals; Postgraduate programs; Conference/workshop
University of Veterinary and Animal Sciences	Pakistan		Antimicrobial resistance; Zoonotic diseases; Biosecurity	Conference/workshop
Chattogram Veterinary and Animal Sciences University	Bangladesh	One Health Institute (OHI); One Health Poultry Hub, Bangladesh (OHPHB)	Antimicrobial resistance; Emerging infectious diseases	Postgraduate programs; conference/workshop
Kerala Veterinary and Animal Sciences University	India	Centre for One Health Education, Advocacy, Research and Training (COHEART); Centre for One Health Kerala (COH-K)	High-priority global public health challenges	Undergraduate and postgraduate programs
University of Nairobi	Kenya	One Health in Eastern and Southern Africa (COHESA)	Food security; Zoonotic diseases; Pastoralism; Environmental degradation; Capacity building	Postgraduate programs
University of Pretoria	South Africa	Hans Hoheisen Wildlife Research Station (HHWRS); Mnisi Community Programme (MCP); Hluvukani Animal Clinic (HAC)	Zoonotic diseases; Wildlife conservation; Antimicrobial resistance	Teaching and research
University of Ibadan	Nigeria	One Health Unibadan	Neglected tropical diseases	Research, teaching, and community engagement
University of Queensland	Australia	Queensland Alliance for One Health Sciences (QAOHS); University of Queensland Veterinary Students' Association (UQVSA) One Health Initiative		Research, Teaching, conference/workshop, and governance

and the Global Virome Project, advance research and conservation worldwide. It also offers extensive education programs incorporating the OH concept at different education levels, including DVM, Master of Preventive Veterinary Medicine, and doctoral degrees in epidemiology, ecosystem health, and public health preparedness [93]. The university offers pathways into OH-related disciplines, such as majors in biology and life sciences, research opportunities, and specialized fellowships, such as the Pathways to OH program, to undergraduate students. In addition, the university has offered hands-on, interdisciplinary training programs such as the Rx One Health Field Institute to prepare students and professionals for emerging GH challenges [94].

4.4.3 University of Minnesota, United States

One Health Initiative is a well-established program at the University of Minnesota (UMN) among the students, staff, and faculty. The initiative was taken globally between 2009 and 2019 when the research team at the College of Veterinary Medicine received a grant from the USAID. The research team co-led the Medical School, School of Public Health, and School of Nursing to build OH university networks in Africa and Southeast Asia to tackle emerging infectious diseases from humans, animals, and the environment [95]. The UMN teams and Tufts University joined forces to provide support for two regional One Health University Networks (OHUNs), the One Health Central and Eastern Africa (OHCEA) network, and the Southeast Asia One Health University Network (SEAOHUN). One Health Workforce (OHW) established by UMN from 2014 to 2019 leveraged these established university networks to create a sustainable transformation in the regional health workforces. Another OH initiative in UMN is the creation of the One Health Systems Mapping and Analysis Resource Toolkit (OH-SMART). OH-SMART is an interactive mapping tool that fosters working processes across organizational and disciplinary lines when preparing or responding to disease outbreaks or other major OH issues [95].

4.4.4 Royal Veterinary College, UK

Royal Veterinary College (RVC) is the house of many OH initiatives in the United Kingdom (UK). It starts from the OH postgraduate program, which educates students about the principles of OH. The course is delivered jointly with the University of London and the London School of Hygiene and Tropical Medicine (LSHTM). At the end of the course, students have full knowledge of OH concepts and methodologies, transdisciplinary interactions, systems approach, socio-ecological systems, food safety, and GH. RVC is one of the major partners of the NEOH, funded by the European Cooperation in Science and Technology (EU COST). The NEOH is an open network that connects people from various disciplines who are interested in OH and evaluation. This network published a book titled "Integrated Approaches to Health – A Handbook for the Evaluation of One Health." This book chapter presents an evidence-based framework for evaluating integrated approaches to health [96].

4.4.5 University of Tokyo, Japan

In response to the pandemic event of 2019, academic and policy activities were enhanced through the emphasis placed on OH both in governance and education by University of Tokyo (UTokyo) [97]. The University expanded its integration of the OH framework in its curriculum as a means of preparing the next generation of health professionals to navigate complex relationships at the human–animal–environment interface [98]. UTokyo's OH model was founded in relation to Japan's unique environmental and PH challenges. It emphasizes the integration of veterinary medicine, PH, and environmental sciences, with a specific focus on zoonoses, environmental pollution, and disaster response [99, 100].

UTokyo established research collaboration organizations intending to create an academic foundation for OH, advancing the field of OH in cooperation with related universities and research institutes and playing a leading international role in Japan [100–102]. This collaborative research cuts across medical, veterinary medical, agricultural, and environmental disciplines. OH, training support is also provided through scholarship opportunities for postgraduate programs and conference/workshop travel grants through the university's collaboration with the SEAOHUN.

4.4.6 University of Veterinary and Animal Sciences, Pakistan

The University of Veterinary and Animal Sciences (UVAS) in Pakistan has a distinguished 137-year history of excellence and is acknowledged as one of the top 10 universities in the country. This institution reached university status in 2002, recognizing the vital importance of the livestock and poultry sectors in the national economy and the growing demand for expertise and research in veterinary and animal sciences. In recent years, UVAS has established itself as a hub for professional development in various fields, including veterinary medicine and animal sciences, food sciences, environmental sciences, zoological sciences, and economics and business management [103].

Through collaborations with various domestic and international academic and research organizations and the private sector, UVAS significantly contributes to economic development through practical research. Its postgraduate programs are centered on the OH approach and explore vital topics such as AMR, zoonotic diseases, and biosecurity. Additionally, the university organizes international conferences, such as the OH Conference, to facilitate interdisciplinary collaboration among scientists, veterinarians, medical professionals, and industry stakeholders. UVAS recently held an international seminar on "Antimicrobial Resistance in a One Health Framework," leading to a brief policy outlining a strategic plan to address this pressing issue within the country [103, 104].

4.4.7 One Health Institute, Chattogram Veterinary and Animal Sciences University, Bangladesh

The OHI in Bangladesh was founded in 2015 at Chattogram Veterinary and Animal Sciences (CVASU) to create a collaborative platform for education, research, and training on OH, addressing public health issues with input from human, animal, and environmental scientists. Preventing emerging infectious diseases is a primary focus of OHI objectives [105]. It is anticipated that by gaining a comprehensive understanding of disease transmission, the public health, veterinary, agricultural, and environmental sectors can cooperate to discover more effective solutions to relevant challenges. Consequently, OHI provides various postgraduate degrees and programs that emphasize the OH concept, including a Master's in Public Health and a Master's in Applied Veterinary Epidemiology, to cultivate skilled public health professionals trained to address any challenges they encounter. To date, 180 students from eight cohorts have been enrolled in Master's programs in Public Health and Applied Veterinary Epidemiology, with five cohorts of MPH graduates having already completed their degrees. The curriculum for both programs was developed on the basis of expert feedback from national and international sources to uphold global standards [105]. Graduates from this institute are expected to contribute significantly to addressing OH issues in Bangladesh and beyond.

Additionally, several important collaborative research projects engaging physicians, veterinarians, and environmentalists focusing on public health matters, such as the seroprevalence of anti-SARS-CoV-2 antibodies among healthcare workers, rotaviral diarrhea in children and AMR in animal products, are currently underway at the institute. Furthermore, we have partnered with various research and academic institutions both nationally and internationally, including the Bangladesh Institute of Tropical and Infectious Diseases (BITID), Institute of Epidemiology, Disease Control and Research (IEDCR), International Centre for Diarrheal Disease Research, Bangladesh (ICDDR,B), Department of Livestock Services, Department of Forest, University of California (USA), One Health Poultry Hub, Bangladesh (OHPHB), and Global Health Development. Annually, the Institute commemorates World One Health Day on November 3 with a range of innovative and awareness-raising activities, such as rallies, seminars, and various competitions for students, including quizzes, poster displays, photography related to the OH concept, discussion panels, and showcases of biodiversity [105].

4.4.8 Kerala Veterinary and Animal Sciences University, India

Kerala Veterinary and Animal Sciences University (KVASU) pioneered the promotion and implementation of OH initiatives in India. Its major initiatives are the Centre for One Health Kerala (COH-K) and the Centre for One Health Education, Advocacy, Research and Training (COHEART). COHEART was established in 2014 and is a key organization that enhances OH programs throughout India. Its primary aim involves addressing high-priority global public health challenges through the collaborative efforts of different disciplines. It imparts education through various courses designed to prepare students and professionals for knowledge and skills to navigate and address complex health issues across the human, veterinary, and environmental health sectors. In addition, COHEART actively undertakes research projects and activities in collaboration with national and international institutions for the development of novel approaches to managing health risks that come from interactions between humans, animals, and the environment [106, 107].

KVASU also offers a one-year postgraduate diploma designed to provide comprehensive information on the various health-related risks faced by health professionals in humans, animals and environmental health. This course enhances the ability of participants to understand the interrelationship among these fields and explore collaborative approaches that can be usefully adopted to mitigate adverse health risks. These programs and initiatives substantially promote OH concepts and practices in the region and beyond through education and research [106, 107].

4.4.9 University of Nairobi, Kenya

The practical application of OH in handling prevalent PH issues in Africa, e.g. food security, zoonotic diseases, pastoralism, and environmental degradation, has been led by the University of Nairobi (UoN) in Kenya [108]. The university has successfully applied the OH model in addressing Nairobi's pressing concerns in the areas of managing wildlife–human conflicts, controlling infectious diseases, and alleviating the impacts of climate change [109, 110].

UoN adopts an integrated OH model, which it provides through a variety of programs, such as the Master of Science in "OH and Emergency Research Ethics" [111]. These programs are borne out of partnerships between diverse professional disciplines, including other stakeholders in the PH sector. They are targeted toward capacity building to strengthen local and regional responses to human and animal health challenges at UoN [108]. The OH model of the UoN, as a matter of emphasis, extends its reach to building a regional capacity for disease response, especially in rural and underserved communities [112, 113].

4.4.10 University of Pretoria, South Africa

The University of Pretoria (UP) is a leading institution in Africa for OH research and education. As previously described for other institutions, UP's OH model integrates veterinary, human, and environmental health professionals to address the challenges of zoonotic diseases, wildlife conservation, and AMR [83]. This university is known for its strong emphasis on field-based research and collaboration with government agencies, NGOs, and international partners, using the OH Quadripartite framework [114]. In southern Africa, UP is one of the driving forces for OH advocacy and the development of practical solutions to health challenges in Africa [86]. UP is currently running a master's program in Global One Health, which is in collaboration with the Department of Biomedical Sciences, Institute of Tropical Medicine (ITM), Antwerp, Belgium. The course allows students to learn about various aspects of OH. The course modules include but are limited to Basic Epidemiology, Introduction to Zoonoses, Introduction to One Health, One Health: Policy, Surveillance and Survey Methodology, Ticks and Tick-borne Diseases, Laboratory Diagnostics, Advanced Epidemiology, General vector-borne Diseases, and Animal Health Management: High Impact and Emerging Diseases [86].

4.4.11 University of Ibadan, Ibadan, Nigeria

The model of the OH approach of the University of Ibadan (UniIbadan) is based on collaborative research projects, joint integrative initiatives, and strategic communication, which involves important stakeholders at both the national and international levels. Although several efforts have been made by institution to develop a structured OH degree program in the past, different OH-tailored events involving several disciplines, such as social demographers, medical doctors and veterinarians, psychologists, environmentalists, nurses, and pharmacists, have been organized [115, 116]. Therefore, UniIbadan's OH model successfully integrates research, teaching, and community engagement activities to contribute to the control and prevention of neglected tropical diseases in Africa and other PH threats.

UniIbadan's OH approach is community-oriented, focusing on sustainable solutions to potential regional, local, and national health issues. Efforts toward fully integrating OH principles into the university's curriculum as a joint program at the undergraduate and postgraduate levels are still very much under development [117, 118].

4.4.12 Queensland Alliance for One Health Sciences, University of Queensland, Australia

QAOHS is a research unit under the School of Veterinary Sciences, UQ, which was launched in 2021. This research unit links international and national governing bodies working on OH issues to researchers in UQ. QAOHIS also holds seminars, events, and symposiums to discuss the interaction among humans, animals, and the environment. The University of Queensland Veterinary Students' Association (UQVSA) also participates in owning an active OH initiative to spread the news of One Health, One World, and One Medicine among veterinary students [119].

4.4.13 Lessons Learned and Key Takeaways

Numerous initiatives must be initiated to educate students, researchers and communities about their significance of OH and OH education. Veterinary schools in high-income regions have more OH initiatives than those in low-resource countries. The majority of OH initiatives focus on postgraduate programs, conferences, and workshops, necessitating the need to include OH in the curriculum of veterinary and other related students [36–39].

4.5 Fostering Interdisciplinary Learning Environments

4.5.1 Building Collaborative Partnerships

The realm of healthcare collaboration includes a range of terms, such as partnerships, coalitions, alliances, networks, interorganizational relationships, collaborative advocacy, and task forces [120]. The concept of intersectoral collaboration was originally introduced at the Alma-Ata conference by the WHO on primary health care in 1978 [121]. It is essential to establish collaborative partnerships between veterinary and related health and environmental institutes to adopt a comprehensive approach to health management [122, 123]. There are a total of 604 groups and organizations recognized globally for their contributions to advancing One Health. This includes 227 academic entities, 94 governmental bodies, 13 intergovernmental organizations, 235 nonprofit organizations, and 34 for-profit private organizations (Figure 4.4) [124].

The disease triangle illustrates the dynamics between pathogens, hosts, and the environment [125]. Animals such as humans and domestic, pet, and wild animals are crucial hosts facilitating the transmission of diseases between animals and humans [126, 127]. A deep understanding of pathogens and their interactions within the host and environment is fundamental for the effective control of pathogen generation, disease pathogenicity, and disease spread [127, 128]. Therefore, it is vital to foster strong partnerships, collaboration, and collective efforts to manage diseases affecting humans, animals, and wildlife.

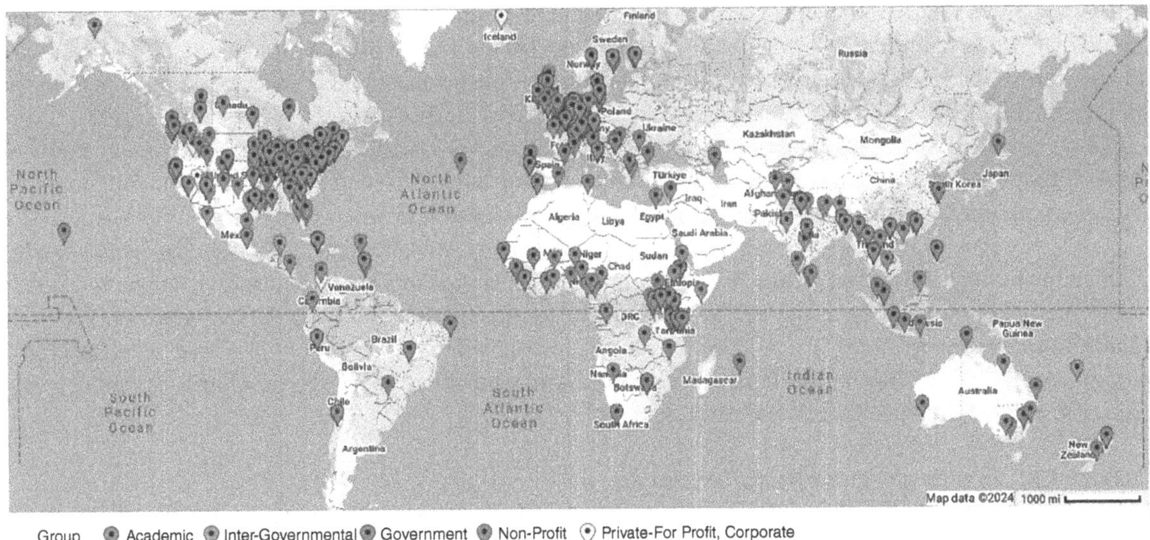

The map was created by the One Health Commission from 2014 to 2024 (www.onehealthcommission.org/) and is included in the chapter with official permission. It can be found at https://tinyurl.com/OHC-WW.

Figure 4.4 Global map of organizations recognized for promoting One Health initiatives [125]. Republished with official permission from the One Health Commission.

The veterinary profession addresses pathogens and the animals they regularly interact with, including pets, companion animals, and animals used for food and other daily necessities [129, 130]. Therefore, establishing robust collaboration between medical schools and other institutions involved in disease prevention, control, and eradication is crucial [131]. Establishing solid connections between veterinary and medical schools might include linking students and faculty from various departments through combined degree programs; interdisciplinary gatherings (such as those involving medical, veterinary, and PH schools); case studies based on real-life scenarios; and opportunities for research or practical training exchanges [5, 132]. It also includes the use of resources such as data, staff, and facilities from the animal and environmental sectors (and vice versa) to improve monitoring, implementation, and capacity for handling sudden outbreaks. Additionally, organizing diverse training, research, and practice projects to evaluate and address the need for better health status, especially at the local level, is crucial in collaboration between veterinary and medical schools [133]. Identifying critical skills for healthcare workers and possibilities for practical training, such as interdisciplinary problem-solving methods, is vital to establishing robust partnerships across medical disciplines [134].

4.5.1.1 Partnership with Medical Schools

Collaboration between veterinary and medical schools is equally vital for promoting an integrated perspective of health system management [135]. Both fields can synergize resources, information, and techniques to collaboratively design a comprehensive disease control strategy that could benefit both human and animal populations [133]. The establishment of partnerships between veterinary and medical schools may support collaborative research, education, and training opportunities; shared resources; and community engagement in novel ways [133].

A variety of collaborative initiatives between veterinary and medical schools are present in different regions worldwide [136]. Beginning in 2023, Bethany College and St. George's University (SGU) in Grenada, West Indies announced a groundbreaking partnership to create pathways for careers in medicine or veterinary science.

Another example comes from the UC Davis, where a solid collaboration between the UC Davis Veterinary School and the UC Davis Medical School was formed around the creation of an integrated institute for OH focused on addressing disease problems occurring at the animal, human, and environmental interfaces [123]. They were also partners in the PREDICT project, which oversees potential zoonotic disease outbreaks worldwide [137].

The vet school and medical school at the University of Pennsylvania established a close collaboration, partnering through the Penn Vet Working Dog Centre to research working dog health and performance and initiating a One Health communication effort to encourage interdisciplinary research in veterinary and medical sciences [138]. Similarly, at Cornell University, the Cornell College of Veterinary Medicine and Weill Medical School created a partnership through the Cornell Feline Health Center and the Institute for Host-Microbe Interactions and Diseases [139]. This pattern of collaboration is also observed at the University of Glasgow and the University of Wisconsin – Madison, among many others. The UTokyo in Japan, Chulalongkorn University in Thailand, the University of Hong Kong, Kasetsart University in Thailand, and other Asian institutions have also developed successful partnerships between veterinary schools and medical schools.

4.5.1.2 Collaboration with Public Health Institutions

The OH Initiative, established in 2006, encourages cooperation among doctors, veterinarians, animal scientists, health policy experts, and environmental and ecological scientists, aiming to increase overall well-being through a multidisciplinary approach. Considering the concept of OH, one must acknowledge that the well-being of humans, animals, and the environment is interconnected and impacts health and disease. Respected institutions such as the American Medical Association (AMA), the American Veterinary Medical Association (AVMA), and the CDC support this approach [140]. The medical and veterinary professions are aligned in promoting collaboration between medical and veterinary schools. Jasani's research in India revealed that 73% of respondents personally identified with the OH concept, 82% believed it should be integrated into medical education and training, and 60% expressed their intention to apply OH principles in their medical practice. Therefore, it is essential to foster partnerships between veterinary schools and PH organizations.

Approximately 60% of new or emerging infectious diseases are zoonotic and are transmitted from animals to humans [141]. This spread can occur through contact with animals, the consumption of animal-based food, owning pets, or other activities involving animals [121, 142]. However, a comprehensive understanding is needed for a veterinarian to effectively prevent these zoonotic diseases and their impact on animals. Veterinarians need to comprehend these diseases from a human standpoint to achieve a country's health prevention objectives successfully [136].

Access to applied research, innovative medical techniques, and a better understanding of PH issues can be achieved through improved collaboration between veterinary schools and PH institutes. Collaborative actions may encompass shared training, seminars, internships for veterinary students in PH facilities, cooperative field monitoring of PH conditions, and the distribution of PH communications via veterinary channels.

Successful partnerships between veterinary schools and PH institutes have been established globally. For example, at UC Davis, collaboration occurs between the School of Veterinary Medicine and the Department of Public Health through the Californian Animal Health and Food Safety Laboratory System. In Scotland, the University of Glasgow's School of Veterinary Medicine collaborates with Public Health Scotland, focusing on interdisciplinary research regarding the epidemiology of PH diseases. Similar partnerships can be found at numerous other universities around the world, such as the UMN, the University of Sydney, the UoN, the UP, Makerere University in Uganda, and CVASU in Bangladesh.

In Asia, partnerships exist between veterinary schools and PH institutes at educational institutions such as the UTokyo in Japan, Mahidol University in Thailand, the University of Hong Kong, Chulalongkorn University in Thailand, Gadjah Mada University in Indonesia, the University of the Philippines, the Chinese University of Hong Kong, Seoul National University in South Korea, and Punjab Agricultural University in India.

While collaborations between veterinary schools and PH institutes exist worldwide, there is a need for more institutional and practical cooperation, along with effective research and infrastructure facilities, to strengthen the concept of OH through veterinary schools [143, 144].

4.5.1.3 Collaboration with Environmental Science Institutions

The epidemiology of diseases is significantly influenced by the coexistence of hosts and pathogens within their environment [145]. Deforestation and other human activities that impact the environment are associated with the rise of infectious diseases [140]. A comprehensive understanding of the environmental factors related to diseases is essential for successful disease investigations [146]. However, factors involved in the combination of animal and human health must be thoroughly understood and addressed in disease prevention strategies. The OH approach necessitates rigorous scrutiny of environmental health and analysis of environmental factors in disease epidemiology. The government and nongovernment authorities responsible for environmental conservation and management are potential sources of solutions for the environmental drivers of diseases [147]. For example, professionals from the Department of Environment and Department of Wildlife, who are directly involved in managing human–animal interactions and wildlife crimes, often encounter unknown zoonotic pathogens originating from the environment and wildlife [148]. Therefore, experiences must be considered when diagnosing diseases in the veterinary and medical science sectors. Given the limited resources in medical and veterinary schools, environmental professionals could play a role in disease control processes by caring for the environmental factors involved in disease emergence. Climate change, deforestation, wildlife trafficking, and other wildlife-related issues may create intricate interactions, requiring environmental professionals to work with professionals from veterinary and medical schools. Successful examples of the integration of environmentalists into VEs and veterinarians into environmental departments exist in the OH consortium in Bangladesh, although extensive movement is needed. However, incorporating environmental issues in the VE system would help develop a collaborative mindset among the professionals of veterinary schools and environmental science institutes. Therefore, enriching the VE system with a stronger focus on environmental, wildlife, and ecological issues related to zoonoses and OH implications is crucial.

4.5.2 Creating Interdisciplinary Courses and Modules

Interdisciplinary subject areas in the curriculum would also be helpful for producing health professionals with composite competencies who can take care of both animal and human problems [149]. Those courses should address health challenges, prevention approaches, and interdisciplinary research themes, including human medical and veterinary medical schools [45, 149]. There are several examples of combined veterinary and medical science courses around the world [129, 149]. For medical and veterinary students, the University of California at Davis offers an interdisciplinary OH Minor in collaboration with studies from both schools. This minor includes zoonoses, animals, the environment, and PH.

In this way, the University of Pennsylvania implemented an OH certificate program that delivers modules on emerging infectious diseases, epidemiology, and comparative medicine to students from veterinary and medical faculties. Moreover, Cornell University designed an interdisciplinary OH course that includes the topics of zoonotic diseases, wildlife health, and GH changes for students in veterinary and medical faculties. In turn, the University of Glasgow provides the OH MSc program, which combines veterinary and medical sciences in infectious disease epidemiology, environmental health, and health policy. Other examples include the DVM/MPH dual degree program at Tufts University, the interdisciplinary OH seminar at the UMN, the comparative pathology-intercalated BSc at the RVC, UK, the OH Modules at the University of Hong Kong, a Master's program in OH at Mahidol University, Thailand, the course of OH at Gadjah Mada University, Indonesia, the course of OH and Zoonoses at Seoul National University, South Korea, and an elective course of OH at the Chinese University of Hong Kong.

These courses cover animal, human, and environmental health issues; disease epidemiology; and disease control mechanisms. To advance the field of OH further, it would be beneficial to develop similar courses tailored to specific geographical needs.

4.5.3 Utilizing Problem-based Learning

PBL was first introduced in 1969 at the medical school of McMaster University in Canada [150]. PBL entails cooperative learning, allowing students to acquire new skills through case-based scenarios, making it a successful method for teaching in small groups [151]. Previously, most medical teaching methods focused on theory-based traditional teaching approaches [152]. However, theoretical teaching methods may not equip students with the necessary skills and understanding to address real-life situations presented in a case [153, 154]. Consequently, PBL is widely acknowledged as one of the most effective methods for medical teaching [155]. Nonetheless, the perception of PBL among faculty is likely influenced by how it is implemented at their institution, which may not always be positive [156].

The implementation of PBL in veterinary schools can be a great example of a one-health approach. By introducing group-based learning in VE, OH can be better promoted [144]. Specifically, at the Faculty of Veterinary Medicine at University College Dublin in Ireland, information is shared with the group, such as real-life scenarios, highlighting the patient's history and clinical signs [156]. Students are then required to collaborate, leveraging their knowledge to create a list of learning issues relevant to the case as part of the team-building process [156].

To address more than 60% of zoonotic diseases that involve common host–pathogen interactions between animals and humans, PBL could be integrated into veterinary schools. Collaborating between veterinary and medical schools to share unique cases in real time could establish a common platform for fostering PBL in an interdisciplinary teaching environment [136]. In the VE system, PBL could be one of the most effective approaches for investigating outbreaks of emerging and reemerging infectious diseases worldwide. Therefore, incorporating PBL in veterinary teaching methods implies advancing the OH approach in the VE system. However, the challenge associated with PBL is that once the methods or curriculum have been developed, most faculty may not be inclined to switch to new methods rather than traditional teaching approaches.

The implementation of PBL in veterinary schools presents challenges; however, the UC Davis School of Veterinary Medicine (USA), the University of Glasgow School of Veterinary Medicine (UK), the University of Sydney Faculty of Veterinary Science (Australia), the Ontario Veterinary College at the University of Guelph (Canada), the RVC, University of London (UK), the University of Melbourne Faculty of Veterinary and Agricultural Sciences (Australia), the Cornell University College of Veterinary Medicine (USA), the Utrecht University Faculty of Veterinary Medicine (Netherlands), the University of Edinburgh Royal (Dick) School of Veterinary Studies (UK), Murdoch University College of Veterinary Medicine (Australia), and CVASU (Bangladesh) have successfully implemented PBL in VE.

4.5.4 Incorporating Fieldwork and Practical Experiences

Collaboration between veterinary schools and medical schools to incorporate fieldwork is inevitable to encourage a mutual learning process in the OH approach [157]. Although all veterinary and medical schools offer internships for hands-on experience through fieldwork, the current practice involves sending vet school graduates to animal care environments such as poultry farms, pet clinics, districts, or subdistrict-level veterinary hospitals. Conversely, medical school internships and field work mainly occur in on-campus medical hospitals. Combining these practices would allow students from both types of schools to gain exposure to each other's field stations and hospitals and become familiar with both medical facilities to address infectious diseases and prevent the epidemiology of infectious diseases [144].

Maintaining joint fieldwork between veterinary and medical schools has proven to be effective in prestigious institutions worldwide [132]. Examples include the National Institutes of Health (NIH) Comparative Biomedical Scientist Training Program in the United States, the Comparative Medicine Program at Johns Hopkins University School of Medicine in the United States, joint programs at the University of Pennsylvania School of Veterinary Medicine and Perelman School of Medicine in the United States, collaborative research projects between the University of Cambridge Department of Veterinary Medicine and School of Clinical Medicine in the UK, the joint efforts of the UTokyo Graduate School of Agricultural and Life Sciences and Graduate School of Medicine in Japan, collaborative initiatives between the National University of Singapore Yong Loo Lin School of Medicine and Faculty of Science in Singapore, joint efforts of the Chinese University of Hong Kong Faculty of Medicine and Jockey Club College of Veterinary Medicine and Life Sciences in Hong Kong, and collaborative work between the Chulalongkorn University Faculty of Veterinary Science and the Faculty of Medicine in Thailand.

Notably, during the COVID-19 surge in Bangladesh, students and faculty from CVASU provided diagnostic support to Chandpur Medical College and Jamalpur Medical College, demonstrating a successful joint effort to address the pandemic. However, it is crucial to identify opportunities for collaborative work, nurture effective leadership with a collaborative mindset, and assess each discipline to develop a cooperative field and research work in veterinary science academic programs, thus promoting a comprehensive "OH" approach.

4.5.5 Promoting Cross-disciplinary Research Projects

Joint research involving veterinary and medical schools is crucial for exploring PH issues [158]. More than 60% of infectious diseases are zoonotic and require a collaborative effort to address them. Importantly, almost 75% of infectious zoonotic diseases originate from wildlife [126]. While our focus is on benefiting humans, we must also consider the well-being of other animals. Therefore, understanding the cross-host transmission, disease epidemiology, and host-specific prevention and control mechanisms is essential.

As veterinarians deal with all animals other than humans, human doctors require their support to understand zoonotic diseases [159]. Similarly, veterinarians need to understand how these diseases can spread to humans to prevent potential zoonosis [129]. Managing wildlife and their habitats is critical in combating 75% of zoonotic diseases originating from wildlife, necessitating the involvement of wildlife, the environment, and forest professionals in research related to zoonosis under the "OH" approach [160].

To facilitate interdisciplinary research targeting "OH," joint research wings could be established in veterinary schools, involving experts from medical schools, veterinary schools, and wildlife and environment sectors [144, 161]. This could be done through a separate research institute or an applied research center under veterinary faculties or postgraduate subjects incorporating research, medicine, and surveillance techniques from veterinary science, medical science, conservation biology, and environmental science. For example, the Coastal Biodiversity, Marine Fisheries, and Wildlife Research Centre at CVASU in Bangladesh is exploring multisubject-related research initiatives.

Efforts such as the "Strategies to Prevent (STOP) Spillover," a US$100 million USAID-funded project in seven countries, are excellent examples of global interdisciplinary research and action initiatives in OH. Interdisciplinary research on OH initiatives can focus on AMR, wildlife conservation, human health, climate change and PH, food safety and PH, wildlife–human interactions and PH, and deforestation and PH [158, 162, 163].

Veterinary schools can further promote these efforts through research projects. Funding and capacity support from state governments, corporate organizations, and international development partners should also be harnessed to promote joint interdisciplinary research in OH. The USAID GH-related security programs are leading examples of global zoonotic disease surveillance and one-health training for humans, veterinary schools, medical professionals, and wildlife conservationists. These are exemplary projects and thus provide a model for other donor organizations that wish to stimulate collaborative, interdisciplinary research through veterinary schools in the OH realm.

4.5.6 Enhancing Communication and Leadership Skills

The development of a robust communication system, which is the cornerstone for successful collaboration between health (animal, human, and environmental) professionals using the OH approach, is necessary. Veterinary schools are also essential for educating OH leaders in the interdisciplinary education and leadership skills necessary to address complex GH threats [164]. For this reason, veterinary schools need to advance in delivering these traits, including communication and leadership skills, in this professional area. It is possible to do this through joint research publications, a unified message system, and a communication protocol between Colleges of Veterinary Medicine (CVMs), medical institutes, environmental institutions, and others. Communication and leadership can also be accomplished by establishing an intersectoral rapid response team for outbreak investigations, including members from veterinary schools, medical schools, and other health professionals [165].

Leadership training for veterinary professionals must provide them with appropriate knowledge in relevant fields and a background to address interdisciplinary problems related to PH. The veterinary curriculum must encode PBL and interdisciplinary field investigation strategies to familiarize individuals with health communication and stakeholder coordination [166]. Moreover, organizing shared seminars, workshops, or conferences may inspire veterinarians to take the initiative in managing health concerns related to their field. Regular bulletins and innovative idea generation on OH issues, or OH issues related to presentations and implementation, are other strategies used successfully to develop leadership skills within the VE system. There are many global initiatives that reveal what is being done and move into the leadership of OH. One such intervention is the Pandemic Prevention Leadership Initiative in LAO PDR by the Wildlife Conservation Society as a model for Developing Adaptive Resilience and Sustainability for Integration (DARSI) deployments and one of its flagship programs focused on catalyzing interdisciplinary leadership across borders around zoonotic research, advocacy, and prevention aimed at bolstering regional capacity building within Southeast Asia. As a result, programs such as these could also be initiated in veterinary schools across the globe to better train future veterinarians in leadership roles within the OH sector.

4.6 Building Institutional Capacity

Owing to its increasing global impact in tackling PH challenges, attempts to develop capacity in OH involve the integration of its principles into VE at a global scale [167]. In fact, as an integral component of the veterinary curricular development core competencies, OH concepts are included [168]. The goal is to develop veterinary professionals with interdisciplinary skills and improve their ability to manage the challenges of GH [169, 170]. OH, integration into veterinary curricula requires a multisystem approach involving multisectoral training, practical learning opportunities, and curriculum restructuring. Advocacies for the inclusion of OH and GH as improvements in the existing VME have increased in recent years [171].

4.6.1 Faculty Training and Development

To accomplish the aim of OH, emerging veterinarians across the globe must be trained in diverse specialties, such as PH, epidemiology, anthropology, microbiology, and environmental health sciences [172]. Therefore, academic staff members in veterinary institutions must undergo relevant training programs to enable them to impart comprehensive OH education to their students. Faculty training and development programs can enhance the knowledge of tutors and keep them abreast of new ideas around the OH concept [173, 174]. The effective incorporation of the principles of OH into the global VE (GVE) curriculum hinges on "Training the Trainers."

In addition, it ensures the smooth introduction of OH subjects and modules by veterinary educators in the Veterinary Educational Establishments (VEEs). Different VEEs have implemented different methods to train faculty members effectively for this purpose [175]. The most effective approach was through regular participation in organized online courses, webinars, conferences, seminars, and workshops focused on OH. Faculty exchange programs to enhance [176] best practices in OH can also be introduced through joint international collaborative training [177]. Some of these initiatives are successful in many application contexts.

The UC Davis, in the United States trained its faculty members on OH teaching to students via a collaborative interdisciplinary approach [176, 178]. The RVC was able to develop a comprehensive OH curriculum through interdisciplinary faculty and research initiatives in the UK [179]. The University of Edinburgh, in its GH Program, offers courses and research projects spread across various disciplines [180]. Similarly, the Malaysia One Health University Network Faculty training program, which is an OH University Network in Malaysia, has increased knowledge and awareness of OH among medical and veterinary faculty members [181].

In addition to these specific examples, there are continental-based programs aimed at developing and training faculty members. In Europe, the Veterinary Continuous Education in Europe (VetCEE) program has enabled veterinary lecturers to incorporate OH concepts into their lecture schedules through CE and the development opportunities it provides for them [182]. The European One Health Training Program (EUOHM) also offers workshops and seminars aimed at enhancing the capabilities of educators in veterinary and PH institutions across the continent [183].

At least some institutions with veterinary degree programs have partnered with government agencies such as the US CDC on the development of in-depth OH curricula, including faculty training programs and professional partnerships [184]. The Afrique One-ASPIRE program also exhibited a commitment to capacity building in the context of OH through an interdisciplinary nexus, as it provided training for faculty from multiple African countries [185].

As part of the holistic capacity development of faculties, each university's veterinary school should consider establishing an Institutional Quality Assurance Capacity (IQAC) unit. This unit could be responsible for training both incoming and existing faculties in various aspects of OH throughout their teaching careers. Additionally, the IQAC could serve as a knowledge hub within the institution, facilitating the gathering and sharing of global OH knowledge with local veterinary faculties and students.

4.6.2 Infrastructure and Resource Allocation

As part of building capacity, infrastructure development and resource distribution are needed for the successful introduction of OH into GVEs [186, 187]. A well-equipped infrastructure aligned with appropriate available resources should be developed to support the implementation of OH education in the veterinary curriculum. The availability of state-of-the-art laboratories and research facilities will provide veterinary students with hands-on experience critical for learning OH [170]. OH should be a critical component of regional and global veterinary curricula with appropriate support from institutions and government agencies.

For example, Institutional Chinese laboratories and research facilities provide students with practical training in zoonotic diseases in advanced OH laboratories [188]. Africa One Health University Network (AFROHUN), an OH African Network, also supports student training by improving infrastructure and resources for instruction in sub-Saharan Africa [189]. Their Veterinary Innovation Partnership developed a cutting-edge simulation center at Cornell University to immerse students in realistic OH scenarios [190]. The Australian Animal Health Laboratory (AAHL) is also an excellent example of the OH research infrastructure in Australia that is committed to studying zoonotic diseases and developing control strategies using advanced diagnostic and research platforms [110]. Asia's Global Hubs for OH research include the International Livestock Research Institute (ILRI), an organization aimed at using the OH approach to improve the livestock sector for performance and sustainability [191, 192]. A comparable One Health Centre with contemporary infrastructure supporting multiple research and education also operates at the Brazilian University of Sao Paulo [193].

To ensure the effective allocation of infrastructure and resources for OH capacity building, institutions must partner with the private and public sectors to significantly invest in building and maintaining modern research facilities and developing digital infrastructure. This will increase the reach and impact of OH in GVE programs.

4.6.3 Policy and Institutional Support

In Europe, the European Union (EU)'s Horizon 2020 program, through policy, successfully implemented funding for numerous projects that support the integration of OH principles in veterinary schools [175]. Australian veterinary schools also enjoy institutional support policies that help develop comprehensive OH curricula [194, 195]. The Pan American Health Organization (PAHO) also developed policies that encourage the integration of OH into veterinary and PH education to ensure a coordinated approach to zoonoses in Latin America [196].

In Canada, comprehensive policies on OH implementation were prepared through a broad stakeholder involvement process in combination with the National Microbiology Lab [197]. Pathak et al. [198] explored the Indian Council of Agricultural Research (ICAR), which also introduced measures for stimulating OH research and education that focused on combining the capabilities of veterinary and PH institutions. The establishment of OH offices within academic schools or universities is an outcome of the policy framework developed by the German OH Initiative, which is responsible for transparency in planning, implementing, and nurturing transdisciplinary collaboration among various faculties [199, 200].

4.6.4 Funding and Sustainability

Continued funding is imperative to the future of OH integration within GVE [201]. It allows VEEs to provide appropriate infrastructure, improve research, and deliver high-quality education. Laing et al. [202] even opined that OH research and education are only sustainable if they are funded. However, obtaining funding represents a significant obstacle to the implementation of OH in veterinary school curricula [203].

Various funding mechanisms have been adopted worldwide to solve this issue. In Canada, for example, the government and private sector, through partnership funding, have successfully collaborated to support some health professional training [204]. Multiyear major funding grants from external development banks such as the World Bank across Southeast Asia have supported OH in VE [205]. In a similar report by Stroud et al. [206], the NIH and the CDC have generously funded OH research, supporting integrated curricula and scientific resources across the United States.

VEEs in low- and middle-income settings need to allocate funds for OH educational programs as well, given the large financial backing already from the government(s) or nongovernmental organizations (NGOs). Importantly, OH educational programs need continuous funding to achieve global sustainability. Additionally, globally, USAID has been funding the strengthening of the OH system through its GH security program [207].

4.7 Research and Innovation in One Health

4.7.1 Promoting Interdisciplinary Research

Encouraging interdisciplinary studies serves as the bedrock in moving OH's agenda forward. As stated before, OH is based on the participation of experts from different areas, such as veterinary and human medicine, environmental sciences, and social sciences [208], to solve emerging health challenges that no longer fit into the recognized disciplinary categories.

The Southern African Centre for Infectious Disease Surveillance (SACIDS) integrated veterinary and human medical expertise to improve disease surveillance and control in the southern region of Africa [209, 210]. Interdisciplinary collaborations among veterinary, medical, and environmental scientists, catalyzed by the LSHTM, have made substantial contributions to understanding zoonotic diseases in the UK [211]. Additionally, India has used the interdisciplinary nature of science to address complicated health challenges through the joint efforts of experts from different fields [212]. Similarly, the Eco-Health Alliance in the United States conducted interdisciplinary research on the wildlife-ecosystem relationship and human health [213].

4.7.2 Innovative Research Methodologies

Innovative research methodologies are also needed to advance OH. These are required to provide previous approaches or strategies for disease prevention and control with deeper insights into complex health challenges [214, 215]. The integration of OH into VE will be improved by applying these cutting-edge research methodologies. While any point-in-time example is essential, these include the use of simulators and video games for surgical tasks. In addition, the use of live animals has also been omitted entirely in line with OHs' principles, which favor humane and eco-friendly learning methods [216]. Educational platforms need to be developed to encourage experiential learning of OH principles through the practical application of relevant methodologies [190]. This comprises the inclusion of effective OH programs in preclinical and clinical curricula.

One example is the use of genomic sequencing and big data analytics to follow spillover zoonotic transmission events in South Korea, providing information on disease dynamics as well as informing PH responses [217, 218]. In Brazil, the use of ecological modeling techniques by the Oswaldo Cruz Foundation to study vector-borne diseases has significantly improved the understanding and control of diseases such as dengue and Zika [219]. In the United States, the application of metagenomics and advanced diagnostic tools has revolutionized the detection and surveillance of zoonotic pathogens, thereby encouraging early intervention and control measures [220]. Japanese researchers are leveraging artificial intelligence and machine learning to analyze large datasets for the prediction and modeling of zoonotic diseases. Another example is the use of genomic sequencing by the OH Research Team of the University of Edinburgh, UK, to monitor AMR genes at the human–animal–environment interface. In Australia, the use of drones with sensors and cameras was pioneered to support wildlife disease surveillance [221–225].

4.7.3 Case Studies of Impactful One Health Research

Case studies of impactful OH research provide lessons from the past and demonstrate the effectiveness of the OH approach. These case studies demonstrate how OH integration can influence the next generation of veterinarians to become change agents in GH.

Several reports have demonstrated the success of using OH research to combat GH events. One such method was the early detection of the Hendra virus in Australia, which led to the development of horse vaccines [226, 227]. The collaborative efforts between veterinary schools and several medical schools under the One Health East African Research Training (OHEART) program addressed the prevention, treatment, and control of zoonoses such as Rift Valley fever and Brucellosis in Kenya [228]. In addition, the multidisciplinary response of medical (human and veterinary) professionals and environmental scientists helped contain the Ebola outbreak in the West African region in 2014 [229, 230].

Many veterinary institutions have adopted different initiatives to incorporate OH strategies into their training programs to ensure that OH principles are well mastered by students. An example is the PH intervention and practical field research programs offered through integrated OH concepts in the veterinary curriculum by the University of Melbourne in Australia [231]. Purdue University in the United States recognized the role of veterinary medical institutions in shaping their students to be prepared for diverse health opportunities and challenges outside the world. The College of Veterinary Medicine of the institution, therefore, consciously introduced the OH approach to producing global veterinarians with collaborative potential [232]. Studies have also shown that educational programs focused on OH can significantly impact students' attitudes toward AMR and antibiotic therapy, emphasizing the importance of incorporating OH principles into veterinary curricula [233]. Similar to the OHEART initiative, a more specific OHCEA exists in Rwanda, which, with support from USAID, formed a network between veterinary and PH schools to build professionals with multidisciplinary skills in response to disease outbreaks [170].

These findings are evidence of the importance of previous OH engagements in different claims of society and educational institutes. Despite these benefits, a recent study revealed that a high percentage of veterinarians and their medical counterparts have not received appropriate training on OH principles [234]. This limited the application of this approach in their practices. Therefore, there is a need to integrate OH at the grassroots level of training young veterinarians to achieve more robust results, with a primary focus on reducing GH challenges through VE.

4.8 Global Perspectives on One Health Education

4.8.1 Regional Case Studies: Africa, Asia, Europe, and the Americas

There are a significant number of case studies that incorporate OH into veterinary studies. In Asia, numerous regional milestones highlight the importance of OH principles and the urgency of implementing them. Initiatives in India are centered on incorporating OH into the medical and VE curricula. Institutions such as the ICAR encourage research and training that spans multiple disciplines to combat zoonotic diseases such as AI and rabies. Even as early as 2021, they took the initiative to establish an OH consortium, which brought together 27 different organizations working on human, animal, and wildlife health issues. It is believed that the consortium would be able to provide the opportunity for specialists working in the disciplines of human, animal, and wildlife health to begin working together across disciplinary lines. Their consortium support includes joint investigations of diseases at the field and laboratory levels, early warning of zoonotic diseases to respective authorities, and holistic responses to any outbreak. In addition to establishing a laboratory network at both the centrally managed and field levels, this collaboration aims to enhance preparedness against disease outbreaks and strengthen the health system [120]. Countries such as Thailand and Vietnam prioritize OH in controlling diseases such as dengue fever and foodborne diseases [235]. Moreover, Bangladesh and Nepal emphasize community engagement and awareness in OH practices, especially in improving the existing knowledge and practices of local-level service providers in controlling zoonoses. In Bangladesh, initiatives are being implemented to educate farmers and healthcare workers on safe livestock farming and disease prevention. Both initiatives highlight the importance of targeted communication interventions to bridge the gap between perceptions and practices in farming communities [236].

Furthermore, case studies from Africa also demonstrated the effectiveness of bottom-up approaches. These include the community people in enhancing pandemic preparedness, which provides valuable policy lessons for the Global North [237]. However, an in-depth review of OH governance in 146 countries worldwide revealed notable variations in governance capacity, demonstrating the need for enhanced governance models and immediate measures to address regional gaps in governance effectiveness [238].

OH, has seen increasing popularity across the Americas in recent years, leading funding for educational and research initiatives to expand quickly [239]. Other activities to foster OH include certificate programs and online courses. Several studies have also revealed an alarming trend in which individuals flag themselves as having experience in a case under the umbrella of OH without even full knowledge of what it means. However, there is a need to build capacity and consider ethical dimensions in delivering OH approaches in Latin America. This highlights the necessity of practicing and sustaining this concept in this region. In a different case, during an investigation of an animal disease outbreak in Ethiopia, community engagement and partnership were considered integral parts of such incidents. However, this research also revealed deficiencies in policies concerning ethical issues during AH emergencies. This underscores the need for ethical standards and policies around OH research ethics in Africa, which should be improved capacity wise to make more informed ethical decisions. The research team, composed of scholars from several regions, also raised awareness about the need to act on interventions required for OH ethics policy recommendations [240].

Conversely, when searching with the search phrase "OH" in connection to Denmark, only a few references were shown among connecting scientific papers and those that did show connections. The results of using this keyword provided a relatively small number of articles, many of which were not directly related to OH. The realization of this limit surfaced when many publications were retrieved. This limited finding encompasses the lack of publications and documentation in this section, which implies further documentation and enhanced research as well as publication under OH, as well as incorporating that into many more institutions [241].

4.8.2 Adapting One Health Education to Local Contexts

In this context, integrating OH at different educational levels is crucial if a future workforce for OH is to be created. A few universities in Bangladesh, such as CVASU, Sher-e-Bangla Agricultural University (SAU), and Sylhet Agricultural University (SyAU), have incorporated studying theory into their relevant courses at the undergraduate level. Furthermore, specialized postgraduate-level higher degree programs in OH are currently being implemented in the South Asian Association for Regional Cooperation (SAARC) region. For example, the Centre for OH Education, Advocacy, and Research Training Programs by Kerala University in India and an established Master of Applied Epidemiology Program in Sri Lanka have gained attention [242]. The Academic Institutions of CVASU and SAU in Bangladesh have implemented master's programs for veterinary students in epidemiology, PH, and OH. The National Institute of Preventive and Social Medicine is another PH institution in Bangladesh that offers a master's program in epidemiology.

Thus, in 2017, Bangladesh successfully developed the OH Institute within CVASU with aspirations for an interdisciplinary postgraduate training program. Nevertheless, their current partnership remains narrow, akin to PH. Hence, the intentional deployment of the OH concept in educational systems is essential. CVASU has also established the Coastal Biodiversity, Marine Fisheries, and Wildlife Research Centre to promote interdisciplinary research in OH at the local level. Thailand and Vietnam are perfect examples of this kind of OH strategy. Chatterjee et al. [243] conducted a research-based, thematic analysis regarding incorporating OH into the existing curricula for human health and veterinary students in Vietnam and Thailand. This study also revealed that the OH concept had already been successfully implemented as an educational module in Vietnam. Moreover, Thailand took a different approach by using more flexible term-curricular adaptation to fit into the designed target groups. This includes shorter or more intense field-level in-service programs, including graduate students and full-time participants.

The United States has recently started to address the building of its OH human resources by integrating this concept into undergraduate and graduate-level courses. For example, the University of Alaska Fairbank, Netherlands, offered through the OH Master's Program, has various educational curricula designed to teach all related aspects of OH comprehensively. The University of Arizona offers a master's degree program in the OH Program on human, animal, and environmental health. The Auburn University College of Veterinary Medicine also offers public and OH programs at the intersection between AH and human diseases. The University of Washington gives a graduate certificate in the integrated PH. At the same time, they provide cooperative field training so that an OH workforce can compare favorably with all other workforces in the future.

4.8.3 International Collaboration and Exchange Programs

For OH initiatives to advance, international cooperation is fundamental. Cooperative efforts and knowledge sharing, with enhanced capacity building across international frontiers. Since there are no borders to the spread of zoonotic infections, prevention detection and response are essential. Many interesting projects have emerged in recent years from around the world.

The Dutch National Institute for Public Health and the Environment (RIVM) works closely together with institutions in other countries and has agreed on ways to cooperate with the European Food Safety Authority. They also have open lines of communication that can be used at any time for serious health threats. The RIVM aims to promote social health, which ensures a robust environment that future generations will love. In addition to performing independent scientific research, RIVM works with important partners to identify the right kind of research to be conducted and inform results for future reference by the government, professionals, or the public.

Moreover, RIVM is also committed to maintaining a healthy living environment and protecting health in society. They also work closely with different Dutch institutes to prepare the nation for emerging zoonoses and AMR [244].

In Europe, the One Health European Joint Program (OHEJP) was organized to stimulate collaboration and address key zoonotic foodborne infections, AMR, and emerging microbiological hazards. The program started in January 2018 and ended on the last day of 2022. RIVM was also closely involved. The One Health EJP plans to establish a permanent European One-Health infrastructure by linking and synchronizing health institutes for humans, animals, and food. This was achieved through joint programming of research agendas that addressed the requirements of national policymakers and stakeholders. This initiative included 38 highly regarded food, veterinary, and medical laboratories and institutes from 19 European Member States and the Med-Vet-Net Association. Each participating country included a reference laboratory from the PH sector and another from the food/veterinary sector. Some organizations from the Netherlands included Wageningen Bioveterinary Research WUR, the Netherlands Centre for One Health (NCOH), and RIVM [244].

Moreover, the African CDC adopted a transdisciplinary approach to create safer and healthier Africa for humans, animals, plants, and their shared environment, which was established in 2028. To address the health risks that affect overall well-being at the human–animal–environment interface, they introduced a plan called "Agenda 2063: Africa We Want."

SEAOHUN and AFROHUN are two well-known names in the One Health University network. In 2011, SEAOHUN was established with the support of USAID and its OH Workforce project. The goal was to develop a skilled next-generation workforce in the field of OH. The development of this network is made possible by additional funding from the Korea International Cooperation Agency (KOICA) and the US Department of State (DOS) via the Lower Mekong Initiative (LMI). SEAOHUN has significantly increased its network membership, now consisting of over 112 universities across eight countries. This expansion includes the four founding countries of Indonesia, Malaysia, Thailand, and Vietnam, as well as Cambodia, Lao PDR, the Philippines, and Myanmar. By fostering connections among university members from various disciplines, their educational programs encourage collaboration on projects and activities across different countries. They have implemented various educational initiatives, such as creating an OH curriculum, PBL cases for teaching, evidence-based advocacy for OH research, student clubs dedicated to OH, and scholarship and fellowship programs [245].

Furthermore, owing to the assistance provided by USAID, AFROHUN was established. This achievement was made possible through the efforts of the leadership Initiative of Public Health in East Africa (LIPHEA) and the Health Alliance, led by Makerere University School of Public Health (MakSPH) in Uganda, in collaboration with Muhimbili University of Health and Allied Sciences (MUHAS), School of Public Health in Tanzania, since 2005. AFROHUN has successfully established collaborations with 10 countries and 27 institutions and has formed connections with 19 universities. Furthermore, this connection provides training to an impressive number of individuals, including 9837 students, 300 faculty members, and 286 professionals seeking in-service training [246].

4.9 Policy and Advocacy

4.9.1 Role of Veterinary Associations and Organizations

Through advocacy, education, research, and collaborative endeavors, veterinary organizations and associations play crucial roles in the promotion and implementation of policies pertaining to OH [247].

Veterinary associations play a significant role in the development of policies that are in line with the ideals of OH. These organizations push for rules and legislation that address issues that are at the intersection of human, animal, and environmental health by engaging with legislators and advocating for them. The AVMA, for example, often collaborates with both the federal government and state governments to formulate regulations that aim to limit the spread of zoonotic illnesses, improve the welfare of animals, and guarantee the safety of food [248].

Through its collaboration with the AMA, the American Public Health Association (APHA), the OH Commission, and various other veterinary associations, the AVMA has effectively led the OH strategy into the future. The AVMA has also played a significant role in the adoption of federal legislation about OH, and it will continue to make efforts to advance OH in addition to these other endeavors [249].

Additionally, veterinary associations encourage collaboration between veterinary and medical services to improve the efficiency and effectiveness of disaster response efforts. Farnham and Hueston [250] state that in addition to performing collaborative work, these organizations also play an important role in bringing issues related to OH to the attention of the public. Veterinary associations educate the public about the importance of integrated health approaches through campaigns, conferences, and publications. This contributes to the development of a society that is better informed, which in turn helps support and comprehend the necessity of OH efforts with greater understanding. One of the best examples is the International Veterinary Students Association (IVSA), which has connected almost 38,000 students from over seventy countries. The main goal of IVSA is to increase the overall standard of VE worldwide [251].

Veterinary organizations frequently take the initiative and provide financial support for research to bridge the gap between human, animal, and environmental health. In regard to advocating these joint research initiatives, these organizations play a significant role because they involve the participation of a wide range of professionals, including veterinarians, physicians, and environmental scientists. There are a few noteworthy collaborations that may be mentioned in relation to the research field. An example of this would be the One Heath Poultry Hub project, which receives funding from the Global Challenges Research Fund and is supported by the UK Research and Innovation. The program is a development research initiative that is driven by impact and is now operating in Bangladesh, India, Sri Lanka, and Vietnam. This is a true example of an interdisciplinary and intersectoral OH approach since it brings together leading laboratory, clinical, veterinary, and social scientists, as well as competent communications specialists, program support personnel, and external stakeholders. The purpose of this research is to investigate the reasons why certain behaviors and activities are adverse, as well as how the rapid expansion of poultry production increases the risk of infectious diseases. In addition, they are putting novel disease management initiatives through their paces as part of robust networks of local, regional, and international stakeholders [252].

One of the most important roles that veterinary associations play is to assist in the formation of partnerships with other health and environmental organizations. These partnerships facilitate the sharing of resources, the interchange of knowledge, and the coordination of responses to health concerns. In the same way that the WHO and the FAO work together to address GH concerns, the World Veterinary Association (WVA) partners with both organizations. Additionally, it acknowledges the contrasts and similarities between OH and other organizations, such as EcoHealth, Planetary Health, Population Health, Conservation Medicine, Oceans Health, and One Welfare. The WVA envisages all these organizations to be associated and interconnected [253]. The Quadripartite introduced the One Health Joint Plan of Action (OH JPA) in 2022 and was also endorsed by the WVA, as it concurs with the definition of One Health provided by the One Health High-Level Expert Panel (OHHLEP). Preparedness to address infectious and noninfectious diseases as well as other health threats, which includes the reduction of zoonotic disease spillover, must continue for veterinary associations that sustain veterinarians considering integrative, collaborative OH methods [254, 255]. It also promotes training and capacity-building, such as the establishment of OH centers of excellence that support public education, research, and training while fostering collaboration between local decision-makers, such as community leaders and policymakers, with respect to values.

Perhaps the best example of a veterinary association in support of OH advocacy is the Global Alliance for Rabies Control (GARC). The GARC was founded in 2007 and works together with the UK-based Alliance for Rabies Control (Alliance for Rabies Control, 2017). The partners of the GARC included the WHO, WOAH, FAO, CDC, and the United States, along with other vaccine manufacturers and NGOs, in 2008 [256]. Working with partner organizations, the GARC collaborates with veterinary organizations around the world to eliminate rabies through mass vaccination campaigns, educates PHs about prevention and offers technical support for policy changes. For example, the GARC established the Pan-African rabies control network in 2015 [257], which consists of 37 different nations. The network supports these countries in developing and implementing effective strategies to eliminate rabies, as well as tracking their progress toward elimination. They also support other networks relevant in terms of protection expertise, such as the Association of Southeast Asian Nations (ASEAN), which also has good capacity-building abilities [258]. This combined approach has already led to a marked decrease in the rabies burden in several regions.

At the local level, there are ample opportunities for veterinary associations and professional groups to contribute to policymaking. For example, in the Bangladesh Forest Department, only a few veterinary officers primarily oversee safe parks, despite the large number of animals requiring regular care and the need for a preventive diagnosis facility. The role of veterinary associations was not adequately considered in the department's restructuring and the inclusion of veterinarians in its operations. Similar situations exist in neighboring countries such as India, Nepal, Pakistan, Bhutan, and Myanmar. However, veterinary organizations must provide support at the local level to ensure the health of both the environment and wildlife, which may be challenging areas for these organizations to address.

4.9.2 Roles of Development Partners and Organizations

To address interconnected health concerns effectively, the contributions made by development partners are complex and crucial. OH programs receive substantial funding from organizations such as the World Bank, which are known for their contributions to GH initiatives. As a result of the World Bank's involvement in GH, particularly in developing countries, there have been shifts in PH policy as well as the development of models for healthcare systems [259]. By demonstrating leadership in the governance of GH and highlighting the significance of resilience and readiness at the interface between humans, animals, and the environment, the World Bank contributes to the fight against disease threats that have the potential to become endemic, emerging, or pandemic, which also includes the fight against AMR [260].

Over fifty countries have received assistance from the USAID since 2005 to improve their ability to monitor the spread of highly pathogenic avian influenza (HPAI) H5N1 among wild birds, domestic poultry, and humans; implement a rapid and effective containment strategy for the virus when it is discovered; and provide assistance to countries through capacity building. The Emerging Pandemic Threats (EPT) project was launched in 2009 by pandemic influenza and other emerging threat units. This activity was performed to generate readiness for other viruses that may emerge as potential pandemics. This supplement to ongoing USAID work on HPAI was carried out in twenty countries and included four separate initiatives that supported and complemented each other. They were named Predict, Prevent and Prepare, Detect localized outbreaks, and Respond with time. The EPT global program aims to build regional, national, and local capabilities for the early detection of disease, laboratory-based disease diagnosis, rapid response mechanisms, and risk reduction. To that end, the EPT global program leverages animal and human health experts on its team.

In this context, One Health University Networks is entrusted with creating and delivering curricula for model programs that equip professionals to work collaboratively across sectors when combating complex GH challenges as part of the USAID OHW-NG project. Since its launch in 2011, SEAOHUN has been united with the vision of USAID to build a resilient and sustainable OH workforce capable of combating current and emerging infectious diseases for both current and future generations. SEAOHUN, in collaboration with stakeholders at the country level, is a partner in the STOP Spillover project by USAID, which aims to understand and respond to challenges associated with zoonotic viral diseases such as COVID-19 and mitigate the risk of spillover from animals [261]. It supplements the OHW-NG effort. USAID started a new OH System Strengthening project in 2024 to strengthen efforts to prevent and control infectious diseases in Bangladesh. Implemented by Development Alternatives Incorporated in association with a consortium of the Center for Natural Resource Studies, CVASU, Eastern Mediterranean Public Health Network, and mPower Social Enterprises [262].

In April 2010, the WOAH, the FAO, and the WHO published a document that was referred to as the "Tripartite Concept Note." This document established a long-term strategy to foster global collaboration, with the goals of sharing responsibility and coordinating worldwide initiatives to address the health hazards that occur because of interactions between humans, animals, and the natural environment [263]. The main goal of this document was to accomplish these goals by establishing a strategy that would foster global collaboration. The Quadripartite Collaboration on OH was established in March 2022 by the WOAH, the FAO, and the United Nations Environment Program (UNEP). To address the complex interrelationships among human health, AH, and the environment, this collaboration aims to leverage the expertise of both parties to combat newly developing diseases, zoonotic infections, foodborne illnesses, and environmental concerns. Currently, these organizations provide ongoing training to strengthen local communities' capabilities in disease detection, response, and prevention [264]. In addition, they impart their technical experience and offer advice to other nations to facilitate the formulation and execution of OH policies and plans.

Agencies from the UK and overseas collaborating in research projects, such as those for the OH initiative, the Southeastern Regional Centre of Excellence for Emerging Infections and Biodefense in the United States, have facilitated and organized conferences focused on research and education frameworks to establish OH. Their priority concerns have been framed in terms of new infectious diseases, health consequences of the environment, and workforce development for tomorrow [265]. The Rx One Health Summer Institute is another example of a transdisciplinary collaboration between the United States and East African partners, which has been used as an experiential model of training that advances the concept. Programs also feature community-based and problem-oriented learning [266]. The Institute for One World Health of San Francisco represents a nonprofit pharmaceutical company that is dedicated to the discovery, development, and marketing of new drugs for treating diseases that mainly affect people in developing nations. As an example of putting the OH concept into practice, this organization demonstrates how to address GH challenges [267].

4.9.3 Influencing Policy at the National and International Levels

A platform can influence policy at the national and international levels in many different ways. The Global Health Security Agenda (GHSA) is a pivotal type of policy that targets OH advocacy and aims to reach the level of the country and other models at international levels. The comprehensive GHSA approach, facilitated by international collaboration, reflects OH in motion while influencing policy globally. This global containment started in 2014 to improve world preparedness against infectious disease threats through the application of an OH approach [268].

The GHSA created the Global Health Security Index in 2019, drawing on publicly available data sources based on numerous other sources, including government publications and data from different international agencies. This index sought to capture the multifaceted realm of opportunities within countries for biological threats [269]. This context included a country's geopolitical considerations, health system, and ability of the government to contain outbreaks.

The GHSA has produced some truly remarkable stories to cover a variety of countries, including Bangladesh, Uganda, Indonesia, Kenya, the United States, and others. Through joint external evaluation and biosafety support measures, the integration of the OH approach into national policies, OH capacity building and training, the construction of an OH platform, and the creation of integrated disease surveillance systems have assisted them in their capacity to be prepared [270].

A comprehensive OH Action Plan was endorsed by the EU to address AMR, a part of the EU's extensive OH Action Plan against AMR. In addition, the EU has allocated funds for the development of novel medicines, alternatives to antibiotics, and surveillance of AMR as a part of substantial research. This initiative aimed at increasing public awareness is carried out by the European Commission to educate the public and experts on the appropriate use of antibiotics [271].

Within the South Asian region, Bangladesh served as a model for the incorporation of the OH concept into the level of national policy formulation. To date, Bangladesh has released two strategic documents on OH to integrate

OH in every relevant sector, especially those addressing zoonotic disease threats [272]. To date, Bangladesh has adopted the OH approach to combat health risks such as AI, Nipah virus, and AMR. Additionally, regarding the institutionalization of OH, Bangladesh has built a government-level coordination mechanism known as the OH Secretariat, which incorporates human, animal, and environmental health team members. The main role of the secretariat is to coordinate and facilitate activities related to OH in Bangladesh [273].

Different countries have formulated various policies to address wildlife rescue and conservation that are aligned with OH approaches. However, proper implementation of these policies is not always ensured. For example, in Bangladesh, the proper rescue and treatment of wildlife necessitates the involvement of trained veterinarians. Unfortunately, in many cases, wildlife is handled by forest officers who lack veterinary certification and training. This results in inadequate care and treatment for the animals, creating OH concerns. Therefore, stringent monitoring is crucial to ensure the effective implementation of policies aimed at strengthening wildlife rescue and conservation efforts in the country.

4.9.4 Advocacy Strategies for One Health Integration

In addition to the One Health University network and disease surveillance system that has been established, there is a requirement for capacity building and training to speed up OH advocacy. The Field Epidemiology Training Program (FETP) is one of them. The CDC makes this possible by providing considerable training opportunities for the PH and AH sectors in the SAARC and the ASEAN regions. This training involves a series of workshops, on-the-job training, and mentorship sessions focusing on competencies for health professionals in the human, animal, or environmental sectors. The CDC trained more than 18,000 disease detectives in over 80 countries through the FETP initiative between 1980 and 2020 [274]. In Bangladesh, 186 fellows have graduated from the program [275]. These guys focus on PH and AH. During outbreaks of various diseases (e.g. anthrax, Nipah, and lead poisoning), graduates serve as the major source of care for those affected by these diseases. Importantly, as noted by Seffren et al. [184], this training program should be carried out to strengthen the PH workforce of a country and thereby scale up regional and global disease detection networks during an emergency.

In addition, the integrated disease surveillance and response (IDSR) framework is an example of practical cooperation. The main goal of this framework is to make surveillance and laboratory data more usable, which will assist PH managers and decision-makers in improving the detection of and response to the leading causes of disease, death, and disability in African countries. Since its conception in 1988, the CDC has been at the forefront of designing, developing, implementing, monitoring, and evaluating the IDSR. Working in conjunction with the WHO/AFRO, the IDSR team at the CDC was able to spearhead the creation of the IDSR framework and the design and development of the Technical Guidelines for Integrated Disease Surveillance and the IDSR Training Modules. This was made possible by support from USAID. In addition, the CDC programs across the agency examined and approved summary guidelines for the framework's 40 priority diseases. These include those diseases, syndromes, and ailments addressed by the International Health Regulations (IHRs) [276].

To effectively advocate for the integration of OH, various techniques must be employed, including involving a wide range of stakeholders, using preexisting structures, and using evidence-based approaches. These examples from different parts of the world illustrate the potential of coordinated efforts to improve health outcomes, build capacity, and influence policy by implementing the OH concept.

4.10 Future Directions in One Health Education

The OH education system is set to evolve to address GH challenges by integrating the OH concept into undergraduate and graduate curricula for studying interdisciplinary collaboration and communication skills. Advanced training programs will focus on disease surveillance, outbreak response, and environmental health assessment.

Global collaboration and networking will be expanded to address these transboundary health issues. OH education is expected to undergo significant changes in the next decade due to emerging trends and innovations. Key areas include integrating digital health technologies, big data analytics, blockchain, global collaborations, genomics, environmental sustainability, climate adaptation strategies, and OH policy and governance. These innovations aim to enhance remote diagnostics, disease surveillance, transparency, and personalized health interventions while addressing emerging diseases and health risks associated with climate change and habitat loss. Future challenges include the complexity of GH threats; addressing emerging infectious diseases, zoonoses, and AMR; and navigating the impacts of urbanization, globalization, and ecosystem changes on health outcomes. Interdisciplinary training and capacity building are essential for bridging gaps between human health, AH, environmental sciences, and social sciences in education and practice. Along with this, equitable access to education and the ability to address social justice disparities in healthcare, food security and environmental health are also expected to be major issues. Addressing emerging infectious diseases, navigating urbanization, and fostering collaboration across diverse sectors are essential. The vision for the next decade is to advance OH, a holistic approach to addressing GH challenges, promoting sustainability and resilience. This will involve leveraging cutting-edge technology, empowering communities through education, influencing policy development, and investing in interdisciplinary research. Finally, OH education can significantly contribute to global security and sustainability in the coming decade by embracing emerging technologies, studying global partnerships, and advocating future inclusive policies [28].

The OH approach emphasizes the interconnectedness of different disciplines in PH education, regardless of the university program [277]. This has led to an increase in OH-related textbooks for university students in medicine and veterinary medicine, with a focus on zoonotic diseases, epidemics, and toxicants [278, 279]. The focus has shifted from food-producing animals to pet ownership, emphasizing the importance of recognizing each other's expertise. OH, has also led to suggestions for a new education on the basis of the philosophy of OH. Calvin Schwabe proposed a new curriculum for veterinary schools, focusing on the population, people, and biology. A more modern attempt would place these areas and students in schools of PH. However, establishing such a curriculum within established disciplines could lead to ambiguity, where one discipline uses another discipline's knowledge without exchange in the opposite direction [280].

An interdisciplinary matrix could help avoid this risk. Schwabe suggested that a new curriculum should be built up by truly interdisciplinary research departments rather than by attempting to collaborate with existing departments. By focusing on the interconnectedness of different disciplines, a new curriculum can be developed and applied in various educational contexts [281, 282].

4.11 Conclusion

The complex relationships among human-animal-environmental health are addressed in this chapter under the GVE. This chapter evolved over the past 50 years of the traditional veterinary curriculum; instead of combining theoretical and clinical training, the gaps and limitations of this curriculum often fail to integrate OH principles. With the advancement of time, the transformation took place in the GVE, which resulted in the existing curriculum, including innovative teaching methods featuring PH and environmental science and the inclusion of modern technology for OH education. Along with the development and creation of interdisciplinary learning, that is, courses and modules, policymakers, development partners, and numerous associations of the veterinary sector promote OH integration for building collaborative partnerships, utilizing PBL, endorsing cross-disciplinary research projects, and incorporating fieldwork to enhance practical experiences, overall improvement in communication and leadership skills.

For the integration of OH, the collaboration of healthcare professionals is vital, as they are involved in veterinary and related health and environmental institutions. To understand the disease triangle, dynamics among hosts, pathogens, and the environment, the interactions of pathogens are determined for efficient control of their growth and propagation as well as disease pathogenicity and spread. The collaboration between veterinary and medical schools is also crucial to making OH education popular in Asia, Africa, Europe, and the Americas. Different veterinary and medical schools, such as SGU, Bethany College, the ICAR, and the UC, Davis, are creating career pathways and incorporating OH principles such as digital health technologies, blockchain, genomics, strategies for climatic adaptation and disease problems at animal, human, and environmental interfaces into veterinary and medical education curricula with a vision to promote sustainability, leverage technology and invest in interdisciplinary research.

Abbreviations

AAHL: Australian Animal Health Laboratory; AAVMC: Association of American Veterinary Medical College; AFROHUN: Africa One Health University Network; AH: Animal Health; AI: Avian Influenza; AMA: American Medical Association; AMR: Antimicrobial Resistance; APHA: American Public Health Association: ASEAN; Association of Southeast Asian Nations; AVMA: American Veterinary Medical Association; AVMA COE: American Veterinary Medical Association Council on Education; BITID: Bangladesh Institute of Tropical and Infectious Diseases; BSc: Bachelor of Science; BVSc: Bachelor of Veterinary Science; CDC: Centers for Disease Control and Prevention; CE: Continuing Education; COHEART: Centre for One Health Education, Advocacy, Research and Training; COH-K: Centre for One Health Kerala; CVASU: Chattogram Veterinary and Animal Sciences University; CVMs: Colleges of Veterinary Medicine; DARSI: Developing Adaptive Resilience and Sustainability for Integration; DOS: US Department of State; DVM: Doctor of Veterinary Medicine; EU: European Union; EU COST: European Cooperation in Science and Technology; EUOHM: European One Health Training Program; FAO: Food and Agriculture Organization; FETP: Field Epidemiology Training Program; GARC: Global Alliance for Rabies Control; GH: Global Health; GHSA: Global Health Security Agenda; GVE: Global Veterinary Education; HPAI: Highly Pathogenic Avian Influenza; ICAR: Indian Council of Agricultural Research; ICDDR,B: International Centre for Diarrheal Disease Research, Bangladesh; IDSR: Integrated Disease Surveillance and Response; IEDCR: Institute of Epidemiology, Disease Control and Research; IHRs: International Health Regulations; ILRI: International Livestock Research Institute; IQAC: Institutional Quality Assurance Capacity; ITM: Institute of Tropical Medicine; IVSA: International Veterinary Students Association; KOICA: Korea International Cooperation Agency; KVASU: Kerala Veterinary and Animal Sciences University; LIPHEA: Initiative of Public Health in East Africa; LMI: Lower Mekong Initiative; LSHTM: London School of Hygiene and Tropical Medicine; MakSPH: Makerere University School of Public Health; MUHAS: Muhimbili University of Health and Allied Sciences; NCOH: The Netherlands Centre for One Health; NEOH: Network for Evaluation of One Health; NGOs: Nongovernmental Organizations; NIH: National Institutes of Health; OH: One Health; OHC: One Health Commission; OH JPA: One Health Joint Plan of Action; OHCEA: One Health Central and Eastern Africa; OHEART: One Health East African Research Training; OHEJP: One Health European Joint Program; OHHLEP: One Health High-Level Expert Panel; OHI: One Health Initiative; OHI: One Health Institute; OHPHB: One Health Poultry Hub, Bangladesh; OH-SMART: One Health Systems Mapping and Analysis Resource Toolkit; OHUNs: One Health University Networks; OHW-NG: One Health Workforce Next Generation; OHW-NG: One Health Workforce-Next Generation; PAHO: Pan American Health Organization; PBL: Problem-based Learning; PH: Public Health; PREDICT: Predicting Infectious Disease Transmission; QAOHS: Queensland Alliance for One Health Sciences; RIVM: Dutch National Institute for Public Health and the Environment; RVC: Royal Veterinary College; SAARC: South Asian Association for Regional Cooperation; SACIDS: Southern African Centre for Infectious Disease Surveillance; SAU: Sher-e-Bangla Agricultural University; SyAU: Sylhet Agricultural University; SEAOHUN: Southeast Asia One Health University Network; SGU: St. George's University; SSPs: Shared Socio-economic Pathways; STOP: Strategies to Prevent; UC Davis: University of California, Davis;

UK: United Kingdom; UMN: University of Minnesota; UNEP: United Nations Environment Program; UniIbadan: University of Ibadan; UoN: University of Nairobi; UP: University of Pretoria; UQ: University of Queensland; UQVSA: University of Queensland Veterinary Students' Association; US: United States; USAID: United States Agency for International Development; UTokyo: University of Tokyo; UVAS: University of Veterinary and Animal Sciences; VE: Veterinary Education; VEEs: Veterinary Educational Establishments; VetCEE: Veterinary Continuous Education in Europe; VMAI: Veterinary Medical Associations of Interest; VME: Veterinary Medical Education; WHO: World Health Organization; WOAH: World Organization for Animal Health; WVA: World Veterinary Association.

Author Contributions

Conceptualization and outline preparation: D.H. and S.Z.T.B; Data collection and curation: D.H., R.O.A, O.G.B., O.A.O., E.J.E, and S.Z.T.B; Figure preparation: D.H.; Table preparation: D.H, R.O.A., A.A.B, and S.Z.T.B; Supervision: D.H. and S.Z.T.B; Validation: D.H., R.O.A., and S.Z.T.B.; Writing- original draft preparation: D.H., R.O.A., N.U., E.J.E., O.A.O., O.G.B., A.A.B., M.M.A., A.D., and S.Z.T.B.; Writing- review and editing: D.H., R.O.A., O.A.O., N.U., E.J.E., and S.Z.T.B. All the authors contributed to the book chapter and approved the submitted version for publication.

Conflicts of Interest

The authors declare no conflict of interest.

Acknowledgments

We extend our heartfelt gratitude to the One Health Commission (OHC) and the One Health Initiative (OHI) for permitting us to use Figures 4.1 and 4.4 in this publication. Your support and collaboration have been invaluable in bringing this work to fruition.

Dedication

This book chapter, "Integrating One Health into Global Veterinary Education," is dedicated to the students, frontline fighters, and professionals of One Health. Your unwavering commitment to the interconnected health of humans, animals, and the environment inspires us all. May this work serve as a testament to your dedication and beacon for future generations.

References

1 One Health Commission. *Definitions of One Health*. https://www.onehealthcommission.org/en/why_one_health/what_is_one_health/ (accessed 30 August 2024).
2 World Health Organization. *One Health*. https://www.who.int/news-room/questions-and-answers/item/one-health (accessed 30 August 2024).

3 Centers for Disease Control and Prevention. *About Zoonotic Diseases*. https://www.cdc.gov/one-health/about/about-zoonotic-diseases.html?CDC_AAref_Val=https://www.cdc.gov/onehealth/basics/zoonotic-diseases.html (accessed 30 August 2024).

4 Baum, S.E., Machalaba, C., Daszak, P., et al. Evaluating one health: are we demonstrating effectiveness? *One Health*. 2017; 3: 5–10. https://doi.org/10.1016/j.onehlt.2016.10.004.

5 Lerner, H. and Berg, C. The concept of health in One Health and some practical implications for research and education: what is One Health? *Infect. Ecol. Epidemiol.* 2015; 5(1): 25300. https://doi.org/10.3402/iee.v5.25300.

6 One Health Initiative. *The One Health Umbrella*. https://onehealthinitiative.com/the-one-health-umbrella/ (accessed 26 November 2024).

7 Armistead, W.W. A fresh approach to veterinary curriculum design. *J. Am. Vet. Med. Assoc.* 1964; 15(144): 1093–1104.

8 Armistead, W.W. Educating tomorrow's veterinarians. *J. Am. Vet. Med. Assoc.* 1965; 1(146): 931–936.

9 Armistead, W.W. Blueprint for a modern Veterinary College. *J. Am. Vet. Med. Assoc.* 1970; 156(11): 1580–1582.

10 Armistead, W.W. Veterinary college organization and curriculum: a look at alternatives. *J. Am. Vet. Med. Assoc.* 1970; 156(12): 1911–1916.

11 Pritchard, W.R. Veterinary medical education for the next decade. *Can. Vet. J.* 1966; 7(3): 55–61.

12 Soltys, M.A. Suggested changes in veterinary education. *Can. Vet. J.* 1968; 9(1): 3–6.

13 Waldhalm, S.J. Yes, veterinaria, there is a knowledge explosion. *Can. Vet. J.* 1989; 30(8): 628–631.

14 Talbot, R.B., McGovern, P.T., Carrig, C.B., and McGrath, C.J. Preparation versus delivery. *J. Vet. Med. Educ.* 1983; 10(1): 16–18.

15 Oyler, F.L.E. and Freeman, L.E. Basic sciences curriculum design—breaking from tradition. *J. Vet. Med. Educ.* 1983; 9(2): 37–38.

16 Turnwald, G.H. and Walkington, J. Design and implementation of curriculum change. *Sci. Tech. Rev.* 2009; 28(2): 789–796. https://doi.org/10.20506/rst.28.2.1922.

17 Eyre, P. Veterinary education with career emphasis: a partnership with private, public, and corporate veterinary practice. *J. Am. Vet. Med. Assoc.* 1992; 200(3): 311–315.

18 O'Neill, E.H. Veterinary medicine in the context of change in the health professions. In: *Proceedings of the XXIV World Veterinary Congress—Symposium on Veterinary Education in the 21st Century*, Rio de Janeiro, Brazil; 1991.

19 Howell, N.E., Lane, I.F., Brace, J.J., and Shull, R.M. Integration of problem-based learning in a veterinary medical curriculum: first-year experiences with Application-Based Learning Exercises at the University of Tennessee College of Veterinary Medicine. *J. Vet. Med. Educ.* 2002; 29(3): 169–175. https://doi.org/10.3138/jvme.29.3.169.

20 Cardinet 3rd, G.H., Gourley, I.M., BonDurant, R.H., et al. Changing dimensions of veterinary medical education in pursuit of diversity and flexibility in service to society. *J. Am. Vet. Med. Assoc.* 1992; 201(10): 1530–1539.

21 Hooper, B.E. Ongoing curricular change in veterinary medical colleges. *J. Vet. Med. Educ.* 1994; 21(2): 125–9. https://scholar.lib.vt.edu/ejournals/JVME/V21-2/hooper.html.

22 Gordon, S., Gardner, D., Weston, J., et al. Fostering the development of professionalism in veterinary students: challenges and implications for veterinary professionalism curricula. *Educ. Sci.* 2021; 11(11): 720. https://doi.org/10.3390/educsci11110720.

23 Espinosa García-San Román, J., Quesada-Canales, Ó., Arbelo Hernández, M., et al. Veterinary education and training on non-traditional companion animals, exotic, zoo, and wild animals: concepts review and challenging perspective on zoological medicine. *Vet. Sci.* 2023; 10(5): 357. https://doi.org/10.3390/vetsci10050357.

24 Gordon, S., Parkinson, T., Byers, S., et al. The changing face of veterinary professionalism—implications for veterinary education. *Educ. Sci.* 2023; 13(2): 182. https://doi.org/10.3390/educsci13020182.

25 Sacchini, S. and Castro-Alonso, A. Veterinary medical education: challenges and perspectives. *Vet. Sci.* 2023. https://doi.org/10.3390/books978-3-7258-1399-5.

26 Pohl, R., Botscharow, J., Böckelmann, I., and Thielmann, B. Stress and strain among veterinarians: a scoping review. *Ir. Vet. J.* 2022; 75(1): 15. https://doi.org/10.1186/s13620-022-00220-x.

27 Stetina, B.U. and Krouzecky, C. Reviewing a decade of change for veterinarians: past, present and gaps in researching stress, coping and mental health risks. *Animals*. 2022; 12(22): 3199. https://doi.org/10.3390/ani12223199.

28 Samad, M.A. Current status and challenges for globalisation of veterinary medical education for the "One Health" programme. *Sci. Tec. Rev*. 2017; 36(3): 741–765. https://doi.org/10.20506/rst.36.3.2711.

29 Lane, I.F., Root Kustritz, M.V., and Schoenfeld-Tacher, R.M. *Veterinary Curricula Today: Curricular Management and Renewal at AAVMC Member Institutions*, University of Toronto Press Inc; 2017. https://doi.org/10.3138/jvme.0417.048.

30 Murray, A.L. and Sischo, W.M. Addressing educational challenges in veterinary medicine through the use of distance education. *J. Vet. Med. Educ.* 2007; 34(3): 279–285. https://doi.org/10.3138/jvme.34.3.279.

31 Sasidhar, P.V.K. and Reddy, P.G. SWOT analysis of veterinary and animal science education in India: implications for policy and future directions. *J. Agric. Educ. Ext.* 2012; 18(4): 387–407. https://doi.org/10.1080/1389224X.2012.684801.

32 Fanning, S., Whyte, P., and O'Mahony, M. Essential veterinary education on the development of antimicrobial and anti-parasitic resistance: consequences for animal health and food safety and the need for vigilance. *Sci. Tech. Rev*. 2009; 28(2): 575–582. http://doi.org/10.20506/rst.28.2.1905.

33 American Association of Veterinary Medical Colleges. North American Veterinary Medical Education Consortium. *American Association of Veterinary Medical Colleges (AAVMC)*. [Online]. http://www.aavmc.org/assets/data-new/files/navmec/navmecmeeting1report.pdf (accessed 30 August 2024).

34 Machalaba, C., Uhart, M., Ryser-Degiorgis, M.P., and Karesh, W.B. Gaps in health security related to wildlife and environment affecting pandemic prevention and preparedness, 2007–2020. *Bull. World Health Organ*. 2021; 99(5): 342–350. http://doi.org/10.2471/BLT.20.272690.

35 del P. Palacios-Díaz, M. and Mendoza-Grimón, V. Environment in veterinary education. *Vet. Sci*. 2023; 10(2): 146. https://doi.org/10.3390/vetsci10020146.

36 Hussein, H.A. Brief review on Ebola virus disease and one health approach. *Heliyon*. 2023; 9(8): e19036. https://doi.org/10.1016/j.heliyon.2023.e19036.

37 Adesola, R.O., Akinniyi, H.T., and Lucero-Prisno III, D.E. An evaluation of the impact of anti-rabies programs in Nigeria. *Ann. Med. Surg*. 2023; 85(2): 358–364. https://doi.org/10.1097/MS9.0000000000000250.

38 Mukherjee, R., Gunjan, K., Himanshu, K., et al. Advancing influenza prevention through a one health approach: a comprehensive analysis. *J. Hazard. Mater. Adv*. 2024; 14: 100419. https://doi.org/10.1016/j.hazadv.2024.100419.

39 Ogunleye, S.C., Akinsulie, O.C., Aborode, A.T., et al. The re-emergence and transmission of monkeypox virus in Nigeria: the role of one health. *Front. Public. Health*. 2024; 11: 1334238. https://doi.org/10.3389/fpubh.2023.1334238.

40 Jordan, T. and Lem, M. One health, one welfare: education in practice veterinary students' experiences with community veterinary outreach. *Can. Vet. J*. 55(12): 1203, 2014.

41 McConnell, I. One Health in the context of medical and veterinary education. *Rev. Sci. Tech*. 2014; 33(2): 651–657. https://doi.org/10.20506/rst.33.2.2304.

42 Nzietchueng, S., Kitua, A., Nyatanyi, T., and Rwego, I.B. Facilitating implementation of the one health approach: a definition of a one health intervention. *One Health*. 2023; 16: 100491. https://doi.org/10.1016/j.onehlt.2023.100491.

43 De La Rocque, S., Caya, F., El Idrissi, A.H., et al. One Health operations: a critical component in the international health regulations monitoring and evaluation framework. *Sci. Tech. Rev*. 2019; 38(1): 303–314. https://doi.org/10.20506/rst.38.1.2962.

44 Togami, E., Gardy, J.L., Hansen, G.R., et al. Core competencies in one health education: what are we missing? NAM Perspectives. Discussion Paper. Washington, DC: National Academy of Medicine; 2018. https://doi.org/10.31478/201806a.

45 Rüegg, S.R., Nielsen, L.R., Buttigieg, S.C., et al. A systems approach to evaluate One Health initiatives. *Front. Vet. Sci.* 2018; 5: 23. https://doi.org/10.3389/fvets.2018.00023.

46 Laing, G., Duffy E., Anderson, N., et al. Advancing One Health: updated core competencies. *CABI One Health.* 2023(2023): ohcs20230002. https://doi.org/10.1079/cabionehealth.2023.000.

47 Frankson, R., Hueston, W., Christian, K., et al. One health core competency domains. *Front. Public Health.* 2016; 4: 192. https://doi.org/10.3389/fpubh.2016.00192.

48 Prata, J.C., Ribeiro, A.I., and Rocha-Santos, T. An introduction to the concept of One Health. In: *One Health: Integrated Approach to 21st Century Challenges to Health*, 1–31. Academic Press; 2022. https://doi.org/10.1016/B978-0-12-822794-7.00004-6.

49 Leddin, D. The impact of climate change, pollution, and biodiversity loss on digestive health and disease. *Gastro. Hep Adv.* 2024; 3(4): 519–534. https://doi.org/10.1016/j.gastha.2024.01.018.

50 Ario, A.R., Djoudalbaye, B., Olatinwo, S. et al. National interagency collaboration for public health. In: *Modernizing Global Health Security to Prevent, Detect, and Respond* (ed. S.J.N. McNabb, A.T. Shaikh and C.J. Haley), 37–51. Academic Press; 2024. https://doi.org/10.1016/B978-0-323-90945-7.00006-3.

51 Leopold, S.R. Dormant ethnobotany: a case study of decline in regional plant knowledge in the bull run mountains of Virginia. Antioch University Dissertations and Theses; 2011. https://aura.antioch.edu/etds/803.

52 Cerda, J.R. and Webb, T.L. Wildlife conservation and preserving biodiversity: impactful opportunities for veterinarians? *J. Am. Vet. Med. Assoc.* 2023; 261(7): 1077–1085. https://doi.org/10.2460/javma.23.02.0094.

53 Hajar, R. Animal testing and medicine. *Heart Views.* 2011; 12(1): 42. https://journals.lww.com/hrtv/fulltext/2011/12010/animal_testing_and_medicine.11.aspx.

54 Alves, R.R.N. and da S. Policarpo, I. Animals and human health: where do they meet? In: *Ethnozoology* (ed. R.R. Nóbrega Alves and U.P. Albuquerque), 233–259. Academic Press; 2018. https://doi.org/10.1016/B978-0-12-809913-1.00013-2.

55 Chaddock, M. Academic veterinary medicine and One Health education: it is more than clinical applications. *J. Vet. Med. Educ.* 2012; 39(3): 241–246. https://doi.org/10.3138/jvme.0612-062.

56 Allela, L., Bourry, O., Pouillot, R., et al. Ebola virus antibody prevalence in dogs and human risk. *Emerg. Infect. Dis. J.* 2005; 11(3): 385. https://doi.org/10.3201/eid1103.040981.

57 Nielsen, N.O., Waltner-Toews, D., Nishi, J.S., and Hunter, D.B. Whither ecosystem health and ecological medicine in veterinary medicine and education. *Can. Vet. J.* 2012; 53(7): 747.

58 Bing-You, R., Hayes, V., Varaklis, K., et al. Feedback for learners in medical education: what is known? A scoping review. *Acad. Med.* 2017; 92(9): 1346–1354. https://pmc.ncbi.nlm.nih.gov/articles/PMC3377457/.

59 Wilkerson, L. and Irby, D.M. Strategies for improving teaching practices: a comprehensive approach to faculty development. *Acad. Med.* 1998; 73(4): 387–396. https://doi.org/10.1097/00001888-199804000-00011.

60 Westberg, J. and Jason, H. *Collaborative Clinical Education: The Foundation of Effective Health Care.* Springer Publishing Company [Online]; 1992. https://dokumen.pub/collaborative-clinical-education-the-foundation-of-effective-health-care-1nbsped-9780826197924-9780826180308.html (accessed 26 November 2024).

61 Irby, D.M. What clinical teachers in medicine need to know. *Acad. Med.* 1994; 69(5): 333–342. https://doi.org/10.1097/00001888-199405000-00003.

62 Strand, P., Edgren, G., Borna, P., et al. Conceptions of how a learning or teaching curriculum, workplace culture, and agency of individuals shape medical student learning and supervisory practices in the clinical workplace. *Adv. Health Sci. Educ.* 2015; 20(2): 531–557. https://doi.org/10.1007/s10459-014-9546-0.

63 Steinert, Y., Mann, K., Anderson, B., et al. A systematic review of faculty development initiatives designed to enhance teaching effectiveness: a 10-year update: BEME Guide No. 40. *Med. Teac.* 2016; 38(8): 769–786. https://doi.org/10.1080/0142159X.2016.1181851.

64 Irby, D.M. Excellence in clinical teaching: knowledge transformation and development required. *Med. Educ.* 2014; 48(8): 776–784. https://doi.org/10.1111/medu.12507.

65 Smith, J.A., Frawley, J., Pechenkina, E., et al. Identifying strategies for improving VET to higher education transitions for Indigenous learners. *Swinburne Rep.* 2017; https://doi.org/10.25916/sut.26295541.v1.

66 Goodwin, A.L., Smith, L., Souto-Manning, M., et al. What should teacher educators know and be able to do? Perspectives from practicing teacher educators. *J. Teach. Educ.* 2014; 65(4): 284–302. https://doi.org/10.1177/0022487114535266.

67 Peluso, M.J. and Hafler, J.P. Medical students as medical educators: opportunities for skill development in the absence of formal training programs. *Yale J. Biol. Med.* 2011; 84(3): 203–209. https://pmc.ncbi.nlm.nih.gov/articles/PMC3178849/.

68 Huston, T. and Weaver, C.L. Peer coaching: professional development for experienced faculty. *Innov. High. Educ.* 2008; 33(1): 5–20. https://doi.org/10.1007/s10755-007-9061-9.

69 Devlin, M. and Samarawickrema, G. The criteria of effective teaching in a changing higher education context. *High. Educ. Res. Develop.* 2010; 29(2): 111–124. https://doi.org/10.1080/07294360903244398.

70 Gardner, S.S. From learning to teach to teaching effectiveness: nurse educators describe their experiences. *Nurs. Educ. Perspect.* 2014; 35(2): 106–111. https://journals.lww.com/neponline/fulltext/2014/03000/from_learning_to_teach_to_teaching_effectiveness_.8.aspx

71 Harden, R.M. and Crosby, J. AMEE Guide No 20: the good teacher is more than a lecturer- the twelve roles of the teacher. *Med. Teach.* 2000; 22(4): 334–347. https://doi.org/10.1080/014215900409429.

72 Magnier, K.M., Wang, R., Dale, V.H.M., and Pead, M.J. Challenges and responsibilities of clinical teachers in the workplace: an ethnographic approach. *J. Vet. Med. Educ.* 2014; 41(2): 155–161. https://doi.org/10.3138/jvme.0813-111R1.

73 Horefti, E. The importance of the One Health concept in combating zoonoses. *Pathogens* 2023; 12(8): 977. https://doi.org/10.3390/pathogens12080977.

74 Chu, Y.H. and Li, Y.C. The impact of online learning on physical and mental health in university students during the COVID-19 pandemic. *Int. J. Environ. Res. Public Health.* 2022; 19(5): 2966. https://doi.org/10.3390/ijerph19052966.

75 Liu, J., Lai, S., Rai, A.A., et al. Exploring the potential of big data analytics in urban epidemiology control: a comprehensive study using CiteSpace. *Int. J. Environ. Res. Public Health.* 2023; 20(5): 3930. https://doi.org/10.3390/ijerph20053930.

76 Open University. Health Education, Advocacy and Community Mobilisation Module: 16. Evaluation of Health Education Programmes. *Open University.* https://www.open.edu/openlearncreate/mod/oucontent/view.php?id=174&printable=1 (accessed 30 August 2024).

77 Mississippi Department of Education. *Health Education Assessment.* https://www.mdek12.org/OHS/HealthEducation/Assessment (accessed 30 August 2024).

78 Centers for Disease Control and Prevention. HECAT: Appendix 6: Understanding Health Education Assessment. https://www.cdc.gov/healthyyouth/hecat/pdf/hecat_append_6.pdf (accessed 30 August 2024).

79 Buléon, C., Mattatia, L., Minehart, R.D., et al. Simulation-based summative assessment in healthcare: an overview of key principles for practice. *Adv. Simul.* 2022; 7(1): 42. https://doi.org/10.1186/s41077-022-00238-9.

80 Fountain, S. and Gillespie, A. Assessment strategies for skills-based health education with a focus on HIV prevention and related issues (Draft 2003). UNICEF Education Section, New York; 2013. https://healtheducationresources.unesco.org/sites/default/files/resources/HIV_AIDS_186.pdf (accessed 30 August 2024).

81 dos S. Ribeiro, C., van de Burgwal, L.H.M., and Regeer, B.J. Overcoming challenges for designing and implementing the One Health approach: a systematic review of the literature. *One Health* 2019; 7: 100085. https://doi.org/10.1016/j.onehlt.2019.100085.

82 Varer Akpinar, C. and Durmaz, S. Medical interns' attitudes towards One Health approach. *Turk. J. Biochem.* 2022; 47(1): 137–144. https://doi.org/10.1515/tjb-2021-0078.

83 Yussuf, B., Ballantyne, P.G., Richards, S., et al. *Report of the Regional Workshop on Building the Capacities of Higher Educational Institutions to Educate, Train, and Empower the Next Generation Workforce to Tackle One*

Health Issues, Gaborone, Botswana, *22-24 November 2022*. Nairobi, Kenya: ILRI; 2022. https://hdl.handle.net/10568/127429.

84 Allen-Scott, L.K., Buntain, B., Hatfield, J.M., et al. Academic institutions and One Health: building capacity for transdisciplinary research approaches to address complex health issues at the animal-human-ecosystem interface. *Acad. Med.* 2015; 90(7): 866–871. https://doi.org/10.1097/ACM.0000000000000639.

85 Doherty, R.F. *Ethical Dimensions in the Health Professions-E-Book: Ethical Dimensions in the Health Professions-E-Book*. Elsevier Health Sciences; 2020. eBook ISBN: 9780323673655.

86 Aqil, J. *A Mixed-Method Evaluation of the One Health-Ness at the Faculty of Veterinary Science, University of Pretoria*. University of Pretoria; 2021. http://hdl.handle.net/2263/95835.

87 Sikkema, R. and Koopmans, M. One Health training and research activities in Western Europe. *Infect. Ecol. Epidemiol.* 2016; 6(1): 33703. https://doi.org/10.3402/iee.v6.33703.

88 Rabinowitz, P.M., Natterson-Horowitz, B.J., Kahn, L.H., et al. Incorporating one health into medical education. *BMC Med. Educ.* 2017; 17: 1–7. https://doi.org/10.1186/s12909-017-0883-6.

89 Dellar, M., Geerling, G., Kok, K., et al. Creating the Dutch One Health shared socio-economic pathways (SSPs). *Reg. Environ. Change.* 2024; 24(1): 16. https://doi.org/10.1007/s10113-023-02169-1.

90 Erkyihun, G.A. and Alemayehu, M.B. One Health approach for the control of zoonotic diseases. *Zoonoses* 2022; 2(1): 963. https://doi.org/10.15212/ZOONOSES-2022-0037.

91 Utrecht University. *One Health - Life Sciences*. https://www.uu.nl/en/research/life-sciences/research/one-health (accessed 30 August 2024).

92 UC Davis. *About the One Health Institute at UC Davis*. Davis: University of California. https://ohi.vetmed.ucdavis.edu/about (accessed 01 December 2024).

93 UC Davis. *Education*. Davis: University of California. https://ohi.vetmed.ucdavis.edu/education (accessed 01 December 2024).

94 UC Davis. *Rx One Health*. Davis: University of California. https://ohi.vetmed.ucdavis.edu/education/rx-one-health#:~:text=Novel%20pathogens%2C%20climate%20change%2C%20biodiversity,field%20course%2C%20visit%20their%20website (accessed 01 December 2024).

95 UMN. *One Health: A World-Changing Approach*. University of Minnesota (UMN). https://twin-cities.umn.edu/news-events/one-health-world-changing-approach (accessed 03 December 2024)

96 RVC. One Health: Ecosystems, Humans and Animals. *Royal Veterinary College (RVC)*. https://www.rvc.ac.uk/study/postgraduate/one-health (accessed 03 December 2024).

97 Sakurai, Y., Ishikura, Y., Nakano, R., et al. University administrators' visions for the recovery of international student exchange in a post-COVID-19 world. *High. Learn. Res. Commun.* 2023; 13(1): 50–69. https://doi.org/10.18870/hlrc.v13i1.1396.

98 Essack, S.Y. Environment: the neglected component of the One Health triad. *Lancet Planet. Health.* 2018; 2(6): e238–e239. https://doi.org/10.1016/S2542-5196(18)30124-4.

99 Kumar, A. Disaster response under "One Health" approach: contribution of veterinary public health. In: *Management of Animals in Disasters*, 245–261. Springer; 2022. https://doi.org/10.1007/978-981-16-9392-2_21.

100 Isiko, J., Khaitsa, M.L., Ekiri, A., and Sischo, W. Engaging Intergovernmental Organizations in the training of students on global animal health, public health and food security. *Pan Afr. Med. J.* 2017; 12(4): 12. https://doi.org/10.11604/pamj.supp.2017.27.4.12368].

101 Baba, Y., Shichijo, N., and Sedita, S.R. How do collaborations with universities affect firms' innovative performance? The role of "Pasteur scientists" in the advanced materials field. *Res. Policy.* 2009; 38(5): 756–764. https://doi.org/10.1016/j.respol.2009.01.006.

102 Yarime, M., Trencher, G., Mino, T., et al. Establishing sustainability science in higher education institutions: towards an integration of academic development, institutionalization, and stakeholder collaborations. *Sustain. Sci.* 2012; 7: 101–113. https://doi.org/10.1007/s11625-012-0157-5.

103 UVAS. *Virtual One Health International Conference 2020 (25-26 November)*. https://uvas.edu.pk/NEWS/2021/Final%20Abstract%20Book%20OHC%2011-12-2020.pdf (accessed 01 December 2024).

104 UVAS. *Antimicrobial Resistance AMR: Current Status and Future Road Map for Pakistan*. https://uvas.edu.pk/doc/Departments/ep/Antimicrobial%20Resistance%20-%20Current%20Status%20and%20Future%20Road%20Map%20for%20Pakistan.pdf (accessed 01 December 2024).

105 CVASU. *One Health Institute*. https://cvasu.ac.bd/office/one-health-institute (accessed 01 December 2024).

106 One Health Commission. *COHEART KVASU*. https://www.onehealthcommission.org/documents/filelibrary/resources/whos_who/52519_COHEART_WhosWhotemplate_9B2E61CE68D14.pdf (accessed 01 December 2024).

107 KVASU. *Academics: Post Graduate Diploma in One Health*. https://www.kvasu.ac.in/one-health-1 (accessed 01 December 2024).

108 Bukachi, S.A., Onono, J., Onyango-Ouma, W., et al. Opportunities, gaps, and challenges in the implementation of the One Health approach in Kenya. *One Health Cases* 2024 (2024): ohcs20240019. https://doi.org/10.1079/onehealthcases.2024.0019.

109 de Nooijer, P. and Abagi, O. *Final Evaluation of the IUC partner programme with the University of Nairobi (UoN), Kenya*. Kenya: University of Nairobi (UoN); 2009. https://cdn.vliruos.be/vliruos/bd4ff133102ceed7c4762763bef05095.pdf.

110 Kelly, T.R., Machalaba, C., Karesh, W.B., et al. Implementing One Health approaches to confront emerging and re-emerging zoonotic disease threats: lessons from PREDICT. *One Health Outlook* 2020; 2: 1–7. https://doi.org/10.1186/s42522-019-0007-9.

111 University of Nairobi. *Master of Science in One Health and Emergency Research Ethics (Mohere)_Department of Public Health Pharmacology and Tox*. University of Nairobi. 2024. https://phpt.uonbi.ac.ke/admission-content-type/master-science-one-health-and-emergency-research-ethics-mohere.

112 Estambale, B., Mutua, E., Ochieng, A., et al. Stakeholder analysis for One-Health preparedness and operationalization in Kenya: the One-Health scorecard approach. 2024. https://doi.org/10.21203/rs.3.rs-4350683/v1.

113 Richards, S., Knight-Jones, T., Angombe, S., et al. Towards institutionalization of One Health in Eastern and Southern Africa. *One Health Cases* 2024 (2024): ohcs20240007. https://doi.org/10.1079/onehealthcases.2024.0007.

114 Michel, A.L. *Faculty Day, Faculty of Veterinary Science*. University of Pretoria. 2014, https://repository.up.ac.za/handle/2263/49075?show=full.

115 Showande, S.J. and Ibirongbe, T.P. Interprofessional education and collaborative practice in Nigeria–Pharmacists' and pharmacy students' attitudes and perceptions of the obstacles and recommendations. *Curr. Pharm. Teach. Learn.* 2023; 15(9): 787–800. https://doi.org/10.1016/j.cptl.2023.07.013.

116 Olugasa, B.O. Opportunities for field research and short course in human-animal disease surveillance in West Africa. *Control and Prevention of Zoonoses*. 2014. https://www.researchgate.net/profile/Babasola-Olugasa/publication/324264149_Rabies_elimination_as_a_one-health_model_for_the_tropics_can_this_be_a_solution_to_the_protracted_problem_in_West_Africa/links/5b126e540f7e9b4981038b7f/Rabies-elimination-as-a-one-health-model-for-the-tropics-can-this-be-a-solution-to-the-protracted-problem-in-West-Africa.pdf.

117 Olayinka, I. *Strengthening Academic Linkages and Collaboration in Universities*. Calabar, Cross River State: The Graduate School, University of Calabar; 2004. http://ir.library.ui.edu.ng/handle/123456789/5428.

118 Babalobi, O.O. *The Role of One Health in Managing Emerging and Re-Emerging National Health Challenges*. 2016. http://ir.library.ui.edu.ng/handle/123456789/7981.

119 UQ. *About Queensland Alliance for One Health Sciences (QAOHS)*. https://veterinary-science.uq.edu.au/queensland-alliance-one-health-sciences (accessed 03 December 2024)

120 Yasobant, S., Lekha, K.S., and Saxena, D. Risk assessment tools from the One Health perspective: a narrative review. *Risk Manag. Healthc. Policy* 2024; 17: 955–972. https://doi.org/10.2147/RMHP.S436385.

121 World Health Organization. *A Health Perspective on the Role of the Environment in One Health*. World Health Organization (WHO); 2022. https://www.who.int/europe/publications/i/item/WHO-EURO-2022-5290-45054-64214.

122 Nyström, M.E., Karltun, J., Keller, C., and Gäre, B.A. Collaborative and partnership research for improvement of health and social services: researcher's experiences from 20 projects. *Health Res. Policy Syst*. 2018: 16(46): 1–17. https://doi.org/10.1186/s12961-018-0322-0.

123 Mazet, J.A.K., Clifford, D.L., Coppolillo, P.B., et al. Health in action a "One Health" approach to address emerging zoonoses: the HALI project in Tanzania. *PLOS Med*. 2009; 6(12); e1000190. https://doi.org/10.1371/journal.pmed.1000190.

124 One Health Commission. *Full Map of "All" Groups and Organizations Identified Around the World as Actively Working to Further One Health*. https://www.onehealthcommission.org/en/resources__services/whos_who_in_one_health/ (accessed 26 November 2024).

125 Scholthof, K.G. The disease triangle: pathogens, the environment, and society. *Nat. Rev. Microbiol*. 2007; 5: 152–156. https://doi.org/10.1038/nrmicro1596.

126 Karesh, W.B., Dobson, A., Lloyd-smith, J.O., et al. Zoonoses 1 Ecology of zoonoses: natural and unnatural histories. *Lancet* 2012; 380(9857): 1936–1945. https://doi.org/10.1016/S0140-6736(12)61678-X.

127 Taylor, L.H., Latham, S.M., and Woolhouse, M.E.J. Risk factors for human disease emergence. *Philos. Trans. R. Soc. Lond. B: Biol. Sci*. 2001; 356(1411): 983–989. https://doi.org/10.1098/rstb.2001.0888.

128 Casadevall, A. and Pirofski, L. Host-pathogen interactions: redefining the basic concepts of virulence and pathogenicity. *Infect. Immun*. 1999; (8): 3703–3713. https://doi.org/10.1128/iai.67.8.3703-3713.1999.

129 Day, M.J. One Health: the importance of companion animal vector-borne diseases. *Parasit. Vectors* 2011; 4(49): 2–7. https://doi.org/10.1186/1756-3305-4-49.

130 Mcewen, S.A. and Fedorka-Cray, P.J. Antimicrobial use and resistance in animals. *Clin. Infect. Dis*. 2002; 34(Suppl 3): 93–106. https://doi.org/10.1086/340246.

131 Frenk, J., Chen, L., Bhutta, Z.A., et al. Health professionals for a new century: transforming education to strengthen health systems in an interdependent World Citation Health professionals for a new century: transforming education to strengthen health systems in an interdependent world. *Lancet*; 2010. https://doi.org/10.1016/S0140-6736(10)61854-5.

132 King, L.J., Anderson, L.R., Blackmore, C.G., et al. Executive summary of the AVMA One Health Initiative Task Force report. *J. Am. Vet. Med. Assoc*. 2008; 233(2): 259–261. http://doi.org/10.2460/javma.233.2.259.

133 Rabinowitz, P. and Conti, L. Links among human health, animal health, and ecosystem health. *Annu Rev. Public Health*. 2013; 34(1): 189–204. https://doi.org/10.1146/annurev-publhealth-031912-114426.

134 Machalaba, C., Berrian, A.M., Berthe, F.C.J., et al. Applying a One Health approach in global health and medicine: enhancing involvement of medical schools and global health centers. *Ann. Glob. Health*. 2021; 87(1): 1–11. https://doi.org/10.5334/aogh.2647.

135 Osburn, B., Scott, C., and Gibbs, P. One World – One Medicine – One Health: emerging veterinary challenges and opportunities. *Sci. Tech. Rev*. 2015; 28(2): 481–486. http://doi.org/10.20506/rst.28.2.1884.

136 Zinsstag, J., Schelling, E., and Tanner, M. From "one medicine" to "one health" and systemic approaches to health and well-being. *Prev. Vet. Med*. 2011; 101(August 2009): 148–156. http://doi.org/10.1016/j.prevetmed.2010.07.003.

137 Dary-Acevedo, L., Aguirre. A., Aguirre, L.F., et al. *Reducing Pandemic Risk, Promoting Global Health*. PREDICT, USAID; 2021.

138 Burgess, B.A. and Morley, P.S. Veterinary hospital surveillance systems. *Vet. Clin. North Am. Small Anim. Pract*. 2014; 45(2): 235–242. https://doi.org/10.1016/j.cvsm.2014.11.002.

139 Fewster-Thuente, L. and Velsor-Friedrich, B. Interdisciplinary collaboration for healthcare professionals. *Nurs. Adm. Q*. 2008; 32(1): 40–48. https://doi.org/10.1097/01.NAQ.0000305946.31193.61.

140 Jasani, S. Using a one health approach can foster collaboration through transdisciplinary teaching using a One Health approach can foster collaboration through. *Med. Teach.* 2018: 1–3. https://doi.org/10.1080/0142159X.2018.1484080.

141 Rahman, T., Sobur, A., Islam, S., et al. Zoonotic diseases: etiology, impact, and control. *Microorganisms.* 2020; 8(9): 1405. https://doi.org/10.3390/microorganisms8091405.

142 Esposito, M.M., Turku, S., Lehrfiel, L., and A. Shoman. The impact of human activities on zoonotic infection transmissions. *Animals.* 2023; 13(10): 1646. https://doi.org/10.3390/ani13101646.

143 Zinsstag, J., Schelling, E., Wyss, K., and Mahamat, M.B. Potential of cooperation between human and animal health. *Lancet.* 2005; 366(9503): 2142–2145. https://doi.org/10.1016/S0140-6736(05)67731-8.

144 Rwego, I.B., Babalobi, O.O., Musotsi, P., et al. One Health capacity building in sub-Saharan Africa. *Infect. Ecol. Epidemiol.* 2016; 6: 34032. https://doi.org/10.3402/iee.v6.34032.

145 Jones, K.E., Patel, N.G., Levy, M.A., et al. Global trends in emerging infectious diseases. *Nature.* 2008; 451: 990–994. https://doi.org/10.1038/nature06536.

146 Gubler, D.J., Reiter, P., Ebi, K.L., et al. Climate variability and change in the United States: potential impacts on vector- and rodent-borne diseases. *Environ. Health Perspect.* 2001; 109(Suppl 2): 223–233. https://doi.org/10.1289/ehp.109-1240669.

147 Pruss-Ustun, A., Corvalán, C.F., and World Health Organization. *Preventing Disease Through Towards an Estimate of the Environmental Burden of Disease.* World Health Organization; 2006. https://www.who.int/publications/i/item/9241593822.

148 Wood, J.L.N., Leach, M., Waldman, L., et al. A framework for the study of zoonotic disease emergence and its drivers: spillover of bat pathogens as a case study. *Philos. Trans. R. Soc. B: Biol. Sci.* 2012; 367(1604): 2881–2892. https://doi.org/10.1098/rstb.2012.0228.

149 Kahn, L.H., Kaplan, B., and Steele, J.H. Confronting zoonoses through closer collaboration between medicine and veterinary medicine (as "one medicine"). *Vet. Ital.* 2007; 43(1): 5–19. https://www.izs.it/vet_italiana/2007/43_1/5.htm.

150 Barrows, H.S. and Tamblyn, R.M. *Problem-Based Learning: An Approach to Medical Education* Vol. *1*. Medical Education, Springer Publishing Company; 1980.

151 Albanese, M.A. and Mitchell, S.M.A. Problem-based learning: a review of literature on its outcomes and implementation issues. *Acad. Med.* 1993; 68(1): 52–81. https://journals.lww.com/academicmedicine/abstract/1993/01000/Problem_based_Learning__A_Review_of_Literature_on.20.aspx.

152 Cooke, M., Irby, D.M., and O'Brien, B.C. Educating physicians: a call for reform of medical school and residency. *J. Chiropr. Educ.* 2011; 25(2): 193.

153 Prince, M. Does active learning work? A review of the research. *J. Eng. Educ.* 2004; 93(3): 223–231. https://doi.org/10.1002/j.2168-9830.2004.tb00809.x.

154 Schmidt, H.G. and Rotgans, J.I. The process of problem-based learning: what works and why. *Med. Educ.* 2011; 45(8): 792–806. https://doi.org/10.1111/j.1365-2923.2011.04035.x.

155 Dolmans, D.H.J.M., De Grave, W., Wolfhagen, I.H.A.P., and Van Der Vleuten, C.P.M. Current perspectives problem-based learning: future challenges for educational practice and research. *Med. Educ.* 2005; 39(7): 732–741. https://doi.org/10.1111/j.1365-2929.2005.02205.x.

156 Lane, E.A. Problem-based learning in veterinary education. *J. Vet. Med. Educ.* 2008; 35(4): 631–636. https://doi.org/10.3138/jvme.35.4.631.

157 Courtenay, M., Conrad, P., Wilkes, M., et al. Interprofessional initiatives between the human health professions and veterinary medical students: a scoping review. *J. Interprof. Care.* 2014; 1820(4): 323–330. https://doi.org/10.3109/13561820.2014.895979.

158 Robinson, T.P., Bu, D.P., Carrique-mas, J., et al. Antibiotic resistance is the quintessential One Health issue. *Trans. R. Soc. Trop. Med. Hyg.* 2016; 110(7): 377–380. https://doi.org/10.1093/trstmh/trw048.

159 Fraser, D. Understanding animal welfare. *Acta Vet. Scand.* 2008; 50(1): S1. https://doi.org/10.1186/1751-0147-50-S1-S1.

160 Daszak, P. Emerging infectious diseases of wildlife- threats to biodiversity and human health. *Science* 2000; 287(5452): 443–449. https://doi.org/10.1126/science.287.5452.443.

161 Gebreyes, W.A., Dupouy-camet, J., Newport, M.J., et al. The global one health paradigm: challenges and opportunities for tackling infectious diseases at the human, animal, and environment interface in low-resource settings. *PLoS Negl. Trop. Dis.* 2014; 8(11): e3257. https://doi.org/10.1371/journal.pntd.0003257.

162 Pongsiri, M.J., Roman, J., Ezenwa, V.O., et al. Biodiversity loss affects global disease ecology. *Bioscience.* 2009; 59(11): 945–954. https://doi.org/10.1525/bio.2009.59.11.6.

163 Foley, J.A. Global consequences of land use. *Science.* 2005; 309(5734): 570–574. https://doi.org/10.1126/science.1111772.

164 Bordier, M., Delavenne, C., Thuy, D., and Nguyen, T. One Health surveillance: a matrix to evaluate multisectoral collaboration. *Front. Vet. Sci.* 2019; 6: 109. https://doi.org/10.3389/fvets.2019.00109.

165 Raftery, P., Hossain, M., and Palmer, J. An innovative and integrated model for global outbreak response and research – a case study of the UK Public Health Rapid Support Team (UK-PHRST). *BMC Public Health* 2021; 21: 11378. https://doi.org/10.1186/s12889-021-11433-0

166 Weinberg, A.D. and Frankson, R. One Health core competency domains. *Front. Public health.* 2016; 4: 192. https://doi.org/10.3389/fpubh.2016.00192.

167 Roopnarine, R. *Factors That Influence the Development of Interprofessional Education and One Health for Medical, Veterinary and Dual Degree Public Health Students at an Offshore Medical School.* The University of Liverpool (United Kingdom) ProQuest Dissertations and Theses; 2020. https://www.proquest.com/openview/d47b6bf98fa7a4699c6718c5865b5df2/1?pq-origsite=gscholar&cbl=18750&diss=y.

168 Estrada, A.H., Behar-Horenstein, L., Estrada, D.J., et al. Incorporating inter-professional education into a veterinary medical curriculum. *J. Vet. Med. Educ.* 2016; 43(3): 275–281. https://doi.org/10.3138/jvme.0715-121R.

169 Sullivan, A., Ogunseitan, O., Epstein, J., et al. International stakeholder perspectives on One Health training and empowerment: a needs assessment for a One Health Workforce Academy. *One Health Outlook* 2023; 5(1): 8. https://doi.org/10.1186/s42522-023-00083-4.

170 Amuguni, H.J., Mazan, M., and Kibuuka, R. Producing interdisciplinary competent professionals: integrating One Health core competencies into the veterinary curriculum at the University of Rwanda. *J. Vet. Med. Educ.* 2017; 44(4): 649–659. https://doi.org/10.3138/jvme.0815-133R.

171 Kochevar, D.T. Fifty years of evolving partnerships in veterinary medical education. *J. Vet. Med. Educ.* 2015; 42(5): 403–413. https://doi.org/10.3138/jvme.0815-136R.

172 Destoumieux-Garzón, D., Mavingui, P., Boetsch, G., et al. The one health concept: 10 years old and a long road ahead. *Front. Vet. Sci.* 2018; 5: 14. https://doi.org/10.3389/fvets.2018.00014.

173 Meredith, A., Anderson, N., Malik, P., et al. Capacity building for wildlife health professionals: the Wildlife Health Bridge. *One Health Impl. Res..* 2022; 27: 68–78. https://doi.org/10.20517/ohir.2022.03.

174 Doucet, M. and Bélisle, M. Developing and implementing a competency-based veterinary medicine program at the Université de Montréal. *J. Vet. Med. Educ.* 2024(aop): e20230172. https://doi.org/10.3138/jvme-2023-0172.

175 Iatridou, D., Bravo, A., and Saunders, J. One Health interdisciplinary collaboration in veterinary education establishments in Europe: mapping implementation and reflecting on promotion. *J. Vet. Med. Educ.* 2021; 48(4): 427–440. https://doi.org/10.3138/jvme-2020-0019.

176 Conrad, P.A., Mazet, J.A., Clifford, D., et al. Evolution of a transdisciplinary "One Medicine-One Health" approach to global health education at the University of California, Davis. *Prev. Vet. Med.* 2009; 92(4): 268–274. https://doi.org/10.1016/j.prevetmed.2009.09.002.

177 Wilkes, M.S., Conrad, P.A., and Winer, J.N. One Health-One Education: medical and veterinary inter-professional training. *J. Vet. Med. Educ.* 2019; 46(1): 14–20. https://doi.org/10.3138/jvme.1116-171r.

178 Lane, S.L. Integrated environmental education: introducing One Health concepts into veterinary technician education. Master's thesis. Montreat College; 2015. https://www.proquest.com/openview/257de0b8618b6aedfd282afa14d01748/1?pq-origsite=gscholar&cbl=18750.

179 Rooke, F. Excellence is expected: quality monitoring and improvement in veterinary medicine. Doctoral dissertation. University of Nottingham; 2023. https://eprints.nottingham.ac.uk/id/eprint/73907.

180 Ali, S.H. and Keil, R. *Networked Disease: Emerging Infections in the Global City*. John Wiley and Sons; 2008. https://doi.org/10.1002/9781444305012.

181 Pribadi, M.P., Nasharudin, N.A.M., and Hassan, L. Evaluating the effectiveness of One Health training programmes among medical, veterinary, ecology, and allied health students. *Int. J. Acad. Res. Bus. Soc. Sci.* 2022; 12(6): 1187–1202. http://doi.org/10.6007/IJARBSS/v12-i6/13942.

182 Kareskoski, M. Accreditation in continuing veterinary education: development of an accreditation system and selection of accreditation criteria. *Front. Vet. Sci.* 2023; 10: 1181961. https://doi.org/10.3389/fvets.2023.1181961.

183 Kahn, L.H. Educating undergraduates on one health. *J. Am. Vet. Med. Assoc.* 2012; 240(2): 144.

184 Seffren, V., Lowther, S., Guerra, M., et al. Strengthening the global one health workforce: veterinarians in CDC-supported field epidemiology training programs. *One Health* 2022; 14: 100382. https://doi.org/10.1016/j.onehlt.2022.100382.

185 Zinsstag, J., Pelikan, K., Gonzalez, M.B., et al. Value-added transdisciplinary One Health research and problem solving. In: *Handbook of Transdisciplinarity: Global Perspectives*, 333–350. Edward Elgar Publishing; 2023. https://doi.org/10.4337/9781802207835.00031.

186 Vink, W.D., McKenzie, J.S., Cogger, N., et al. Building a foundation for "One Health": an education strategy for enhancing and sustaining national and regional capacity in endemic and emerging zoonotic disease management. In: *One Health: The Human-Animal-Environment Interfaces in Emerging Infectious Diseases: Food Safety and Security, and International and National Plans for Implementation of One Health Activities* vol. 366, (ed. J. Mackenzie, M. Jeggo, P. Daszak and J. Richt), 185–205. Heidelberg, Berlin: Springer; 2012. https://doi.org/10.1007/82_2012_241.

187 Bhatia, R. *National Framework for One Health*. Food and Agriculture Organization; 2021. https://openknowledge.fao.org/handle/20.500.14283/cb4072en.

188 Liu, J.S., Li, X.C., Zhang, Q.Y., et al. China's application of the One Health approach in addressing public health threats at the human-animal-environment interface: advances and challenges. *One Health* 2023; 17: 100607. https://doi.org/10.1016/j.onehlt.2023.100607.

189 Mwangi, W., de Figueiredo, P., and Criscitiello, M.F. One Health: addressing global challenges at the nexus of human, animal, and environmental health. *PLoS Pathog*. 2016; 12(9): e1005731. https://doi.org/10.1371/journal.ppat.1005731.

190 Fletcher, O.J., Hooper, B.E., and Schoenfeld-Tacher, R. Instruction and curriculum in veterinary medical education: a 50-year perspective. *J. Vet. Med. Educ.* 2015; 42(5): 489–500. https://doi.org/10.3138/jvme.0515-071.

191 Nguyen-Viet, H., Doria, S., Tung, D.X., et al. Ecohealth research in Southeast Asia: past, present and the way forward. *Infect. Dis. Poverty* 2015; 4(5): 1–13. https://doi.org/10.1186/2049-9957-4-5.

192 Nguyen-Viet, H., Lam, S., Nguyen-Mai, H., et al. Decades of emerging infectious disease, food safety, and antimicrobial resistance response in Vietnam: the role of One Health. *One Health* 2022; 14: 100361. https://doi.org/10.1016/j.onehlt.2021.100361.

193 Pettan-Brewer, C., Martins, A.F., de Abreu, D.P.B., et al. From the approach to the concept: one health in Latin America-experiences and perspectives in Brazil, Chile, and Colombia. *Front. Public Health.* 2021; 9: 687110. https://doi.org/10.3389/fpubh.2021.687110.

194 Gibbs, S.E.J. and Gibbs, E.P.J. The historical, present, and future role of veterinarians in One Health. *Curr. Top. Microbiol. Immunol.* 2013; 365: 31–47. https://doi.org/10.1007/82_2012_259.

195 McGreevy, P., Thomson, P., Dhand, N.K., et al. VetCompass Australia: a national big data collection system for veterinary science. *Animals* 2017; 7(10): 74. https://doi.org/10.3390/ani7100074.

196 Cediel Becerra, N.M., Olaya Medellin, A.M., Tomassone, L., et al. A survey on One Health approach in Colombia and some Latin American countries: from a fragmented health organization to an integrated health response to global challenges. *Front. Public Health.* 2021; 9: 649240. https://doi.org/10.3389/fpubh.2021.649240.

197 Mubareka, S., Amuasi, J., Banerjee, A., et al. Strengthening a One Health approach to emerging zoonoses. *Facets* 2023; 8: 1–64. https://doi.org/10.1139/facets-2021-0190.

198 Pathak, H., Mishra, J.P., and Mohapatra, T. Indian agriculture after independence. *Indian Council Agric. Res., New Delhi* 2022; 110(001): 426. https://krishi.icar.gov.in/jspui/bitstream/123456789/78946/1/IndianAgricultureafterIndependence_Fisherieschapter_2022-2-12.pdf.

199 Laaser, U., Stroud, C., Bjegovic-Mikanovic, V., et al. Exchange and coordination: challenges of the global One Health movement. *South Eastern Eur. J. Public Health* 2022. https://doi.org/10.11576/seejph-6076.

200 Zinsstag, J., Hediger, K., Osman, Y.M., et al. The promotion and development of One Health at Swiss TPH and its greater potential. *Diseases* 2022; 10(3): 65. https://doi.org/10.3390/diseases10030065.

201 Bock, B., Hacking, N., and Miele, M. *Coordinated European Animal Welfare Network (EuWelNet)-Deliverable 4 (2014)*; 2014. https://www.euwelnet.eu/media/1138/excecutive_summary_final_english.pdf.

202 Laing, G., Duffy, E., Anderson, N., et al. Advancing One Health: updated core competencies. *CABI One Health.* 2023 (2023): ohcs20230002. https://doi.org/10.1079/cabionehealth.2023.0002.

203 Brown, G.W., Rhodes, N., Tacheva, B., et al. Challenges in international health financing and implications for the new pandemic fund. *Glob. Health* 2023; 19(1): 97. https://doi.org/10.1186/s12992-023-00999-6.

204 Uchtmann, N., Herrmann, J.A., Hahn, E.C., and Beasley, V.R. Barriers to, efforts in, and optimization of integrated One Health surveillance: a review and synthesis. *EcoHealth* 2015; 12: 368–384. https://doi.org/10.1007/s10393-015-1022-7.

205 Beckham, T.R., Brake, D.A., and Fine, J.B. Strengthening One Health through investments in agricultural preparedness. *Health Secur.* 2018; 16(2): 92–107. https://doi.org/10.1089/hs.2017.0069.

206 Stroud, C., Kaplan, B., Logan, J.E., and Gray, G.C. One Health training, research, and outreach in North America. *Infect. Ecol. Epidemiol.* 2016; 6(1): 33680. https://doi.org/10.3402/iee.v6.33680.

207 Paranjape, S.M. and Franz, D.R. Implementing the global health security agenda: lessons from global health and security programs. *Health Secur.* 2015; 13(1): 9–19. https://doi.org/10.1089/hs.2014.0047.

208 Murtaugh, M.P., Steer, C.J., Sreevatsan, S., et al. The science behind One Health: at the interface of humans, animals, and the environment. *Wiley Online Lib.* 2017; 1395(1): 12–32. https://doi.org/10.1111/nyas.13355.

209 Rweyemamu, M.M., Mmbuji, P., Karimuribo, E., et al. The Southern African Centre for infectious disease surveillance: a one health consortium. *Emerg. Health Threats J.* 2013; 6(1): 19958. https://doi.org/10.3402/ehtj.v6i0.19958.

210 Hanin, M.C.E., Queenan, K., Savic, S., et al. A One Health evaluation of the southern African centre for infectious disease surveillance. *Front. Vet. Sci.* 2018; 5: 33. https://doi.org/10.3389/fvets.2018.00033.

211 Musvuugwa, T. Grappling with (re)-emerging infectious zoonoses: risk assessment, mitigation framework, and future directions. *Int. J. Disaster Risk Reduc.* 2022; 82: 103350. https://doi.org/10.1016/j.ijdrr.2022.103350.

212 Sharma, A. and Zodpey, S.P. Transforming public health education in India through networking and collaborations: opportunities and challenges. *Indian J. Public Health.* 2013; 57(3): 155–160. https://doi.org/10.4103/0019-557X.119833.

213 Comizzoli, P., Pagenkopp Lohan, K.M., Muletz-Wolz, C., et al. The interconnected health initiative: a Smithsonian framework to extend one health research and education. *Front. Vet. Sci.* 2021; 8: 629410. https://doi.org/10.3389/fvets.2021.629410.

214 DiClemente, R., Nowara, A., Shelton, R., and Wingood, G. Need for innovation in public health research. *Am. J. Public Health.* 2019; 109(S2): S117–S120. https://doi.org/10.2105/AJPH.2018.304876.

215 Singh, S., Sharma, P., Pal, N., et al. Holistic one health surveillance framework: synergizing environmental, animal, and human determinants for enhanced infectious disease management. *ACS Infect. Dis.* 2024; 10(3): 808–826. https://pubs.acs.org/doi/10.1021/acsinfecdis.3c00625.

216 Chen, C., Ragle, C.A., Lencioni, R., and Fransson, B.A. Comparison of 2 training programs for basic laparoscopic skills and simulated surgery performance in veterinary students. *Vet. Surg.* 2017; 46(8): 1187–1197. https://doi.org/10.1111/vsu.12729.

217 Polonsky, J.A., Baidjoe, A., Kamvar, Z.N., et al. Outbreak analytics: a developing data science for informing the response to emerging pathogens. *Philos. Trans. R. Soc. B.* 2019; 374(1776): 20180276. https://doi.org/10.1098/rstb.2018.0276.

218 Stockdale, J.E., Liu, P., and Colijn, C. The potential of genomics for infectious disease forecasting. *Nat. Microbiol.* 2022; 7(11): 1736–1743. https://doi.org/10.1038/s41564-022-01233-6.

219 Castro, L.R. Vectors of health: epidemics, ecologies, and the reinvention of mosquito science in Brazil. Doctoral dissertation. Massachusetts Institute of Technology; 2021. https://dspace.mit.edu/bitstream/handle/1721.1/139970/castro-luisarc-phd-sts-2021-thesis.pdf.

220 Ko, K.K.K., Chng, K.R., and Nagarajan, N. Metagenomics-enabled microbial surveillance. *Nat. Microbiol.* 2022; 7(4): 486–496. https://doi.org/10.1038/s41564-022-01089-w.

221 Lammie, S.L. and Hughes, J.M. Antimicrobial resistance, food safety, and one health: the need for convergence. *Annu. Rev. Food sci. Technol.* 2016; 7(1): 287–312. https://doi.org/10.1146/annurev-food-041715-033251.

222 Carlson, C.J., Farrell, M.J., Grange, Z., et al. The future of zoonotic risk prediction. *Philos. Trans. R. Soc. B.* 2021; 376(1837): 20200358. https://doi.org/10.1098/rstb.2020.0358.

223 Robinson, J.M., Harrison, P.A., Mavoa, S., and Breed, M.F. Existing and emerging uses of drones in restoration ecology. *Methods Ecol. Evol.* 2022; 13(9): 1899–1911. https://doi.org/10.1111/2041-210X.13912.

224 Guo, W., Lv, C., Guo, M., et al. Innovative applications of artificial intelligence in zoonotic disease management. *Sci. One Health.* 2023; 2: 100045. https://doi.org/10.1016/j.soh.2023.100045.

225 Mechan, F., Bartonicek, Z., Malone, D., and Lees, R.S. Unmanned aerial vehicles for surveillance and control of vectors of malaria and other vector-borne diseases. *Malaria J.* 2023; 22(1): 23. https://doi.org/10.1186/s12936-022-04414-0.

226 Abdus Samad, M. Current status and challenges for globalisation of veterinary medical education for the "One Health" programme. *Rev. Sci. Tech.* 2017; 36(3): 741–765. https://doi.org/10.20506/rst.36.3.2711.

227 Steele, S.G., Booy, R., Manocha, R., et al. Towards One Health clinical management of zoonoses: a parallel survey of Australian general medical practitioners and veterinarians. *Zoonoses Public Health* 2021; 68(2): 88–102. https://doi.org/10.1111/zph.12799.

228 Vanlangendonck, C., Mackenzie, J., and Osterhaus, A. Highlights from science policy Interface sessions at the one health congress 2020. *One Health Outlook* 2021; 3(1): 1. https://doi.org/10.1186/s42522-020-00033-4.

229 Guenin, M.J., De Nys, H.M., Peyre, M., et al. A participatory epidemiological and One Health approach to explore the community's capacity to detect emerging zoonoses and surveillance network opportunities in the forest region of Guinea. *PLOS Negl. Trop. Dis.* 2022; 16(7): e0010462. https://doi.org/10.1371/journal.pntd.0010462.

230 Maudling, R. How can One Health contribute to pandemic prevention? Looking at Ebola through a One Health lens. *CABI One Health* 2022(2022): ohcs20220004. https://doi.org/10.1079/cabionehealth20220004.

231 Reid, S.A., McKenzie, J., and Woldeyohannes, S.M. One Health research and training in Australia and New Zealand. *Infect. Ecol. Epidemiol.* 2016; 6(1): 33799. https://doi.org/10.3402/iee.v6.33799.

232 Smith, W. and San Miguel, S.F. A global veterinary education program for North American veterinary students: a description of Purdue University Best Practices. *J. Vet. Med. Educ.* 2020; 47(4): 408–413. https://doi.org/10.3138/jvme.1018-130r.

233 Sobierajski, T., Wanke-Rytt, M., Chajecka-Wierzchowska, W., et al. One Health in the consciousness of veterinary students from the perspective of knowledge of antibiotic therapy and antimicrobial resistance: a multi-centre study. *Front. Public Health.* 2023; 11: 1165035. https://doi.org/10.3389/fpubh.2023.1165035.

234 Özgüler, Z. and Aslan, D. Knowledge and perceptions of physicians and veterinarians about One Health in Türkiye. *Eastern Mediterranean Health J.* 2023; 29(10): 767–774. https://doi.org/10.26719/emhj.23.082.

235 Ounsaneha, W., Parunawin, W., Laosee, O., et al. Household environmental practice for prevent and control dengue fever toward One Health framework in an endemic area of Central Region, Thailand. *EnvironmentAsia* 2022; 15(2): 33–34. https://tshe.org/main/ea-journal-content?id=4.

236 Chowdhury, S., Aleem, M.A., Khan, M.S.I., et al. Major zoonotic diseases of public health importance in Bangladesh. *Vet. Med. Sci.* 2021; 7(4): 1199–1210. https://doi.org/10.1002/vms3.465.

237 Corredor Jimenez, J., Grimm, H.M., Ceesay, L.O., and Wondirad, M. Lessons not (yet) learned: what African Countries could teach the Global North about One Health during the Pandemics. *J. Comp. Policy Anal.: Res. Pract.* 2023; 25(5): 487–505. https://doi.org/10.1080/13876988.2023.2187698.

238 Li, O.Y., Wang, X., Yang, K., et al. The approaching pilot for One Health governance index. *Infect. Dis. Poverty.* 2023; 12(1): 16. https://doi.org/10.1186/s40249-023-01067-2.

239 Pettan-Brewer, C., Vezeau, N., Barbosa, D.S., and Biondo, A.W. One Health predatory symposiums and publishers in Brazil and Latin America: how to recognize and find solutions to avoid them? *CABI One Health.* 2023(2023): ohcs20230002. https://doi.org/10.1079/cabionehealth.2023.0002.

240 Nguta, J.M., Belaynehe, K.M., Arruda, A.G., et al. "One Health" research ethics in emergency, disaster and zoonotic disease outbreaks: a case study from Ethiopia. In: *Ethics, Integrity and Policymaking: The Value of the Case Study* (ed. D. O'Mathúna and R. Iphofen), 151–164. Cham: Springer International Publishing; 2022. https://doi.org/10.1007/978-3-031-15746-2_12.

241 Benedetti, G., Jokelainen, P., and Ethelberg, S. Search term "One Health" remains of limited use to identify relevant scientific publications: Denmark as a case study. *Front. Public Health.* 2022; 10: 938460. https://doi.org/10.3389/fpubh.2022.938460.

242 McKenzie, J.S., Dahal, R., Kakkar, M., et al. One Health research and training and government support for One Health in South Asia. *Infect. Ecol. Epidemiol.* 2016; 6(1): 33842. https://doi.org/10.3402/iee.v6.33842.

243 Chatterjee, P., Chauhan, A.S., Joseph, J., and Kakkar, M. One Health/EcoHealth capacity building programs in South and South East Asia: a mixed method rapid systematic review. *Hum. Resour. Health.* 2017; 15(1): 72. https://doi.org/10.1186/s12960-017-0246-8.

244 RIVM. *One Health International Collaboration.* https://www.rivm.nl/en/one-health/international-collaboration (accessed 30 August 2024).

245 Southeast Asia One Health University Network. *One Health Education.* https://www.seaohun.org/oh-education (accessed 31 August 2024).

246 Africa One Health University Network. *About Us.* https://afrohun.org/about-us/ (accessed 31 August 2024).

247 van Herten, J. and Meijboom, F.L.B. Veterinary responsibilities within the One Health framework. *Food Ethics* 2019; 3(1): 109–123. https://doi.org/10.1007/s41055-019-00034-8.

248 Gibbs, S.E.J. and Gibbs, E.P.J. The historical, present, and future role of veterinarians in One Health. In: *One Health: The Human-Animal-Environment Interfaces in Emerging Infectious Diseases: The Concept and Examples of a One Health Approach* (ed. J.S. Mackenzie, M. Jeggo, P. Daszak and J.A. Richt), 31–47. Berlin, Heidelberg: Springer Berlin Heidelberg; 2013. https://doi.org/10.1007/82_2012_259.

249 American Veterinary Medical Association. *One Health.* https://www.avma.org/resources-tools/one-health (accessed 30 August 2024).

250 Farnham, M.W. and Hueston, W.D. Continuing Education and Incorporation of the 'One Health' Concept: 12th Conference of the OIE Regional Commission for the Middle East. *World Organization for Animal Health (OIE)*; 2013. http://www.oie.int/publications-and-documentation/compendium-of-technical-items/.

251 International Veterinary Students Association. *Mission Statement.* https://www.ivsa.org/mission-statement (accessed 31 August 2024).

252 One Health Poultry Hub. *One Health.* https://www.onehealthpoultry.org/search/?fwp_search=one+health (accessed 30 August 2024).

253 World Veterinary Association. *WVA Position Statement on One Health.* https://worldvet.org/wp-content/uploads/2024/03/WVA-PS-on-One-Health.pdf (accessed 30 August 2024).

254 Moro, M. Integrating the veterinarian scientist to the One Health concept. In: *Adult Vaccinations: Changing the Immunization Paradigm* (ed. J.-P. Michel and S. Maggi), 111–113. Cham: Springer International Publishing; 2019. https://doi.org/10.1007/978-3-030-05159-4_18.

255 Shaheen, M.N.F. The concept of one health applied to the problem of zoonotic diseases. *Rev. Med. Virol.* 2022; 32(4): e2326. https://doi.org/10.1002/rmv.2326.

256 Lembo, T., Attlan, M., Bourhy, H., et al. Renewed global partnerships and redesigned roadmaps for rabies prevention and control. *Vet. Med. Int.* 2011; 2011(1): 923149. https://doi.org/10.4061/2011/923149.

257 Scott, T.P., Coetzer, A., de Balogh, K., et al. The Pan-African Rabies Control Network (PARACON): a unified approach to eliminating canine rabies in Africa. *Antivir. Res.* 2015; 124: 93–100. https://doi.org/10.1016/j.antiviral.2015.10.002.

258 Global Alliance for Rabies Control. *Alliance for Rabies Control: 2021 Annual Report.* https://rabiesalliance.org/about/arc (accessed 30 August 2024).

259 Harman, S. The World Bank and health. In: *Global Health Governance: Crisis, Institutions, and Political Economy*, vol. 10 (ed. A. Kay and O.D. Williams), 227–244. Springer; 2009. https://doi.org/10.1057/9780230249486_11.

260 Berthe, F.C.J., Bouley, T., Karesh, W.B., et al. *One Health: Operational Framework for Strengthening Human, Animal, and Environmental Public Health Systems at their Interface.* The World Bank; 2018. https://documents1.worldbank.org/curated/fr/703711517234402168/pdf/123023-REVISED-PUBLIC-World-Bank-One-Health-Framework-2018.pdf.

261 USAID. *Strengthening One Health Workforce in Southeast Asia.* https://www.usaid.gov/sites/default/files/2022-10/FS_SEAOHUN_Dec_2021.pdf (accessed 30 August 2024).

262 US Embassy in Bangladesh. *New US "One Health" Project to Bolster Response to Infectious Disease and Pandemic Threats in Bangladesh.* https://bd.usembassy.gov/new-u-s-one-health-project-to-bolster-response-to-infectious-disease-and-pandemic-threats-in-bangladesh/ (accessed 30 August 2024).

263 FAO-OIE-WHO. *The FAO-OIE-WHO Collaboration: A Tripartite Concept Note.* https://www.who.int/publications/m/item/the-fao-oie-who-collaboration (accessed 30 August 2024).

264 World Organization for Animal Health. *WOAH Assumes Chair of Quadripartite Secretariat Outlining Vision for One Health Collaboration.* https://www.woah.org/en/woah-assumes-chair-of-quadripartite-secretariat-outlining-vision-for-one-health-collaboration/ (accessed 30 August 2024).

265 Gargano, L., Gallagher, P., Barrett, M., et al. Issues in the development of a research and education framework for One Health. *Emerg. Infect. Dis. J.* 2013; 19(3): e121103. https://doi.org/10.3201/eid1903.121103.

266 Berrian, A.M., Wilkes, M., Gilardi, K., et al. Developing a global One Health workforce: the "Rx One Health Summer Institute" approach. *EcoHealth.* 2020; 17(2): 222–232. https://doi.org/10.1007/s10393-020-01481-0.

267 Pitt, S.J. and Gunn, A. The one health concept. *Br. J. Biomed. Sci.* 2024; 81: 12366. https://doi.org/10.3389/bjbs.2024.12366.

268 USAID. *Global Health Security Agenda.* https://www.usaid.gov/sites/default/files/2023-07/USAID%20Global%20Health%20Security%20Agenda_July_23.pdf (accessed 30 August 2024).

269 GHS Index. *Global Health Security Index.* https://ghsindex.org/wp-content/uploads/2019/10/2019-Global-Health-Security-Index.pdf (accessed 30 August 2024).

270 Global Health Security Agenda. *GHSA Stories of Impact.* https://globalhealthsecurityagenda.org/stories-of-impact/ (accessed 30 August 2024).

271 European Commission. *EU Action on Antimicrobial Resistance.* https://health.ec.europa.eu/antimicrobial-resistance/eu-action-antimicrobial-resistance_en (accessed 30 August 2024).

272 IEDCR. *Strategic Framework for One Health Bangladesh.* https://www.iedcr.org/pdf/files/One Health/Strategic_framework_for_One_Health_Bangladesh-26 Jan.pdf (accessed 30 August 2024).

273 Esha, E.J. *Briefing: What More Is Needed to Make One Health a Reality in Bangladesh*? https://www.onehealthpoultry.org/publications/what-more-is-needed-to-make-one-health-a-reality-in-bangladesh/ (accessed 30 August 2024).

274 Centers for Disease Control and Prevention. *Field Epidemiology Training Program (FETP)*. https://www.cdc.gov/globalhealth/healthprotection/fetp/index.htm (accessed 30 August 2024).

275 TEPHINET. *Spotlight on the Bangladesh Field Epidemiology Training Program*. https://www.tephinet.org/news/spotlight-bangladesh-field-epidemiology-training-program (accessed 30 August 2024).

276 Centers for Disease Control and Prevention. *Integrated Disease Surveillance and Response (IDSR)*. https://www.cdc.gov/globalhealth/healthprotection/idsr/index.html (accessed 30 August 2024).

277 Gibbs, E.P.J. The evolution of one health: a decade of progress and challenges for the future. *Vet. Rec.* 2014; 174(4): 85–91. https://doi.org/10.1136/vr.g143.

278 Kahn, L.H. Who's in Charge? Leadership during epidemics, bioterror attacks, and other public health crises. *Emerg. Infect. Dis.* 2010; 16(6): 1050–1051. https://doi.org/10.3201/eid1606.100345.

279 Peter, L.A.C. and Rabinowitz, M. Human-animal medicine: clinical approaches to zoonoses, toxicants, and other shared health risks. *Emerg. Infect. Dis.* 2010; 16(6): 1050. https://doi.org/10.3201/eid1606.100367.

280 Kahn, L.H. The need for one health degree programs. *Infect. Ecol. Epidemiol.* 2011; 1(1): 7919. https://doi.org/10.3402/iee.v1i0.7919.

281 Lerner, H. Philosophical roots of the one medicine movement: an analysis of some relevant ideas by Rudolf Virchow and Calvin Schwabe with their modern implications. *Stud. Philos. Eston.* 2013; 6: 97–109. https://doi.org/10.12697/spe.2013.6.2.07.

282 Barbara Natterson-Horowitz, B. and Bowers, K.E. *Zoobiquity: The Astonishing Connection Between Human and Animal Health*. New York: Vintage Books; 2013. https://archive.org/details/zoobiquityastoni0000natt_v4h1.

5

Advanced Veterinary Sciences for Sustainable Agriculture and Global Food Security

Abdullah Ahmed Butt[1]* *and Zahra Ahmed*[2]

[1] *Department of Food Science and Technology, Government College University, Faisalabad, Pakistan*
[2] *Department of Pharmacology, King Edward Medical University, Lahore, Pakistan*

*Corresponding author: abdullahahmad100233@gmail.com

TABLE OF CONTENTS

5.1 Introduction
5.1.1 Impacts of Animal Diseases on Food Production and Global Food Security
5.2 Technological Innovations in Veterinary Medicine and Agriculture
5.2.1 Advancements in Diagnostics and Disease Surveillance
5.2.2 Emerging Technologies for Disease Prevention and Control
5.3 One Health Approach: Integrating Veterinary and Human Health
5.3.1 One Health: Relevance to Agriculture and Food Security
5.4 Nutrition and Feed Management for Livestock Health
5.4.1 Importance of Balanced Nutrition for Animal Health and Productivity
5.4.2 Innovations in Feed Formulation and Delivery Systems
5.4.3 Sustainable Feed Production Practices
5.5 Disease Control and Biosecurity Measures
5.5.1 Strategies for Preventing and Managing Infectious Disease in Livestock
5.5.2 Biosecurity Protocols for Farms and Food Production Facilities
5.5.3 Role of Vaccination in Disease Control and Eradication
5.6 Climate Change and Veterinary Challenges
5.6.1 Impact of Climate Change on Animal Health and Agriculture
5.6.2 Adaptation Strategies for Livestock Farming in Changing Environmental Conditions
5.6.3 Mitigation Measures to Reduce the Environmental Footprint of Animal Agriculture
5.7 Veterinary Extension and Capacity Building
5.7.1 Importance of Education and Training in Veterinary Sciences for Sustainable Agriculture
5.7.2 Extension Services to Disseminate Best Practices and Innovations
5.7.3 Capacity Building Initiatives for Veterinary Professionals in Developing Countries
5.8 Challenges and Future Directions
5.8.1 Identifying Challenges in Veterinary Medicine and Agriculture
5.8.2 Opportunities for Future Research and Collaboration
5.8.3 Exemplary Projects Showcasing the Application of Advanced Veterinary Sciences
5.8.4 Lessons Learned and Recommendations for Future Interventions
5.9 Conclusion
References

One Health Integration: Global Perspectives on Animal Health and Sustainable Agriculture. First Edition.
Edited by Pratik Subhash Gaikwad, Vivek Harishankar Shukla and Pintu Choudhary.

Companion Website: https://www.wiley.com/go/pratikgaikwad/onehealth

5.1 Introduction

Ushering us into an era when the synergy among advanced veterinary sciences and sustainable agricultural practices emerges as a catalyst to secure food for all, thus contributing to global resilience in food systems, we are forced into an era of unprecedented challenges. Veterinary science is a wide field incorporating many areas and utilizing many techniques to maximize health and productivity of livestock which are crucial components of existing agricultural systems [1]. The prime goal is to preserve and preserve the health status of animal populations to boost the performance and welfare of animal populations. Its scope covers diseases that may affect farm animals (e.g., infections such as foot and mouth disease (FMD), avian influenza, metabolism disorders, nutritional deficiency, etc.,) [2]. State-of-the-art diagnostic modalities – molecular diagnostics and genomic sequencing, capable of highly sensitive detection that pertains to a variety of diseases have helped transform from late-stage disease management toward early-stage disease evaluation leading to preventative interventions. These methods provide a means to unambiguously identify pathogens, as well as evaluate genetic variations contributing both to disease resistance and susceptibility. The use of innovative vaccine design advancements like recombinant DNA technology and advanced adjuvant formulations have resulted in reduced burden on animal health from infectious diseases through more efficacious, longer-lasting vaccines.

The health of livestock is directly linked to food security in those healthy animals can produce more and better-quality products, such as meat, milk, and eggs; as well as other animal-derived foods. Not only used to feed a growing world, but high productivity also promotes the economic opportunities of farmers and society in rural development [3]. Similarly, veterinary sciences are fundamental to food safety; these ensure that food products of animal origin are not contaminated with toxic pathogens and contaminants [4]. Proper disease control practices and biosecurity also help to reduce the occurrence of zoonotic diseases (diseases that can be spread from animals to humans), which plays a role in protecting public health. Examples include the monitoring and control of bovine tuberculosis, brucellosis, or avian influenza to prevent outbreaks capable of wiping out animals as well as human populations (Figure 5.1). In addition, connecting veterinary sciences to sustainable farming practices supports the environmental sustainability of farming [5]. Well-treated animals use fewer resources (and space), and they need less feed, water, veterinary pharmaceuticals, etc., in production which lowers their environmental footprint. Precision livestock farming (PLF), a practice that incorporates data-powered technology to check the health of animals and enhance resource conservation is an example of linking veterinary science with sustainable agriculture [6]. All these practices support the productivity, health, and well-being of these cattle while adding to soil conservation and grazing management goals. Advanced veterinary sciences are the key factors for ensuring stable and sustainable agriculture and food production worldwide. Veterinary science is essential for keeping livestock healthy and productive, which in turn supports the supply of safe and nutritious food while helping to protect public health as well as ensuring that agriculture systems are supportive. With hundreds of pages, this chapter does not provide a detailed viewpoint on the specific developments in veterinary medicine for obvious reasons but instead offers an insight into new approaches and cooperation required to meet today's multifaceted challenges. We must continue working together with veterinary professionals, farmers, policymakers, and researchers to create food systems that are sustainable enough to feed an ever-expanding global population while securing the future for all.

5.1.1 Impacts of Animal Diseases on Food Production and Global Food Security

Animal diseases have deeply affected food production and global food security, with different implications for the availability of adequate nutritious quality foods as well as the economic stability and health status of communities worldwide. Animal diseases, including both endemic and epidemic ones, are major constraints to agricultural productivity, public health, as well as food system resilience within the community. Therefore, it is important to determine these impacts for implementing measures towards risk mitigation and sustainable production of crops.

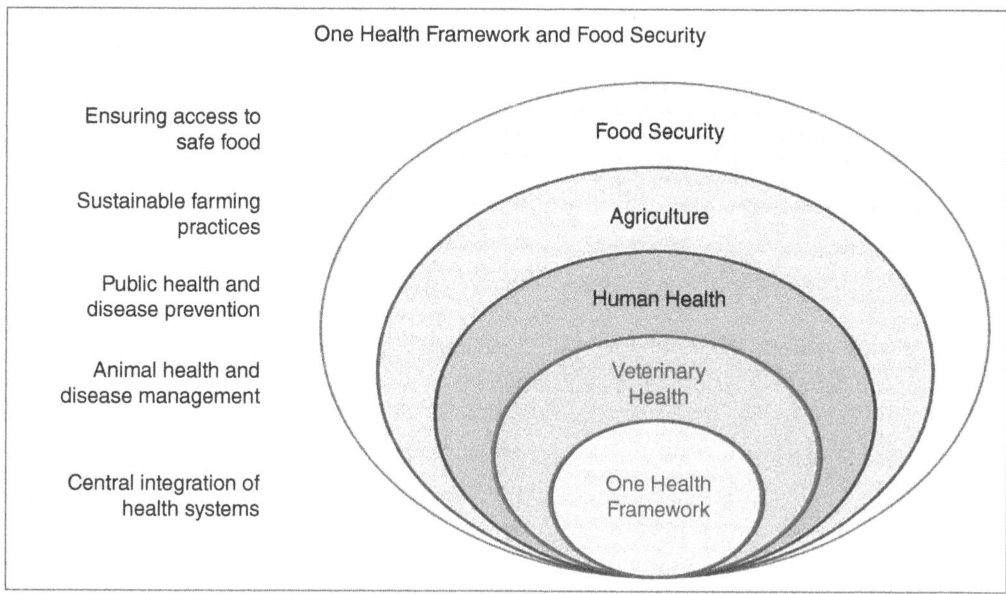

Figure 5.1 Interconnectedness of veterinary and human health within the One Health framework.

One important consequence of animal diseases is that they directly or indirectly decrease the productivity of animals (meat, milk, eggs, etc.,) [7]. Harmful effects of infectious diseases such as FMD, avian influenza, and African swine fever are also recorded due to high morbidity and mortality rates in the affected animal population [8]. Namely, in the case of an outbreak such as FMD, there may be catastrophic production losses to cattle and swine following a large decrease in meat and milk supplies. Bird flu outbreaks can also wipe out most poultry flocks, leading to greatly reduced egg production and poultry meat. These are translated into direct food losses and therefore less availability of cheap food, which hits hard on many regions suffering from a heavy dependence on livestock products for their nutrition or income (Table 5.1).

In addition to the direct losses of animals, animal diseases can have broad economic effects. Controlling the infectious diseases of livestock is expensive, involving vaccination programs; quarantine and culling strategies for infected or high-risk animals; isolation techniques (i.e., biosecurity); etc., [19]. Although measures need to be taken because of control over devastating diseases, they place economic stress on farmers and budgets for governments. The most vulnerable are small-scale farmers in developing countries, as they may not have the necessary resources to properly prepare for and deal with disease outbreaks and could lose their livelihoods as a result. This economic burden carries through to the wider agricultural industry and impacts trade as well as market activity. Disease outbreaks often create trade disruptions by imposing additional restrictions on the movement and export of livestock and animal products, hence incurring heavy economic losses both at national (domestic) levels as well as internationally.

From zoonosis like avian influenza, bovine tuberculosis and brucellosis, which can snag human populations in their deadly spider's pits of disease till death do us part. The link between animal and human health is a reminder of the need for a One Health perspective that combines veterinary, medical, and environmental sciences to tackle zoonotic disease transmission dynamics. As a result, it is vitally important that animal diseases be managed effectively to protect both livestock and public health while keeping the food supply safe. The havoc that animal diseases play on the environment adds to this confusing mix. Animals that are diseased often have lower fed efficiency, which means it takes more food and other resources for them to make the same amount of output as healthy animals. Because of this inefficiency, animals eating maize emit more greenhouse gases per

Table 5.1 Overview of key veterinary diseases and their impact on food security.

Diseases	Impact on food security	Most affected areas	References
FMD	Reduces milk and increases mortality of calves	Africa, Asia, South America	[9]
Avian Influenza	Reduction in poultry production	Southeast Asia, Europe, North America	[10]
African Swine Fever	Culling and economic impacts	Sub-Saharan Africa, Asia	[11]
Bovine Spongiform Encephalopathy (BSE)	Reduced beef production and market losses	Europe, North America	[12]
Peste des Petits Ruminants (PPR)	High mortality in sheep and goat	South Asia, Middle East	[13]
Rift Valley Fever	Milk and meat shortage	Africa, Middle East	[14]
Newcastle Disease	Impacts rural food security	Africa, Asia	[15]
Brucellosis	Milk contamination	Developing countries like India	[16]
Trypanosomiasis	Reduced meat and milk yield	Sub-Saharan Africa	[17]
Mastitis	Decrease milk yield and quality	In dairy rich regions	[18]

unit of animal product than if they were fed something else in the same region, which unduly magnifies what are already large environmental footprints from livestock [20]. Furthermore, the management of sick animals either due to culling or natural mortality, also creates extra complications as it carries a risk of possible soil and water pollution. Therefore, a One Health approach aimed at a global strategy for the prevention of animal diseases spread is required to provide better methods of worldwide support. Scientific progress in the field of veterinary sciences with the discovery and development of better diagnostic tools, vaccines, and therapeutic options are important for precise detection to prevent or treat early animal diseases [21]. Improved biosecurity and surveillance would help to not eliminate the introduction of infectious agents. The need to foster collaboration across stakeholders including farmers, veterinarians, researchers, as well as policymakers and international organizations is also imperative for the development and implementation of successful disease control strategies.

Worldwide, animal disease results in direct losses to food production and knock-on effects on global food security; acting as a drag on not only livestock productivity but other major economies of significance including public health, economy, and environmental sustainability. Their management and control depend substantially on a comprehensive strategy by using state-of-the-art veterinary science, robust biosecurity implementations, as well as cross-sectoral/border cooperation. The risks animal diseases pose can be reduced by our actions, potentially making global food systems more resilient and sustainable to better deliver dietary resources at a time of expanding requirement.

5.2 Technological Innovations in Veterinary Medicine and Agriculture

Yet today, the juncture of veterinary medicine and agriculture is changing rapidly as technologies advance. In a world facing various global issues, including climate change and population growth in the context of constrained resources such as water, energy, and raw materials markets, then scaling up veterinary scientific discovery into innovation is increasingly critical. But not only are these technological innovations boosting the health and productivity of livestock (like their crop counterparts they also add to sustainability and resilience in agricultural systems, which is critical if we want, as a civilization, genuine global food security). Advances known across veterinary medicine have revolutionized numerous diagnostic technologies critically employed to detect and treat many animal illnesses aptly early, including molecular diagnostics and genomic sequencing. They make a candidate diagnostic test that provides high-resolution pathogen identification, tracks disease spread, and crafts customized intervention plans to optimize the survivability of animals. Concomitantly, new vaccines or developments in conventional vaccine technologies via recombinant DNA and novel adjuvant systems have been deployed to increase the general efficacy while improving overall biosecurity and maintaining our efforts toward disease control within specific livestock populations [22].

This perfectly blends the technology used with agriculture, and this is an epic example of it in the rise of PLF as a battery-backed data-driven tool to optimally utilize resources at lower prices for better animal husbandry practices. By way of example, PLFs prosper from the near real-time information related to animal health (physiological status), behavior, or environmental aspects made possible by automated feeding devices, wearables, and remote monitoring technology. This information can inform future decisions predict the impact removal would have on animal welfare, and better targeting of limited interventions. Additionally, the introduction of artificial intelligence (AI) and machine learning algorithms into PLF improves predictability via predictive analytics as well as early warning capabilities for optimal livestock sustainability/productive outcomes [23]. Innovations in animal management and genetics efforts are well underway along with the latest research developments. The ability to predict complex traits via genomic selection and the advent of new biotechnologies including *CRISPR-Cas9* gene editing will allow genetic modification for desirable trait expression in livestock, such as disease resistance, growth rates, and reproductive efficiency. Technology has the potential to increase genetic gain in breeding programs leading to more robust, higher-producing livestock breeds that can thrive in different and changing environments.

Also, there is the potential of blockchain technology in the livestock supply chain industry, especially transparency traceability food safety. Blockchain can be used by us to have all your animal health histories, conventional and organic production practices, as well as movement on the chain ensuring food supply integrity from farm gate to plate [24]. This technology is especially useful in managing food fraud and guarantees animal welfare standards and health regulations. New technological innovations in veterinary medicine and agriculture are beginning to reshape the potential competitive landscape of animal health, as well as transforming agricultural food production practices. These developments not only result in the optimization and sustainable intensification of animal husbandry but at built-in solving strategies for challenges related to world food supply as well as environmental sustainability. In this chapter, we delve into the broad spectrum of technological innovations and how these may be utilized, what benefits they can provide for animal health and production as well as their implications for veterinary medicine and agriculture in the future. This report provides a key assessment of these technologies helping to demystify their transformative impacts in building more resilient food systems that can continue meeting the needs of a growing world population in the face of global challenges.

5.2.1 Advancements in Diagnostics and Disease Surveillance

Diagnostics and disease surveillance is a major leap in veterinary medicine using advanced technologies to tackle animal health challenges in today's agriculture industry. In recent years, molecular diagnostics have been widely used for the identification and characterization of pathogens with rapidity specificity at the genetic level: polymerase chain reaction (PCR) technique based on their DNA targets or another diagnosis approach such as LAMP loop-mediated isothermal amplification. Early intervention by using these techniques helps to control the spread of infectious diseases and reduces reliance on broad-spectrum antimicrobials, which is a key strategy in combatting antimicrobial resistance (AMR). Through the use of next-generation sequencing (NGS), we can achieve an even deeper understanding by uncovering pathogen variants, resistance genes, and transmission paths at a genomic level [24]. Knowledge of this genomic is critical for new anti-viral, vaccines, and/or monoclonal antibodies. Wearable biosensors and Internet of Things (IoT) devices are becoming powerful tools for livestock management providing continuous real-time monitoring of physiological parameters like temperature, heart rate, or activity [25]. This allows the detection of subtle modifications that precede clinical symptoms, and to intervene promptly with veterinary advice. AI-powered machine learning algorithms are turning the massive amount of data produced by these technologies into patterns and forecasting disease outbreaks with a high level of accuracy. Such predictive power is essential to take preventive measures and diminish disease effects on the livestock population. Disease surveillance through the mapping using geographic information systems (GIS) and remote sensing techniques of disease prevalence along with environmental factors that affect disease transmission namely climate conditions, and landscape features [26]. The integration of these emerging diagnostic and surveillance tools into veterinary diagnostics genuinely has the potential to transform disease control in agriculture, for healthier livestock, fewer economic losses/quality assurance issues, as well as global food security.

5.2.2 Emerging Technologies for Disease Prevention and Control

A new generation of technologies aimed at preventing diseases, stopping them from being on track when they strike, and working rapidly to contain outbreaks is transforming veterinary medicine and agriculture: providing the means to help keep animals healthy – a pathway also critical to our food security. Among these are the innovations generating new vaccines containing recombinant DNA sequences; synthetic biology tools, and next-generation adjuvant systems that can modify responses to an extent unheard of with conventional immunization. Not only do these vaccines provide superior immunity against a broad spectrum of pathogens including those not covered by conventional vaccines but they can be rapidly developed in response to new and emerging diseases. This includes how the super-fast and adaptable mRNA vaccines, similar to those used for COVID-19, which are now being fashioned to be utilized in livestock, can provide rapid responses as well. This technology allows the fast production of vaccines against strains of pathogenic agents, with less time between disease outbreak and control. As well as the vaccination, gene editing by CRISPR-Cas9 is used to generate disease-resistant livestock. It is possible to improve the innate immunity of animals by targeting certain genes that are known to be involved in susceptibility to infection [27]. It will not only benefit animals' health but this also measure along with reducing the usage of antibiotics and resulting in facilitating good farm practices which reduce AMR. An example of this is genetic editing to produce resistance against Porcine Reproductive and Respiratory Syndrome (PRRS) in pigs, a disease that has major economic consequences for the swine industry. These genetic interventions have the potential to increase herd health and productivity sustainably.

Nanotechnology is also an emerging area that can save lives from diseases. One prominent piece of technology often discussed in the context of enhancing drug delivery is nanoparticles. Nanoparticles can encapsulate either antigens or drugs, shielding them from degradation and facilitating their uptake into immune cells [28]. This improves the impact of vaccines and therapies, therefore providing improved health outcomes. Additionally, intrinsically antimicrobial polymers applied at the surface of various materials can be used to achieve results that cannot simply be achieved using nanotechnology-based diagnostic tools such as nano-biosensors for accurate and early diagnosis of diseases. Until now, biosecurity technologies have been a significant player in disease evolution. This includes the use of automated disinfection systems like UV light and ozone generators to sanitize animal housing and equipment that collectively dampens pathogen loads in the environment [29]. Continuous smart monitoring of animal behaviors and environmental factors, to which data analytics on the other end is increasingly being AI-driven through an arsenal of technologies like drones fitted with small cameras. These systems can identify a deviation in the regular movement pattern or signs of discomfort that at worst may suggest disease presence and provide for premature adjustments (Table 5.2). By incorporating these technologies into disease control, the approach of veterinary medicine and agriculture is changing forever. Using this technology, animal health can be managed much more proactively and accurately due to persistent monitoring of your data. This contributes to healthier livestock populations and more sustainable farming techniques by minimizing the use of chemicals on their land while optimizing resource utilization. These are rapidly shifting technologies that

Table 5.2 Emerging technologies in veterinary medicine for sustainable agriculture.

Technology	Application	Role in food security	References
Molecular Diagnostics	Disease diagnosis	Minimize losses in livestock due to early detection of disease	[30]
Precision Livestock Farming (PLF)	Disease monitoring and management	Reduce mortality rates	[31]
Vaccinology	Disease prevention	Improved disease immunity	[32]
Genomic Selection	Breeding programs	Developments of resilient livestock breeds	[33]
CRISPR-Cas9 Gene Editing	Genetic improvement	Enhance disease resistance	[34]
Artificial Intelligence (AI)	Data analytics	Predicts disease outbreaks	[35, 36]

will only become more accessible; their utilization on a global scale is essential to ensure the security of our food sources and prevent new diseases at home before they arrive from abroad.

5.3 One Health Approach: Integrating Veterinary and Human Health

The idea of One Health is a holistic approach emphasizing the interrelated and interconnected nature of human health, animal health, and the environment. It is grounded in an understanding that human, animal, and environmental health are interconnected and must be addressed as such. Such an approach promotes interdisciplinary collaboration among veterinary medicine, human health/ecology/environmental health/scientists (MDs and PhDs). At the heart of One Health is an understanding that zoonotic infections such as Ebola, avian influenza, and COVID-19 come from animals before spilling over into human populations – compelling neighboring surveillance efforts by veterinary and health sectors alongside with rapid detection to follow up response strategies. It also should and does include pollutants in water, air, and soil: climate change impacts on human health (including animal health); and AMR among common infectious bacteria of relevance to both humans and animals. By working at the interface of human and animal health along with three pillars – more natural ecosystem; more antibiotic treatment alternatives to reduce reliance on conventional antibiotics, 3 R's in practice (responsible use sensible regulations including bans); vaccinate animals also for public good among others, enhanced global collaboration is needed. One Health vision aims to bring together veterinarians, ecologists, physicians, scientists, and policymaker's communities worldwide to enable practices that will not only foster healthy living activities by reducing disease but environmental changes affecting environmental costs as well.

5.3.1 One Health: Relevance to Agriculture and Food Security

The idea of One Health and its connection to agriculture and food security indicates the great combination of various fields that share a common goal, which is to ensure global health as well as sustainability. It is a holistic One Health approach that underlines the interrelated nature of human health, animal health, and environmental health. This highlights the spillover between these fields and their translational ramifications more broadly, emphasizing mutual vulnerabilities across them that provide a clear rationale for some joined-up thinking around cross-cutting determinants of health. One Health recognizes what has always been true: that veterinary medicine and keeping our livestock as healthy and productive as possible is at least as important perhaps even more important than human health when it comes to ensuring food security, particularly in light of the current problems unfolding across Africa with African Swine Fever. For human nutrition and livelihoods around the world, livestock is a crucial source of protein, dairy, and other agricultural produce [37]. Second, the health of people is connected to that of animals and our planet; this principle informs One Health which promotes a holistic approach where coordination between veterinary medicine (which has historically been more familiar with zoonoses) together human medical practice and environmental science are needed for surveillance and prevention. The emergence of these zoonotic diseases, such as avian influenza, Ebola, and COVID-19 can cause great harm to animal welfare and human health [38]. All three are integral components to help reduce these risks and keep food supplies safe while protecting the public.

In addition, One Health acknowledges that environmental effects affect health outcomes beyond species. Problems such as climate change, habitat loss/alteration, pollution, and AMR may not only impact ecosystem stability but also ultimately harm agricultural productivity including food security [39]. The decline in health and resilience of environmental resources can lead to higher disease susceptibility, as well as decrease agricultural yields due to the reduced ability for these varied natural wild foods that livestock can rely upon. Solving these problems involves researchers working together in many disciplines and creating sustainable processes for the health of ecosystems that allow food production to be resilient. By embedding the principles of One Health, it paves the way for working together in ways that other sectors (agriculture/health/veterinary/public health/policy) may have never done before to help all come up with really resilient responses to global issues. One Health service serves people and the environment by promoting long-term equity in safe and tasty food for current as well as coming generations, while also preserving both biodiversity and health through balanced ecosystems on a global scale.

5.4 Nutrition and Feed Management for Livestock Health

Providing holistic care and sustainable production, nutrition and feed management practices are also essential worldwide for domestic animals. It is an intricate and comprehensive relationship as it determines not only the growth and maintenance of animals but also their resistance to pathogens on the one hand; and quality, functionality and/or physiological effects of the products they produce. Likewise, a rationally planned balanced diet specifically designed to satisfy the nutritional requirements of different species, ages, and production phases is crucial for reaching optimal growth rates or reproductive efficiency according to each need. The supply of essential nutrients such as protein, carbohydrates, fat, vitamins, and minerals will play a significant role in metabolic functions, maintaining immune competence which thereby optimizes the utilization of feed resources. Feed management practices apply to all stages of the feed life cycle, beginning with free-choice feeding in the diet and ending at storage level or delivery. Feeding ingredients are sustainably sourced, as well as required to be of high quality and supplemented (where necessary) that will provide livestock with all the nutrients for health and productivity [40]. Adopting diets that match the nutrition requirements of animals in terms of feed available will limit costs and environmental impacts but demand a lot more care. Innovations such as precision feeding systems and nutritional modeling improve the farmers' ability to deliver precise diets tailored to individual animal requirements, reduce food wastage per unit of production volume (feed efficiency), and thus minimize land occupation.

Transitable feed management also should have lower poststorage losses and be safe for efficient feeding to the animals which forms as a part of effective feed management strategies. Adequate storage and handling procedures also protect animals, from mold toxins as well as spoilage which would affect farm economics [41]. Feed management practices (besides nutritional considerations) contribute to sustainability by reducing waste and improving input resources with livestock operations. The section defines the fundamental principles of nutrition and feed management in livestock production, exploring the scientific basis for their development and technological advances to allow practical implementation required to improve animal health, welfare, and productivity. By making a union of our solid science with good new practices, we can enable farmers to farm better and produce a more efficient livestock product that supports global food security as well as environmentally resilient stewardship.

5.4.1 Importance of Balanced Nutrition for Animal Health and Productivity

A good nutrition is the most basic and important segment of health supporting animal productivity in all livestock populations across any agricultural system worldwide. Never undervalue the role that a carefully prepared as well as quite balanced diet plays in contributing to an animal's overall healthy life. This precision in intensity has implications for livestock performance, with growth rates and reproductive efficiency as well as overall metabolic function all predicted to be differentially affected by this immunological approach. Amino chains, sugars, and fats are a few of the many different other molecules animals need to live in; they contribute not only to forging support inside bodies but also help process glucose. Now, while proteins are building blocks for muscle growth and repair, carbs and fats provide energy to keep us running. Also, vitamins and minerals, cofactors of many biochemical reactions, also act as bone development, immune health zone system, and reproductive factors.

However, appropriate nutrition also increases the natural resistance of livestock and provides for higher animal productivity in terms of both quality (e.g., meat or eggs) and quantity. For instance, omega 3 diets can increase the nutritional value of eggs for consumers [42]. The formulation of diets that contain perfect nutrients for different species, ages, and production stages is an area that focuses on the ideal balance needed to achieve such equilibrium. This can be an important element for using genetics background, how the environment was made available specifically to that diet, and other target production objectives when decisions are taken toward this goal. New technology associated with feed production and nutrition also raises the bar for diet customization capabilities, precision feeding systems can be utilized to precisely deliver specified rations, and nutritional modeling tools allow immediate adjustments on the fly when it comes time to hone diets down even finer just that one last bit needed by a scarce margin of productivity gain while using every morsel and respecting the upper limits to cow intake [43]. Besides contributing to animal health and performance, adequate nutrition is essential for improving feed efficiency in a sustainable way of crop use. This is also critical for improving environmental sustainability (e.g., lowering greenhouse gas emissions and nutrient losses) of livestock production systems. Last, the sustainability of livestock systems is also related to strategic feed management techniques (e.g., minimizing feeding wastage and incorporating local resources into animal diets). Farmers, of course, are working for animal welfare and economic sustainability by striving to have a balanced diet – but here they are playing the front role in global food solidarity with efficient production livestock systems using (that something important that all scares us) limited resources.

5.4.2 Innovations in Feed Formulation and Delivery Systems

Improved feed formulation as supported through Feed Management Systems (FMS) and Computerized/Electronic Varied Feeders (CVF) are the major mandates toward determined nutrition in livestock farming, an essential apparatus for health, productivity, and sustainability essentials [44]. The nutritional needs of the various types and life stages of livestock that we raise, and what our end products (stock for reproducing or producing – like milk/egg production) require have been elucidated to a very detailed level by advancements in agricultural research over many years. This perception provides a foundation for tailoring feed formulations to best meet these needs and thus optimize animal growth, reproduction, and metabolic tasks. So, by innovating in feed ingredients other than protein resources provided from soybean meals using things like insect meals or algae-derived proteins as alternative nutritional profiles, we can decrease our reliance on those traditional feeds and what that provides is diversification for further environmental impact reductions.

Using this technology could help reduce the common infectious pathogens, and improve gut health and absorption efficiency of nutrients by supplementation of livestock with a functional additive like probiotics-fortification on animal feed or diet [45]. Probiotics, for example, supply the gut with a bunch of helpful microbial communities that consume some food before it goes through to your cells (specific immune system). These added enzymes break down the larger recalcitrant carbohydrates and proteins into forms that can be more easily digested, thus increasing nutrient uptake while improving feed efficiency. These advances not only improve animal health and performance but also help decrease feed costs, as well as minimize nutrient losses in the environment [46]. Together with new feed materials, advances in feed treatment technologies are key to increasing nutrient availability and digestibility. Pelleting, extrusion, and micronization processes contribute to the improvement of physical–chemical properties in the feed improving palatability as well as nutrient absorption along the digestive tract. Pelleting for example can help with feed digestibility as it will break down the cell walls and reduce particle size, while extrusion provides better starch gelatinization and protein denaturation so more nutrients are available but also controlled antinutritional factors. Feed delivery systems that are automated and digitalized also allay the feed management challenge. These feeding systems are equipped with sensors and monitoring devices to allow automated, real-time adjustments in feed delivery as animals (pigs or poultry) consume them on an individual basis that contribute to a specific physiological status ensuring consistent nutrient intake which at the same time minimizes any feed wastage [47]. The inbuilt data analytics offer a lot of information about the feeding patterns and behavior of each animal, allowing farmers to tailor their feed management strategy according to this feedback loop to optimize health/performance/resource efficiency This set of scientific achievements in the system formulation and feeding/feed delivery can play a crucial part in sustainable agricultural practices, as they promote better livestock feed use efficiency for productivity and cut down potential environmental knock-ons associated with feed management/production. Using these technologies, farmers are better poised to combat the global food challenges of feeding a growing worldwide supply while promoting animal welfare and being stewards of environmental protection in livestock production.

5.4.3 Sustainable Feed Production Practices

The adoption of sustainable feed production practices into new agricultural strategies designed to keep livestock healthy, productive, and environmentally sound is globally imperative. The problem with sustainable feed production is how to balance the nutritional needs of animals vs. all other environmental impacts linked to or due to sourcing, growing, and processing of feeds. Key to these efforts is the implementation of methods aimed at achieving environmental neutrality through the entire feed production chain by mitigation against environmental deterioration, natural resource conservation, and reduction in greenhouse gas emissions. Sourcing feed ingredients from well-managed agricultural systems is a key factor in sustainable feed production. It focuses on the use of locally grown and regionally suitable feed crops, minimizing transportation costs a substantial portion of the carbon footprint in food production and supporting local communities [48]. In addition, agroecological practices including crop rotations and cover crops, accompanied by vegetative buffer strips between croplands prevent soil erosion which also supports plant diversity [49]. These practices contribute to the sustainability of feed production as well as help counteract many of the downsides associated with massive monocultures, such as top soil erosion, loss of soil fertility due to nutrient release from organic matter decomposition, and water pollution.

Precision agriculture employs advanced technologies to minimize the use of resources and reduce environmental impacts in feed production. Precision agriculture employs data-driven applications stemming from remote sensing, GIS, and sensor technologies to record soil fertility, crop vitality, and water management [50]. This can give way to better-nuanced applications of fertilizers and irrigation, cutting down on nutrient runoff while preserving water resources. In addition, the help of precision agriculture body optimizes precise nutrient levels for genetic species and stage growth and surrounding parameters leading to the formulation of accurate feed. When we can balance feed compositions perfectly to the exact needs of an animal type, then farmers will achieve better feed production and limit waste byproducts thereby enhancing livestock operations with sustainability. Sustainable feed production. Specifically for aquaculture, as it is known that animal-based feed requires about 10 kg of aquatic ingredients to yield only one kg of fish or shrimp, promotion can contribute towards sustainably sourced ingredient supply and use small scale operations and destroy efficient resource reuse (i.e., closed

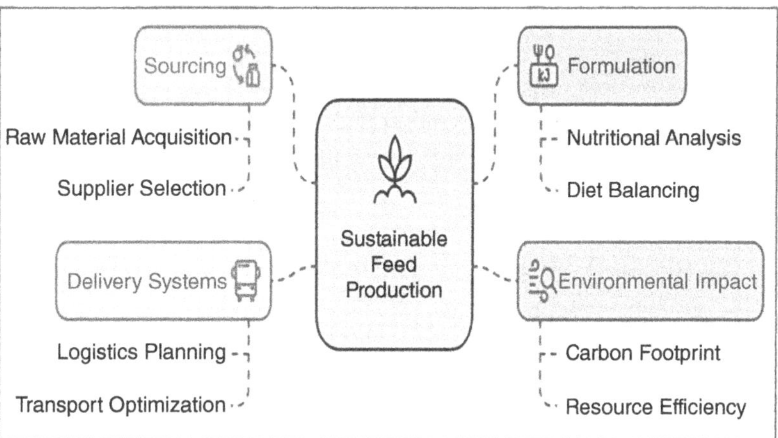

Figure 5.2 Sustainable feed production cycle.

loop farming). This includes the development of various feed processing practices such as pelleting and extrusion which improve digestibility intake by birds and decrease projectabilities [51]. Overall, the recycling and repurposing of agricultural byproducts/food waste into animal feed also aid in sustainability aims as it decreases landfill volume and functions to close nutrient cycles within an agroecosystem.

Utilizing advances in science and sustainable practices can help the feed industry to contribute to the nutrition, and safety of animal diets, reducing environmental impacts while ensuring the resilience of agricultural production systems (Figure 5.2).

5.5 Disease Control and Biosecurity Measures

Biosecurity and disease prevention are key elements of present-day animal agriculture in general as well to an important extent modern livestock production is coupled with fringes on food safety issues or subsequent economic losses from hitched-up zoonotic diseases. Disease outbreaks are devastating to livestock health and reduce productivity (milk production) morbidity/mortality, causing economic losses for farmers and the agri-industrial sectors. It comprises a system, or measures used to reduce the transmission of diseases among populations that are groups like herd health management. These protocols include disinfection, mandatory quarantine for all incoming animals, ban on outsiders entering facilities, and vaccination strategies that adapt to endemic diseases. Surveillance for early detection and rapid response to limit the scope of a disease outbreak are also crucial components of an effective policy. Farmers protect their animals, food production systems and contribute to global sustainable agriculture – farmers by implementing stringent biosecurity measures and disease control strategies.

5.5.1 Strategies for Preventing and Managing Infectious Disease in Livestock

Livestock infectious diseases pose major threats to animal health, agricultural productivity, and global food security alike; prevention strategies for livestock infections are imperative. India has holistically devised these strategies, combining the best practices of proactive biosecurity measures with efficient disease management protocols. Instinctively core biosecurity practices, already present include stringent hygiene protocols, controlled access to facilities, and quarantine procedures designed to block or hold back the acceptance and spread of pathogens [52]. Vaccination strategies addressing individual disease threats enhance herd immunity, making livestock populations significantly less subjected to infection, and are directly beneficial in reducing the spread of diseases [53].

Early detection (using surveillance systems) allows for timely intervention and outbreak containment to avert global spread. Finally, rapid diagnostic technologies with PCR assays and serological testing can help identify pathogens in time to inform a targeted response. Coordinated efforts between veterinarians, producers, and government agencies are required to promote a holistic approach towards biosecurity and disease mitigation measures aiming at preparedness for emergent challenges while keeping sustainable livestock production systems worldwide.

5.5.2 Biosecurity Protocols for Farms and Food Production Facilities

Ensuring biosecurity measures in farms and food production facilities is a key strategy for the prevention of introduction and transmission of infectious diseases in livestock, including in intact zoo sanitary situations that help protect animal health as well as ensure both the safety of the consumed meat economy stability within the agricultural system. Based on this, protocols have been put in place that incorporate unbending measures to reduce the risks of disease transmission from external sources and between animals within a facility. Key biosecurity measures consist of good hygiene practices such as equipment, vehicles, and site cleaning/disinfection [54]. Disinfection of possible pathogen reservoir areas such as feed storage facilities and water systems are effective protocols to reduce the risk of survival, spread, and perpetuating infections [55]. Table 5.3 compares biosecurity measures across different regions, highlighting the variations in practices and their effectiveness.

With defining implemented biosecurity measures, control access is the most important tool to mitigate the entrance of pathogens into farms and production sites. Limited color-coded access by personnel, visitors, and vehicles also slows the entry of contamination from external environments that can bring diseases without checking into these vulnerable livestock populations. Additionally, creating biosecurity zones within facilities provides additional means of disease control through separation or compartmentalization among the many production areas.

Quarantine of new animals allows you to intercept all incoming livestock, and scrub them down as tightly as possible without drowning the animal in strong chemicals and/or nutrients if that's what they need (although ideally none of us should have such a low point on our nutritional requirements). This comprised of health screens, and

Table 5.3 Comparison of biosecurity measures across regions.

Regions	Biosecurity protocols	Effectiveness	Challenges	Implementation	References
North America	Disinfection systems, and traceability	Highly effective in commercial settings	Cost of implementation	Common in large farms	[57]
Europe	Comprehensive disease monitoring, zoning	Occasional outbreaks	Resource allocation	Implemented with strong regulatory support	[58]
Southeast Asia	Vaccination campaigns, quarantine protocols	Moderately effective	Lack of uniform enforcement	Being implemented in urban areas	[59]
South America	Vaccination, and farm hygiene practices	Effective for specific diseases	Weak enforcement of regulations	Moderate implementation	[60]
Middle East	Quarantine protocols, import restrictions	Moderately effective	Conflict zones hinder enforcement	Gaps in enforcement	[61]
South Asia	Vaccination, hygiene improvement	Moderately effective	Unregulated backyard farming	Low enforcement	[62]

testing and supervised waiting for detection and quarantine of individuals potentially carrying the virus. Surveillance and monitoring programs monitor the health of animals ensuring early detection of diseases [56]. Rapid diagnostic technologies such as PCR assays and serological tests have paved the way for confirming disease presence quickly, assisting rapid response to control outbreaks with the prevention of further transmission. Compliance with rigorous biosecurity measures is not only critical for animal health and disease prevention but also important to maintain trust in food production systems. Adhering to such stringent biosecurity standards ensures that farmers and food producers are contributing to the broader picture of global food security, one farm at a time. These technologies are imperative for reducing the economic damage from outbreaks of disease and since they contribute to fairly, consistent livestock production, so that confidence can continue the part of consumers about safety and reliability level food.

5.5.3 Role of Vaccination in Disease Control and Eradication

Today, vaccines are considered key tools in modern agriculture implementing prophylactic strategies aimed at the control and eradication of communicable diseases; animal welfare concerns are now being the actual support anchors to the fourth arm (sustainable intensification of livestock production), which need to step over direct economic issues twined with that specific front called disease economics. These programs are specifically designed to stimulate livestock immune systems and provide vaccination against particular infectious diseases most prevalent in specific regions or production practices. Veterinarians vaccinate animals with vaccines containing live-attenuated or killed pathogens, making the immune system respond to noninfectious components of the infectious particles and build an arsenal that will prevent infections when exposed [32]. In livestock systems, vaccination is bivalent. First off, it increases the health of each animal by decreasing disease severity and susceptibility. This supports not only animal welfare but also ongoing productivity in the livestock populations that food production systems depend on. Second, vaccines add to the herd immunity concept where if a large proportion of animals within your population are immune against it there may be limited risk for disease transmission. This communal defense is important in guarding against outbreaks and disease transmission among larger populations of animals.

Vaccination is an essential part of a disease control plan that provides another layer of protection in conjunction with biosecurity measures designed to help prevent pathogens from entering and transmitting between production phases. Vaccination schedules are to be made specifically concerning the epidemiological characteristics of target diseases, like frequency and severity of disease outbreaks in specific regions and type of animals at risk as well as magnitude or status/states on immunity level/susceptibility prevalent among population that would enable strategical approach fitting those existing scenario [63]. Control of vaccine-type disease through monitoring of paralytic poliomyelitis establishes the necessary baseline for evaluating vaccination and guiding needed adaptations in protocol to maintain defense against propagating pathogens or developing infectious challenges. In turn, serve as a fundamental element of global eradication campaigns for certain infectious diseases that have significant international health and economic impacts on farm livestock (vaccination). This is particularly so when designing eradication programs for contagious diseases (e.g., FMD or avian influenza) where vaccinating as many farm animals at risk of infection to reduce the reservoir hosts and hopefully prevent future outbreaks is a successful control measure that can incorporate less than optimal vaccines that may still provide some direct protection ox indirect immunity through herd effects. These initiatives promote global trade by demonstrating disease control and sanitary standards as well as helping to safeguard regional livestock populations. For each of these examples, vaccination is the bedrock in disease control tottered by no more than a high rise. Effective vaccination programs not only serve to safeguard animal welfare and food safety but can also promote the practice of sustainable agriculture by farmers, and veterinary practitioners and bolster global initiatives aimed at maintaining worldwide food security. Vaccination is thus an essential component for sustainable and secure herd production systems globally as it is one of our powerful tools against infectious diseases.

5.6 Climate Change and Veterinary Challenges

Climate change not only represents one of the biggest challenges for veterinary science and livestock management (as well as, by extension, human health and welfare) but also impacts the animal production system in terms of efficiency or environmental sustainability. The direct risks to livestock of heat stress and the indirect effects on vector-borne diseases (such as tick fever) from altered disease-transmission dynamics are seen with rising global temperatures. In addition, these types of environmental changes might influence animal physiology and behavioral patterns as well as spatiotemporal variations in infectious disease transmission. Certified professional veterinarians in their up-gradation to bring solutions for these challenges and create a new change which is the most innovative adaptive strategy to be able to no climate change effects on livestock. The section that follows will discuss the intricate web of climate change and a veterinary medical world with dangers to emerging animal health, novel methodologies for disease control, in addition to things we must do – sustainably.

5.6.1 Impact of Climate Change on Animal Health and Agriculture

Climate change directly affects animal health and agriculture thereby providing an interventionistic pathway for addressing the complex trans-sectional burden of zoonotic diseases, warranting scientific knowledge and inventive solutions from veterinary professionals. Global warming and changes in world climate places important impacts on animal health, productivity, and disease dynamics [64]. One of the most important problems is heat stress, which has devastating effects on animal welfare and physiological parameters because long exposure to warm temperatures disrupts growth rates and reproduction retardation in addition due to suppressive immune function occurs. When experiencing heat stress, animals will modify their behavior to try and cool off (in the case of birds that might involve panting and moving into shade), but sometimes prolonged or extreme exposure can overwhelm these adaptive mechanisms [65].

Differences in precipitation are additionally fascinating when we contemplate domestic animals and disease transmission. That is why a bamboozle area event may have great synergistic effects, for instance producing more rainfall that causes waterlogging in the pastures and abundant light or nutrients competition of bamboo, getting unfavorable conditions that reduce cows' diet quality as they are experiencing few but enough resource supply [66]. One of the very real outcomes is a significant elevation in incidence rates to acquired immune dysfunction that has been functionally, and structurally diminished by malnutrition subsequently predisposing them susceptible to deadly infectious diseases due to pathogens operating thus pathophysiologically eurphoricity underlie environmental mimicking stressors. Climate change could increase the range of diseases such as West Nile virus and Rift Valley fever, which are mainly transmitted by mosquitoes, while heartwater disease easily passes from animals to humans through ticks (and their close contact with both animal hosts) (Figure 5.3). It is the reason behind veterinary science academics but provides other reasons by stating that animal health and agriculture must address climate change impacts.

Improved disease detection systems monitor the burden and geography of diseases accurately so that early warning may help identify where additional health areas are needed for transmission reduction plans. This can include devising custom vaccination schedules to prevent infectious disease outbreaks and enhance the herd immunity of herds. It is diagnostic reading in understanding and predicting progress in the tools of diagnosis, itself a vital part of any prophylactic control strategy that might anticipate future outbreaks like phylloxera provided adaptation by producers and regulators. Indeed, encourage new housing and ventilation practices for heat stress-resilient livestock; balanced feed diets by adjusted nutritional requirements due to each growth phase needs, besides systems with integrated monthly services toward sustainable landscape management. This then improves farm resilience to shocks at the same time as fostering more sustainable biodiversity across farming landscapes that will provide ecological services on which agriculture also depends.

Closer interdisciplinary and multiscale collaboration among veterinarians, farmers, researchers, and policymakers is essential to develop innovation that can perform under demonstrably challenging conditions of a

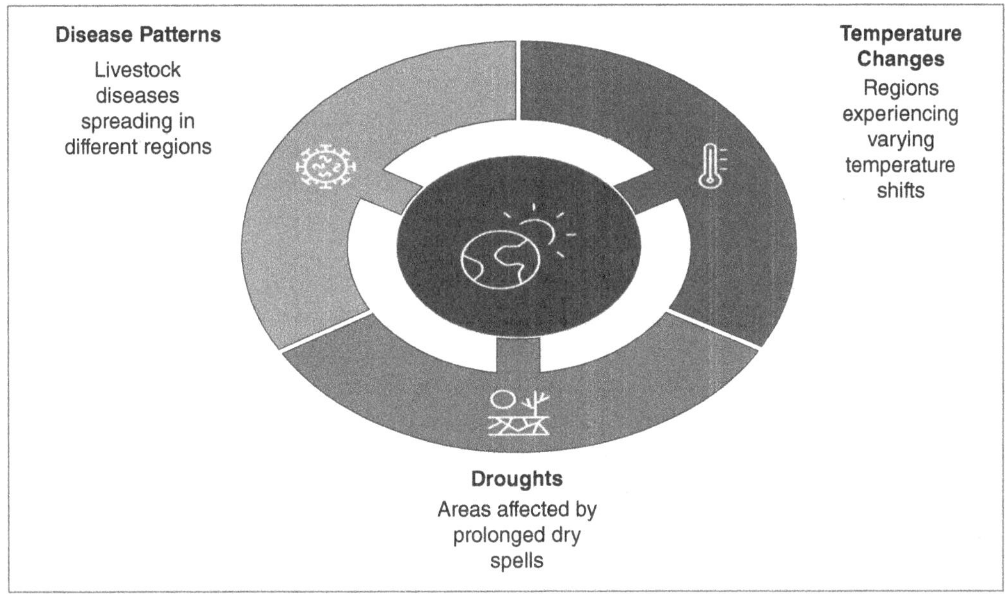

Figure 5.3 Climate-related challenges affecting livestock.

changing climate faced by livestock systems while addressing the sustainability question potentially together with productivity because they are often co-dependent.

5.6.2 Adaptation Strategies for Livestock Farming in Changing Environmental Conditions

As such, it is of utmost importance to adopt livestock farming practices due to changes in environmental conditions especially when climate change and other environmental impacts threaten agricultural sustainability. Increasing global temperature and fluctuating rainfall patterns affect the health, productivity of livestock, and resilience systems within various agriculture systems globally. Farmers and agricultural professionals are responding to this by practicing various adaptation strategies to reduce the risks while optimizing management practices. Breeding and genetic selection, the second important tactic is to enhance the breeding/GW methods. Hence, selective breeding of livestock or traits like heat resistance, disease threats, and nutrient use efficiency can therefore be made to accommodate breeds that fit the given region. This makes animals more resistant to the environment and increases productivity in different conditions. Feeding and nutrition management improvement are vital for the said purpose. Changes in feed formulation are necessary as environmental variability modifies grazing patterns and the availability of water and forage [67]. This, together with precision feeding technologies to optimize feed efficiency and fortify the diet with essential nutrients enables us to restrict changes in dietary composition caused by shifting environmental conditions.

The non-core part is effective water management and conservation practices. Methods such as rainwater harvesting, effective irrigation techniques, and recycling of water can also be employed to maximize the potential for your animals in case they are needed during a drought [68]. Sustainable water management helps maintain the welfare of livestock and the integrity of environmental ecosystems; it is an element that influences not only land use but contributes to ensuring a habitat in which animal health thrives. One of the major contributions to reducing stress and comfort living in livestock, especially during heat waves or cold snaps is adaptive housing and shelter solutions [69]. The animals' health and well-being production in turn enhanced when facilities are appropriately upgraded to be open to the climate (owing, for example, design enhancement interventions such as improved ventilation systems) or closed off from extremes (e.g., provision of shade structures insulated shelters).

Adapting to the environment retains immense importance and so do strategies for disease prevention and health management. In the face of a climate-induced increase in disease burden, biosecurity measures need to be strengthened, and more comprehensive vaccination programs must become a priority for prevention; meanwhile, investments should shift toward enhancing surveillance capacity. The earlier the disease is noticed, and actions are taken to react, the less spread of it we will see and therefore lesser economic loss. The resilience of rangelands is also largely influenced by proper animal grazing and pasture management practices. Practices like rotational grazing, species diversification in pastures, and effective stocking rates are used to restore soil health, maintain ground cover from a good mix of plant varieties, and increase carbon storage [70]. These practices also help maintain ecosystem resilience to natural variations in the environment. The adaptive capacity is also amplified with climate-resilient infrastructure and technology blend. Infusion of resources into energy efficiency buildings, renewable technologies, and weather forecast devices improve systems to save costs at operational levels and cut across climate change effects. Such infrastructure is the lifeblood of farm operations, enabling farms to adapt in response to changes brought about by climate change. Education and knowledge exchange are key areas for stimulating the uptake of climate-smart agricultural practices. Training and capacity building, adaptive strategies, and technologies for sustainable farm production will put tremendous knowledge in the hands of farmers, thereby enabling them to make informed decisions on how best practices could be deployed or adopted within their farms. Policy support and financial incentives from governments and organizations can largely help adaptation endeavors. To help with such adaptive farming practices, it is necessary to have policies that promote climate-resilient agriculture along with financial incentives for sustainable practices and research and development initiatives.

Incorporating these adaptation strategies into livestock farming practices will help in making farms more resilient, reducing risks due to climate change, and contributing toward sustainable agricultural development. The successful upscaling of climate-smart practices therefore requires concerted efforts among stakeholders, research institutions, and policymakers to identify farm-level changes that can offer the greatest potential for long-term solutions on a global scale in livestock farming under diverse evolving environmental threats.

5.6.3 Mitigation Measures to Reduce the Environmental Footprint of Animal Agriculture

Animal agriculture is increasingly under pressure to decrease its environmental footprint. We must mitigate the sector's contribution to climate change, its effect on land degradation, and its role in draining resource pools. Animal agriculture, including livestock farming, is a well-recognized major source of greenhouse gas emissions (methane, nitrous oxide, and carbon dioxide). Emissions from many parts of livestock production occur including enteric fermentation in ruminants, manure management, and feed production [71]. Many strategies and technologies are available to lower the environmental impact of this sector, and while this is not a panacea for either global food security or environmental impact, it is a start in the right direction.

The most direct and effective way to reduce the environmental footprint of animal agriculture is to reduce methane emissions from ruminants. In the process of enteric fermentation in ruminants (e.g., cows and sheep), methane is produced along the digestive tract. Dietary interventions that alter the fermentation process have been developed as several mitigation strategies to reduce methane production. Some feed additives, such as tannins, fats, or 3-nitrooxypropanol (3-NOP) can inhibit the microbes notable for methane production in the rumen [72]. In addition, the efficiency with which livestock is fed, it is optimal in terms of protein content and digestibility, can also reduce the overall methane produced per unit of each livestock product. Genetically improving livestock to reduce methane emissions is also an area of new research, with some breeds outpacing others in terms of reducing methane emissions. Improving manure management practices is also an important key strategy. Manure is a big source of methane and nitrous oxide, which are gases that are both potent greenhouse gases. Traditional manure management systems, such as open lagoons or direct land applications, permit the emission of large amounts of these gases into the atmosphere. By cutting emissions to anaerobic digestion for manure to produce biogas as a form of renewable energy, such gases could be dramatically reduced in emissions and shifted to more sustainable practices. In reducing methane and nitrous oxide emissions, composting or controlling manure storage systems are also used. In addition, manure can also be spread onto crops as fertilizer in safe amounts for a source of needed nutrients for crops while reducing dependence on synthetic fertilizers that require a large amount of energy input and also produce greenhouse gases [73]. There is another way to solve the ecological footprint of animal agriculture: grow under the agroecological principles of resource efficiency, biodiversity, and ecosystem services. Also included in this are practices like rotational grazing, which increases soil health, decreases the risk of overgrazing, and sequesters carbon in the soil. The concept of herding multiple different kinds of animals together simultaneously can increase the way nutrients cycle, especially at the grass level, and reduce the requirement for inputs like synthetic fertilizer. Numerous environmental benefits accrue from integrating trees into livestock systems: where trees and livestock coexist in agroforestry (or across integration of trees into livestock systems), carbon sequestration, water retention, and biodiversity enrichment are realized. These practices not only help in keeping the environmental footprint in color but can also add to building resilience to climate change.

But another big area that can significantly cut the amount of environmental damage from livestock farming is the much less efficient production of feed. Land, water, and energy are used up in the production of animal feed like grain and soy, with the energy often a fossil fuel, and deforestation and habitat loss can and do occur. In place of feed ingredients that do more harm than good, such as heavy inputs of fossil fuel-based products, shifting to more sustainable feed ingredients, including byproducts of other agricultural processes, will reduce the need for land conversion and lower the environmental costs of feed production. Other sources of alternative protein, including insect meal, algae, or even fermented microbial proteins, can also help to reduce the ecological impact of feed production. Precision agriculture technologies can also help in the optimal use of inputs of fertilizer, water, and pesticides, reducing the environmental burden of growing feed crops. The emerging mitigation strategy of cultured meat, also referred to as lab-grown meat, is another. Cultured meat is meat that has been grown in a conditioned environment outside of an animal. The potential for this technology to significantly reduce the environmental impact of meat production exists due to its elimination of the need for land for grazing and therefore water use, in addition to minimizing greenhouse gas emissions from traditional livestock farming. Cultured meat is still in its early stages of commercialization but could make an important contribution to a future sustainable food system. Reducing the environmental footprint involves the reduction of animal production and fundamentally improving the overall efficiency of animal production. Through good livestock health, good livestock genetics, and good livestock management, the farmer can produce more meat, milk, and eggs on less resources. Current PLF technologies, that is, the sensor and wearable devices, enable real-time monitoring of the health and the behavior of the animals which farmers can exploit to optimize feeding practices, decrease the lost food, and increase productivity [74]. But better health management can reduce our need for antibiotics and other inputs and therefore reduce the environmental footprint even more. Finally, policy interventions and economic incentives are necessary to facilitate the adoption of sustainable practices in animal agriculture. Subsidies, tax breaks, or carbon credits can and should be used by governments to incentivize practices including carbon sequestration, improved feed efficiency, and methane reduction. Such international frameworks as the Paris Agreement are also important in guiding countries to develop targets for emissions reduction in agriculture. Such policies allow the agricultural sector to get in line with global climate goals, toward the objective of more sustainable food systems.

5.7 Veterinary Extension and Capacity Building

5.7.1 Importance of Education and Training in Veterinary Sciences for Sustainable Agriculture

Pillars to advance sustainable agriculture and secure long-term food security are education and training in veterinary sciences. From climate change and resource scarcity to the race toward feeding a growing population, veterinarians are taking an increasingly important role in maintaining animal health, improving productivity, and reducing the environmental impact of livestock farming, worldwide. Veterinary professionals need to be equipped with the latest knowledge and skills to meet the evolving requirements of modern agriculture and to add to more sustainable farming practices. Taking part in the mandatory One Health course, the integration of which is one of the key aspects of veterinary education is one of the key aspects of veterinary education. To prevent and manage zoonotic diseases foodborne illnesses and environmental degradation, it is necessary to educate veterinarians to consider these interdependencies. With knowledge about the wider ecological and public health impacts of their work, veterinarians can develop the best interventions that are not only protecting animal health but also people populations and the environment [75]. Integrated approach training programs provide veterinarians with the opportunity to work more readily with individuals from public health, environmental science, and agriculture backgrounds and develop multidisciplinary responses to more complex problems.

Education and training of veterinarians can be employed to teach them how to support the genetic improvement of more resilient livestock breeds, more efficient feeding systems, and disease management strategies that reduce the need for chemical intervention. If veterinarians who have advanced knowledge in such things as precision medicine, genomics, or sustainable feed systems can offer evidence-based solutions that increase livestock productivity, the primary goal of the whole activity, while not causing environmental damage, is the secondary goal. Instead, training veterinarians on how to incorporate these innovative practices into their day-to-day jobs will allow them to help farmers adopt sustainable practices such as rotational grazing, integrated pest management, or the use of fewer antibiotics. Furthermore, regular continued education of vet professionals through specialized training programs or workshops is essential to maintain the veterinary professionals on new emerging diseases, trendy treatment protocols as well as cutting-edge technology [76]. Scientific discovery and technological innovation develop at lightning speed, leaving behind those who are looking for up-to-date information on diagnostic tools, vaccines, and breeding techniques to provide competent care and support in the agricultural sector. Additionally, veterinary ethics and welfare education ensures that veterinarians will be able to strike a balance between animal productivity and animal welfare that meets social norms of acceptable practices of animal husbandry.

In rural and largely constrained environments where veterinary services are sparse, education and training particularly are critical to building operations capacity for improving local food security and bolstering smallholder farmers. By building tailored training programs that respond to local challenges, such as climate-specific disease risk, resource limitation, and traditional farming behavior, we will help farmers adopt best practices to improve animal health and productivity. Depending on the location, advancing toward broader public health objectives in this way also helps to increase the number of well-trained veterinary professionals, and if the veterinarian is situated in these regions, his or her central role in disease surveillance and prevention, education, and food safety can be quite important. To a broader field of agricultural policy development, education in veterinary sciences also makes an important contribution. As experts in animal health and agriculture, veterinarians are consulted frequently for guidance on the regulatory frameworks and policies that govern animal welfare, biosecurity, and food safety. This solid educational background enables veterinary professionals to engage in evidence-based discussion of policy and to advocate for sustainable means of agricultural practice within a global context tied to the broader goals of global food security.

5.7.2 Extension Services to Disseminate Best Practices and Innovations

Best practices and innovations related to veterinary medicine and agriculture, from which extension services play a critical role in disseminating, serve to promote the adoption of sustainable methods that are likely to augment animal health and agricultural productivity. They act as a link between research institutes, government bodies, and farmers to exchange knowledge, technology, and skills down to the grassroots. Extension services provide the latest advances to empower farmers, livestock keepers, and veterinary professionals to manage their farms more optimally, to better ensure animal welfare, and to contribute to environmental sustainability. The major function of extension services is to train and technical assist farmers with new veterinary practices and agricultural innovations. It means encouraging farmers to learn how biosecurity measures, disease control measures, sustainable feed, and nutrition practices can protect their crops. On the ground, in rural places, extension workers do what people sometimes believe is impossible; they demonstrate how effective these techniques can be, help farmers brainstorm solutions to problems they are encountering, and guide farmers as they adopt new technologies, like PLF and digital health monitoring, as well as genetic selection to develop disease-resistant breeds. Extension services enhance the increase in the uptake of best practices which are directly linked to productivity and sustainability through hands-on training and field demonstration [77]. Additionally, extension services play an important role in finding local and regional solutions. For example, extension workers can help farmers in areas impacted by climate change choose adaptive strategies, such as breeding heat-tolerant livestock, improving water usage, and improving land management. In the course, these also assist farmers in traversing such complexity in sustainable agriculture which advises them on crop and livestock integration, conservation tillage, agroforestry, and other practices that ensure ecological balance. Extension services ensure that innovations are locally appropriate because recommendations are tailored to local conditions making it more likely the innovations will be adopted. An important task of extension services is to foster the exchange of knowledge and experience among the farmers. Extension services enable such communities to talk about becoming farmers by providing opportunities for farmers to learn about each other and discuss problems and solutions through workshops, farmer field schools, and so on, bringing together and encouraging the sharing of solutions to tie communities and promote collaborative problem-solving. They also enable farmers to learn from early adopters of new technologies merely by observing precedents from these local champions of innovation. It enables peer-to-peer learning, it builds trust and it speeds the adoption of new practices across whole agricultural communities [78]. One of its roles is to facilitate the implementation of government policies and programs that seek to promote agricultural sustainability and food security through extension services.

Extension workers help farmers comply with national and international standards for animal health, food safety, and environmental conservation by providing critical information about subsidies, regulations, and new legislation. Furthermore, they serve as the channels through which the reaction of the farmers to government policies is channeled, thus allowing the government to capture and respond to farmers' views and suggestions so that the government's interventions can be more effective. As digital technologies are increasingly employed in agriculture, extension services have started to use digital tools to reach and impact the farmers better [79]. Real-time information, disease alerts and technical support to farmers are increasingly being provided through mobile applications, online platforms and remote advisory services for farmers in remote areas. In addition to helping to extend the geographical reach of extension services, these technologies also provide relatively cheap delivery of training and technical assistance. For instance, mobile apps can help a farmer track an animal's health, keep track of feeding practices, and get market information, which in turn aid the farmer with making informed decisions and improving farm management. It also helps extension services to raise awareness of the longer-term effects of agriculture on global food security, public health, and the environment. Through the extension program integration of One Health principles, extension services assist farmers to understand how animal health, human health, and ecosystem health are related. It is this holistic approach, attempting more sustainable farming practices that consider what is good for the planet in the long term, and what is good for even its inhabitants.

5.7.3 Capacity Building Initiatives for Veterinary Professionals in Developing Countries

Veterinary professionals in developing countries need capacity-building initiatives to tackle the multiplicity of challenges these countries face when trying to achieve sustainable agriculture, improved animal health, and food security. The veterinary workforce in many developing regions is generally small and poorly trained, and therefore cannot effectively control livestock diseases, increase productivity, or promote food safety. Capacity-building initiatives support veterinarians in developing the skills, knowledge, and capability to add value to the health of animals, so their health impacts the livelihoods of farmers and communities. Capacity building in veterinary sciences is one of the primary goals to increase the professional education and training involved in the training of veterinarians [80]. These can be done using advanced training programs, workshops, and exchange programs with institutions in developed countries. However, these programs tend to train veterinarians in the latest knowledge in disease prevention, diagnostics, treatment protocols, and new technologies in veterinary treatment. These initiatives build upon existing research and best industry practices to ensure that veterinary professionals are equipped with up-to-date evidence-based solutions to the problems faced by farmers in developing countries. Capacity building also covers the improvement of accessibility of veterinary services, which is an important element of veterinary health services to the underserved. Veterinary care is largely provided in urban areas, cut off from professional assistance in many developing countries. The training of community-based animal health workers/paraprofessionals could be translated into support services for their veterinary services in remote places. Doctors can play an important role here and can, by providing basic training in animal health and disease management, serve as the first line of support in terms of stopping outbreaks, allowing farmers to intervene on time to, for example, prevent diseases from spreading and save animals from cruelty. These workers in addition also play a major role in the delivery of health education to farmers, given that they raise awareness of good practices in animal husbandry, biosecurity, and nutrition. A key aspect of capacity building in developing countries is to strengthen the existing veterinary infrastructure [81]. Many regions lack adequate facilities for handling animals, have little or no diagnostic tools, and cannot even afford vaccines and medications. To enable effective disease surveillance and treatment, disease surveillance capacity-building initiatives (e.g., improving infrastructure, e.g., providing mobile veterinary clinics, establishing veterinary diagnostic laboratories, or improving supply chains of veterinary products) are required. In this context, partnerships with international organizations, government, and the private sector are crucial mechanisms for raising the required resources and expertise to fill these gaps. Moreover, greater coordination and even faster response to outbreaks of transboundary animal diseases is strengthened through greater coordination, and the development of an even faster response, through the strengthening of national and regional veterinary networks. An important component of capacity building is the promotion of research and development (R&D) in veterinary sciences customized to the situation in developing countries. However, the bulk of the veterinary research done in developed countries does not apply directly to the different issues that arise in resource-limited settings. Capacity-building initiatives geared to locally relevant R&D tend to generate context-specific solutions, for example, vaccines and appropriate treatments for diseases endemic to a given geographic area, as well as low-cost animal husbandry techniques to increase productivity without sacrificing animal welfare. By promoting collaboration between veterinary professionals, agricultural researchers, and policymakers, R&D efforts led by these partners can be efficient and sustainable in their implementation, aligning with real-world farmer needs. Among other things, capacity-building initiatives involve training in the areas of public health and zoonotic diseases. Zoonotic diseases pose a particular threat to many developing countries because of the transmission of diseases from animals to humans. Avian influenza, FMD, and rabies are among such diseases which pose considerable threats to public health and food security [82]. Capacity-building initiatives carry the potential to enhance veterinary professionals' knowledge and skills regarding surveillance (including reporting) and measures for the control of zoonotic disease thereby safeguarding human and animal health. Additionally, One Health-trained veterinarians who understand the connections between human, animal, and environmental health are more likely to prevent and manage outbreaks that both compromise agricultural and public health systems. Finally, leadership and management skills need to be fostered in veterinary professionals to engender the long-term sustainability of veterinary services in developing countries. Leadership development, veterinary management, and policy advocacy initiatives are capacity-building efforts aimed at providing veterinarians with the capacity to play leadership roles in national agricultural development, health, and policy advocacy. Additionally, these initiatives enhance the development of networks and partnerships aimed at knowledge exchange and resource mobilization as well as collaboration between countries and international organizations for enhanced veterinary services in developing regions.

5.8 Challenges and Future Directions

5.8.1 Identifying Challenges in Veterinary Medicine and Agriculture

Veterinary medicine and agriculture face complex challenges that directly influence global food security. It is among the most urgent problems: emerging and reemerging diseases. There are highly pathogenic avian influenza and African swine fever pathogens that will kill livestock populations, shut down food production, and cause huge economic losses. Thus, rapid economic spread and virulent spread of infectious diseases take place as a result of infectious disease permitting a rapid globalization of society through techniques such as trade, animal movement, and more generally, trade. Thus, sophisticated diagnostics, vigilant surveillance, and appropriate disease control are necessary to minimize risk. The other serious threat to human health and animal health is AMR [83]. Resistant strains of bacteria are caused by the overuse and misuse of antibiotics in the animal agriculture sector and render traditional treatment less effective. The trouble is how to coddle infection while reducing the chance of high mortality and economic losses in livestock. Effective countermeasures to AMR should include disciplined use of antimicrobials, search for alternatives, and enhanced systems to evaluate the effectiveness of antimicrobial therapy.

Together all this adds up climate change makes it not only more difficult but less likely to successfully raise animals and keep them healthy, which becomes much more of a challenge as temperatures rise, the weather gets more erratic, and we see the manifest extremes of productivity and disease in animals across the globe. Among the more obvious direct impacts of a changing climate are heat stress altered disease distribution and water availability. These challenges require that our adaptation strategies include breeding resilient livestock, boosting water and feed efficiencies, and practicing sustainable agriculture, to ensure stable food supplies. The increasing global demand for animal protein is also raising resource scarcity and necessitating sustainable feeding strategies. For example, traditional feed ingredients such as soy and maize are tremendously intensive regarding natural resources and cause environmental degradation. Sustainable feed alternatives, optimization of feed conversion efficiency, and reduction of food waste are needed to square livestock production with environmental conservation. Access to veterinary services, often advanced technologies and credit, is persistently hampered by economic barriers, for small-scale farmers in developing countries. Constrained by this productivity tends to be lower, and food security is at more risk of disease outbreaks. Increasing market pathways, financial support, and veterinarian infrastructure are essential to the livelihood resilience of resilient livestock systems that are economically viable and resilient for coping with challenges.

Additional hurdles faced are knowledge gaps in veterinary medicine, especially in rural and developing regions. Animal health management managed according to best practices can be hampered by a lack of access to updated training and education. Capacity building, extension services, and hands-on training are necessary to prepare veterinary professionals and livestock producers to respond to emerging agricultural challenges. In regions such as Northern Vietnam where resources and infrastructure are scarce, the challenge of maintaining robust biosecurity on farms and in food production facilities is great. To prevent disease transmission, effective biosecurity measures are needed; however, the gaps in implementation and compliance can further the spread of infections [84]. To protect food supplies as well as promote animal health, our work needs to enhance surveillance systems, enforce biosecurity protocols, and raise awareness among farmers. While technological advancements have promised to improve animal health and productivity, costs and institutional and infrastructural shortcomings impede adoption. Precision farming tools, genomic technologies, and digital monitoring systems present a way to significantly boost agricultural efficiency, but access to these innovations must be broadened so they can realize their full potential in a wide range of farm settings. It is a concept of One Health, which emphasizes the interconnection of the health of humans, animals, and the environment, reflecting on the significance of veterinary medicine in public health. An integrated approach is required to address zoonotic diseases, foodborne pathogens, and the ecological impact of agriculture. Integration of these intersecting health risks to maintain food safety requires effective collaboration among veterinarians, public health officials, and environmental scientists. Veterinary and agricultural challenges are complicated by sociocultural factors and policy limitations. Failure can occur due to modern, sustainable approaches not being put in place as selective and traditional practices, cultural beliefs and inadequate policies restrict their use. To overcome these barriers, culturally sensitive outreach, policy reforms of targeted immediacy, and economic incentives in which agricultural practices are aligned with long-term environmental and health goals are required.

5.8.2 Opportunities for Future Research and Collaboration

Innovations in veterinary sciences show transformations to agricultural systems which face greater and greater pressures from population growth, climate change, and disease threats. The most effective translation of veterinary advancements for their impact on the society and environment may depend on a research agenda that is driven by interdisciplinary approaches that bring together animal health, environmental sustainability, and socio-economic stability, and partnerships that expand resources, technology, and expertise. Future research efforts include creating precision medicine as well as diagnostic tools targeting livestock. Genomic sequencing, biomarker identification, and digital monitoring systems are advancing in ways that make it possible to perform highly targeted disease interventions and deliver personalized health management to animals. By pinning down certain disease susceptibility or resilience genes, veterinary scientists hope to breed livestock that are naturally healthier, more productive, and ecologically tenable. This approach would help reduce over-reliance on antibiotics and other chemicals in support of antibiotic stewardship minimize AMR and improve the safety of food.

Future vaccine development research also has the potential to contribute to disease prevention and control strategies for zoonotic and economically disruptive diseases. New frontier areas of highly efficacious and scalable immunization against pathogens that threaten both animal and human populations include novel vaccine technologies like mRNA platforms and nanoparticle-based vaccines [85]. While further research into thermostable vaccines and alternative delivery methods such as oral or nasal formulation could help make vaccines more accessible in remote or resource-limited areas, ease of manufacturing and handling vaccines like this may be minimal forcing the WHO to reconsider requirements for thermostable vaccines. That said, when it comes to this area of collaboration, there would be international collaboration, which would enable frontrunners in this space to share their innovations with both developed and developing regions. Feed innovation and sustainable nutrition are important research directions to mitigate the environmental impact of livestock farming, at the level of animal health and productivity. Feeding research into sources of alternative feed, among them insect protein, algae, and byproducts from the agricultural process, can drastically diminish dependence on traditional feedstocks such as soy and maize, spreading deforestation and biodiversity loss. Agricultural scientists, veterinarians, and environmental experts working together may develop new formulations to optimize nutrient profiles, increase digestibility, and reduce greenhouse gas emissions to form a more sustainable production of livestock. Also, future research will have to address the climate resilience of animal agriculture. Breeding for heat tolerance and developing cooling technologies for livestock are necessary climate change adaptation strategies to prevent the compromise of animal health and productivity in a changing climate [86]. To proactively manage emerging threats, we will need to learn about the effects of climate change on disease vectors and pathogen behavior. Understanding these complex interactions and developing effective adaptation measures will depend heavily on multinational partnerships and data-sharing initiatives.

Research and collaboration in the future will be guided by the framework of the One Health approach with a focus on the connections between human, animal, and environmental health. Zoonotic diseases, food-borne pathogens, and the health of ecosystems can be addressed integrally through the combination of veterinary sciences with public health and environmental studies. Collaboration between veterinary and medical professionals is needed further for the development of prediction models for disease outbreaks, joint surveillance, and the development of interdisciplinary response strategies. In addition, a collaborative model may lead to stronger policies and practices aimed at advancing sustainable agriculture and promoting the health of people. Finalizing the research and translating it into practice can be difficult, even in developed countries, where resources may be lacking for the rapidly advancing care and technologies in veterinary. Expanding training programs, scholarships and knowledge exchange initiatives can provide the next generation of veterinarians with the skills to meet the needs of the future, in terms of implementing sustainable practices and dealing with new challenges. Investing in education, researching, and supporting veterinary extension services can ensure that recent advancements from research and policymakers are available to small-scale farmers and large contributors to local food systems and rural economies. Opportunities for research in the realm of policy and regulation also exist in the development of frameworks that promote sustainable practices and protect animal welfare. Collaborative studies on the impact of policy, trade regulations, and economic incentives could help to bring agricultural practices closer to sustainable development goals. To establish regulatory environments that support innovation, promote the safety of food while prioritizing the well-being of life forms produced for food, and foster ethical standards in animal production, these regulatory environments require a partnership between governments, academia, and industry.

5.8.3 Exemplary Projects Showcasing the Application of Advanced Veterinary Sciences

The possibility of using scientific innovations to improve animal health, agriculture, and food security is demonstrated through examples of exemplary projects that demonstrate how advanced veterinary sciences are being applied. These projects showcase how the integration of modern veterinary practices, technologies, and multidisciplinary approaches can facilitate solving some of the most important challenges of livestock production and disease control and create a more resilient and secure food system. There is such a great example of it, which is the development of PLF technologies, for example. This real-time monitoring of the health and behavior of livestock in PLF is enabled using sensors, data analytics, and automation. Suppose, for example, in some countries, smart collars, wearable sensors, and biometric monitors are used to capture a broad suite of parameters for animal monitoring, including body temperature, heart rate, activity level, etc. What these systems do is allow farmers to detect early signs of illness or distress before it gets to the point of antibiotics and other veterinary drugs. Additionally, the data that these systems produce can be used to improve feeding practices and reduce waste, while also increasing the overall efficiency of livestock production. AI and machine learning integration make it possible to create predictive models to predict disease outbreaks or health issues that can later be used as a management tool for animal health [87].

Genomics and molecular diagnostics have proven useful in the battle against transboundary animal diseases (TADs) in a notable project. The Food and Agriculture Organization (FAO) and the World Organization for Animal Health (OIE) in the context of the Global Genomic Surveillance Program track and control through genomic tools diseases like FMD, avian influenza, and African swine fever. Sequencing genomes of pathogens and finding genetic markers associated with pathogenicity and transmission help scientists improve diagnostics, surveillance, and vaccine development. Other genomic approaches also allow the identification of disease hot spots which can lead to more focused and comprehensive interventions (hot spots) in at-risk areas. Such advanced veterinary science applications not only boost disease control efforts but also play a role in the resilience of the overall livestock farming systems to thwart major epidemics of disease that affect such large swathes of the livestock herd and can feed into widespread epidemics that could virtually wipe out both animal populations and food supplies. Vaccination programs to control zoonotic diseases are another good project where the application of veterinary sciences has been used to increase food security [88]. One example is the African rabies vaccination project, which has shown success in the decrease of rabies incidence both in animals and humans. In many parts of the continent, dogs have proved to be a major vector for rabies that is transmitted from dogs to humans. With local governments and their veterinary counterparts, the World Health Organization (WHO) and the OIE have joined forces in rolling out mass dog vaccination campaigns. As a result, rabies incidence has been greatly reduced, animal health has improved, and the risk of humans is reduced. Utilization of veterinarians' knowledge and mass vaccination of cattle against rabies helped this project not only improve public health but also reduce adverse effects on livestock by vaccination.

An example that stands out is the genomic application for mainstream genetic improvement and breeding to improve livestock resilience in the field. The US Dairy Herd Improvement Program (DHIP) offers genomic selection of dairy cattle in terms of health, productivity, and longevity, taking cow breeding into a stone age and a bronze age at once. In addition, the program has also been selecting animals with superior genetic traits for resistance to disease, reproductive efficiency, and milk production using the program's genomic information and using them to improve herd management and reduce the dependency on antibiotics in dairy farming. Similar genomic-based breeding programs have already been used by other livestock species including cattle, pigs, and chickens to improve disease resistance, for example to mastitis, FMD, and avian influenza [89]. These programs are imperative in building more resilient and sustainable livestock populations that help farmers boost productivity and shrink the ecological and economic footprint of disease outbreaks. Additionally, integrated pest and disease management (IPDM) systems are also promoted as a means of promoting sustainable animal agriculture [90]. These systems are managed by management that use a holistic approach to livestock health and well-being, in that it uses veterinary care, application of the environment, and the practice of natural pest control. IPDM systems have been used by farmers in India to control ticks and other ectoparasites on cattle because such ectoparasites cause loss of productivity in cattle because of disease transmission. The advantage of these integrated systems was the use of complementary tools: biological controls, insect growth regulators, and focused veterinary interventions that together reduced the use of chemical pesticides and improved animal health. Not only does the approach minimize the ecological burden of pest management but also makes the economics of livestock farming more feasible by improving the health and production of animals.

Besides these projects, cultured meat technology is beginning to receive greater attention in its use as an innovative solution to lower the environmental footprint of meat production. There are companies and research institutes throughout the world researching the development of lab-grown meat, which is growing animal cells in bioreactors to produce muscle tissue without having to raise and kill animals. By doing this, we could massively reduce land use, water use, and greenhouse gas emissions from traditional livestock farming. While there is still a long way to go to get there, this development is in its infancy but a demonstration of the potential of veterinary science to work toward creating more sustainable, ethical meat production. Tissue engineering, cellular biology, and bioprocessing technologies are most likely to contribute to the development of cultured meat, which might one day serve to fulfill the global need for protein in the best possible way.

5.8.4 Lessons Learned and Recommendations for Future Interventions

Valuable lessons and insights gained in advancing veterinary sciences for sustainable agriculture and global food security have been generated, which can guide future interventions. Many new innovative technologies and practices have been proven to foster improvements in animal health, production of food, and minimize environmental impact, but there is still work to be done. Therefore, these lessons learned and recommendations for future interventions are important to boost the long-term sustainability and resilience of global agriculture systems. A key lesson learned here is that we cannot allow ourselves to ignore the fact that animal health, the environment, and the well-being of people are interdependent, and thus must be treated as one system. PLF technologies have not only demonstrated significant promise for the improvement of animal health and productivity but are also advancing other precision agriculture (Pe2Ag) technologies [91]. Nevertheless, these systems have to be integrated within a larger framework including quality infrastructure, appropriate management practices, and farmers' education. Such technologies can only have their full potential realized without a holistic approach. Future work on such interventions should place focus on the integration of human capital with technology, such that farmers and veterinary professionals can use these technologies and manage them well. The second and probably more important lesson is to revamp veterinary education and training, especially in developing countries. However, there still exists a gap in knowledge and skills in many regions of the world concerning food security, although postprogressive veterinary medicine and agricultural advances have made great strides in their development. Targeted training programs and extension services to capacity building the veterinarians, farmers, and other stakeholders are imperative to fill this gap and make the veterinarians, farmers, and others take up the forthcoming challenges. Future interventions should devote energy and resources to the development of curricula for the utilization of the most current technologies in animal health care, disease prevention sustainable farming practices, and continued professional development opportunities for practicing veterinarians. The one important lesson is about early detection systems and surveillance systems that help prevent transboundary and zoonotic diseases from spreading. Genomic tools, molecular diagnostics, and surveillance networks have been successfully deployed for identifying disease outbreaks and rapidly responding to contain current and future outbreaks [92]. Nevertheless, there is a need for further effort to advance global coordination in disease surveillance systems, particularly in resource-poor areas. To prevent future outbreaks and ensure food security, strengthening regional disease monitoring systems and international collaborations while encouraging data sharing becomes imperative. However, the One Health approach, which looks at the linkages between human, animal, and environmental health, should continue to be built into disease control strategies so that more unification and holistic approaches can be taken to maximize control of the disease.

Another major issue impacted by lessons learned is that of sustainability. The evidence of promising reductions in the environmental impact of animal agriculture from promoting sustainable feed production, efficient manure management, and innovative livestock management practices however is not enough; greater focus should be put on the development and promotion of alternative sources of protein like plant-based proteins, insects, and cultured meat [93]. These alternatives represent ways of supplying the increasing global demand for protein without further damaging natural resources. The areas where research and development must be accelerated for the sake of future interventions to make sustainable food choices more accessible and economically feasible have been focused on. In addition, education and awareness campaigns can encourage shifts in what consumers demand for protein intake, including more sustainable protein sources. Another key takeaway has been the role of vaccination in preventing disease and helping to secure food security. Targeted vaccination interventions, such as for rabies in Africa or FMD in Asia, have proven that reducing the incidence of disease and improving the productivity of livestock, as well as reducing the risk of transmission to humans, in zoonotic disease response can be achieved through targeted vaccination strategies [32]. But this effort must be taken to other diseases and areas and directed by those of disease that threatens smallholder farmers in developing countries. Future interventions will need to focus on the development of affordable and easily deployable vaccines and improving supply chains to assure equitable access to vaccinations in resource-poor settings.

There is another valuable lesson to learn from this is the need for a system-based approach to livestock farming that will consider the health, productivity, and environmental aspects together. We have seen agroecological practices, such as rotational grazing, agroforestry, and Integrated Pest Management delivering improvements in soil health, and biodiversity and reducing the carbon footprint of livestock; nevertheless, adoption of these practices is generally limited in industrial farming systems. To solve this, future interventions need to target providing farmers with financial and technical support to move to more environmentally sustainable practices, and policies and promote environmentally friendly farming practices. Third, one of the most important recommendations for future interventions is the important need promoted by collaboration between researchers, policymakers, and farmers. No single stakeholder can address the complex challenges to food security, animal health, and sustainability. Both solutions are going to require multidisciplinary collaboration among veterinarians, agricultural scientists, environmentalists, policymakers, and the farmers themselves to make them both effective and equitable.

5.9 Conclusion

There is a need for a research agenda that considers vigorous capacity-building measures for veterinary professionals in developing countries and that would ensure sustainable progress of sustainable agriculture now and in the context of global food security. This occurs when veterinarians are presented with education programs, practical training, and additional education opportunities, which will enable them to manage animal health issues in line with current best practices that function for optimal disease risk prevention and mitigation and improvement of relevel agricultural return. For instance, they do not only achieve healthcare; they foster creativity, resilience, and social harmony among rural farm workers. The odds that the veterinary profession, both broadly and overseas, will relieve equitable development by boosting the broader adoption of best husbandry practices; enhancing general livestock welfare; and securing future resilience in the line of natural or financial harm are substantial. Such continued investment examinations and collaboration will be essential; to both hoped-for vital, inclusive healthcare system and to ensure that animal breeding is possible well into the next generation.

References

1 Spencer, T.E., Wells, K.D., Lee, K., et al. Future of biomedical, agricultural, and biological systems research using domesticated animals. *Biol. Reprod.* 2022; 106: 629–638. https://doi.org/10.1093/biolre/ioac019.

2 Ashraf, A and Imran, M. Causes, types, etiological agents, prevalence, diagnosis, treatment, prevention, effects on human health and future aspects of bovine mastitis. *Anim. Health Res. Rev.* 2020; 21: 36–49. https://doi.org/10.1017/S1466252319000094.

3 Delgado, C.L. and Siamwalla, A. Rural economy and farm income diversification in developing countries. In: *Food Security, Diversification and Resource Management: Refocusing the Role of Agriculture*? 126–143: Routledge; 2018.

4 Garcia, S.N, Osburn, B.I., and Jay-Russell, M.T. One Health for food safety, food security, and sustainable food production. *Front. Sustain. Food Syst.* 2020; 4: 1. https://doi.org/10.3389/fsufs.2020.00001.

5 Rose, D.C, Sutherland, W.J., Barnes, A.P., et al. Integrated farm management for sustainable agriculture: lessons for knowledge exchange and policy. *Land Use Policy* 2019; 81: 834–842. https://doi.org/10.1016/j.landusepol.2018.11.001.

6 Benjamin, M. and Yik, S. Precision livestock farming in swine welfare: a review for swine practitioners. *Animals* 2019; 9: 133. https://doi.org/10.3390/ani9040133.

7 Espinosa, R., Tago, D., and Treich, N. Infectious diseases and meat production. *Environ. Resour. Econ.* 2020; 76: 1019–1044. https://doi.org/10.1007/s10640-020-00484-3.

8 Sánchez-Vizcaíno. J.M., Laddomada, A., and Arias, M.L. African swine fever virus. *Dis. Swine*. 2019: 443–452. https://doi.org/10.1002/9781119350927.ch25.

9 Abubakar, M., Syed, Z., Manzoor, S., and Arshed, M.J. Deciphering molecular dynamics of foot and mouth disease virus (FMDV): a looming threat to Pakistan's dairy industry. *Dairy*. 2022; 3: 123–136. https://doi.org/10.3390/dairy3010010.

10 Rehman, S., Effendi, M.H., Witaningruma, A.M., et al. Avian influenza (H5N1) virus, epidemiology and its effects on backyard poultry in Indonesia: a review. *F1000Res.* 2023; 11: 1321. https://doi.org/10.12688/f1000research.125878.2.

11 Brown, V.R., Miller, R.S., McKee, S.C., et al. Risks of introduction and economic consequences associated with African swine fever, classical swine fever and foot-and-mouth disease: a review of the literature. *Transbound. Emerg. Dis.* 2021: 68: 1910–1965. https://doi.org/10.1111/tbed.13919.

12 De Menezes, T.C., Countryman, A.M., Hagerman, A.D., and Galvão de Miranda, S.H. Economy-wide effects of bovine spongiform encephalopathy in Brazil. *J. Agric. Resour. Econ.* 2024; 49: 489–513. https://doi.org/10.22004/ag.econ.342181.

13 Fathelrahman, E.M., Reeves, A., Mohamed, M.S., et al. Epidemiology and cost of peste des petits ruminants (Ppr) eradication in small ruminants in the United Arab Emirates—disease spread and control strategies simulations. *Animals* 2021; 11: 2649. https://doi.org/10.3390/ani11092649.

14 O'Neill, L., Gubbins, S., Reynolds, C., et al. The socioeconomic impacts of Rift Valley fever: a rapid review. *PLoS Negl. Trop. Dis.* 2024; 18: e0012347. https://doi.org/10.1371/journal.pntd.0012347.

15 Amoia, C.F.A.N.G., Nnadi, P.A., Ezema, C., and Couacy-Hymann, E. Epidemiology of Newcastle disease in Africa with emphasis on Côte d'Ivoire: a review. *Vet. World.* 2021; 14: 1727. https://doi.org/10.14202/vetworld.2021.1727–1740.

16 Dubey, S., Brahmbhatt, M., Nayak, J., et al. Brucellosis and its public health significance in India: a review. *LSD Virus* 2022; 20: 24–30.

17 Gelaye, A. and Fesseha, H. Bovine trypanosomiasis in Ethiopia: epidemiology, diagnosis and its economic impact—a review. *Open Access J. Biogeneric Sci. Res.* 2020; 2: 1–10. https://doi.org/10.46718/JBGSR.2020.02.000059.

18 Hameed, T., Tareen, M.A., Younus, M., et al. Assessing the impact of subclinical mastitis on dairy cattle in Balochistan. *Pak-Euro. J. Med. Life Sci.* 2022; 5: 589–596. https://doi.org/https://doi.org/10.31580/pjmls.v4i2.1433.

19 Doeschl-Wilson, A., Knap, P., Opriessnig, T., and More, S.J. Livestock disease resilience: from individual to herd level. *Animal* 2021; 15: 100286. https://doi.org/10.1016/j.animal.2021.100286.

20 Xu, X., Sharma, P., Shu, S., et al. Global greenhouse gas emissions from animal-based foods are twice those of plant-based foods. *Nat. Food.* 2021; 2: 724–732. https://doi.org/10.1038/s43016-021-00358-x.

21 Charlier, J., Barkema, H.W., Becher, P., et al. Disease control tools to secure animal and public health in a densely populated world. *Lancet Planet. Health.* 2022; 6: e812–e824. https://doi.org/10.1016/S2542-5196(22)00147-4.

22 Francis, M.J. Recent advances in vaccine technologies. *Vet. Clin: Small Anim. Pract.* 2018; 48: 231–241. https://doi.org/10.1016/j.cvsm.2017.10.002.

23 García, R., Aguilar, J., Toro, M., et al. A systematic literature review on the use of machine learning in precision livestock farming. *Comput. Electron. Agric.* 2020; 179: 105826. https://doi.org/10.1016/j.compag.2020.105826.

24 Kampan, K., Tsusaka, T.W., and Anal, A.K. Adoption of blockchain technology for enhanced traceability of livestock-based products. *Sustainability* 2022; 14: 13148. https://doi.org/10.3390/su142013148.

25 Akhigbe, B.I., Munir, K., Akinade, O., et al. IoT technologies for livestock management: a review of present status, opportunities, and future trends. *Big Data Cogn. Comput.* 2021; 5: 10. https://doi.org/10.3390/bdcc5010010.

26 Kumar, H.C., Hiremath, J., Yogisharadhya, R., et al. Animal disease surveillance: its importance & present status in India. *Indian J. Med. Res.* 2021; 153: 299–310. https://doi.org/10.4103/ijmr.IJMR_740_21.

27 Islam, M.A., Rony, S.A., Rahman, M.B., et al. Improvement of disease resistance in livestock: application of immunogenomics and CRISPR/Cas9 technology. *Animals* 2020; 10: 2236. https://doi.org/10.3390/ani10122236.

28 Malachowski, T. and Hassel, A. Engineering nanoparticles to overcome immunological barriers for enhanced drug delivery. *Eng. Regen.* 2020; 1: 35–50. https://doi.org/10.1016/j.engreg.2020.06.001.

29 Yuferev, L., Sokolov, A., and Mironyuk, S.S. UV-based indoor disinfecting system. In: *Advanced Agro-Engineering Technologies for Rural Business Development*, 65–95. IGI Global; 2019. https://doi.org/10.4018/978-1-5225-7573-3.ch003.

30 Chu, H., Liu, C., Liu, J., et al. Recent advances and challenges of biosensing in point-of-care molecular diagnosis. *Sens. Actuators B: Chem.* 2021; 348: 130708. doi: 10.1016/j.snb.2021.130708.

31 Schillings, J., Bennett, R., and Rose, D.C. Exploring the potential of precision livestock farming technologies to help address farm animal welfare. *Front. Anim. Sci.* 2021; 2: 639678. https://doi.org/10.3389/fanim.2021.639678.

32 Sander, V.A., Sánchez López, E.F., Mendoza Morales, L., et al. Use of veterinary vaccines for livestock as a strategy to control foodborne parasitic diseases. *Front. Cell. Infect. Microbiol.* 2020; 10: 288. https://doi.org/10.3389/fcimb.2020.00288.

33 Sinha, P., Singh, V.K., Bohra, A., et al. Genomics and breeding innovations for enhancing genetic gain for climate resilience and nutrition traits. *Theor. Appl. Genet.* 2021; 134: 1829–1843. https://doi.org/10.1007/s00122-021-03847-6.

34 Wang, S., Qu, Z., Huang, Q., et al. Application of gene editing technology in resistance breeding of livestock. *Life* 2022; 12: 1070. https://doi.org/10.3390/life12071070.

35 AlZubi, A.A. Artificial intelligence and its application in the prediction and diagnosis of animal diseases: a review. *Indian J. Anim. Res.* 2023; 57. https://doi.org/10.18805/IJAR.BF-1684.

36 Bauskar, S.R, Madhavaram, C.R., Galla, E., et al. Predicting disease outbreaks using AI and big data: a new frontier in healthcare analytics. *Eur. Chem. Bull.* 2022; 11(12). https://doi.org/10.53555/ecb.v11:i12.17745.

37 Garcia, S.N., Osburn, B.I., and Cullor, J.S. A one health perspective on dairy production and dairy food safety. *One Health.* 2019: 7: 100086. https://doi.org/10.1016/j.onehlt.2019.100086.

38 Marchant-Forde, J.N. and Boyle, L.A. COVID-19 effects on livestock production: a one welfare issue. *Front. Vet. Sci.* 2020; 7: 585787. https://doi.org/10.3389/fvets.2020.585787.

39 Mugadza, A.A. The disastrous effects of deforestation and forest degradation in the climate vulnerability era. *CIFILE J. Int. Law.* 2022; 3: 12–40. https://doi.org/10.30489/cifj.2022.324393.1049.

40 Dineshbabu, G., Goswami, G., Kumar, R., et al. Microalgae–nutritious, sustainable aqua-and animal feed source. *J. Funct. Foods.* 2019; 62: 103545. https://doi.org/10.1016/j.jff.2019.103545.

41 Kępińska-Pacelik. J. and Biel, W. Mycotoxins—prevention, detection, impact on animal health. *Processes* 2021; 9: 2035. https://doi.org/10.3390/pr9112035.

42 Javed, A., King, A.J., Imran, M., et al. Omega-3 supplementation for enhancement of egg functional properties. *J. Food Process. Preserv.* 2019; 43: e14052. https://doi.org/10.1111/jfpp.14052.

43 González, L., Kyriazakis, I., and Tedeschi, L. Precision nutrition of ruminants: approaches, challenges and potential gains. *Animal* 2018; 12: s246–s261. https://doi.org/10.1017/S1751731118002288.

44 Føre, M., Frank, K., Norton, T., et al. Precision fish farming: a new framework to improve production in aquaculture. *Biosyst. Eng.* 2018; 173: 176–193. https://doi.org/10.1016/j.biosystemseng.2017.10.014.

45 Boyko, T., Chaunina, E., Buzmakova, N., and Zharikova, E., Biologically active additives for cows as a factor in the production of environmentally friendly products in animal husbandry. In: *IOP Conference Series: Earth and Environmental Science*, 012063; 2021. https://doi.org/10.1088/1755-1315/624/1/012063.

46 Pearlin, B.V., Muthuvel, S., Govidasamy, P., et al. Role of acidifiers in livestock nutrition and health: a review. *J. Anim. Physiol. Anim. Nutr.* 2020; 104: 558–569. https://doi.org/10.1111/jpn.13282.

47 Halachmi, I., Guarino, M., Bewley, J., and Pastell, M. Smart animal agriculture: application of real-time sensors to improve animal well-being and production. *Annu. Rev. Anim. Biosci.* 2019; 7: 403–425. https://doi.org/10.1146/annurev-animal-020518-114851.

48 Balehegn, M., Duncan, A., Tolera, A., et al. Improving adoption of technologies and interventions for increasing supply of quality livestock feed in low- and middle-income countries. *Glob. Food Sec.* 2020; 26: 100372. https://doi.org/10.1016/j.gfs.2020.100372.

49 Shah, K.K., Modi, B., Pandey, H.P., et al. Diversified crop rotation: an approach for sustainable agriculture production. *Adv. Agric.* 2021; 2021: 8924087. https://doi.org/10.1155/2021/8924087.

50 Soussi, A., Zero, E., Sacile, R., et al. Smart sensors and smart data for precision agriculture: a review. *Sensors* 2024; 24: 2647. https://doi.org/10.3390/s24082647.

51 Liermann, W., Bochnia, M., Berk, A., et al. Effects of feed particle size and hydro-thermal processing methods on starch modification, nutrient digestibility and the performance and the gastrointestinal tract of broilers. *Animals* 2019; 9: 294. https://doi.org/10.3390/ani9060294.

52 Scollo, A., Perrucci, A., Stella, M.C., et al. Biosecurity and hygiene procedures in pig farms: effects of a tailor-made approach as monitored by environmental samples. *Animals* 2023; 13: 1262. https://doi.org/10.3390/ani13071262.

53 Smith, D.R. Herd immunity. *Vet. Clin. Food Anim. Pract.* 2019; 35: 593–604. https://doi.org/10.1016/j.cvfa.2019.07.001.

54 McCarthy, M., O'Grady, L., McAloon, C., and Mee, J.F. A survey of biosecurity and health management practices on Irish dairy farms engaged in contract-rearing. *J. Dairy Sci.* 2021; 104: 12859–12870. https://doi.org/10.3168/jds.2021-20500.

55 Collett, S.R., Smith, J.A., Boulianne, M., et al. Principles of disease prevention, diagnosis, and control. *Dis. Poul.* 2020: 1–78. https://doi.org/10.1002/9781119371199.ch1.

56 Bordier, M., Uea-Anuwong, T., Binot, A., et al. Characteristics of One Health surveillance systems: a systematic literature review. *Prev. Vet. Med.* 2020; 181: 104560. https://doi.org/10.1016/j.prevetmed.2018.10.005.

57 Delpont, M., Salazar, L.G., Dewulf, J., et al. Monitoring biosecurity in poultry production: an overview of databases reporting biosecurity compliance from seven European countries. *Front. Vet. Sci.* 2023; 10: 1231377. https://doi.org/10.3389/fvets.2023.1231377.

58 Souillard, R., Allain, V., Dufay-Lefort, A.C., et al. Biosecurity implementation on large-scale poultry farms in Europe: a qualitative interview study with farmers. *Prev. Vet. Med.* 2024; 224: 106119. https://doi.org/10.1016/j.prevetmed.2024.106119.

59 Oyuchua, M., Siengsanan-Lamont, J., Le, K.K., et al. The importance and challenges of implementing and maintaining biorepositories for high-consequence veterinary and One Health pathogens in South-East Asia. *Appl. Biosaf.* 2024; 29: 35–44. https://doi.org/10.1089/apb.2023.0006.

60 Da Silva, R.A., Arenas, N.E., Luiza, V.L., et al. Regulations on the use of antibiotics in livestock production in South America: a comparative literature analysis. *Antibiotics* 2023; 12: 1303. https://doi.org/10.3390/antibiotics12081303.

61 AL-Eitan, L.N., Ali, H.O., Kharmah, H.S.A., et al. Addressing poxvirus challenges in the middle east to enhance biosafety and biosecurity measures. *J. Biosaf. Biosecur.* 2024; 6: 142–156. https://doi.org/10.1016/j.jobb.2024.06.003.

62 Thamali, K. and Jayawardana, N. The current status of national biosafety regulatory systems in South Asia. *Environ. Susten. Food Safety: Need Vibrant Policy Init. Sri Lanka*. 2022 198: 198.

63 Ulziibat, G., Raizman, E., Lkhagvasuren, A., et al. Comparison of vaccination schedules for foot-and-mouth disease among cattle and sheep in Mongolia. *Front. Vet. Sci.* 2023; 10: 990043. https://doi.org/10.3389/fvets.2023.990043.

64 Zinsstag, J., Crump, L., Schelling, E., et al. Climate change and One Health. *FEMS Microbiol. Lett.* 2018; 365: fny085. https://doi.org/10.1093/femsle/fny085.

65 Chauhan, S.S., Rashamol, V., Bagath, M., et al. Impacts of heat stress on immune responses and oxidative stress in farm animals and nutritional strategies for amelioration. *Int. J. Biometeorol.* 2021: 65: 1231–1244. https://doi.org/10.1007/s00484-021-02083-3.

66 Fenger, F., Casey, I., Holden, N., and Humphreys, J. Access time to pasture under wet soil conditions: effects on productivity and profitability of pasture-based dairying. *J. D. Sci.* 2022; 105: 4189–4205. https://doi.org/10.3168/jds.2021-20752.

67 Godde, C., Dizyee, K., Ash, A., et al. Climate change and variability impacts on grazing herds: insights from a system dynamics approach for semi-arid Australian rangelands. *Glob. Chang. Biol.* 2019; 25: 3091–3109. https://doi.org/10.1111/gcb.14669.

68 Voulvoulis, N. Water reuse from a circular economy perspective and potential risks from an unregulated approach. *Curr. Opin. Environ. Sci. Health.* 2018; 2: 32–45. https://doi.org/10.1016/j.coesh.2018.01.005.

69 Hristov, A., Degaetano, A., Rotz, C., et al. Climate change effects on livestock in the Northeast US and strategies for adaptation. *Clim. Change* 2018; 146: 33–45. https://doi.org/10.1007/s10584-017-2023-z.

70 Alemu, A.W., Kröbel, R., McConkey, B.G., and Iwaasa, A.D. Effect of increasing species diversity and grazing management on pasture productivity, animal performance, and soil carbon sequestration of re-established pasture in Canadian Prairie. *Animals* 2019; 9: 127. https://doi.org/10.3390/ani9040127.

71 Tongwane, M.I. and Moeletsi, M.E. Provincial cattle carbon emissions from enteric fermentation and manure management in South Africa. *Environ. Res.* 2021; 195: 110833. https://doi.org/10.1016/j.envres.2021.110833.

72 Yu, G., Beauchemin, K.A., and Dong, R. A review of 3-nitrooxypropanol for enteric methane mitigation from ruminant livestock. *Animals* 2021; 11: 3540. https://doi.org/10.3390/ani11123540.

73 O'Brien, P.L. and Hatfield, J.L. Dairy manure and synthetic fertilizer: a meta-analysis of crop production and environmental quality. *Agrosyst. Geosci. Environ.* 2019; 2: 1–12. https://doi.org/10.2134/age2019.04.0027.

74 Monteiro, A., Santos, S., and Gonçalves, P. Precision agriculture for crop and livestock farming—brief review. *Animals* 2021; 11: 2345. https://doi.org/10.3390/ani11082345.

75 Nieuwland, J. and Meijboom, F.L. One Health: how interdependence enriches veterinary ethics education. *Animals* 2019; 10: 13. https://doi.org/10.3390/ani10010013.

76 Verma, S., Malik, Y.S., Singh, G., et al. *Core Competencies of a Veterinary Graduate.* Springer; 2024. https://doi.org/10.1007/978-981-97-0433-0.

77 Osumba, J.J., Recha, J.W., and Oroma, G.W. Transforming agricultural extension service delivery through innovative bottom–up climate-resilient agribusiness farmer field schools. *Sustainability* 2021; 13: 3938. https://doi.org/10.3390/su13073938.

78 Cooreman, H., Vandenabeele, J., Debruyne, L., et al. A conceptual framework to investigate the role of peer learning processes at on-farm demonstrations in the light of sustainable agriculture. *Int. J. Agric. Extension* 2018; 6: 91–103.

79 Norton, G.W. and Alwang, J. Changes in agricultural extension and implications for farmer adoption of new practices. *Appl. Econ. Perspect. Policy.* 2020; 42: 8–20. https://doi.org/10.1002/aepp.13008.

80 Wilkes, M.S., Conrad, P.A., and Winer, J.N. One health–One Education: medical and veterinary inter-professional training. *J. Vet. Med. Educ.* 2019; 46: 14–20. https://doi.org/10.3138/jvme.1116-171r.

81 Opoola, O., Mrode, R., Banos, G., et al. Current situations of animal data recording, dairy improvement infrastructure, human capacity and strategic issues affecting dairy production in sub-Saharan Africa. *Trop. Anim. Health Prod.* 2019; 51: 1699–1705. https://doi.org/10.1007/s11250-019-01871-9.

82 Yadav, M.P., Singh, R.K., and Malik, Y.S. Emerging and transboundary animal viral diseases: perspectives and preparedness. *Emerg. Transbound. Anim. Vir.* 2020; 1–25. https://doi.org/10.1007/978-981-15-0402-0_1.

83 White, A. and Hughes, J.M. Critical importance of a one health approach to antimicrobial resistance. *EcoHealth.* 2019: 16: 404–409. https://doi.org/10.1007/s10393-019-01415-5.

84 Subasinghe, R., Alday-Sanz, V., Bondad-Reantaso, M.G., et al. Biosecurity: reducing the burden of disease. *J. World Aquacult. Soc.* 2023; 54: 397–426. https://doi.org/10.1111/jwas.12966.

85 Matić, Z. and Šantak, M. Current view on novel vaccine technologies to combat human infectious diseases. *Appl. Microbiol. Biotechnol.* 2022; 106: 25–56. https://doi.org/10.1007/s00253-021-11713-0.

86 Cheruiyot, E.K., Haile-Mariam, M., Cocks, B.G., and Pryce, J.E. Improving genomic selection for heat tolerance in dairy cattle: current opportunities and future directions. *Front. Genet.* 2022; 13: 894067. https://doi.org/10.3389/fgene.2022.894067.

87 Guo, W., Lv, C., Guo, M., et al. Innovative applications of artificial intelligence in zoonotic disease management. *Sci. One Health* 2023; 100045. https://doi.org/10.1016/j.soh.2023.100045.

88 Roth, J.A. and Galyon, J. Food security: the ultimate one-health challenge. *One Health* 2024; 100864. https://doi.org/10.1016/j.onehlt.2024.100864.

89 Pal, A. and Chakravarty, A. Disease resistance for different livestock species. *Genet. Breed. Dis. Res. Livest.* 2019: 271. https://doi.org/10.1016/B978-0-12-816406-8.00019-X.

90 Riudavets, J., Moerman, E., and Vila, E. Implementation of integrated pest and disease management in greenhouses: from research to the consumer. In: *Integrated Pest and Disease Management in Greenhouse Crops* (ed. M. Gullino, R. Albajes, and P. Nicot), 457–485. Springer Nature; 2020. https://doi.org/10.1007/978-3-030-22304-5_16.

91 Papakonstantinou, G.I., Voulgarakis, N., Terzidou, G., et al. Precision livestock farming technology: applications and challenges of animal welfare and climate change. *Agriculture* 2024; 14: 620. https://doi.org/10.3390/agriculture14040620.

92 Zhang, L., Guo, W., and Lv, C. Modern technologies and solutions to enhance surveillance and response systems for emerging zoonotic diseases. *Sci. One Health* 2024; 3: 100061. https://doi.org/10.1016/j.soh.2023.100061.

93 Fatima, N., Emambux, M.N., Olaimat, A.N., et al. Recent advances in microalgae, insects, and cultured meat as sustainable alternative protein sources. *Food Hum.* 2023; https://doi.org/10.1016/j.foohum.2023.07.009.

6

Global Zoonotic Diseases and Public Health: A One Health Perspective

Delower Hossain[1,2], Shamsaldeen Ibrahim Saeed[3,4], Daniel Jesuwenu Ajose[5], Chidozie Freedom Egbu[6,7], Ridwan Olamilekan Adesola[8], Oluwaseun Adeolu Ogundijo[9], Olamilekan Gabriel Banwo[8], Fernando Ulloa[10], and Sabiha Zarin Tasnim Bristi[2]*

[1] *Department of Medicine and Public Health, Faculty of Animal Science and Veterinary Medicine, Sher-e-Bangla Agricultural University (SAU), Dhaka, Bangladesh*
[2] *Department of Veterinary Medicine and Animal Sciences (DIVAS), Università degli Studi di Milano (UNIMI), Lodi, Italy*
[3] *Nanotechnology in Veterinary Medicine Research Group, Faculty of Veterinary Medicine, Universiti Malaysia Kelantan (UMK), Pengkalan Chepa, Kelantan, Malaysia*
[4] *Department of Microbiology, Faculty of Veterinary Science, University of Nyala, Sudan*
[5] *Department of Microbiology, School of Biological Sciences, Faculty of Natural and Agricultural Sciences, North-West University, Mmabatho, South Africa*
[6] *Department of Agriculture and Animal Health, College of Agriculture and Environmental Sciences, University of South Africa, Roodepoort, South Africa*
[7] *Department of Agricultural Science Education, Faculty of Vocational and Technology, Alvan Ikoku Federal University of Education, Owerri, Imo State, Nigeria*
[8] *Department of Veterinary Medicine, Faculty of Veterinary Medicine, University of Ibadan, Ibadan, Nigeria*
[9] *Department of Veterinary Public Health and Preventive Medicine, University of Ibadan, Ibadan, Nigeria*
[10] *Escuela de Graduados, Facultad de Ciencias Veterinarias, Universidad Austral de Chile, Valdivia, Chile*

*Corresponding author: delowervet@sau.edu.bd, delower.hossain@unimi.it

TABLE OF CONTENTS

6.1 Introduction
6.2 Emerging Trends in Global Zoonotic Diseases
6.2.1 Distribution of Zoonotic Diseases Globally
6.2.2 Factors Driving the Emergence and Spread of Zoonotic Diseases
6.2.3 Epidemiology of Emerging and Re-emerging Zoonotic Diseases (December 2019–January 2025)
6.2.3.1 Highly Pathogenic Avian Influenza
6.2.3.2 Coronavirus Disease 2019
6.2.3.3 Dengue Fever
6.2.3.4 Monkeypox
6.2.3.5 Chikungunya Virus Disease
6.2.3.6 Salmonellosis
6.2.3.7 Human Metapneumovirus Infection
6.2.4 Challenges in Predicting and Controlling Zoonoses
6.2.5 Economic and Societal Effects of Zoonotic Disease Outbreaks
6.3 One Health Strategies for Disease Surveillance and Prevention
6.3.1 Principles of the One Health Approach
6.3.2 Interconnectivity of the One Health Component Parts
6.3.3 Multidisciplinary Approaches to Disease Surveillance and Prevention
6.3.4 Integrated Surveillance Systems for Rapid Diagnosis and Swift Action of Zoonoses

One Health Integration: Global Perspectives on Animal Health and Sustainable Agriculture. First Edition.
Edited by Pratik Subhash Gaikwad, Vivek Harishankar Shukla and Pintu Choudhary.

Companion Website: https://www.wiley.com/go/pratikgaikwad/onehealth

6.4 Collaborative Approaches in Pandemic Preparedness
6.4.1 Understanding the Risk of Zoonotic Disease Pandemics
6.4.2 International Frameworks for Pandemic Preparedness and Response
6.4.3 Importance of Multisectoral Collaboration in Pandemic Response
6.4.4 Role of Interdisciplinary Collaboration in Pandemic Preparedness
6.4.5 Vaccine Development and Distribution
6.4.6 Public Awareness and Community Engagement Initiatives
6.5 Social and Ecological Dimensions of Zoonotic Diseases
6.5.1 Impact of Socio-economic Factors on Zoonotic Disease Transmission
6.5.2 Role of Environmental Factors in Zoonotic Disease Emergence and Spread
6.5.2.1 Extreme Weather Conditions
6.5.3 Role of Cultural Practices and Behavior Changes in Zoonotic Disease Emergence and Spread
6.5.3.1 Increased Farming of Wildlife
6.5.3.2 Livestock Farming and Pet Ownership
6.5.3.3 Live Animal Market Practices (Wet Markets)
6.5.3.4 Globalization, Industry, and Technology
6.5.4 Importance of Sustainable Land Use and Wildlife Conservation in Disease Prevention
6.6 Case Studies and Examples of Global Zoonoses Control and OH Integration
6.6.1 Successful One Health Interventions
6.6.1.1 Rabies Control in Latin America
6.6.1.2 The Hendra Virus in Australia
6.6.1.3 Avian Influenza Control in Southeast Asia
6.6.1.4 Rift Valley Fever in Kenya
6.6.1.5 Ebola Virus Disease in West Africa
6.6.2 Lessons Learned from Previous Zoonotic Outbreaks
6.6.2.1 Ebola
6.6.2.2 COVID-19
6.6.2.3 Avian Influenza (H5N1)
6.6.2.4 Dengue Fever
6.6.2.5 Chikungunya Virus Disease
6.6.2.6 Severe Acute Respiratory Syndrome
6.6.2.7 Middle East Respiratory Syndrome
6.6.2.8 Monkeypox
6.6.2.9 Swine Flu (H1N1)
6.7 Challenges and Opportunities
6.7.1 Barriers to Implementing One Health
6.7.2 Strategies for Overcoming Challenges
6.7.2.1 Exemplary Governance and Leadership
6.7.2.2 Good Teamwork and Coordination
6.7.2.3 Training and Capacity Building
6.7.2.4 Robust Collaborations and Cooperative Efforts
6.7.2.5 Strengthening of Diagnosing Skills and Surveillance Capabilities
6.7.2.6 Financial Assistance
6.8 Conclusion
Abbreviations
Author Contributions
Conflicts of Interest
References

6.1 Introduction

The World Health Organization (WHO) defines zoonosis as the transmission of infectious diseases that occur naturally between humans and animals or between animals and other vertebrate animals [1]. More than 60% of human diseases have zoonotic origins [2]. Numerous microorganisms, including bacteria, viruses, fungi, protozoa, and parasites, have been implicated as causative agents of many zoonotic diseases [3]. The occurrence, recurrence, spread, and patterns of zoonoses have been significantly impacted by several factors, including anthropogenic influences, urbanization, animal and human migration (travel and tourism), the nature of the vector, and changing climates [3].

Zoonoses affect both human and animal health in a variety of ways. Over 75% of emerging and new human illnesses are zoonotic and connected to domestic and wild animals [4]. Despite being difficult to measure, the effects of zoonoses can be evaluated using metrics such as disease incidence, morbidity, death, and economic loss [3]. The livestock sector in any nation might suffer enormous financial losses due to animal mortality caused by zoonotic diseases. Without death, these diseases can impact animal productivity and health. This leads to decreased availability of high-protein animal products such as milk, meat, and eggs, affecting human nutrition and health [5].

The recent coronavirus disease 19 (COVID-19) pandemic has dramatically harmed the world economy. Every area of society has been incredibly affected by COVID-19, including the financial, travel, hospitality, sports, health, and education sectors [6]. According to the World Bank, millions of people are predicted to live in extreme poverty because the pandemic has slowed economic growth [7]. Other zoonotic outbreaks have been recorded after the incidence of COVID-19, such as Monkeypox (Mpox), Zika, Usutu, Marburg disease, salmonellosis, rabies, arboviral diseases, avian influenza (H5N1), and anthrax [6, 8–14]. In an era of unprecedented global connectivity and rapid change, a collaborative multidisciplinary effort is needed to address this complex health problem.

The One Health (OH) approach, which integrates human, animal, and environmental health information, has been widely adopted globally in the last decade and has shown substantial benefits that are widely acknowledged [15]. The Food and Agricultural Organization (FAO), the World Organization for Animal Health (WOAH) (formerly Office International des Epizooties, OIE), and the WHO tripartite (FAO-OIE-WHO) exemplify OH collaboration to enhance human, animal, and environmental health synergies and strengthen global health security through concerted international efforts [16]. This multidisciplinary collaboration leverages the unique skills and resources of each group to improve human, animal, and environmental health using the "OH approach."

Additionally, the adoption of the OH concept will enable the formulation of disease prevention and control programs for humans as well as animals with the engagement of many stakeholders. Similarly, the OH concept will contribute to advances in knowledge and discovery and optimize the efficiency of clinical care, public health (PH), and medical education programs as well as disease management programs for both humans and animals [17]. This chapter aims to discuss many political features of modern zoonotic research, guidelines, initiatives, and best practices in different countries associated with OH structures and demanding situations.

6.2 Emerging Trends in Global Zoonotic Diseases

Emerging patterns in zoonotic diseases around the world underscore the increasing frequency and complexity of these diseases, driven by various factors. It also emphasizes the pressing necessity for integrated surveillance and control techniques, along with the challenges and socioeconomic impacts of zoonotic disease epidemics.

6.2.1 Distribution of Zoonotic Diseases Globally

Emerging zoonotic diseases pose a significant challenge to PH, animal health, welfare, and food security. It can cause substantial economic impacts due to increased mortality, cost of treatment and control, reduced productivity, loss in trade, and decreased gross domestic product (GDP) [18]. Currently, over 60% of pathogens known to affect humans are zoonotic, and the majority of these (71.8%) originate in wildlife (e.g. severe acute respiratory syndrome [SARS], coronavirus disease, and Ebola virus). These pathogens are rising at an alarming rate [19] and can be transmitted to humans through direct or indirect contact [20]. Several pathogens, including bacteria, viruses, fungi, protozoa, parasites, and other pathogens, can cause zoonotic diseases [3] such as anthrax, brucellosis, leptospirosis, tuberculosis, salmonellosis, plague, rabies, SARS, Ebola, human immunodeficiency virus (HIV), avian influenza, toxoplasmosis, giardiasis, trypanosomiasis, leishmaniasis, and ringworms [3]. In the past 10 years, the precise cost of zoonotic diseases has been calculated to exceed $20 billion, with additional losses of approximately $200 billion to the economies that have been impacted [21]. Table 6.1 shows the distribution and transmission of major zoonotic diseases globally.

6.2.2 Factors Driving the Emergence and Spread of Zoonotic Diseases

The emergence, re-emergence, and distribution of zoonotic diseases are believed to be driven primarily by several factors, including climate change, urbanization, animal migration and trade, travel and tourism, vector biology, anthropogenic factors, and natural factors [50]. Recent zoonotic disease spillover to humans, such as Zika and Ebola, has been discovered primarily in and around areas where forests have been cleared. Deforestation damages the environment, making it unsuitable for human habitation, where Zika, Ebola, and Mpox have emerged as new

Table 6.1 Distribution and transmission of major zoonotic diseases.

Disease	Distribution	Agents	Transmission	References
VIRUSES				
COVID-19	Worldwide	Coronavirus 2 (severe acute respiratory syndrome coronavirus 2, SARS-CoV-2)	Respiratory droplets	[22]
Avian influenza	Worldwide	Influenza type-A viruses	Direct contact with or consuming contaminated animals' product	[23]
Ebola	Africa	Ebola viruses	Contact with infected blood and bodily fluids	[24]
Rabies	Worldwide	Rabies virus	Bites from infected dogs	[25]
Dengue fever (DF)	Worldwide	Dengue virus (DENV)	Mosquitoes	[26]
Marburg	Africa	Marburg virus	Direct contact	
West Nile fever (WNF)	Worldwide	Flavivirus	Mosquitoes	[27]
Rift Valley fever (RVF)	African and Middle East	Phlebovirus	Mosquitoes	[28]
Crimean-Congo hemorrhagic fever	Southeast Asia, Africa, Middle East, and Mediterranean European Countries	Arbovirus	Direct contact with affected animals or bites from infected ticks	[29]
Zika fever	Latin America, Southeast Asia, part of Africa	Flavivirus	Mosquitoes	[30]
Nipah virus infection	Southeast Asia	Henipavirus	Direct contact with infected animals	[31]
Chikungunya virus disease (CHIKVD)	Worldwide	Alphavirus	Transmitted by mosquitoes (*Aedes* spp.)	[32]
Monkeypox (Mpox)	Africa	Monkeypox virus (MPXV)	Body fluids or skin lesions of infected animals/humans	[33]

Disease	Distribution	Agents	Transmission	References
Human metapneumovirus (hMPV) infection	China, India, Bangladesh, USA, UK, Australia, Malaysia, Kazakhstan, Philippines	Human metapneumovirus (hMPV)	Respiratory droplets that spread through the air from a sick person to others or contact with contaminated surfaces	[34, 35]
BACTERIA				
Q fever	Worldwide	*Coxiella burnetii*	Inhalation	[36]
Brucellosis	Worldwide	*Brucella abortus Brucella melitensis, Brucella suis, Brucella canis*	Contact with infected body fluid and consuming unpasteurized milk from infected animals	
Campylobacteriosis	Worldwide	*Campylobacter* spp.	Contact with diseased animals and consuming contaminated meat, eggs, and milk	[37]
Bovine tuberculosis	Worldwide	*Mycobacterium bovis*	Aerosol or unpasteurized milk consumption of infected animals	[38]
Leptospirosis	Worldwide	*Leptospira interrogans*	Urine from carrier animals	[39]
Anthrax	Worldwide	*Bacillus anthracis*	Direct exposure to environmental or bioterrorist-released spores, contaminated animal products, or infected or dead animals	[39]
Salmonellosis	Worldwide	*Salmonella enterica, Salmonella bongor*	Ingestion of feces-contaminated food or water	[40]
Rickettsiosis	Worldwide	*Rickettsia* spp.	Ticks	[41]
PROTOZOA				
Leishmaniasis	Worldwide	*Leishmania infantum*	Transmitted by sand fly	[42]
Toxoplasmosis	Worldwide	*Toxoplasma gondii*	Exposure to infected animals or contaminated food or water	[43]
Cryptosporidiosis	Worldwide	*Cryptosporidium parvum*	Exposure to infected animals or contaminated food or water	[44]
Trypanosomiasis	Worldwide	*Trypanosoma evansi*	Transmitted by biting insects and vampire bats	[45]
FUNGI				
Dermatophytosis/ ringworm/tinea	Worldwide	*Microsporum* spp., *Trichophyton* spp.	Direct contact with infected animals	[46]
Aspergillosis	Worldwide	*Aspergillus* spp.	Inhalation	[47]
Cryptococcosis	Worldwide	*Cryptococcus neoformis*	Inhalation	[48]
Histoplasmosis	Worldwide	*Histoplasma capsulatum var. capsulatum*	Inhalation	[49]

infectious diseases. Deforestation causes a decline in biodiversity, and the degraded biodiversity, combined with the impact of climate change, results in close contact between humans and zoonotic diseases of wildlife origins. Owing to climate change and deforestation, the planet has become warmer and more humid, which increases the risk of infectious disease transmission under hot and dry climate conditions. In the end, infectious diseases restricted to tropical zones spread to other regions, causing outbreaks of deadly diseases with massive global health and socioeconomic impacts [51].

Additionally, rapid growth and intensified animal farming and production with limited biosecurity measures, extensive misuse of antimicrobials leading to the development of antimicrobial resistance (AMR), deforestation, and industrialization are great drivers contributing to the emergence and re-emergence of zoonotic diseases globally [52, 53]. Moreover, one other factor that contributes significantly to the emergence and spread of zoonotic disease is poverty. For instance, the recent Ebola outbreak in West Africa was reported to spread widely and rapidly among poor communities such as Monrovia and Conakry [54]. Impoverished societies usually live in close contact with animals, and a lack of healthcare and clean water contributes to the spread of zoonotic outbreaks [51]. Table 6.2 shows the major factors responsible for the emergence and spread of zoonotic diseases globally.

Table 6.2 Factors contributing to the occurrence and spread of zoonotic diseases.

Specific factors	Discussion	Pathogens emergency	References
Anthropogenic land-use changes	Anthropogenic land-use changes are the changes humans cause to land and its other ecosystems. They are one of the drivers of zoonotic disease emergencies.	Ebola virus, Nipah virus, Rabies virus, *Leishmania* spp., *Borrelia* spp. MERS-CoV, SARS-CoV-2, and *Rickettsia* spp.	[55]
Trafficking, migration, and eating of wild animals	Wild animals serve as reservoirs of zoonotic diseases. The relationship between wild animals and humans is very close. More than one billion contacts (either direct or indirect) occur between humans and wild animals. Illegally trading, eating, or migrating wild animals contributes to this closeness, facilitating the spread of zoonotic diseases to humans from wild animals.	RVF virus, West Nile virus (WNV), highly pathogenic avian influenza (HPAI) virus, SARS-CoV-2 virus	[55, 56]
Travel and tourist	International or local travel contributes to the spread of zoonotic disease from endemic to nonendemic regions. Tourists are susceptible to infection because of their weak immune systems (due to traveling stress), which makes it easier for them to transmit zoonotic diseases to their family or community.	SARS-CoV-2 virus, *Leptospira* spp., and Chikungunya virus (CHIKV)	[53]
Agricultural intensification	The increase in human population has led to the intensification of agriculture. Farmers build dams to wet their crops to increase production yield. Meanwhile, the dam serves as a breeding place for mosquitoes that transmit zoonotic diseases to humans.	*Escherichia coli (E. coli) O157:H7*, and methicillin-resistant *Staphylococcus aureus*	[53]
Urbanization, deforestation, and habitat fragmentation	An increased human population contributes to expanding the human environment, the wild animal community, and natural habitats, increasing emerging zoonotic diseases. Deforestation and urbanization lead to decreased biodiversity. The higher the biodiversity, the lower the burden of diseases, and vice versa.	*Plasmodium knowlesi*, Tick-borne pathogens, Ebola virus, *Borrelia* spp.	[53, 57]

Specific factors	Discussion	Pathogens emergency	References
Pathogen adaptation and change	Different traits of zoonotic pathogens make them survive in harsh environments.	CHIKV and AMR	[53]
Breakdown of public health measures	Various PH measures are available to safeguard the spread of zoonotic pathogens, such as handwashing, biosecurity, sanitation, etc. The bridge in any of these measures will lead to exposure to zoonotic pathogens, especially in endemic regions.	*Vibro cholerae* and Nosocomial pathogens	[52]
Companion and food animals	Many zoonotic pathogens have been transferred through the proximity of humans with their pets and farm animals. The International Union for the Conservation of Nature confirmed that 99% of zoonoses are transmitted from domestic animals to humans.	*Salmonella* spp., *E. coli O157:H7, Leishmania* spp., *Haemobartonella* spp., Measles virus and *Campylobacter* spp.	[58, 59]
Host susceptibility	Zoonotic pathogens are adapted to various hosts, but recently, there have been reports of cross-transfer of zoonotic diseases based on the level of susceptibility. Some diseases also contribute to humans' exposure to zoonotic diseases because of their significant influence on the immune system.	HIV/acquired immune deficiency syndrome (AIDS), Leishmaniasis, Bacillary angiomatosis, Peliosis, and *Cryptosporidium* spp.	[60]
Political factors	Zoonotic disease transmission can occur due to the occurrence of civil or world wars as a result of the destruction of healthcare centers and natural communities.	Crimean-Congo hemorrhagic fever virus, Ebola virus, HPAI virus	[53]
Climate changes	Climate changes, such as harsh weather, flooding, wind patterns, disastrous storms, and land and ocean temperatures, contribute to the increased transmission of zoonotic diseases. The high prevalence of vector-, food-, and water-borne zoonotic diseases has been recorded in regions with any climate change phenomena.	AMR, vector-borne pathogens, DENV, and malaria	[61–63]

Furthermore, Figure 6.1 represents a map that could visually illustrate the first global outbreak of significant zoonotic diseases and their distribution.

6.2.3 Epidemiology of Emerging and Re-emerging Zoonotic Diseases (December 2019–January 2025)

This section of the chapter highlights the epidemiology of notable reported emerging and re-emerging zoonotic diseases from December 2019 to January 2025.

6.2.3.1 Highly Pathogenic Avian Influenza

Highly pathogenic avian influenza (HPAI) is a highly contagious zoonotic disease caused by influenza viruses (alpha influenza virus, under the family Orthomyxoviridae) [23]. The HPAIs are enveloped, segmented, negative-sense, and single-stranded RNA viruses. These viruses consist of eight gene segments that encode a minimum of 11 structural and nonstructural/regulatory proteins. The disease caused by the virus is a highly contagious respiratory disease of poultry and birds, resulting in high morbidity and mortality and causing substantial financial losses to the poultry sector [23, 64]. H5N1 serotypes are of global concern due to their high pathogenicity, particularly clade 2.3.4.4b, which emerged in 2013 and has since spread across Asia, African Europe,

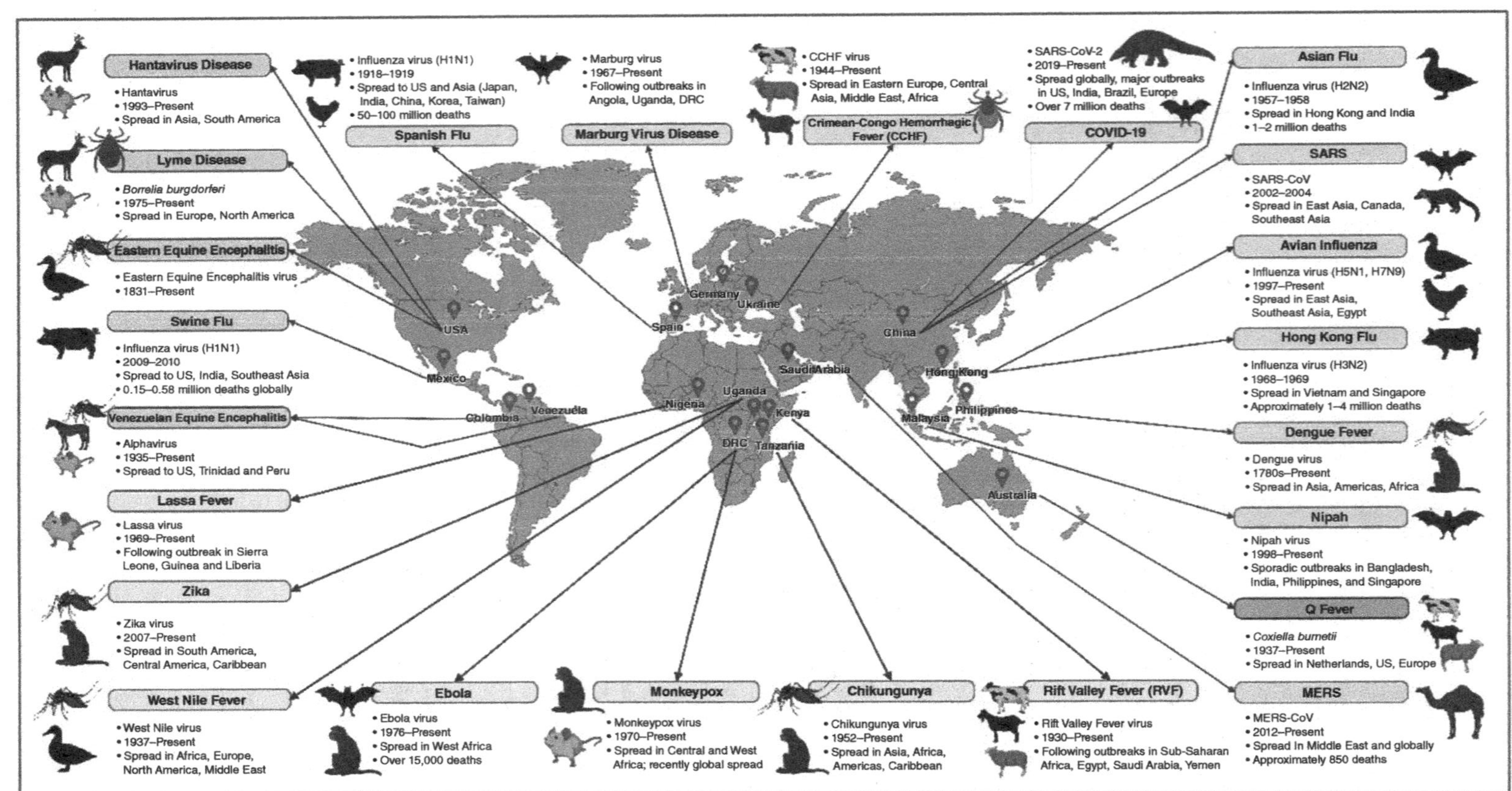

Figure 6.1 Global map of first zoonotic disease outbreaks.

and America, leading to outbreaks in various poultry and animal species [23, 64]. Over the course of more than 20 years, sporadic human infections with the HPAI A (H5N1) virus have been reported in 23 countries. Infections present a broad spectrum of clinical severity and have an aggregate case fatality exceeding 50%. In 2020 and 2021, HPAI A (H5N1) clade 2.3.4.4b viruses were transmitted in wild birds globally, leading to outbreaks in poultry and other animal species [23, 65]. In March 2024, several outbreaks of HPAI A (H5N1) clade 2.3.4.4b viruses were also reported in dairy cows, and positive samples of unpasteurized milk were reported from different cities within the United States of America (USA) [66].

6.2.3.2 Coronavirus Disease 2019

COVID-19 is a highly contagious respiratory disease caused by SARS-CoV-2 and is transmitted via aerosols [67]. The virus was first detected in Wuhan, Hubei Province, China, in 2019 and then spread worldwide. On March 12, 2020, the WHO declared COVID-19 a pandemic, and as of June 9, 2024, it had infected 775.62 million people and caused approximately 20 million deaths [68, 69]. SARS-CoV-2, SARS-CoV, and Middle East respiratory syndrome coronavirus (MERS-CoV) cause severe respiratory illness, with fatality rates of 2.9%, 9.6%, and 36%, respectively [67].

SARS-CoV-2 is highly similar to bat SARS-like coronaviruses [70] and might be a reservoir host. Patients with COVID-19 develop symptoms ranging from mild to severe illness, and the most common symptoms include fever, cough, and dyspnea. In some cases, patients develop gastrointestinal-associated symptoms such as vomiting, nausea, diarrhea, and abdominal pain [71]. After the pandemic hit, pharmaceutical companies started to develop vaccines, which became available at the end of 2020. The vaccine tremendously reduced the spread of SARS-CoV-2 and saved lives. Unfortunately, owing to the emergence of Omicron variants, vaccine efficacy has been reduced [68].

6.2.3.3 Dengue Fever

Dengue fever (DF) is a mosquito-borne viral infection caused by dengue viruses (DENVs) belonging to the Flaviviridae family. DENVs are positive-sense RNA viruses transmitted by mosquitoes [72]. Each year, millions of humans get infected through bites from infected female Aedes species mosquitoes. Patients with dengue often develop high fever with other symptoms, such as eye and muscle pain, nausea, and vomiting. In the most common cases, the disease is asymptomatic, and the immune system successfully controls virus replication within a few days. In severe cases, dengue can progress to a more critical disease termed dengue hemorrhagic fever (DHF) or fatal dengue shock syndrome (DSS) [72].

The most recent outbreak was reported in 2024 in several countries, including European countries and America, in addition to Asia and Africa [73]. Climate change is the greatest driver for the emergence of dengue in Europe. According to the Pan-American Health Organization's latest estimates, approximately 4.6 million people in the Americas are estimated to have been infected with DF in the first four months of 2024 alone. In the absence of a universally accepted prophylactic vaccine or therapeutic drug, treatment is mainly restricted to supportive measures. In endemic areas, the most successful way to fight and control dengue infection is through mosquito control [72].

6.2.3.4 Monkeypox

Mpox is a potential fetal zoonotic disease caused by the MPXV and is endemic in forested areas in central and western Africa. It is a double-stranded DNA (dsDNA) virus belonging to the Orthopoxvirus (OPXV) genus within the Poxviridae family. Transmission from animals to humans usually occurs via contact with bodily fluids or skin lesions of infected animals/humans. Additionally, people became infected through sexual contact with the infected person. Patients with Mpox often develop symptoms, including high fever, headache, skin rash, and muscle aches. The most recent outbreak of Mpox was reported in 25 of 26 provinces, including urban areas, in the Democratic Republic of the Congo (DRC) by June 2024, according to data released by the Centers for Disease

Control and Prevention (CDC) [74]. There is no specific vaccine for MPXV available. However, smallpox vaccines have been reported to result in 85% cross-immunity against MPXV due to their shared antigenic characteristics. Multisectoral OH approaches are needed to fight MPXV [33].

6.2.3.5 Chikungunya Virus Disease

Chikungunya virus disease (CHIKVD) is a viral infection caused by the CHIKV, Togaviridae, which is transmitted by mosquito bites of *Aedes albopictus* and *Aedes aegypti* [73]. The virus was first identified in a patient in Tanzania in 1952, followed by sporadic cases recorded in Africa and Asia. Recently, CHIKV has spread globally, affecting millions of people annually in all tropical and subtropical countries [75]. The transmission of infection to humans occurs through mosquito bites, and the infection is transmitted from person to person via direct contact with the bodily fluids of infected people. The disease is characterized by high fever, rash, muscle, and joint pain. In severe cases, renal and neurological symptoms develop [50]. The first significant outbreak of CHIKV was reported in Kenya in 2004. Since then, the virus has spread globally, and several outbreaks have been reported worldwide, including in European countries [50]. As of 30 April 2024, approximately 240 000 CHIKVD and over 90 deaths have been reported worldwide. CHIKVD cases were reported in 18 countries, with 11 from the Americas, six from Asia, and one from Africa, according to the European Centre for Disease Prevention and Control [75]. There is no specific therapy for CHIKVD; in most cases, the infection is self-limited within a few weeks. However, a vaccine is available and recommended for people at risk and traveling to endemic areas.

6.2.3.6 Salmonellosis

Salmonellosis is a global foodborne disease caused by Gram-negative bacteria of the genus *Salmonella*. It is estimated that each year, approximately 90 million people are infected with salmonellosis worldwide, with approximately 155 000 deaths [76]. The most recent outbreak in May 2024 in 29 states in the USA reported an outbreak of zoonotic Salmonella linked to contact with backyard poultry. The infection occurs via direct or indirect contact with infected animals, particularly poultry. Salmonella are highly diverse bacteria found in the digestive tract of animals and humans, and they live widely in the environment [77]. More than 2600 *Salmonella* serovars have been identified. Salmonella is a common cause of acute human bacterial gastroenteritis, and the symptoms and mortality rates vary depending on the serotype and host characteristics, such as age, sex, immune status, and nutrition. Salmonella can be divided into typhoidal and nontyphoidal *Salmonella* serovars (NTSs), all of which can cause diseases in animals and/or humans with different levels of severity. Typhoidal serovars are highly adapted to the human host, where NTSs are known as zoonotic agents. The most common NTSs are *S. enteritidis* and *S. typhimurium*, which are considered the most important serovars with the greatest impact on PH and are responsible for more than 70% of human infections [76]. Two critical aspects are essential for the prevention and control of salmonellosis: reducing the incidence rate in animals by practicing biosecurity and protecting people from infection. These are key aspects. Salmonellosis prevention at the food chain level necessitates a thorough strategy at the farm, manufacturing, distribution, and consumer levels. Handling food properly, preventing cross-contamination, and cooking it thoroughly can help lower risk and ensure food safety [33, 76].

6.2.3.7 Human Metapneumovirus Infection

The recent outbreak of human metapneumovirus (hMPV) in China has brought renewed focus to respiratory pathogens and the challenges they pose to public health., hMPV, first was identified in the Netherlands in 2001. hMPV typically causes mild respiratory symptoms such as fever, cough, runny or stuffy nose, nasal congestion, gasp for breath, sore throat, body ache, headache, and fatigue, with an incubation period of 3–6 days [34, 35, 78]. However, vulnerable groups like infants, elderly, and immunocompromised individuals are at risk of severe complications [78]. Unlike COVID-19, hMPV is not a novel virus, and healthcare systems are better equipped to manage its outbreaks. hMPV is a single-stranded, enveloped, non-segmented, negative-stranded RNA virus that belongs to the subfamily *Pneumovirinae* [34, 35, 78]. The hMPV genome (nearly 13 kb) contains 8 genes that encode nine proteins, namely nucleoprotein (N), phosphoprotein (P), matrix protein (M), fusion protein (F), matrix-2 proteins (M2-1 and M2-2), small hydrophobic (SH) protein, glycoprotein (G), and large (L) polymerase protein. According to the genetic features of the F and G genes, hMPV strains prevalent worldwide could be classified into 4 genotypes (A1, A2, B1, and B2) and further divided into 6 lineages (A1, A2a, A2b, A2c, B1, and B2) [34]. hMPV is thought to have originated from zoonotic transmission. It shares a close genetic similarity with avian metapneumovirus C and is believed to have diverged from it between 200 and 400 years ago, following its transmission from birds to humans [79, 80]. The hMPV primarily spreads through respiratory droplets that spread through the air from a sick person to others or contact with contaminated surfaces [35, 78]. Although it is not a new virus, its impact during the current outbreak, particularly in northern China, children under 14 years and over 65 years old, has drawn significant attention [34, 78, 81, 82]. Studies have shown that the prevalence of hMPV is higher in children (<5 years, 85%) compared to the elderly (>65 years, 3.2%), middle-aged adults (25–65 years; 2.0%), and teenagers (14–25 years; 0.9%) [34, 81].

The outbreak started in late 2024, with a significant increase in cases by mid-December, causing hospitals to become overcrowded, similar to the initial phase of the COVID-19 pandemic. Social media reports and videos reveal hospitals grappling with various respiratory viruses, such as hMPV, influenza A, *Mycoplasma pneumoniae*, and persistent COVID-19 cases [83, 84]. Chinese health authorities have downplayed the threat of the recent hMPV outbreak, attributing it to typical seasonal patterns. The Chinese Center for Disease Control and Prevention (CCDC) reported that hMPV accounted for 6.2% of positive respiratory disease tests during 16–22 December 2024, which is consistent with normal winter trends [85, 86]. They have emphasized that hMPV is a well-known virus with widespread immunity in the population [85].

Testing for hMPV is well-established, and medical professionals are familiar with its treatment and prevention protocols [34, 35, 87]. Several different molecular diagnosis methods have been developed to perform hMPV molecular detection. The most prominent of these methods are the reverse transcription polymerase chain reaction (RT-PCR), the real-time quantitative reverse transcription polymerase chain reaction (RT-qPCR), and the reverse transcription loop-mediated isothermal amplification reaction (RT-LAMP) [34, 35, 87]. Currently, there is no specific antiviral treatment or vaccine for hMPV. Management emphasizes supportive care, which includes hydration, fever reduction, and, in severe cases, oxygen therapy or mechanical ventilation [35, 87].

To address the outbreak, China's National Disease Control and Prevention Administration has introduced a monitoring system for pneumonia cases of unknown origin [86]. Authorities have also issued public health recommendations, including frequent handwashing with soap and water for at least 20 seconds, staying away from sick people, covering mouth and nose when coughing and sneezing, avoiding touching your eyes, nose, and mouth with unwashed hands, improved ventilation, and mask-wearing in crowded areas [87]. Although these measures are typical for respiratory viruses, the magnitude of the outbreak has increased public anxiety. The memories of the COVID-19 pandemic have intensified concerns, with many people confusing hMPV for a new and unknown virus.

Several countries reported confirmed cases during the 2024–2025 hMPV outbreak, although specific data on deaths remain limited. China showed a significant increase in cases and recorded 6.2% of laboratory tests were positive for hMPV, while Malaysia confirmed 327 cases [88]. Kazakhstan reported 301 cases, and the Philippines had 284 cases (5.2% of laboratory tests) [88, 89]. India recorded 7 cases across multiple states, and Romania confirmed 2 cases [88, 90, 91]. In the USA, 1.94% of weekly tests were positive for hMPV (28 000 confirmed cases) as of late December 2024, while the UK and Mexico reported a positivity rate of 4.5 and 5.4% during the same period, respectively [91, 92]. Additionally, Australia recorded a positivity rate of 7.8% among individuals with fever and cough symptoms by mid-December 2024 [93]. Recently, Bangladesh confirmed the detection of the first case of hMPV in a 30-year-old woman [94]. However, the WHO has not raised alarms, emphasizing that the increase in cases aligns with seasonal trends in the Northern Hemisphere [95]. Experts have drawn clear distinctions between hMPV and COVID-19, nothing that the former is a well-researched virus with widespread immunity, unlike the novel coronavirus that emerged in 2019 [95].

The outbreak has also highlighted gaps in surveillance and the need for international collaboration. Experts have called for China to share more data on the outbreak to support global research efforts. Vaccine development for hMPV is underway, with promising candidates targeting both hMPV and Respiratory Syncytial Virus (RSV). Oxford Vaccine Group and AstraZeneca are optimistic about the progress in this area [96, 97].

The hMPV outbreak emphasizes the importance of robust public health systems and continuous monitoring. While it does not constitute a global health emergency like COVID-19, it offers an opportunity for health systems worldwide to enhance their response strategies. As winter progresses in the Northern Hemisphere, following preventive measures and strengthening surveillance will be crucial to control the spread of hMPV and other respiratory viruses [95]. Advancements in vaccine development and treatment methods will enhance our ability to manage such outbreaks effectively in the long run.

6.2.4 Challenges in Predicting and Controlling Zoonoses

Many countries, particularly developing countries, face considerable challenges in predicting and controlling zoonoses. This is due to various factors, including a lack of healthcare infrastructure, limited resources, and the capacity to implement policies to eliminate and control zoonotic outbreaks [98].

Among the greatest challenges is the lack of a legal framework and policy for zoonotic preparedness, surveillance, control, and prevention. Other challenges include a lack of well-trained healthcare workers, a lack of public awareness, insufficient collaboration and coordination between PH veterinary and government agencies, and weak research and diagnostic facilities [98].

6.2.5 Economic and Societal Effects of Zoonotic Disease Outbreaks

Zoonotic disease not only causes serious PH concerns globally but also poses a significant socioeconomic impact at the global level. These diseases have the potential to spread across borders. Many zoonotic infections have gained prominence in the PH context. Zoonosis outbreaks have a significant socioeconomic impact on humans and animals, including the cost of treatment, diagnosis, and control measures such as the use of vaccination, social distancing, lockdown in cities, quarantining, culling infected animals, bans on exportation and national movement, reducing animal production, and increasing motility and mortality rates. Consequently, this has led to enormous economic devastation [24]. For example, the H5 subtype of bird flu can infect at least 1 billion people and cause between 2 and 7 million deaths, according to a recent WHO estimate [99]. The World Bank estimates that a severe avian flu pandemic among humans could cost the global economy approximately 3.1% of the world's GDP approximately US$1.25 trillion in the world's GDP of US$40 trillion [100].

The most recent impact of the COVID-19 pandemic on socioeconomic systems and human relationships has caused an unprecedented global crisis in our recent history, causing more than double the impact of the 2008 financial crisis [101]. The isolation, social distancing, and travel restrictions imposed by several countries around the globe to control the spread of COVID-19 have had an impact on the business sector, reducing the economic growth and employment rates worldwide. Consequently, reducing GDP growth rates leads to higher inequality and poverty rates [101]. Millions of people are losing their jobs. Many enterprises have been forced to close, most have imposed an indefinite hiring freeze, and many governments have adopted draconian quarantine measures [102]. According to estimates, there were 495 million job losses globally in the second quarter of 2020, a significant decrease from the 195 million projected in April for the same period, which reflects deteriorating circumstances in many regions of the world [102].

6.3 One Health Strategies for Disease Surveillance and Prevention

Humans and animals (especially domesticated ones) are susceptible to several pathogenic microorganisms because of their coexistence in the same habitat. Some recent outbreaks, such as Ebola, yellow fever, measles, and COVID-19, have been attributed to animal hosts and, as such, have been termed zoonotic diseases [103, 104]. Humans and animals can come into contact with tainted food or drug-resistant microbes through direct interaction. Among the pertinent issues that are beyond the purview of one sector to control and resolve are environmental contamination, ecological devastation, AMR (resulting from the inappropriate use of antimicrobials), and foodborne illness (resulting from contaminated foods, animal products, and water) [105]. A few fundamental disease prevention and control methods are immunization, maintaining hygiene, and public education. Nonetheless, a synchronized OH approach is needed across the human, animal, and environmental health sectors to address these challenges effectively.

6.3.1 Principles of the One Health Approach

Multiple fundamental concepts serve as the foundation for the OH paradigm. First, how individuals, animals, and the environment are interconnected regarding health is understood. Others realize that the two components' respective states of health can be affected by the third state, highlighting how important it is for professionals from various health areas to work together and communicate and support the use of a multidisciplinary strategy that incorporates specialists from the social sciences, environmental science, PH, veterinary medicine, and medicine [106]. In addition, the United Nations has established 17 Sustainable Development Goals (SDGs), of which five, namely, Zero Hunger (Goal 2), Good Health and Well-being (Goal 3), Clean Water and Sanitation (Goal 6), Life Below Water (Goal 14), and Life on Land (Goal 15), including the principles of OH [107]. Therefore, it is imperative to adopt an integrated and cohesive strategy to reduce and eliminate health risks associated with OH components.

To improve the health of all individuals, the OH strategy facilitates collaborative disease surveillance, outbreak management, and prevention of zoonotic diseases while also improving food safety and security and reducing the prevalence of antibiotic-resistant infections [108–110]. Overall, this approach improves laboratory diagnostic systems, disease monitoring and surveillance systems, networks for early response and detection of zoonoses, and data exchange with every stakeholder by promoting strong collaboration and coordination among relevant sectors.

6.3.2 Interconnectivity of the One Health Component Parts

The spread of diseases across and among the OH units is made possible by their relationship. All fields that generally address the health of people, animals, and the environment are included under the umbrella term "OH." The term also includes the interactions between people, other animals, plants, and the entire ecological system. Thus, health professionals, PH workers, biologists, and environmental science specialists must cooperate closely with OH research [111].

A greater understanding of various health impacts and remedies is made possible by the OH approach. By examining the issue from multiple angles from human, animal, and environmental health perspectives, researchers can find influencing elements they would not have otherwise seen, leading to better-informed intervention design [112]. Therefore, to formulate a research study that effectively employs the OH strategy, investigators must consider a framework that combines components from human, animal, and environmental health, along with the various intersections between each (Figure 6.2).

The interconnection of the environment, animals, and humans has a widespread impact across all domains. One of the harmful consequences of this relationship is the transmission of zoonotic diseases. Urban wildlife relocation is partly caused by natural habitat loss and environmental degradation. These animals discharge pathogens that they commonly harbor due to increased stress from human interactions [113, 114]. Similarly, microbial

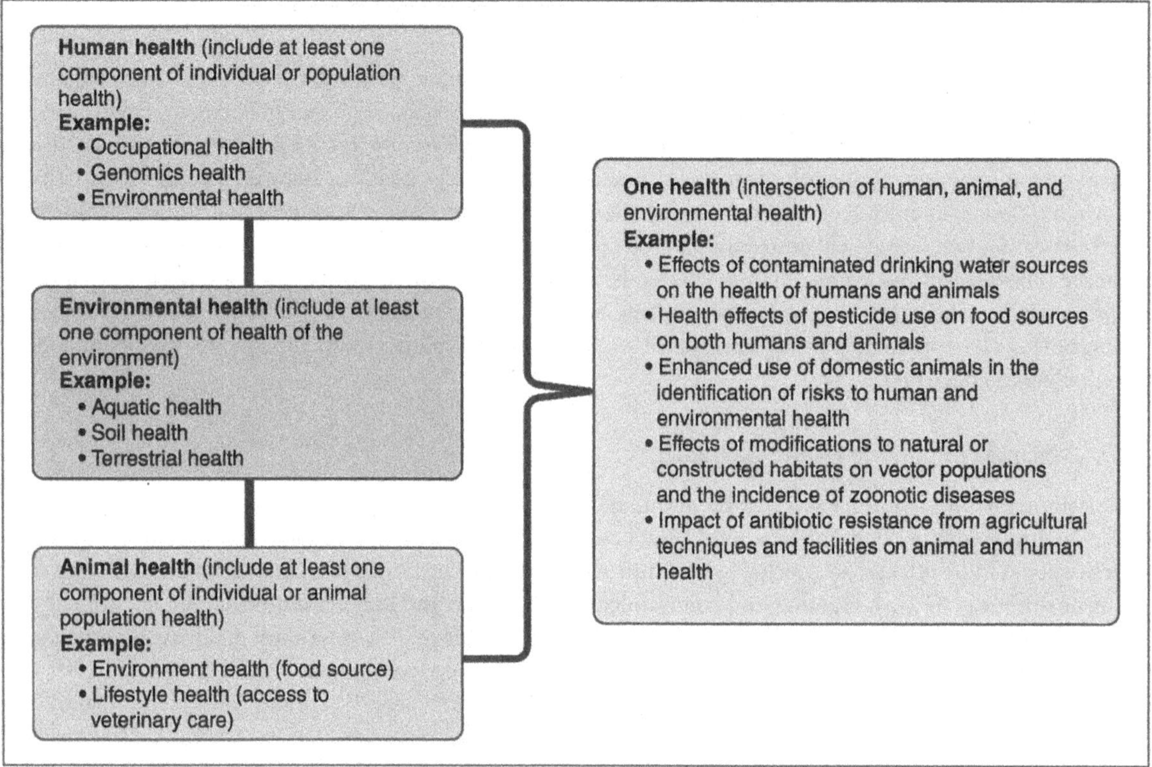

Figure 6.2 One Health research framework.

organisms that never coexist will be transferred from animals to humans, and vice versa, owing to global warming forcing these animals to relocate. Some infections have the potential to cause dangerous conditions. Zoonotic diseases, including dengue, Zika fever, and anthrax, are among the estimated 58% of infectious diseases that have spread more widely due to climate change [115]. Additionally, reports have revealed specific emerging and re-emerging zoonotic pathogens, such as lyssavirus and the food-borne bacterial pathogen *Staphylococcus haemolyticus* [116, 117].

Intersectoral integration and/or collaboration are strongly needed to address this intricate and interrelated health issue based on interactions among humans, animals, and the environment. This would lessen the burden and enable the effective future prevention and management of all zoonotic illnesses. The OH strategy and its coordination mechanisms can help attain this goal. By bringing together pertinent governmental entities, the OH model not only effectively organizes all key stakeholders in the animal, human, environmental, and other relevant sectors but also may significantly improve the health sector and its development objectives [118].

6.3.3 Multidisciplinary Approaches to Disease Surveillance and Prevention

There is a new urgency for transdisciplinary research to address the complex health and environmental needs of today. The OH approach is increasingly useful as a tool for conceptualizing and acknowledging the continuing changes in relationships involving humans, animals, and the environment. This approach requires more collaboration and interdisciplinary work between different sectors of veterinary, human, domestic animal health, and ecological medicine to prevent or respond to emerging risks [119]. A systematic framework for incorporating elements from all three health domains into the early stage of research is important because conceptualization and planning are critical stages in collaboration.

Scientific knowledge from various disciplines may influence strategies for successfully integrating surveillance systems. This approach considers social and ecological variables in addition to the scientific components of health. For instance, the prevention and management of vector-borne diseases in an increasingly industrialized world must consider the effects of both natural and artificial environmental changes on disease vector proliferation patterns. Researchers can collaborate across disciplines in climate change research to integrate various data sources, develop cross-cutting approaches, and address questions regarding the broader impacts of environmental health on human health and animal welfare [112]. Additionally, planetary health is another emerging area of transdisciplinary scientific and health research. The field of planetary health recognizes that maintaining natural systems is essential to human existence and well-being. The OH method is based on the same principle, which also encourages development and innovation in procedures, laws, and technological advancements that support environmental preservation and responsible stewardship [120]. Figure 6.3, illustrating the OH model,

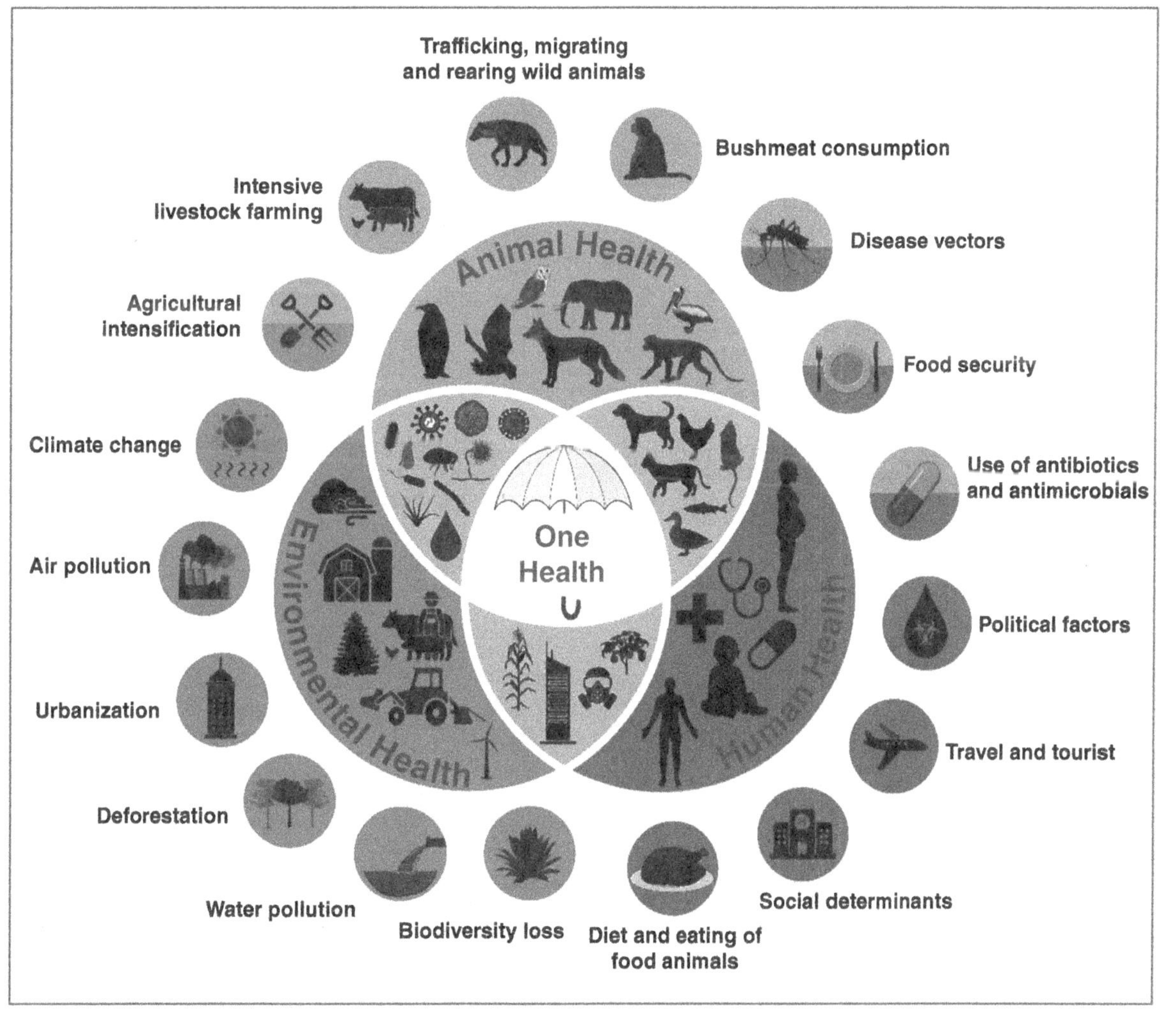

Figure 6.3 One Health model showing interconnectedness among human, animal, and environmental health.

could depict the interconnections among human, animal, and environmental health, demonstrating their interactions within a surveillance and response framework.

6.3.4 Integrated Surveillance Systems for Rapid Diagnosis and Swift Action of Zoonoses

A number of international OH initiatives, such as the OH congress and conferences [121], the quadripartite memorandum of understanding [122], the operational framework for strengthening OH systems [123], and the management of zoonotic infections using the OH approach [124, 125], among others, have been created and are being utilized to help nations manage common health threats, boost international well-being, and abide by International Health Regulations (IHRs) (Table 6.3). These initiatives also help design schemes, execution programs, guidelines, and law enactment [126].

The establishment of the workforce and technical working groups, emergency preparedness and response systems, cooperative surveillance, prioritizing of major zoonotic diseases, efficient communication, and information sharing, and enhanced laboratory capacity are some of the most successful OH strategies that are frequently used to manage and prevent diseases [108]. Consequently, the quadripartite agreement was signed in March 2022 by integrating the United Nations Environment Program (UNEP) into the previously formed tripartite agreement by the FAO, WOAH, and WHO.

Table 6.3 One Health strategy for the surveillance and prevention of zoonotic diseases.

Strategy	Outcome/recommendation	References
Global summit on bird flu	Fostering the integration of human and animal health systems to better prepare for pandemics in the interest of OH.	[110]
Collaboration of FAO, WOAH, WHO, UNICEF, World Bank and UNESCO	Created a coordinated strategy framework entitled "Contributing to One World, OH" to address the resurgence of infectious illnesses.	[110]
Tripartite agreement among FAO, WOAH, and WHO	Decided to collaborate on treating rabies, tuberculosis, antibiotic resistance, and MERS-CoV. This agreement aims to facilitate the sharing of responsibilities and the coordination of global health efforts that involve the interactions between humans, animals, and ecosystems. It recommends and promotes a sustained tactical direction for international collaboration in this area.	[127]
OH's operational framework for enhancing the health systems (people, animals, and the environment)	Designed to give OH orientation and assist the OH components in comprehending and using the strategy.	[126]
Inaugural OH congress	The importance of incorporating several fields, such as economics, behavioral sciences, food security, and safety, as well as the significance of cooperating to promote an OH approach, were all covered during the conference.	[121]
OH Collaboration: World Medical and Veterinary Association	Two organizations inked a memorandum of cooperation to combine a cohesive strategy for dealing with shared health risks and efficiently advancing global health. Their agreement centers on zoonoses, including education, antibiotic resistance, and rabies control.	[128]
Measures for control of zoonotic diseases using the OH approach	To assist nations, international organizations, stakeholders, and non-governmental entities in achieving their goals using a comprehensive and inclusive method, the WHO has a historical OH approach action companion document. This document aims to address NTDs by providing a roadmap for the years 2021–2030.	[124, 125]

UNICEF- United Nations International Children Emergency Fund, UNESCO- United Nations Educational, Scientific and Cultural Organization

6.4 Collaborative Approaches in Pandemic Preparedness

The collaborative approaches to pandemic preparedness are outlined below.

6.4.1 Understanding the Risk of Zoonotic Disease Pandemics

Yasobant et al. reported that 61% of emerging infectious diseases worldwide are zoonotic since humans and animals are closely connected with environmental factors such as deforestation and climate change [129]. Thus, establishing an effective risk assessment requires risk detection plus exposure evaluation combined with dose–response evaluation and, finally, risk characterization. These components facilitate the determination of both the probability and impact related to the likelihood of transmission of zoonotic disease outbreaks. For instance, the Global Early Warning System (GLEWS) was established by the FAO, WOAH, and WHO to evaluate the likelihood of disease-causing agents being transmitted between wild and domestic animals (Table 6.4) [130].

Similarly, hazards are equally influenced by temperature, cleanliness, and proximity to animal habitats, and water pollution has been shown to facilitate the spread of zoonotic infections [131]. Therefore, having access to fresh drinking water and a proper waste disposal system are essential for decreasing these risks. It is crucial to create a thorough OH risk assessment tool that includes many elements related to humans, animals, and the environment. The assessment tool should comprehensively evaluate hazards and enable prompt identification and response to mitigate zoonotic disease outbreaks.

6.4.2 International Frameworks for Pandemic Preparedness and Response

The COVID-19 pandemic has exposed international frameworks, revealing their strengths and notable gaps within the global health system. The IHR is a core international framework, a legally binding treaty for WHO member states [138]. The articles of the IHR are designed to assist international action for the prevention and control of PH hazards that could affect human populations internationally. Based on the IHR, countries must develop

Table 6.4 Risk assessment tools.

Tool Name	Objective	Origin	References
Tool for Influenza Pandemic Risk	To establish a consistent and clear method for evaluating the danger of influenza viruses that might cause a global pandemic.	WHO	[132]
Influenza Risk Assessment Tool	To evaluate influenza disease risk	CDC	[133]
Joint Risk Assessment Operational Tool	Assists nations in determining the prevalence of zoonotic diseases.	FAO, WOAH, WHO	[134]
GLEWS+ Risk Assessment	Evaluates the likelihood of COVID-19 being transmitted from humans to animals.	WHO	[135]
Measles Programmatic Assessment Tool	To quickly stop the spread of the measles virus, which is endemic	WHO	[136]
Disease Attribute Intelligence System Tool	Evaluate the potential hazards presented by newly developing infectious diseases in humans.	Health Analysis and Information Action	[137]

core PH capacities and report disease outbreaks and PH events to the WHO. The IHR includes a broad scope but has been characterized as weak because of a lack of compliance, funding, and political commitment. Many countries face difficulties in meeting their IHR obligations, such as timely reporting and the ability to respond effectively promptly to outbreaks [139]. This underscores the necessity of more strong and efficient enforcement management, and we need to allocate resources sustainably for that purpose.

Hence, the COVID-19 pandemic has led to a need for the establishment of a new global convention to address pandemics. This accord, promoted by the Heads of 26 countries and the WHO's Director-General, seeks to establish an organized and compelling universal framework that ensures improved preparedness, response, and responsibility in future pandemics. The accord addresses equal vaccine distribution, diagnostics, and treatments; global regulatory surveillance and monitoring systems; and enhanced collaborative approaches across national and international strata [140]. This further suggests that ad hoc arrangements are inadequate at ameliorating the challenges facing global health exigencies.

Furthermore, the pandemic influenza preparedness (PIP) framework was embraced by WHO member states in 2011. The PIP aimed to enhance the global exchange of influenza viruses that have potential pandemic attributes and increase vaccination availability for resource-poor countries during pandemic exigencies [141]. The PIP framework enabled a precedent for equal risk and benefit sharing during the administration of pandemic threats, emphasizing the need for global unity and collaboration among all countries.

Similarly, the Sendai Framework for Disaster Risk Reduction 2015–2030 delivers a universal goal addressing every facet of disaster risk management and pandemics. The Sendai Framework highlights disaster risk governance, investment in disaster risk reduction for resilience, and disaster preparedness for effective response, not health, as a primary consideration [142]. It endorses a multi-hazard approach; the dual-level coordination proposed by bilateral cooperation with regional and national stakeholders is essential when handling natural and biological hazards.

6.4.3 Importance of Multisectoral Collaboration in Pandemic Response

For program financing, policy-making processes, among other national emergency responses, fall under government institutions. Health underscores the need to think progressively about health implications in the all-policies (HiAPs) public policy approach. According to Ramirez-Rubio et al., HiAP looks toward creating synergies to promote a better health situation for all citizens; it also seeks to avoid poor health outcomes while improving population health and equity [143]. Transportation, education, and finance, among other sectors, are involved, which facilitates coherently and cooperatively addressing health problems.

Nongovernmental organizations (NGOs) go a long way in bridging government gaps by being able to promptly roll out initiatives and relate with people within a given locality. In Brazil, the National Commission operates under the President's Office to bring together central ministries, local governments, civil society, and research institutions, showcasing the successful cooperation of many stakeholders [144]. This teamwork guarantees that initiatives are more thorough and successfully reach disadvantaged groups.

Researchers produce data and evidence that provide information for policy-making and practical application. They are crucial in monitoring, detecting rising dangers, and creating inventive remedies.

6.4.4 Role of Interdisciplinary Collaboration in Pandemic Preparedness

The multistakeholder spatial decision support system (MS-SDSS) is advantageous for addressing the difficulties presented by the COVID-19 pandemic [145]. The MS-SDSS enhances disease spread monitoring and potential outbreak evaluation, enabling interaction between first responders and PH professionals. Hence, enhancing continual care services to patients through data sharing among stakeholders in the healthcare sector, including patients, medical doctors, medical officers, and policymakers. To combat the spread of this virus, many countries have used trials before its advent in addition to border closures, social distancing methods, and public awareness programs, among other measures such as testing before symptoms occur. Good examples of managing pandemics include Taiwan's proactive tests, border control measures, public awareness campaigns, and relief efforts. This highlights the efficacious application of multilayer governance, which includes local governments, enterprises, and insurance companies. In the same vein, South Korea utilized its emergency response system, ensuring timely and effective coordination with networks of stakeholders, including government bodies, in addition to scientific officials [145].

It is against this backdrop that any efficacy of interdisciplinary coordination in pandemic preparation will be contingent on coordinating research, data and community engagement systematically. Furthermore, employing technology-driven decision-support systems enables an understanding of the dynamics of disease transmission, which is essential for effective mitigation measures.

6.4.5 Vaccine Development and Distribution

The symphony between vaccine development and distribution takes center stage in pandemic preparedness and response. With preexisting coronavirus research and cutting-edge messenger ribonucleic acid (mRNA) technology, the scientific community has managed to produce a vaccine within a year [146]. This is different from typical vaccine development, which takes 10–15 years. However, this swift evolution was not accompanied by obstacles. It was necessary to perform fast clinical trials for vaccine safety and effectiveness, which raised doubts about the issue of repercussions in the long run. Furthermore, the development and distribution of vaccines worldwide has introduced significant logistical challenges. For example, facilities for producing sterile items such as vaccines must be designed with certain unique features [147].

In addition, the vaccine distribution highlighted issues of fairness and accessibility. High-income countries can easily obtain large amounts of vaccines, ignoring low-income countries. This gap emphasized the need for a more coherent and fair approach to address global health emergencies, which organizations aimed at bridging by providing vaccines to such nations. Despite these efforts, limitations persist within the current global health infrastructure, calling attention to revising international cooperation and resource sharing for future pandemics [146].

6.4.6 Public Awareness and Community Engagement Initiatives

Public consciousness and local involvement stand as pivotal pillars in readiness for pandemics. Hafez et al. noted that an assortment of activities falls under the broad definition of community interventions, framed within community information, consultation, involvement, collaboration, and empowerment (CICICE) [148]. These range from informing communities about pandemic risks and ensuring that they are empowered to act independently to support preparedness. Such interventions aim to facilitate easy access and absorption of information on epidemic and pandemic threats, weaving strong social networks with adequate social capital at the grassroots level, mobilizing material resources within communities, and allowing communities to decide on resource allocation toward resilience. The components of the intervention should work together based on cooperation between different bodies.

A practical approach to public awareness is the application of risk communication methods. These include but are not limited to public information campaigns and social media messaging, community outreach work, and peer-to-peer interventions. All these methods are aimed at promoting trust and social capital within communities. With respect to PH messaging, trust building is crucial because it affects community openness. It was essential to use effective communication and engagement tactics to acquire community confidence and ensure compliance with health measures during the Ebola outbreak [148].

Crucial to early identification and response are community-based epidemic monitoring and surveillance systems. Community health workers (CHWs) play an essential role in many of these initiatives as intermediaries between patients and healthcare providers. CHWs' participation in providing services, counseling, and navigating healthcare systems strengthens communities. In addition, community responses during pandemics rely on programs encouraging volunteering and supporting community groups. These diverse approaches highlight the need to include communities as active participants in pandemic reactions and preparations rather than only as information receivers.

6.5 Social and Ecological Dimensions of Zoonotic Diseases

The major effects of socioeconomic and ecological factors on zoonotic disease transmission are described below.

6.5.1 Impact of Socio-economic Factors on Zoonotic Disease Transmission

While disasters impact health systems and epidemiological factors, poverty and low socioeconomic levels are thought to be the primary drivers of people's vulnerability to disease [149]. Farmers will not invest in enhancing biosecurity if they do not directly profit financially from doing so [150, 151]. These findings suggest a dual relationship between disease knowledge, economic conditions, and disease persistence. The risk of livestock disease is related to a farmer's socioeconomic status [152]. To prevent disease, one must possess a thorough understanding of the epidemiological context and pertinent risk factors or indicators, which include health protocols and housing and management policies that affect the social dynamics of farms [153]. Earlier studies indicated that knowledge developed multiple disease management and control practices and strategies, increased awareness of the disease, and improved the sociocultural profile of farmers [154].

Lassa fever is a disease for which most infections are maintained and transmitted by rodents rather than circulating from human to human [155]. Recent socioeconomic changes due to housing and agricultural modifications leading people into closer contact with these preferred ecological habitats of rodents have increased the chance that such zoonotic pathogens can spill over to humans.

There is a strong correlation between the spread of disease, unlawful free-ranging pigs, and human socioeconomic situations [152]. With respect to African swine fever (ASF), this strong correlation between culture, animal husbandry practices, and disease transmission is even more evident. Research conducted in pig farming communities with limited resources has shown that socioeconomic issues are essential barriers to controlling ASF [150]. The cost and unsuitability of animal health and production inputs make farms in socioeconomically challenging areas particularly susceptible to disease [152]. Unplanned and unsustainable patterns of urban expansion have brought about numerous new environmental and health risks. Urbanization can influence the spread of pandemics through several different mechanisms, but the most common mechanisms are related to high population density, poor sanitation, poverty, substandard living conditions (particularly in slums), and alterations in behavior or lifestyle that accelerate the transmission of infectious diseases.

Zachreson et al. [156] demonstrated how fast urbanization impacts the timing, incidence, and bimodality of influenza pandemics in Australia via a census-calibrated model. In Tanzania, there was a correlation between increased risk of zoonotic diseases and factors such as education, occupation, place of residence, and ethnicity. Although little is known about the prevalence of zoonotic diseases in the nation, poor individuals who live near animals, particularly impoverished livestock caretakers, are nonetheless frequently afflicted with these illnesses [157].

Using COVID-19 as a case study, Oztig and Askin [158] proposed a connection between the amount of human movement and the frequency of COVID-19 cases in nations with high levels of air travel. Additionally, they discovered that, in contrast to other countries, those with higher population densities and higher percentages of older people were more likely to be afflicted by COVID-19.

Even if the majority of research has connected livestock health to the health of individual animals and management techniques, human elements are not considered because agricultural sustainability has had a more significant influence on modern sociology. Studies have linked social behaviors to the spread of bovine tuberculosis, underscoring the importance of animal and social dynamics in disease transmission [159, 160].

6.5.2 Role of Environmental Factors in Zoonotic Disease Emergence and Spread

The most recognized factors in the emergence of disease are ecological changes, including those caused by agricultural or economic development. Ecological factors typically cause emergence by bringing individuals into contact with a host or natural reservoir that is home to an infection that was previously unknown to humans. This can occur through growing closer to or, more frequently, by altering the environment to support a higher microbe population or its natural host. Taking Lyme disease as an example, reforestation increased the number of deer and deer ticks, the disease vector, which in turn increased the likelihood that Lyme disease would spread to the USA and Europe. A more significant population was positioned close to the vector because of the migration of people into these regions. According to Sutherst [161], climate and environmental changes have accelerated the global emergence of zoonotic diseases. The UNEP has reported that most new or re-emerging infectious diseases affecting human beings are zoonotic in nature and are related to significant changes in climate and environmental determinants [162].

Numerous earlier studies have demonstrated a connection between past pandemics and changes in environmental and climatic conditions. In the tropics, climate change readily increases the spread of zoonotic viruses and carriers, thus promoting the quick transfer of viruses from carrier to host species [163]. Studies have also revealed that modifications in temperature and precipitation because of climate change can produce genetic fluctuations inside the evolutionary makeup of virus types. A similar example occurred in North America following the emergence of the West Nile virus (WNV); a temperature-mediated adaptive mutation facilitated its survival and spread at relatively high temperatures [164]. Studies carried out in the case of COVID-19 have shown varying results, with some showing a positive relationship [165] between COVID-19 and temperature and between COVID-19 and relative humidity [166], others showing a negative relationship, and others showing no relationship at all [167]. The COVID-19 transmission rate decreased as the temperature increased, according to Shi et al. [168]. The same investigation confirmed that there was no significant correlation between the incidence of COVID-19 and absolute humidity. Many newly discovered zoonoses are associated with viruses and are spread by arthropods, which are vectors, as well as reservoir animals [169]. The increase in global temperature over the last few decades and the Intergovernmental Panel on Climate Change (IPCC)'s 2013 estimate of an increase of approximately 3 °C by 2050 have resulted in the spread of human pathogen vectors, such as insects, and reservoirs in unrecorded parts of the world [170]. Therefore, the impact of climate factors, especially an increase in global temperature, can reveal much more about the ecology of disease-causing zoonotic pathogens and how they affect people.

Several scientific reports have addressed the potential for infectious disease outbreaks at Arctic sites in relation to climate change [171, 172]. Based on these findings, it can be concluded that in cold regions, each 1C increase in temperature will support multiple factors for microbiologically diseased pathogens and their vector species. According to Parkinson et al. [171], rising temperatures dramatically impact ecosystems in polar areas, which change the abundance and distribution of arthropod vectors and animal reservoirs. Owing to changes in temperature, humidity, precipitation patterns, and other factors, ecosystems may be directly or indirectly altered by climate change, either improving or worsening the situation for nonhuman species. Through trade, migration, or human migration, vectors or reservoirs can spread, dispersing infections into new areas where climate change may have already created favorable circumstances. A prime example is the spread of the DENV in southern Europe [173].

6.5.2.1 Extreme Weather Conditions

Extreme weather conditions, such as prolonged droughts and floods, have been shown to contribute to the spread of pandemics. Shaman et al. [174] reported that mosquito vectors and avian hosts were introduced to southern Florida by a prolonged period of drought followed by precipitation. Similarly, Paull et al. [175] forecasted that, in areas where human immunity to the virus is minimal, an increase in drought severity over the next 30 years could triple the number of WNV infections. Furthermore, growing dependence on bushmeat due to droughts and desertification increases the risk of zoonotic disease transfer to humans [176]. The high prevalence of infectious diseases spread by vectors has been indirectly connected to floods caused by heavy, erratic rains. For example, heavy rainfall and flooding in Romania (1996–1997), the Czech Republic (1997), Italy (1998), southern Africa (2000), and certain regions of Southeast Asia (2011) resulted in increases in DENV, WNV, and malaria outbreaks [62, 177, 178]. The establishment of relief camps following flood occurrence can also contribute to the spread of infectious diseases owing to high population densities, unsanitary circumstances, inadequate nutrition, limited access to clean water, and floods [179].

6.5.3 Role of Cultural Practices and Behavior Changes in Zoonotic Disease Emergence and Spread

The zoonotic transmission of diseases relies on direct or indirect contact at the animal–human interface, where interactions between species enable cross-species pathogen transfer [180]. Although domestic and wild animals have coexisted with people for millennia, in recent decades, several human-induced factors have increased their interactions with animals and, as a result, the potential for disease spillover [180]. The growing human population and measures taken to reduce poverty, including intensive farming and unsustainable resource extraction, are the leading causes of this increasing intensity in human–animal interactions and associated disease risk. A spillover incident that leads to effective and long-lasting transmission between people can spread swiftly throughout our increasingly globalized planet. The COVID-19 pandemic, which has caused unprecedented worldwide PH, social, and economic crises, has clearly shown this [181]. Certain practices that have contributed to the increase in the animal–human interface that promotes the emergence of zoonotic diseases and their spread, some of which are discussed below, effectively characterize the associations between disease frequency and farmer behaviors, which are influenced by a range of factors, including socioeconomic status, social networks, and demographics. It is not surprising that culture and behavior can impact the epidemiology of animal diseases, given that human populations of animals are regulated [154].

6.5.3.1 Increased Farming of Wildlife

Many mammals, such as deer [182], rodents [183], and fur mammals, are produced under a variety of production systems globally and offer both protein and money. Nevertheless, health monitoring programs are rarely implemented on wildlife farms, despite the presence of intensive farming conditions and minimal genetic diversity [184]. These factors serve as stressors for farmed wildlife species and captive wild animals, compromising their immune systems and increasing the risk of contracting diseases [185]. The case of avian influenza strains on Ostriches in South African farms illustrates this [186].

6.5.3.2 Livestock Farming and Pet Ownership

Livestock and companion animals play a significant role in the intricate pathways that lead to the emergence of zoonotic diseases (EZDs) because of their interaction with both people and wildlife [180]. Global market needs, such as urbanization and population growth, are driving an increase in intensive livestock farming and changing the production and distribution of food [187]. Concurrent human variables, including altered land use, create shared ecosystems that amplify and spillover new EZDs and create wildlife–domestic species interfaces [188]. For example, the emergence of the Nipah virus in Malaysia in 1998 resulted from the dual agriculture of intensive pig farming with mango plantations, which created a bat-pig interface that permitted a spillover of the Nipah virus from bats feeding on mango fruits to pigs in the house below [189]. Recurrent spillover of the virus in pigs led to prolonged virus circulation in pigs, consequently increasing the opportunity for human spillover [190]. This finding demonstrates that large populations of a single livestock species can increase the risk of EZDs in people by facilitating the persistence of a potential pathogen at the livestock–human interface.

Humans' evolving interactions with pets and their environments could have unfavorable outcomes, such as altered feeding regimens, excessive breeding, behavioral issues, and the spread of anthropozoonosis. Risky behaviors, including sleeping with pets, allowing them to lick wounds or faces, owning exotic animals, importing rescue dogs, and having contact with soil, can increase the risk of zoonotic virus transmission in humans [191]. Animals can transmit microorganisms, such as bacteria, viruses, and fungi, through direct contact by biting, licking, scratching, sneezing, or coughing. Microorganisms can also be transmitted through pets or their body fluids or secretions. Additionally, indirect contact can occur through contaminated bedding, food, water, or bites from an arthropod vector [192].

6.5.3.3 Live Animal Market Practices (Wet Markets)

In recent years, wet markets have faced stigma because they are related to the potential introduction of infectious diseases, such as the spread of avian influenza in live bird markets [193]. Additionally, several wet markets (known as wildlife markets) allow people to purchase exotic animals, including reptiles, porcupines, and various other species. The SARS virus outbreak (2002–2003), which resulted in the death of 774 individuals, is believed to have commenced from masked palm civets (*Paguma larvata*) that were being sold at wildlife markets in Guangdong Province, China [194, 195].

Wet markets are frequently associated with unsanitary conditions and the confinement of living animals in overcrowded and unsuitable environments [155, 196]. In addition to the challenge or almost insurmountable task of providing food in a hygienic manner in such environmental settings, another factor that increases the risk of EZDs is the wide range of viruses present in different wildlife populations, such as rodents, monkeys, and bats, which have not been well studied [154, 196]. When wild animals are removed from their native environment and kept in unfavorable housing circumstances, they experience extreme stress, which may lead to immunosuppression and the shedding of the pathogens they may harbor [185, 197].

6.5.3.4 Globalization, Industry, and Technology

There is a close relationship between the two possibilities of disease spreading through the global movement of people and goods and high-density settings. A pathogen found in a small subpopulation may spread more widely if high-intensity animal production is practiced. Hemolytic uremic syndrome (HUS)-causing *E. coli* strains may have originated in relatively small subpopulations of cattle at one point, but they later expanded widely as cattle from various sources were brought together in high-density environments [198].

Bovine spongiform encephalopathy is another plausible example of an industrial process-induced interspecies transmission of a pathogen. This disease most likely resulted from an interspecies transfer of scrapie from sheep to cattle. It first appeared in cattle in the 1980s and was later linked to a novel variant of Creutzfeldt–Jakob disease in humans. The transfer appears to have occurred when modifications to rendering procedures resulted in insufficient rendering of the scrapie agent in sheep byproducts fed to cattle [199].

Humans who bought prairie dogs (*Cynomys* spp.) as companion animals from a supplier in the Midwestern USA in 2003 were found to have cases of Mpox [200, 201]. African rodents carrying the MPXV were kept together with the prairie dogs. Certain prairie dogs that contracted the virus and subsequently fell ill themselves infected their human owners with it. There were 71 documented cases in humans across six states in the USA, 35 of which had laboratory confirmation [201]. This is an example of how globalization allows agents to be introduced from other countries or continents into different continents.

6.5.4 Importance of Sustainable Land Use and Wildlife Conservation in Disease Prevention

Changes in land use caused by humans are the leading causes of many infectious disease outbreaks and emergency events. They also alter how endemic infections spread. Deforestation, road building, agricultural encroachment, dam construction, irrigation, coastal zone degradation, wetland modification, mining, the concentration or expansion of urban environments, and other activities are examples of these land use changes. Some studies have demonstrated that urban sprawl, forest fragmentation, and decreased biodiversity are associated with a greater risk for Lyme disease in the USA's northeast states [202]. The growth of and modifications to farming methods are closely linked to the emergence of Nipah infection in Malaysia [203, 204], European cryptosporidiosis, North America, and several food-borne infections worldwide [205]. Road construction is correlated with bushmeat consumption, which might have been crucial in the emergence of types 1 and 2 human immunodeficiency viruses [206].

Sustainable land use policies that discourage changes in land use, such as road building, deforestation, agricultural encroachment, dam construction, irrigation, etc., will help decrease the emergence of diseases or spillover of diseases from animals to humans.

Wildlife conservation is the practice of protecting wild plant and animal species along with their habitats to preserve healthy wildlife populations, improve biodiversity, and restore natural ecosystems. This practice reduces the risk of spillovers of diseases from the wildlife population to the human populace. Wild animals are maintained in their habitat, preventing significant human–animal interactions, which is one major factor that contributes to the emergence of zoonotic diseases and the re-emergence and spread of zoonoses from wild animals. Wildlife conservation prevents the hunting and capture of wild animals by humans and prevents humans from invading the natural habitat of wild animals, preventing the consumption of wild animals by humans and consequently reducing the frequency of interaction between humans and wild animals, thereby decreasing the risk of the emergence of new zoonotic diseases or the spread of already existing zoonotic diseases from wild animal species to the human population.

Magouras et al. [181] noted that for successful cross-species transmission of diseases, direct or indirect contact between humans and the animals or body fluids of animals is necessary. Sustainable land use and wildlife conservation aim to minimize human–wildlife interactions, thereby reducing the risk of cross-species transmission of diseases.

6.6 Case Studies and Examples of Global Zoonoses Control and OH Integration

This section describes the successful case studies of zoonotic disease control and prevention, lessons learned from previous outbreaks, and successful OH integration toward zoonosis control.

6.6.1 Successful One Health Interventions

As described in previous chapters, the OH approach has been useful in addressing diverse health challenges, especially zoonoses. Although many countries have not keyed into the concept of OH or have failed to adopt it, OH has been successfully deployed to prevent, manage, or control health events globally. This section discusses several successful applications of OH interventions in different regions of the world.

6.6.1.1 Rabies Control in Latin America

Rabies is a fatal global viral disease associated with PH. Although it still ravages many parts of African and Asian countries, Latin America has been able to achieve a significant reduction in human rabies cases, especially in regions of Mexico and Brazil [207, 208]. By adopting mass vaccination campaigns for dogs, which are still regarded as the primary reservoirs for rabies and general enlightenment programs for people, such as the OH approach, there was an over 95% decline in the previously recorded cases of canines and humans [209].

6.6.1.2 The Hendra Virus in Australia

The Hendra virus, which is transmitted by fruit bats, has been used to pose a significant threat to both horses and human populations in Australia [210]. Field and colleagues studied the ecology and transmission dynamics of the causative agent of the Hendra virus, leading to the implementation of the OH strategy, which considers the surveillance and monitoring of bat populations, the vaccination of horses, and public awareness campaigns directed explicitly to susceptible populations of horse owners and equine veterinarians [211]. This approach significantly reduced the incidence of Hendra virus infections. Some researchers even reported zero human cases of the disease by 2014, which was attributable to the effective results of the OH measures [212, 213].

6.6.1.3 Avian Influenza Control in Southeast Asia

Many countries worldwide are actively surveilling avian influenza (H5N1) because of its transboundary potential and mode of spread [214]. The H5N1 serotype has caused severe economic damage to both small- and large-scale poultry farmers globally and has also led to human deaths and hence PH. As one of the most drastically affected areas, Southeast Asia developed the OH framework of interdisciplinary collaboration among environmental health, medical, and veterinary professionals [215, 216]. This has led to enhanced surveillance of poultry and wild birds, vaccination of poultry, culling of infected flocks, and biosecurity measures on farms, which are instrumental in controlling the spread of H5N1 outbreaks, especially in countries such as Thailand and Vietnam [217, 218].

6.6.1.4 Rift Valley Fever in Kenya

As devastating as the RVF virus is concerning livestock and human health in Africa, Kenya has successfully managed RVF outbreaks through an OH approach [219]. The improved prevention and control of RVF, as evidenced by the significant reduction in reported cases of humans and livestock, demonstrated the effectiveness of the encompassing approach. The strategy employed vector control measures against the primary mosquito vectors, mass vaccination campaigns for livestock, public awareness programs to educate the communities on control and preventive measures, and the introduction of effective proactive systems of warning using climatic and environmental data to prevent large-scale outbreaks [220–222].

6.6.1.5 Ebola Virus Disease in West Africa

Several West African countries were affected by viral hemorrhagic fever caused by the Ebola virus between 2014 and 2016 [223]. However, some countries (such as Guinea and Liberia) swiftly implemented detailed OH strategies to control the Ebola outbreak. The approach included identifying and monitoring wildlife reservoirs, enhanced surveillance and rapid response to human cases, and public education campaigns [224]. These measures eventually led to the containment of Ebola virus disease (EVD) and helped strengthen overall health systems in vulnerable populations [225, 226].

Notably, the highlighted case scenarios demonstrate the efficacy of the OH strategy in managing zoonoses, which is achievable through multisectoral collaborations and measures geared toward human, environmental, and animal health. These are selected OH intervention strategies. Several other prominent success stories exist in the use of the OH approach to mitigate zoonotic disease outbreaks.

6.6.2 Lessons Learned from Previous Zoonotic Outbreaks

In this section, we examine past zoonotic disease outbreaks, and the lessons learned, if any, to determine the global health status in the years to come. This will be related to the importance of OH implementation at different levels of society to prevent future epidemics and pandemic health events worldwide.

6.6.2.1 Ebola

In West Africa, Ebola broke out as a re-emerging infectious disease between 2014 and 2016. This outbreak recognized the importance of multisectoral collaboration through the joint efforts of the human, animal, and environmental sectors in mobilizing international resources and expertise, which facilitated the control of the outbreak [223]. The role of community engagement via effective communication and improved awareness campaigns cannot be overemphasized in breaking the chain of transmission. Notably, many of the earlier deaths recorded during the period of the outbreak were due to incorrect information and cultural practices. However, prompt response efforts by joint healthcare workers with targeted public education improved community cooperation and hindered the further spread of the causative organism [224–226].

6.6.2.2 COVID-19

The coronavirus outbreak of the 2019 pandemic remains a benchmark consideration in understanding the importance of a global OH scheme. In the event of the 2020 PH emergency [227], the role of strengthened and continuous surveillance systems in wildlife and domestic animals was brought to the forefront to enhance early detection of zoonotic pathogens, as already circulating SARS-CoV-2 was identified in different animal species [228]. To date, there have been continuous partnerships between virologists, epidemiologists, ecologists, and other experts at the human–animal–environment nexus to increase the understanding of virus transmission dynamics and potential reservoirs rapidly [229–231].

6.6.2.3 Avian Influenza (H5N1)

Outbreaks of the H5N1 strain of the avian influenza virus have provided valuable information for different global communities, both human and animal populations [215]. Currently, much emphasis has been placed on improved biosecurity measures and vaccination programs based on previous influenza disease events. The complete control and prevention of infection in animals contributes immensely to human safety. The improved biosecurity approach is multidimensional and can be used at poultry farms or markets [232]. Regular cleaning and disinfection, movement restriction of live birds, and constant screening protocols have been found to be effective biosecurity measures over time. However, it is limited in acceptability in some countries worldwide because of the need for close monitoring and updates on circulating strains, which may differ globally. Poultry bird vaccination remains an important biosecurity measure to curtail avian influenza [214, 216–218].

6.6.2.4 Dengue Fever

Aside from the environmental control of the vector, *Aedes aegypti* mosquitoes, which involves bush clearing and chemical and biological control, the management of DF has been found to be more effective when there is public awareness and education [233]. Mosquito breeding site elimination and individual health protection via community involvement have drastically controlled outbreaks in endemic countries [234].

6.6.2.5 Chikungunya Virus Disease

CHIKVD, another mosquito-borne disease, highlights the need for coordinated efforts in vector control and disease management [235]. Establishing robust surveillance networks to quickly detect and respond to outbreaks, including monitoring both human cases and mosquito populations, is critical [236]. Good PH messaging has informed communities about preventive and control strategies for CHIKVD, including the correct use of insecticide-treated nets, mosquito repellents, and the removal of stagnant water as breeding sites [237].

6.6.2.6 Severe Acute Respiratory Syndrome

The earliest outbreak of potentially pandemic SARS occurred in 2002–2003, which, for the first time, spiked in Asian regions [238]. However, early international cooperation and sharing of information among health organizations enabled the implementation of plans for action and containment strategies such as quarantine and restrictions on travel that prevented the spread of the SARS-CoV-1 virus [239–241].

6.6.2.7 Middle East Respiratory Syndrome

MERS reminds us of the need for knowledge concerning zoonotic reservoirs and their transmission dynamics [242]. Early identification of camels as the primary reservoir for MERS-CoV was a key step in controlling the disease, leading to measures to reduce human–camel interactions [239]. Further enhancement of infection prevention and control (IPC) measures in healthcare settings later helped to nip nosocomial transmission in the bud [243, 244].

6.6.2.8 Monkeypox

Mpox, caused by the MPXV belonging to the Orthopoxvirus genus, has re-emerged as a significant zoonotic threat, particularly in Africa. After attaining a novel multicountry spread in 2022, different from the 2003 spread to the USA, Mpox reached the status of a "PH emergency of international concern" on 23 July 2022 [227]. Previous preventive measures include monitoring wildlife reservoirs, especially rodents, as a control method; however, recent outbreaks revealed novel transmission routes [245]. This necessitated improved control measures and, thus, OH integration. Recently, intensified vaccination campaigns and public education about avoiding contact with identified animal reservoirs and acts that can encourage disease spread have been effective control strategies [246, 247].

6.6.2.9 Swine Flu (H1N1)

In 2009, the rapid spread of H1N1 influenza reached pandemic potential. Rapid PH interventions involving mass vaccination campaigns and public enlightenment were effective in curbing the impact and continuous spread of the pandemic [232, 248]. Therefore, continually developing, maintaining, and reviewing pandemic preparedness plans, including stockpiling antivirals and vaccines and targeting human and animal populations, is essential [218, 249, 250].

From these disease events, the conclusion remains that through integrated efforts of the OH approach, the human, animal, and environmental health sectors will be better prepared and positioned to handle future impending global zoonotic threats. However, there are contradictions surrounding the implementation of OH strategies. For example, there are conflicts arising from measures such as culling healthy animals to ensure PH safety, a clear definition of the OH mantra, and moral dilemmas within the OH approach. Given these concerns, OH should be globally accepted and implemented to address the complex health threats of zoonoses.

6.7 Challenges and Opportunities

This section underscores the challenges and strategies to overcome in the successful integration of OH approaches in zoonoses control and prevention.

6.7.1 Barriers to Implementing One Health

The primary barriers encountered globally in OH programs include conflicting priorities, mistrust, and divergent interests [251]. A successful OH approach must consist of the following: knowledge sharing, program development, institutional collaboration, civil society engagement, capacity building, sustainable financing, policy formulation, and community engagement [252]. Diverse practitioners in the environmental, animal, and human health fields must collaborate while engaging in interdisciplinary work, such as OH, to achieve holistic goals.

Another significant challenge for OH can also be a lack of cross-sector collaboration. This was shown in a study performed in Tanzania, where the authors identified incorporating certain sectors' operations into those of another instead of focusing on joint efforts [253]. According to a different study, several sectors, particularly the veterinary and environmental sectors, contribute little to coordinating plans and sharing, and their integration is weak [254, 255]. These issues are highlighted because disparate sectors may have distinct goals and policies, which can lead to conflicts and impede cooperation with others. A lack of trust among collaborative partners may arise during OH initiatives. A study has shown the experience of Indians in weak and redundant response systems that have resulted from failure to support the connections between the health of humans and animals and the environment [256].

A lack of policies that support and coordinate the program has hampered the implementation of OH programs. An analysis of Ethiopia's OH strategy, for example, revealed that a significant obstacle is the commitment of the higher government and the leadership's shortcomings [255]. The requirement for more precise regulation regarding public–private partnerships' involvement with OH was also mentioned in the Ethiopian study. Furthermore, in many low-resource nations, such as some African countries, there are frequently no PH systems in place to direct the implementation of OH. This makes the implementation of OH difficult for the sectors involved. There are limited fund sources available for OH programs because of the longer extended period it takes for the OH to reach the surface. Many governments are hesitant to fund projects.

Different sectors of OH require capacity building to carry out their projects, which they do in different ways. The development of competent people at all levels is crucial as part of capacity building, but it is insufficient [257]. Most countries invest more in human health than animal or environmental health [256], which contributes to the lack of resources in these sectors, causing recent outbreaks of zoonotic diseases and other OH issues. Furthermore, there is limited knowledge of OH in some parts of the world [258], which might pose challenges in implementing OH in such regions.

6.7.2 Strategies for Overcoming Challenges

6.7.2.1 Exemplary Governance and Leadership

For OH interventions to be easily implemented, strong upper-level governance and leadership are essential. Policies that permit a multisectoral approach to topics of relevance for all sectors are the foundation for the effectiveness of OH interventions. Governments must offer the required policy support for the successful implementation of OH solutions. Policies should encourage cooperation and collaboration among all sectors while concentrating on enhancing the health of people, animals, and the environment. To improve coordination, it is necessary to develop strategic papers and operationalize the OH secretariat in government parastatals. OH-related contemplation, orientation, and planning were made easier by the availability of reference framework papers and programs. Finding dynamic technical working groups inside a high-level platform can facilitate the adoption of OH strategies. India has institutionalized collaboration frameworks to adopt an OH strategy for disease prevention and management because of its experience with emerging illnesses such as Ebola and avian influenza [256].

6.7.2.2 Good Teamwork and Coordination

Successful OH implementation depends on the ability to coordinate and collaborate effectively at all scales, within and across sectors. This is in line with prior reviews, which reported that joint meetings, interdisciplinary teamwork, and communication are needed to meet the challenges of global health opportunities. In Burkina Faso, a study underlines the necessity of having formal and efficient communication channels between OH sectors [259]. It is also an excellent practice to place OH as the focal point for each ministry or section. The strategy had to have adequate resources, sufficient funds, and easily available partners for finances and technological support.

6.7.2.3 Training and Capacity Building

Capacity building and training for developing a workforce with the technical skills required to implement OH initiatives successfully. For example, healthcare workers should be educated about risk assessment, environmental monitoring and the diagnosis and management of zoonotic diseases. Mentoring and technical assistance programs can be other resources to help build capacity. A study by Mbugi et al. indicated that a detailed understanding of the epidemiology of infectious diseases in both the human and animal sectors is necessary to effectively operationalize the OH approach [253]. As stated previously, workforce education and training constitute the primary means of accomplishing this goal.

6.7.2.4 Robust Collaborations and Cooperative Efforts

Partnerships and collective efforts among different stakeholders are needed and crucial. This demonstrates the effective engagement of stakeholders, who are crucial facilitators for the implementation of OH interventions in low- and middle-income countries. Engaging stakeholders across sectors has the potential to increase collaboration, build momentum, and increase the impact of interventions. The design of effective interventions, such as outbreak investigations and responses, and the identification of obstacles are made more accessible through strong collaboration and partnerships. Rwanda's experience demonstrated that foreign collaboration is very beneficial to a nation, particularly when it encompasses all industries, including PH, medicine, veterinary care, the environment, and agriculture [260]. A study from Ethiopia confirmed that the National One Health Steering Committee (NOHSC) needs the participation of all Member Ministries for Ethiopia to implement the OH policy successfully [261]. Partnerships also facilitate the exchange of information, experience, and resources, all of which help overcome challenges.

6.7.2.5 Strengthening of Diagnosing Skills and Surveillance Capabilities

Strengthening surveillance capacities and revolutionizing diagnostic labs with tools and skills are essential. Whether at the federal, provincial, or subnational level, having a robust laboratory network and an appropriate surveillance system is necessary. One of the main recommendations made at the end of the workshop on OH zoonotic disease prioritization for multisectoral engagement in Burkina Faso was to improve laboratories' ability to diagnose diseases that were prioritized for the human and animal sectors, as well as to strengthen collaboration among the three sectors involved in OH to guarantee diagnostic testing. The OH strategy is quickly institutionalized through awareness of OH and leaders collaborating across sectors and faculties.

6.7.2.6 Financial Assistance

In developing nations, financial support can play a crucial role in facilitating the implementation of OH. An increased number of fund allocations are required for OH programs in several low- and middle-income nations. With respect to a Tanzanian evaluation, OH offers collaborative global health projects the chance to utilize resources more efficiently than if they were just focused on one area [253]. International organizations and donor agencies can close this funding gap and supply the resources required to carry out OH projects successfully. Sufficient funding is necessary to carry out OH initiatives successfully. As such, obtaining adequate funding sources is essential. All sectors engaged in OH activities should obtain sufficient allocation of financial resources. The assistance of financial and technical partners will aid in addressing the budget shortfall.

6.8 Conclusion

The increasing prevalence of animal diseases, emerging infectious diseases, and AMR require greater use of the OH approach. The "One Health" concept embraces the complex relationships among animals, humans, and environmental health and the need for multilateral cooperation to control critical PH issues. Opportunities such as partnerships and public awareness support the OH approach to maximize its use of ongoing challenges such as governance, insufficient resources, and awareness. The interdisciplinary nature of the OH approach is critical to providing a long-term, safe, healthy environment for all. The lack of knowledge and comprehension of OH ideas among stakeholders are one of the most significant challenges impeding the teamwork needed to handle complicated PH concerns. Nevertheless, there are several important drivers, such as increasing the general understanding of OH and fostering excellent communication and collaboration among many stakeholders, such as PH experts, veterinarians, environmentalists, legislators, and the general public. The provision of infrastructure and funds is crucial to fostering multidisciplinary research and education and international collaboration to address global health concerns.

Abbreviations

AIDS: Acquired Immune Deficiency Syndrome; AMR: Antimicrobial Resistance; ASF: African Swine Fever; CCDC: Chinese Center for Disease Control and Prevention; CDC: Centers for Disease Control and Prevention; CHIKV: Chikungunya Virus; CHIKVD: Chikungunya Virus Disease; CHWs: Community Health Workers; CICICE: Community Information, Consultation, Involvement, Collaboration, and Empowerment; COVID-19: Coronavirus Disease 19; DF: Dengue Fever; DENVs: Dengue Viruses; DHF: Dengue Hemorrhagic Fever; dsDNA: Double-stranded DNA; DSS: Dengue Shock Syndrome; EVD: Ebola Virus Disease; EZDs: Emergence of Zoonotic Diseases; FAO: Food and Agricultural Organization; GDP: Gross Domestic Product; GLEWS: Global Early Warning System; HiAPs: Health Implications in the All-policies; HIV: Human Immunodeficiency Virus; hMPV: Human Metapneumovirus; HPAI: Highly Pathogenic Avian Influenza; HUS: Hemolytic Uremic Syndrome; IHRs: International Health Regulations; IPC: Infection Prevention and Control; IPCC: Intergovernmental Panel on Climate Change; MERS-CoV: Middle East Respiratory Syndrome Coronavirus; Mpox: Monkeypox; MPXV: Monkeypox Virus; MS-SDSS: Multistakeholder Spatial Decision Support System; NGOs: Nongovernmental Organizations; NOHSC: National One Health Steering Committee; NTSs: Nontyphoidal *Salmonella* Serovars; OH: One Health; OIE: Office International des Epizooties; OPXV: Orthopoxvirus; PH: Public Health; PIP: Pandemic influenza preparedness; RSV: Respiratory Syncytial Virus; RT-LAMP: Reverse Transcription Loop-Mediated Isothermal Amplification Reaction; RT-PCR: Reverse Transcription Polymerase Chain Reaction; RT-qPCR: Real-Time Quantitative Reverse Transcription Polymerase Chain Reaction; RVF: Rift Valley Fever; SARS: Severe Acute Respiratory Syndrome; SDGs: Sustainable Development Goals; UNEP: United Nations Environment Program; UNESCO: United Nations Educational, Scientific and Cultural Organization; UNICEF: United Nations International Children Emergency Fund; USA: United States of America; WHO: World Health Organization; WNF: West Nile fever; WNV: West Nile virus; WOAH: World Organization for Animal Health.

Author Contributions

Conceptualization and outline preparation: D.H.; Data collection and curation: D.H., S.I.S., D.J.A., C.F.E., R.O.A., O.G.B., and O.A.O.; Figure preparation: D.H., and D.J.A.; Figures 6.1–6.3 were created with Biorender.com; Table preparation: S.I.S., D.J.A., R.O.A., C.F.E., and D.H.; Supervision: D.H.; Validation: D.H., R.O.A., D.J.A., C.F.E., S.I.S., and S.Z.T.B. Writing- original draft preparation: D.H., S.I.S., D.J.A., C.F.E., R.O.A., O.A.O., O.G.B., and S.Z.T.B. Writing-review and editing: D.H., D.J.A., R.O.A., C.F.E., F.U., and S.Z.T.B. All authors contributed to the book chapter and approved the submitted version for publication.

Conflicts of Interest

The authors declare that they have no conflicts of interest.

References

1 WHO. *Zoonoses*. 2020. https://www.who.int/news-room/fact-sheets/detail/zoonoses (accessed 30 August 2024).

2 Weiss, R.A. and Sankaran, N. Emergence of epidemic diseases: zoonoses and other origins. *Fac. Rev*. 2022; 11. https://doi.org/10.12703/r/11-2.

3 Rahman, M.T., Sobur, M.A., Islam, M.S., et al. Zoonotic diseases: etiology, impact, and control. *Microbe*. 2020; 8(9): 1405. https://doi.org/10.3390/microorganisms8091405.

4 Milbank, C. and Vira, B. Wildmeat consumption and zoonotic spillover: contextualising disease emergence and policy responses. *Lancet Planet. Health*. 2022; 6(5): e439–e448, https://doi.org/10.1016/S2542-5196(22)00064-X.

5 Arámbulo, P.V. and Thakur, A.S. Impact of Zoonoses in tropical America *Ann. N.Y. Acad. Sci.* 1992; 653(1): 6–18. https://doi.org/10.1111/j.1749-6632.1992.tb19624.x.

6 Mofijur, M., Fattah, I.M.R., Alam, M.A., et al. Impact of COVID-19 on the social, economic, environmental and energy domains: lessons learnt from a global pandemic. *Sustain. Prod. Consum.* 2021; 26: 343–359. https://doi.org/10.1016/j.spc.2020.10.016.

7 Valensisi, G. COVID-19 and Global poverty: are LDCs being left behind?. *Eur. J. Dev. Res.* 2020; 32(5): 1535–1557. https://doi.org/10.1057/s41287-020-00314-8.

8 Chlebicz, A. and Śliżewska, K. Campylobacteriosis, salmonellosis, yersiniosis, and listeriosis as zoonotic foodborne diseases: a review. *Int. J. Environ. Res. Public Health*. 2018; 15(5): 863. https://doi.org/10.3390/ijerph15050863.

9 Denkyira, S.A., Adesola, R.O., Idris, I., et al. Marburg virus in ghana: a public health threat to Ghanaians and to Africans. *Public Health Chall.* 2022; 1(4). https://doi.org/10.1002/puh2.32.

10 Akinsulie, O.C., Adesola, R.O., Aliyu, V.A., et al. Epidemiology and transmission dynamics of viral encephalitides in West Africa. *Infect. Dis. Rep.* 2023; 15(5): 504–517. https://doi.org/10.3390/idr15050050.

11 Akinsulie, O.C., Adesola, R.O., Bakre, A., et al. Usutu virus: an emerging flavivirus with potential threat to public health in Africa: Nigeria as a case study. *Front. Vet. Sci.* 2023; 10. https://doi.org/10.3389/fvets.2023.1115501.

12 Adesola, R.O., Okeke, V.C., Hamzat, A., et al. Unraveling the binational outbreak of anthrax in Ghana and Nigeria: an in-depth investigation of epidemiology, clinical presentations, diagnosis, and plausible recommendations toward its eradication in Africa. *Bull. Natl. Res. Cent.* 2024; 48(1): 45. https://doi.org/10.1186/s42269-024-01203-4.

13 Adesola, R.O., Akinniyi, H.T., and Lucero-Prisno. D.E., et al. An evaluation of the impact of anti-rabies programs in Nigeria. *Ann. Med. Surg.* 2023; 85(2): 358–364. https://doi.org/10.1097/MS9.0000000000000250.

14 Ogunleye, S.C., Akinsulie, O.C., Aborode, A.T., et al. Chinyere. The re-emergence and transmission of Monkeypox virus in Nigeria: the role of one health. *Front. Public Health* 2024; 11. https://doi.org/10.3389/fpubh.2023.1334238.

15 Sinclair, J.R. Importance of a One Health approach in advancing global health security and the sustainable development goals. *Rev. Sci. Tech. OIE*. 2019; 38(1): 145–154. https://doi.org/10.20506/rst.38.1.2949.

16 WHO, FAO, and WOAH. *Taking a Multisectoral, One Health Approach: A Tripartite Guide to Addressing Zoonotic Diseases in Countries*. 2019. https://iris.who.int/handle/10665/325620 (accessed 30 August 2024).

17 Kaneene, J.B. Miller, R.A. Kaplan, B.J. et al. Preventing and controlling zoonotic tuberculosis: a one health approach. *Vet. Ital.* 2014; 50(1): 7–22. https://doi.org/10.12834/VetIt.1302.08.

18 Barratt, A.S., Rich, K.M., Eze, J.I., et al. Framework for estimating indirect costs in animal health using time series analysis. *Front. Vet. Sci.* 2019; 6(JUN). https://doi.org/10.3389/fvets.2019.00190.

19 Jones, K.E., Patel, N.G., Levy, M.A., et al. Global trends in emerging infectious diseases. *Nature* 2008; 451(7181): 990–993. https://doi.org/10.1038/nature06536.

20 Taylor, L.H., Latham, S.M., and Woolhouse. J., Risk factors for human disease emergence. *Philos. Trans. R. Soc. B, Biol. Sci.* 2001; 356(1411): 983–989. https://doi.org/10.1098/rstb.2001.0888.

21 Narrod, C., Zinsstag J., and Tiongco. M. One health framework for estimating the economic costs of zoonotic diseases on society. *EcoHealth* 2012; 9(2): 150–162. https://doi.org/10.1007/s10393-012-0747-9.

22 Poorolajal. J. Geographical distribution of COVID-19 cases and deaths worldwide. *J. Res. Health Sci.* 2020; 20(3): 1–2. https://doi.org/10.34172/jrhs.2020.24.

23 Graziosi, G., Lupini, C., Catelli, E., and Carnaccini. S. Highly pathogenic avian influenza (HPAI) H5 clade 2.3. 4.4 b virus infection in birds and mammals. *Animals* 2024; 14(9): 1372. https://doi.org/10.3390/ani14091372.

24 Seimenis, A. and Battelli, G. Main challenges in the control of zoonoses and related foodborne diseases in the south mediterranean and middle east region. *Vet. Ital.* 2018; 54(2): 97–106. https://doi.org/10.12834/VetIt.1340.7765.1.

25 Li, G., Zhang, Y., He, H.-L., et al. Evolution and distribution of rabies viruses from a panorama view. *Microbiol. Spectr.* 2023; 11(5): 1–15. https://doi.org/10.1128/spectrum.05257-22.

26 Khetarpal, N. and Khanna. I. Dengue fever: causes, complications, and vaccine Strategies. *J. Immunol. Res.* 2016; 2016(3). https://doi.org/10.1155/2016/6803098.

27 Dauphin, G., Zientara, S., Zeller, H., and Murgue, B. West Nile: worldwide current situation in animals and humans. *Comp. Immunol. Microbiol. Infect. Dis.* 2004; 27(5): 343–355. https://doi.org/10.1016/j.cimid.2004.03.009.

28 Van Den Hurk, S. and Velayudhan. B.T. Rift valley fever, an emerging viral zoonosis worthy of increased attention. *J. Biomed. Res. Environ. Sci.* 2024; 5(4): 312–320. https://doi.org/10.37871/jbres1898.

29 Rekik, S., Hammami, I., Timoumi, O., et al. A review on Crimean–Congo hemorrhagic fever infections in Tunisia. *Vector-Borne and Zoonotic Dis.* 2024; 24(6). https://doi.org/10.1089/vbz.2023.0079.

30 Wang, Z., Wang, P., and An. Zika, J. virus and Zika fever. *Virol. Sin.* 2016; 31(2): 103–109. https://doi.org/10.1007/s12250-016-3780-y.

31 Aditi, and Shariff, M. Nipah virus infection: a review. *Epidemiol. Infect.* 2019; 147: 1–6. https://doi.org/10.1017/S0950268819000086.

32 Constant, L.E.C., Rajsfus, B.F., Carneiro, P.H.T., et al. Overview on Chikungunya Virus infection: from epidemiology to state-of-the-art experimental models. *Front. Microbiol.* 2021; 12(October): 1–20. https://doi.org/10.3389/fmicb.2021.744164.

33 Laidlow, T.A., Stafford, R., Jennison, A.V., et al. A multi-jurisdictional outbreak of salmonella typhimurium infections linked to backyard poultry—Australia, 2020. *Zoonoses Public Health.* 2022; 69(7): 835–842. https://doi.org/10.1111/zph.12973.

34 Feng, Y., He, T., Zhang, B., et al. Epidemiology and diagnosis technologies of human metapneumovirus in China: a mini review. *Virol. J.* 21(1): 59, 2024. https://doi.org/10.1186/s12985-024-02327-9.

35 WHO. Human metapneumovirus (hMPV) infection. *World Health Organization (WHO).* 2025. https://www.who.int/news-room/questions-and-answers/item/human-metapneumovirus-(hmpv)-infection (accessed 14 January 2025).

36 Tan, T., Heller, J., Firestone, S., et al. A systematic review of global Q fever outbreaks. *One Health* 2024; 18(December 2023). https://doi.org/10.1016/j.onehlt.2023.100667.

37 Amin, S., Mahmood, H., and Zorab. H. Ch. 13: Campylobacteriosis. In: *One Health Triad*, 2 (ed. R. Abbas, N. Saeed, M. Younus, L. AguilarMarcelino, and A. Khan), 87–93, Unique Scientific Publisher; 2023. https://doi.org/10.47278/book.oht/2023.46.

38 Bilal, S., Iqbal, M., Murphy, P., and Power. J. Human bovine tuberculosis - remains in the differential. *J. Med. Microbiol.* 2010; 59(11): 1379–1382. https://doi.org/10.1099/jmm.0.020511-0.

39 Suganya, T., Packiavathy, I.A.S.V., Aseervatham, G.S.B., et al. Tackling multiple-drug-resistant bacteria with conventional and complex phytochemicals. *Front. Cell. Infect. Microbiol.* 2022; 12(June): 1–21. https://doi.org/10.3389/fcimb.2022.883839.

40 Lamichhane, B., Mawad, A.M.M., Saleh, M., et al. Salmonellosis: an overview of epidemiology, pathogenesis, and innovative approaches to mitigate the antimicrobial resistant infections. *Antibiotics.* 2024; 13(1). https://doi.org/10.3390/antibiotics13010076.

41 Piotrowski, M. and Rymaszewska, A. Expansion of tick-borne rickettsioses in the world. *Microorganisms.* 2020; 8(12): 1906. https://doi.org/10.3390/microorganisms8121906.

42 Steverding. D. The history of leishmaniasis. *Parasit. Vectors.* 2017; 10(1): 1–10. https://doi.org/10.1186/s13071-017-2028-5.

43 Saadatnia, G. and Golkar, M. A review on human toxoplasmosis. *Scand. J. Infect. Dis.* 2012; 44(11): 805–814. https://doi.org/10.3109/00365548.2012.693197.

44 Xiao, L. and Feng, Y. Zoonotic cryptosporidiosis. *FEMS Microbiol. Immunol.* 2008; 52(3): 309–323. https://doi.org/10.1111/j.1574-695X.2008.00377.x.

45 Desquesnes, M., Dargantes, A., Lai, D.H., et al. Trypanosoma evansi and surra: a review and perspectives on transmission, epidemiology and control, impact, and zoonotic aspects. *Biomed Res. Int.* 2013; 2013. https://doi.org/10.1155/2013/321237.

46 Moskaluk, A.E. and VandeWoude, S. Current topics in dermatophyte classification and clinical diagnosis. *Pathogens.* 2022; 11(9), 2022. https://doi.org/10.3390/pathogens11090957.

47 Rizwan, M., Imran, M.M., Irshad, H., et al. Aspergillosis: an occupational zoonotic disease. *International Journal of Agriculture and Biosciences.* 2023; (Zoonosis Volume 4): 380–391. https://doi.org/10.47278/book.zoon/2023.163.

48 Pal, M. and Dave. P. Crptococcosis: a global fungal zoonosis. *Intas Polivet* 2006; 7: 412–420. Cryptococcosis_A_global_fungal_zoonosis.pdf.

49 Benedict, K. and Mody, R.K. Epidemiology of histoplasmosis outbreaks, United States, 1938–2013. *Emerg. Infect. Dis.* 2016; 22(3): 370–378. https://doi.org/10.3201/eid2203.151117.

50 Petersen, L.R. and Powers, A.M. Chikungunya: epidemiology. *F1000Research.* 2016; 5: 1–8. https://doi.org/10.12688/f1000research.7171.1.

51 Das, G.K. Effects of Deforestation and climate change for zoonosis like coronavirus crisis. *Frontier* 2020; 20–21. https://www.frontierweekly.com/views/dec-20/21-12-20-Effects%20of%20Deforestation%20and%20Climate%20Change.html.

52 Adesola, R.O., Opuni, E., Idris, I., et al. Navigating Nigeria's health landscape: population growth and its health implications. *Environ. Health Insights.* 2024; 18: 11786302241250212. https://doi.org/10.1177/11786302241250211.

53 Naicker, P.R. The impact of climate change and other factors on zoonotic diseases. *Arch. Clin. Microbiol.* 2011; 2(2): 4. https://doi.org/10:3823/226.

54 Eisenstein. M. Disease: Poverty and pathogens. *Nature* 2016; 531(7594): S61–S63. https://doi.org/10.1038/531S61a.

55 Marie, V. and Gordon. M.L. The (re-) emergence and spread of viral zoonotic disease: a perfect storm of human ingenuity and stupidity. *Viruses* 2023; 15(8): 1638. https://doi.org/10.3390/v15081638.

56 Sheikh, P.A. and O'Regan, K.C. *Wildlife Trade, COVID-19, and Other Zoonotic Diseases. Congressional Research Service.* 2021. https://www.everycrsreport.com/reports/IF11494.html (accessed 30 August 2024).

57 Bloomfield, L.S.P., McIntosh, and E. F. Lambin. Habitat fragmentation, livelihood behaviors, and contact between people and nonhuman primates in Africa. *Landsc. Ecol.* 2020; 35(4): 985–1000. https://doi.org/10.1007/s10980-020-00995-w.

58 Kock, R. and Caceres-Escobar, H. *Situation Analysis on the Roles and Risks of Wildlife in the Emergence of Human Infectious Diseases.* Gland, Switzerland: International Union for Conservation of Nature (IUCN); 2022. https://doi.org/10.2305/IUCN.CH.2022.01.en.

59 Wolfe, N.D., Dunavan, C.P., and Diamond, J. Origins of major human infectious diseases. *Nature* 2007; 447(7142): 279–283. https://doi.org/10.1038/nature05775.

60 Jiang, X., Fan, Z., Li, S., and Yin, H. A review on zoonotic pathogens associated with non-human primates: understanding the potential threats to humans. *Microorganisms.* 2023; 11(2): 246. https://doi.org/10.3390/microorganisms11020246.

61 Rupasinghe, R., Chomel, B.B., and Martínez-López. B. Climate change and zoonoses: a review of the current status, knowledge gaps, and future trends. *Acta Tropica* 226: 106225, 2022. https://doi.org/10.1016/j.actatropica.2021.106225.

62 Manzoor, A. and Adesola. R.O. Disaster in public health due to flood in Pakistan in 2022. *Health Sci. Rep.* 2022; 5(6): e903. https://doi.org/10.1002/hsr2.903.

63 Mora, C., McKenzie, T., Gaw, I.M., et al. Over half of known human pathogenic diseases can be aggravated by climate change. *Nat. Clim. Chang.* 2022; 12(9): 869–875. https://doi.org/10.1038/s41558-022-01426-1.

64 Chowdhury, S., Aleem, M.A., Khan, M.S.I., et al. Major zoonotic diseases of public health importance in Bangladesh. *Vet. Med. Sci.* 2021; 7(4): 1199–1210. https://doi.org/10.1002/vms3.465.

65 Mosaad, Z., Elhusseiny, M.H., Zanaty, A.M., et al. Emergence of highly pathogenic avian influenza a virus (H5N1) of clade 2.3. 4.4 b in Egypt, 2021–2022. *Pathogens* 2023 12(1): 90. https://doi.org/10.3390/pathogens12010090.

66 Burrough, E.R., Magstadt, D.R., Petersen, B., et al. Highly pathogenic avian influenza A (H5N1) clade 2.3. 4.4 b virus infection in domestic dairy cattle and cats, United States, 2024. *Emerg. Infect. Dis.* 2024; 30(7): 1335–1343. https://doi.org/10.3201/eid3007.240508.

67 Hu, B., Guo, H., Zhou, P., and Shi, Z. L. Characteristics of SARS-CoV-2 and COVID-19. *Nat. Rev. Microbiol.* 2021; 19(3): 141–154. https://doi.org/10.1038/s41579-020-00459-7.

68 Krammer, F. The role of vaccines in the COVID-19 pandemic: what have we learned? *Semin Immunopathol.* 2023; 45(4): 451–468. https://doi.org/10.1007/s00281-023-00996-2.

69 WHO. WHO COVID-19 dashboard. *World Health Organization (WHO).* https://data.who.int/dashboards/covid19/cases?n=c (accessed 25 July 25 2024).

70 Temmam, S., Vongphayloth, K., Baquero, E., et al. Bat coronaviruses related to SARS-CoV-2 and infectious for human cells. *Nature* 2022; 604(7905): 330–336. https://doi.org/10.1038/s41586-022-04532-4.

71 Ciotti, M., Ciccozzi, M., Terrinoni, A., et al. The COVID-19 pandemic. *Crit. Rev. Clin. Lab. Sci.* 2020; 57(6): 365–388. https://doi.org/10.1080/10408363.2020.1783198.

72 Sinha, S., Singh, K., Ravi Kumar, Y.S., et al. Dengue virus pathogenesis and host molecular machineries. *J. Biomed. Sci.* 2024, 31(1): 1–24. https://doi.org/10.1186/s12929-024-01030-9.

73 Laverdeur, J., Desmecht, D., Hayette, M.-P., and Darcis, G. Dengue and chikungunya: future threats for Northern Europe?. *Front. Epidemiol.* 2024; 4(January): 1–8. https://doi.org/10.3389/fepid.2024.1342723.

74 CDC. Mpox in the Democratic Republic of the Congo - Level 2 - Level 2 - Practice Enhanced Precautions - Travel Health Notices I Travelers' Health I CDC. *Centers for Disease Control and Prevention (CDC).* 2024. https://wwwnc.cdc.gov/travel/notices/level2/monkeypox-democratic-republic-of-congo (accessed 25 July 2024).

75 Saba Villarroel, P.M., Gumpangseth, N., Songhong, T., et al. Emerging and re-emerging zoonotic viral diseases in Southeast Asia: one health challenge. *Front. Public Health.* 2023; 11(June): 1–14. https://doi.org/10.3389/fpubh.2023.1141483.

76 Galán-Relaño, Á., Valero Díaz, A., Huerta Lorenzo, B., et al. Salmonella and salmonellosis: an update on public health implications and control strategies. *Animals* 13(23): 3666, 2023. https://doi.org/10.3390/ani13233666.

77 Nichols, M., Gollarza, L.A., Palacios, A., et al. Salmonella illness outbreaks linked to backyard poultry purchasing during the COVID-19 pandemic: united States, 2020. *Epidemiol. Infect.* 2021; 149(December): 10–12. https://doi.org/10.1017/S0950268821002132.

78 Euronews. What is HMPV, the respiratory virus spreading across China, and should we be worried about it?. *Euronews* https://www.euronews.com/health/2025/01/07/what-is-hmpv-the-respiratory-virus-straining-healthcare-systems-in-china (accessed 14 January 2025).

79 Yang, C.F., Wang, C.K., Tollefson, S.J.R., et al. Genetic diversity and evolution of human metapneumovirus fusion protein over twenty years. *Virol. J.* 6(1): 138, 2009. https://doi.org/10.1186/1743-422X-6-138.

80 Jesse, S.T. Ludlow, M. and Osterhaus, A.D.M.E. Zoonotic origins of human metapneumovirus: a journey from birds to humans. *Viruses* 2022; 14(4): 677. https://doi.org/10.3390/v14040677.

81 Li, J., Wang, Z., Gonzalez, R., et al. Prevalence of human metapneumovirus in adults with acute respiratory tract infection in Beijing, China. *J. Infect.* 2012; 64(1): 96–103. https://doi.org/10.1016/j.jinf.2011.10.011.

82 Van Den Bergh, A., Bailly, B., Guillon, P., et al. Antiviral strategies against human metapneumovirus: targeting the fusion protein. *Antiviral Res.* 2022; 207: 105405. https://doi.org/10.1016/j.antiviral.2022.105405.

83 Gavi. Everything you need to know about human metapneumovirus (HMPV). *Gavi, the Vaccine Alliance.* https://www.gavi.org/vaccineswork/everything-you-need-know-about-human-metapneumovirus-hmpv (accessed 14 January 2025).

84 BBC. What is HMPV and how does it Spread?. *British Broadcasting Corporation (BBC)*. https://www.bbc.com/news/articles/c23vjg7v7k0o (accessed 14 January 2025).

85 Nytimes. What We Know About HMPV, the Common Virus Spreading in China. *The New York Times*. https://www.nytimes.com/2025/01/07/health/hmpv-virus-china.html (accessed 14 January 2025).

86 Hindustan Times. China Steps up Monitoring of Emerging Respiratory Diseases: Report. *Hindustan Times*. https://www.hindustantimes.com/world-news/china-battles-new-mystery-virus-outbreak-five-years-after-covid-pandemic-101735892326018.html (accessed 14 January 2025).

87 CDC. About Human Metapneumovirus. *Centers for Disease Control and Prevention (CDC)*. https://www.cdc.gov/human-metapneumovirus/about/index.html (accessed 14 January 2025).

88 Newsweek. HMPV Outbreak: Full List of Countries With Reported Cases. Newsweek. https://www.newsweek.com/hmpv-outbreak-countries-china-malaysia-india-kazakhstan-2010210 (accessed 14 January 2025).

89 PNA. *DOH reports 284 HMPV Cases in 2024; Monitors Respiratory Virus Trends*. Philippine News Agency. https://www.pna.gov.ph/articles/1241281 (accessed 14 January 2025).

90 Ancheta. Two Cases of HMPV Confirmed in Romania! INSP Recommendations. *Ancheta Online, Romania*. https://anchetaonline.ro/doua-cazuri-de-hmpv-confirmate-in-romania-recomandarile-insp-211445/ (accessed 14 January 2025).

91 Aljazeera. What is HMPV, the Respiratory Virus Surging in China?. *Aljazeera*. https://www.aljazeera.com/news/2025/1/8/what-is-hmpv-the-respiratory-virus-surging-in-china (accessed 14 January 2025).

92 Dailymail. Nearly 28,000 Americans Caught HMPV Virus Last Year... here's Where Infections are Highest and how to Stay Safe. *Daily Mail, UK*. https://www.dailymail.co.uk/health/article-14271789/americans-chinese-hmpv-infections-rates-highest-stay-safe.html (accessed 14 January 2025).

93 ACDC. Australia Monitoring International Increases in Human Metapneumovirus (hMPV). *Australian Centre for Disease Control (ACDC)*. https://www.cdc.gov.au/newsroom/news-and-articles/australia-monitoring-international-increases-human-metapneumovirus-hmpv (accessed 14 January 2025).

94 Daily Star. HMPV Detected in Bangladesh. *The Daily Star*. https://www.thedailystar.net/health/disease/news/hmpv-detected-bangladesh-3797571 (accessed 14 January 2025).

95 WHO. Trends of Acute Respiratory Infection, Including Human Metapneumovirus, in the Northern Hemisphere. *World Health Organization (WHO)*. https://www.who.int/emergencies/disease-outbreak-news/item/2025-DON550 (accessed 14 January 2025).

96 EuroWeekly. What you need to know about the HMPV Virus in China. *Euro Weekly News, Spain*. https://euroweeklynews.com/2025/01/09/what-you-need-to-know-about-the-hmpv-virus-in-china/ (accessed 14 January 2025).

97 Astrazeneca. AstraZeneca to Acquire Icosavax, Including Potential First-in-Class RSV and hMPV Combination Vaccine with Positive Phase II data. *Astrazeneca*. https://www.astrazeneca.com/media-centre/press-releases/2023/astrazeneca-to-acquire-icosavax-including-potential-first-in-class-rsv-and-hmpv-combination-vaccine-with-positive-phase-ii-data.html (accessed 14 January 2025).

98 Sharan, M., Vijay, D., Yadav, J.P., et al. Surveillance and response strategies for zoonotic diseases: a comprehensive review. *Sci. One Health* 2023; 2: 100050. https://doi.org/10.1016/j.soh.2023.100050.

99 Bhatia, R. and Narain. J.P. The challenge of emerging zoonoses in Asia Pacific. *Asia Pac. J. Public Health* 2010; 22(4): 388–394. https://doi.org/10.1177/1010539510370908.

100 World Bank. Project Appraisal Document on a Proposed Loan in the Amount of US$220 million. *World Bank* https://documents1.worldbank.org/curated/en/997191468194073921/pdf/37292.pdf (accessed 25 July 2024).

101 Clemente-Suárez, V.J., Navarro-Jiménez, E., Moreno-Luna, L., et al. The impact of the covid-19 pandemic on social, health, and economy. *Sustainability (Switzerland)*. 2021; 13(11): 1–25. https://doi.org/10.3390/su13116314.

102 Donthu, N. and Gustafsson. A. Effects of COVID-19 on business and research. *J. Bus. Res.* 2020; 117(June): 284–289. https://doi.org/10.1016/j.jbusres.2020.06.008.

103 Ghareeb, O.A. Ebola-A fatal emerging zoonotic disease: a review. *Ann. Rom. Soc. Cell Biol.* 2021; 25(6): 8748–8754.

104 Ray, A.S. and Bhattacharya, K. An overview on the zoonotic Aspects of *COVID-19*. *Proc. Natl. Acad. Sci. India Sect. B Biol. Sci.* 2024; 94(1): 9–13. https://doi.org/10.1007/s40011-023-01445-8.

105 Oluwarinde, B. Ajose, O.D.J. Abolarinwa, T.O.P. et al. Safety properties of escherichia coli O157: H7 specific bacteriophages: recent advances for food safety. *Foods* 2023; 12(21): 3989. https://doi.org/10.3390/foods12213989.

106 Kazim, A. One health: an interconnected approach to human, animal, and environmental health. *Int. J. Res. Anal. Rev.* 2023; 10(3).

107 JPA Health. One World, One Health: Exploring the Connectability between Human, Animal and Environmental Health. *JPA Health.* https://jpa.com/wp-content/uploads/2023/11/one-world-one-health-nov-2023.pdf. (accessed 25 July 2024).

108 Erkyihun, G.A. and Alemayehu, M.B. One health approach for the control of zoonotic diseases. *Zoonoses* 2022; 2(1): 37. https://doi.org/10.15212/ZOONOSES-2022-0037.

109 Africa CDC. One Health Program. *Africa Centers for Disease Control and Prevention (Africa CDC).* https://africacdc.org/programme/surveillance-disease-intelligence/one-health/ (accessed 25 July 2024).

110 CDC. About One Health. *Centers for Disease Control and Prevention* (CDC). https://www.cdc.gov/one-health/about/ (accessed 25 July 2024).

111 Steele, S.G., Toribio, J.-A., Booy, R., and Mor. S.M. What makes an effective One Health clinical practitioner? opinions of Australian one health experts. *One Health* 2019; 8: 100108. https://doi.org/10.1016/j.onehlt.2019.100108.

112 Lebov, J., Grieger, K., Womack, D., et al. A framework for one health research. *One Health* 2017; 3: 44–50. https://doi.org/10.1016/j.onehlt.2017.03.004.

113 Ajose, D.J., Abolarinwa, T.O., Oluwarinde, B.O., et al. Application of plant-derived nanoparticles (PDNP) in food-producing animals as a bio-control agent against antimicrobial-resistant pathogens. *Biomedicines* 2022; 10(10): 2426. https://doi.org/10.3390/biomedicines10102426.

114 Moore, J.H., Gibson, L. Amir, Z.W. The rise of hyperabundant native generalists threatens both humans and nature. *Biol. Rev.* 2023; 98(5): 1829–1844. https://doi.org/10.1111/brv.12985.

115 El-Ansary, H. Perspectives on the interconnectedness of human, animal, and environmental health. *Routledge Handbook of Climate Change and Health System Sustainability.* 2024. https://doi.org/10.4324/9781032701196.

116 Esha, E.J., Fazilani, S.A., Ghosh, S.I., et al. Addressing emerging zoonotic diseases through a one health approach: challenges opportunities. *Zoonosis, USP, Faisalabad.* 2023; 1: 156–167. https://doi.org/10.47278/book.zoon/2023.011.

117 Shoaib, M., Xu, J., Meng, X., et al. Molecular epidemiology and characterization of antimicrobial-resistant Staphylococcus haemolyticus strains isolated from dairy cattle milk in Northwest, China. *Front. Cell. Infect. Microbiol.* 2023; 13. https://doi.org/10.3389/fcimb.2023.1183390.

118 Dasgupta, R., Tomley, F., Alders, R., et al. Adopting an intersectoral One Health approach in India: time for one health committees. *Indian J. Med. Res.*. 2021; 153(3). https://journals.lww.com/ijmr/fulltext/2021/03000/adopting_an_intersectoral_one_health_approach_in.8.aspx

119 Alonso Aguirre, A., Basu, N., Kahn, L.H., et al. Transdisciplinary and social-ecological health frameworks—Novel approaches to emerging parasitic and vector-borne diseases. *Parasite Epidemiol Control.* 2019; 4: e00084. https://doi.org/10.1016/j.parepi.2019.e00084.

120 Whitmee, S., Haines, A., Beyrer, C., et al. Safeguarding human health in the Anthropocene epoch: report of The Rockefeller Foundation–Lancet Commission on planetary health. *Lancet* 2015; 386(10007): 1973–2028. http://dx.doi.org/10.1016/ S0140-6736(15)60901-1.

121 Mackenzie, J.S. and Jeggo, M.H. 1st International one health congress. *EcoHealth.* 2011; 7(1): 1–2. https://doi.org/10.1007/s10393-011-0676-z.

122 WHO. Quadripartite Memorandum of Understanding (MoU) Signed for a New era of One Health Collaboration. *World Health Organization (WHO).* https://www.who.int/news/item/29-04-2022-quadripartite-memorandum-of-understanding-(mou)-signed-for-a-new-era-of-one-health-collaboration (accessed 25 July 2024).

123 Berthe, F.C.J., Bouley, T., Karesh, W.B. *One Health: Operational Framework for Strengthening Human, Animal, and Environmental Public Health Systems at their Interface.* The World Bank. 2018. http://documents.worldbank.

org/curated/en/703711517234402168/Operational-framework-forstrengthening-human-animal-and-environmental-public-health-systems-at-their-interface.

124 WHO. One Health: Approach for Action Against Neglected Tropical Diseases 2021–2030. *World Health Organization (WHO)*. https://iris.who.int/bitstream/handle/10665/351193/9789240042414-eng.pdf?sequence=1#:~:text=The%20approach%20mobilizes%20multiple%20sectors,action%20on%20climate%20change%2C%20and (accessed 25 July 2024).

125 WHO. Ending the Neglect to Attain the Sustainable Development Goals: A Road Map for Neglected Tropical Diseases 2021–2030. *World Health Organization (WHO)*. https://www.who.int/publications/i/item/9789240010352 (accessed 25 July 2024).

126 De La Rocque, S., Caya, F., El Idrissi, A.H. et al. One Health operations: a critical component in the international health regulations monitoring and evaluation framework. *Rev. Sci. Tech.* 2019; 38(1): 303–314. doi. 10.20506/rst.38.1.2962

127 FAO-OIE-WHO. Taking a Multisectoral One Health Approach: A Tripartite Guide to Addressing Zoonotic Diseases in Countries. *Food and Agriculture Organization*, 2019. https://openknowledge.fao.org/items/870b5a92-2fc4-430e-87a9-f8086335acc6 (accessed 25 July 2024).

128 JVMA. One Health. *Japan Veterinary Medical Association (JVMA)*. https://jvma-vet.jp/en/activity/onehealth.html (accessed 25 July 2024).

129 Yasobant, S., Lekha, K.S., and Saxena, D. Risk assessment tools from the one health perspective: a narrative review. *Risk Manag. Healthc. Policy*. 2024; 17(null): 955–972. https://doi.org/10.2147/RMHP.S436385.

130 Bouchot, A. and Bordier. M. The OIE Strategy to address threats at the Interface between humans, animals and ecosystems. In: *Socio-Ecological Dimensions of Infectious Diseases in Southeast Asia* (eds. S. Morand, J.-P. Dujardin, R. Lefait-Robin, and C. Apiwathnasorn), 275–291. Singapore: Springer Singapore; 2015. https://doi.org/10.1007/978-981-287-527-3_16.

131 Alegbeleye, O.O. and Sant'Ana. A.S. Manure-borne pathogens as an important source of water contamination: an update on the dynamics of pathogen survival/transport as well as practical risk mitigation strategies *Int. J. Hyg. Environ. Health*. 2020; 227: 113524. https://doi.org/10.1016/j.ijheh.2020.113524.

132 WHO. Tool for influenza pandemic risk assessment (TIPRA). *World Health Organization (WHO)*, 2016. https://www.who.int/teams/global-influenza-programme/avian-influenza/tool-for-influenza-pandemic-risk-assessment-(tipra) (accessed 25 July 2024).

133 Burke, S.A. and Trock. S.C. Use of influenza risk assessment tool for prepandemic preparedness. *Emerg. Infect. Dis*. 2018; 24(3): 471. https://doi.org/10.3201/eid2403.171852.

134 Abutarbush, S.M., Hamdallah, A., Hawawsheh, M., et al. Implementation of one health approach in Jordan: joint risk assessment of rabies and avian influenza utilizing the tripartite operational tool. *One Health* 2022; 15: 100453. https://doi.org/10.1016/j.onehlt.2022.100453.

135 WHO. SARS-CoV-2 in animals used for fur farming: GLEWS+ risk assessment. *World Health Organization (WHO)*, 2021. https://www.who.int/publications/i/item/WHO-2019-nCoV-fur-farming-risk-assessment-2021.1 (accessed 25 July 2024).

136 Ducusin, M.J.U., de Quiroz-Castro, M., Roesel, L.C., et al. Using the world health organization measles programmatic risk assessment tool for monitoring of supplemental immunization activities in the Philippines. *Risk Anal*. 2017; 37(6): 1082–1095. doi. 10.1111/risa.12404.

137 Adlam. B. *Risk Assessment Tool (DAISY) for Emerging Human Infectious Diseases. Health Analysis and Information for Action (HAIFA)*. 2012. https://haifa.esr.cri.nz/assets/Uploads/Docs/Disease-Attribute-Intelligence-System-Tool.pdf (accessed 30 August 2024).

138 Wamala, J.F., Okot, C., Makumbi, I., et al. Assessment of core capacities for the international health regulations (IHR[2005])–Uganda, 2009. *BMC Public Health*. 2010; 10(1): S9. https://doi.org/10.1186/1471-2458-10-S1-S9.

139 Heymann, D.L., Chen, L., Takemi, K., et al. Global health security: the wider lessons from the west African Ebola virus disease epidemic. *Lancet*. 2015; 385(9980): 1884–1901. https://doi.org/10.1016/S0140-6736(15)60858-3.

140 Burci, G.L., Moon, S., Crosato Neumann, A., and Bezruki, A. *Envisioning an International Normative Framework for Pandemic Preparedness and Response: Issues, Instruments and Options*. 2021. https://www.graduateinstitute.ch/library/publications-institute/envisioning-international-normative-framework-pandemic-preparedness (accessed 30 August 2024).

141 Abubakar, A., Elkholy, A., Barakat, A., et al. Pandemic influenza preparedness (PIP) framework: progress challenges in improving influenza preparedness response capacities in the Eastern Mediterranean Region, 2014–2017. *J. Infect. Public Health*. 2020; 13(3): 446–450. Available: https://doi.org/10.1016/j.jiph.2019.03.006.

142 Johansson, M. Experience of data collection in support of the assessment of global progress in the sendai framework for disaster risk reduction 2015–2030 – a Swedish pilot study. *Int. J. Disaster Risk Reduct*. 2017; 24: 144–150. https://doi.org/10.1016/j.ijdrr.2017.06.008.

143 Ramirez-Rubio, O., Daher, C., Fanjul, G., et al. Urban health: an example of a "health in all policies" approach in the context of SDGs implementation. *Glob. Health*. 2019; 15(1): 87, 2019. https://doi.org/10.1186/s12992-019-0529-z.

144 Amri, M. Chatur, A. and O'Campo, P. An umbrella review of intersectoral and multisectoral approaches to health policy. *Soc. Sci. Med*. 2022; 315: 115469. https://doi.org/10.1016/j.socscimed.2022.115469.

145 Panneer, S., Kantamaneni, K., Pushparaj, R.R.B., et al. Multistakeholder participation in disaster Management—the case of the COVID-19 pandemic. *Healthcare, MDPI*. 2021; 9(2): 203. https://doi.org/10.3390/healthcare90 20203.

146 Injac, R. Global pandemic vaccine development, production and distribution challenges for the world population. *Int. J. Risk Saf. Med*. 2022; 33: 235–248. https://doi.org/10.3233/JRS-227019.

147 Abbas, M.N., Iqbal, W., and Khan, S. Sterile Products. In: *Essentials of Industrial Pharmacy* (ed. S.A. Khan), 177–201. Cham: Springer International Publishing; 2022. https://doi.org/10.1007/978-3-030-84977-1_11.

148 Hafez, S., Ismail, S.A., Zibwowa, Z., et al. Community interventions for pandemic preparedness: a scoping review of pandemic preparedness lessons from HIV, COVID-19, and other public health emergencies of international concern. PLOS *Glob. Public Health* 2024; 4(5): e0002758-. https://doi.org/10.1371/journal.pgph.0002758.

149 Braam, D. Zoonotic disease transmission risks in displacement. *Eur. J. Public Health*. 2020; 30(Suppl 5). https://doi.org/10.1093/eurpub/ckaa166.267.

150 Chenais, E., Boqvist, S., Sternberg-Lewerin, S., et al. knowledge, attitudes and practices related to African swine fever within smallholder pig production in Northern Uganda. *Transbound. Emerg. Dis*. 2017; 64(1): 101–115. https://doi.org/10.1111/tbed.12347.

151 Costard, S., Porphyre, V., Messad, S., et al. Multivariate analysis of management and biosecurity practices in smallholder pig farms in Madagascar. *Prev. Vet. Med*. 2009; 92(3): 199–209. https://doi.org/10.1016/j.prevetmed.2009.08.010.

152 Cappai, S. Rolesu, S. A. Coccollone, A. Laddomada, and F. Loi. Evaluation of biological and socio-economic factors related to persistence of African swine fever in Sardinia. *Prev. Vet. Med*. 2018; 152: 1–11. https://doi.org/10.1016/j.prevetmed.2018.01.004.

153 Proudfoot, K. and Habing. G. Social stress as a cause of diseases in farm animals: current knowledge and future directions. *Vet. J*. 2015; 206(1): 15–21. https://doi.org/10.1016/j.tvjl.2015.05.024.

154 Hidano, A., Enticott, G., Christley, R.M., and Gates, M.C. Modeling dynamic human behavioral changes in animal disease models: challenges and opportunities for addressing bias. *Front. Vet. Sci*. 2018; 5. https://doi.org/10.3389/fvets.2018.00137.

155 Lo, M.Y. Ngan, W.Y., Tsun, S.M., et al. A field study into Hong Kong's wet markets: raised questions into the hygienic maintenance of meat contact surfaces and the dissemination of microorganisms associated with nosocomial infections. *Front. Microbiol*. 2019; 10. https://doi.org/10.3389/fmicb.2019.02618.

156 Zachreson, C., Fair, K.M., Cliff, O.M., et al. Urbanization affects peak timing, prevalence, and bimodality of influenza pandemics in Australia: results of a census-calibrated model. *Sci. Adv.* 2018; 4(12). https://doi.org/10.1126/sciadv.aau5294.

157 Masanja, Y.L. and Van, H.T.H. Patterns of zoonotic diseases and associated socio-economic factors in tanzania: a scoping review. *Tạp chí Nghiên cứu Y học* 2022; 154(6): 108–120. https://doi.org/10.52852/tcncyh.v154i6.768.

158 Oztig, L.I. and Askin. O.E. Human mobility and coronavirus disease 2019 (COVID-19): a negative binomial regression analysis. *Public Health* 2020; 185: 364–367. https://doi.org/10.1016/j.puhe.2020.07.002.

159 Drewe, J.A. Eames, K.T.D. Madden, J.R. and Pearce G.P. Integrating contact network structure into tuberculosis epidemiology in meerkats in South Africa: Implications for control. *Prev. Vet. Med.* 2011; 101(1–2): 113–120. https://doi.org/10.1016/j.prevetmed.2011.05.006.

160 Patterson, S., Drewe, J.A., Pfeiffer, D.U., and Clutton-Brock, T.H. Social and environmental factors affect tuberculosis related mortality in wild meerkats. *J. Anim. Ecol.* 2017; 86(3): 442–450. https://doi.org/10.1111/1365-2656.12649.

161 Sutherst, R.W Global change and human vulnerability to vector-borne diseases. *Clin. Microbiol. Rev.* 2004; 17(1): 136–173. https://doi.org/10.1128/CMR.17.1.136-173.2004.

162 UNEP. *UNEP Frontiers* 2016 *Report: Emerging Issues of Environmental Concern United Nations Environment Programme, Nairobi.* United Nations Environment Program (UNEP), 2016. https://www.unep.org/resources/frontiers-2016-emerging-issues-environmental-concern.

163 Armon, R. and Cheruti, U. *Environmental Aspects of Zoonotic Diseases. Water Intelligence Online.* 11, 2012. https://doi.org/10.2166/9781780400761.

164 Brault. A.C. Changing patterns of West Nile virus transmission: altered vector competence and host susceptibility. *Vet. Res.* 2009; 40(2): 43. https://doi.org/10.1051/vetres/2009026.

165 Prata, D.N., Rodrigues, W., and Bermejo. P.H. Temperature significantly changes COVID-19 transmission in (sub) tropical cities of Brazil. *Sci. Total Environ.* 2020; 729: 138862. https://doi.org/10.1016/j.scitotenv.2020.138862.

166 Sobral, M.F.F., Duarte, G.B., da Penha Sobral, A.I.G., et al. Association between climate variables and global transmission oF SARS-CoV-2. *Sci. Total Environ.* 2020; 729: 138997. https://doi.org/10.1016/j.scitotenv.2020.138997.

167 Yao, Y., Pan, J., Liu, Z., et al. No association of COVID-19 transmission with temperature or UV radiation in Chinese cities. *Eur. Respir. J.* 2020; 55(5): 2000517. https://doi.org/10.1183/13993003.00517-2020.

168 Shi, P., Dong, Y., Yan, H., et al. Impact of temperature on the dynamics of the COVID-19 outbreak in China. *Sci. Total Environ.* 2020; 728: 138890. https://doi.org/10.1016/j.scitotenv.2020.138890.

169 Wang, L.F. and Crameri. G. Emerging zoonotic viral diseases. *Rev. Sci. Tech. de l' OIE.* 2014, 33(2): 569–581. https://doi.org/10.20506/rst.33.2.2311.

170 Caminade, C., McIntyre, K.M., and Jones, A.E. Impact of recent and future climate change on vector-borne diseases. *Ann. N.Y. Acad. Sci.* 2019; 1436(1): 157–173. https://doi.org/10.1111/nyas.13950.

171 Parkinson, A.J. Evengard, B. Semenza, J.C. et al. Climate change and infectious diseases in the Arctic: establishment of a circumpolar working group. *Int. J. Circumpolar Health* 2014; 73(1): 25163. https://doi.org/10.3402/ijch.v73.25163.

172 Waits, A., Emelyanova, A., Oksanen, A., et al. Human infectious diseases and the changing climate in the Arctic. *Environ. Int.* 2018; 121: 703–713. https://doi.org/10.1016/j.envint.2018.09.042.

173 Rocklöv, J. and Dubrow, R. Climate change: an enduring challenge for vector-borne disease prevention and control. *Nat. Immunol.* 2020; 21(5): 479–483. https://doi.org/10.1038/s41590-020-0648-y.

174 Shaman, J., Day, J.F., and Stieglitz. M. Drought-induced amplification and epidemic transmission of west nile virus in southern florida. *J. Med. Entomol.* 2005; 42(2): 134–141. https://doi.org/10.1093/jmedent/42.2.134.

175 Paull, S.H., Horton, D.E., Ashfaq M., et al. Drought and immunity determine the intensity of west nile virus epidemics and climate change impacts. *Proc. R. Soc. B Biol. Sci.* 2017; 284(1848): 20162078. https://doi.org/10.1098/rspb.2016.2078.

176 da Silva Santos, S., de Lucena, R.F.P., de Lucena Soares, H.K., et al. Use of mammals in a semi-arid region of Brazil: an approach to the use value and data analysis for conservation. *J. Ethnobiol. Ethnomed.* 2019; 15(1): 33. https://doi.org/10.1186/s13002-019-0313-4.

177 Han, L.L., Popovici, F., Alexander, J.P., et al. Risk factors for west nile virus infection and meningoencephalitis, Romania, 1996. *J. Infect. Dis.* 1999; 179(1): 230–233. https://doi.org/10.1086/314566.

178 Hubálek, Z. and Halouzka, J. West nile fever–a reemerging mosquito-borne viral disease in Europe. *Emerg. Infect. Dis.* 1999; 5(5): 643–650. https://doi.org/10.3201/eid0505.990505.

179 Okaka, F.O. and Odhiambo, B.D.O. Relationship between flooding and out break of infectious diseasesin Kenya: a review of the literature. *J. Environ. Public Health.* 2018; 2018: 1–8. https://doi.org/10.1155/2018/5452938.

180 Magouras, I., Brookes, V.J., Jori, F., et al. Emerging zoonotic diseases: should we rethink the animal–human interface?. *Front. Vet. Sci.* 2020; 7. https://doi.org/10.3389/fvets.2020.582743.

181 Hossain, D., Ghosh, S., Uddin, N., et al. Individual-level preventive measures during the first wave of COVID-19 pandemic among Bangladeshi residents. *Microbes Infect. Chemother.* 2023; 3: e1907. https://doi.org/10.54034/mic.e1907.

182 Jori, F., Godfroid, J., Michel, A.L., et al. An assessment of zoonotic and production limiting pathogens in Rusa Deer (*Cervus timorensis rusa*) from Mauritius. *Transbound. Emerg. Dis.* 2014; 61: 31–42. https://doi.org/10.1111/tbed.12206.

183 Wang, W., Yang, L., Wronski, T., et al. Captive breeding of wildlife resources—China's revised supply-side approach to conservation. *Wildl. Soc. Bull.* 2019; 43(3): 425–435. https://doi.org/10.1002/wsb.988.

184 Patou, M.L., Chen, J., Cosson, L., et al. Low genetic diversity in the masked palm civet *Paguma larvata* (Viverridae). *J. Zool.* 2009; 278(3): 218–230. https://doi.org/10.1111/j.1469-7998.2009.00570.x.

185 Martin, L.B. Stress and immunity in wild vertebrates: timing is everything. *Gen. Comp. Endocrinol.* 2009; 163(1–2): 70–76. https://doi.org/10.1016/j.ygcen.2009.03.008.

186 Abolnik, C., Olivier, A., Reynolds, C., et al. Susceptibility and status of avian influenza in ostriches. *Avian Dis.* 2016; 60(1s): 286. https://doi.org/10.1637/11110-042815-Reg.

187 Rushton, J. Improving the use of economics in animal health – Challenges in research, policy and education. *Prev. Vet. Med.* 2017; 137: 130–139. https://doi.org/10.1016/j.prevetmed.2016.11.020.

188 Horby, P.W., Hoa, N.T., Pfeiffer, D.U., and Wertheim, H.F.L. Drivers of emerging zoonotic infectious diseases. In: *Confronting Emerging Zoonoses*, 13–26. Tokyo: Springer Japan; 2014. https://doi.org/10.1007/978-4-431-55120-1_2.

189 Daszak, P., Zambrana-Torrelio, C., Bogich, T.L., et al. Interdisciplinary approaches to understanding disease emergence: the past, present, and future drivers of Nipah virus emergence. *Proc. Natl. Acad. Sci* 2013; 110(Suppl 1): 3681–3688. https://doi.org/10.1073/pnas.1201243109.

190 Pulliam, J.R.C., Epstein, J.H., Dushoff, J., et al. Agricultural intensification, priming for persistence and the emergence of nipah virus: a lethal bat-borne zoonosis. *R. Soc. Interface.* 2012; 9(66): 89–101. https://doi.org/10.1098/rsif.2011.0223.

191 Overgaauw, P.A.M. Vinke, C.M. van Hagen, M.A.E. and Lipman. L.J.A. A one health perspective on the human–companion animal relationship with emphasis on zoonotic aspects. *Int. J. Environ. Res. Public Health* 2020; 17(11): 3789. https://doi.org/10.3390/ijerph17113789.

192 Westgarth, C., Pinchbeck, G.L., Bradshaw, J.W.S., et al. Dog-human and dog-dog interactions of 260 dog-owning households in a community in Cheshire. *Vet. Rec.*. 2008; 162(14): 436–442. https://doi.org/10.1136/vr.162.14.436.

193 Chen, Y., Liang, W., Yang, S., et al. Human infections with the emerging avian influenza A H7N9 virus from wet market poultry: clinical analysis and characterisation of viral genome. *Lancet.* 2013; 381(9881): 1916–1925. https://doi.org/10.1016/S0140-6736(13)60903-4.

194 Zhong. N. Management and prevention of SARS in China. *Philos. Trans. R. Soc. B, Biol. Sci.* 2004; 359(1447): 1115–1116. https://doi.org/10.1098/rstb.2004.1491.

195 Adesola, R.O., Waheed, S.A., and Abodunrin, L. Coronavirus: the hidden truth. *World News Nat. Sci.* 2022; 43: 38–59.

196 Sekoai, P.T., Feng, S., Zhou, W., et al. Insights into the microbiological safety of wooden cutting boards used for meat processing in Hong Kong's wet markets: a focus on food-contact surfaces, cross-contamination and the efficacy of traditional hygiene practices. *Microorganisms* 2020; 8(4): 579. https://doi.org/10.3390/microorganisms 8040579.

197 Fischer, C.P. and Romero. L.M. Chronic captivity stress in wild animals is highly species-specific. *Conserv. Physiol.* 2019; 7(1). https://doi.org/10.1093/conphys/coz093.

198 Morse. S.S. Factors and determinants of disease emergence. *Revue Scientifique et Technique de l'OIE*. 2004, 23(2): 443–451. https://doi.org/10.20506/rst.23.2.1494.

199 Wilesmith, J., Ryan, J., and Atkinson. M. Bovine spongiform encephalopathy: epidemiological studies on the origin. *Vet. Rec.* 1991; 128(9): 199–203. https://doi.org/10.1136/vr.128.9.199.

200 Guarner, J., Johnson, B.J., Paddock, C.D., et al. Monkeypox transmission and pathogenesis in prairie dogs. *Emerg. Infect. Dis.* 2004; 10(3): 426–431. https://doi.org/10.3201/eid1003.030878.

201 CDC. *Update: Multistate Outbreak of Monkeypox* – Illinois, Indiana, Kansas, Missouri, Ohio, and Wisconsin. 2003. https://www.cdc.gov/mmwr/preview/mmwrhtml/mm5227a5.htm (accessed 30 August 2024).

202 Schmidt, K.A. and Ostfeld. R.S. Biodiversity and the dilution effect in disease ecology. *Ecology* 2001; 82(3): 609–619. https://doi.org/10.1890/0012-9658(2001)082[0609:BATDEI]2.0.CO;2.

203 Lam, S.K. and Chua. K.B. Nipah virus encephalitis outbreak in Malaysia. *Clin. Infect. Dis.* 2002; 34(Suppl 2): S48–S51. https://doi.org/10.1086/338818.

204 Adesola, R.O., Miranda, A.V., Tran, Y.S.J., et al. Langya virus outbreak: current challenges and lesson learned from previous henipavirus outbreaks in China, Australia, and Southeast Asia. *Bull. Natl. Res. Cent.* 2023; 47(1): 87. https://doi.org/10.1186/s42269-023-01064-3.

205 Rose, J.B., Epstein, P.R., Lipp, E.K., et al. Climate variability and change in the United States: potential impacts on water- and foodborne diseases caused by microbiologic agents. *Environ. Health Perspect.* 2001; 109(Suppl 2): 211–221. https://doi.org/10.1289/ehp.01109s2211.

206 Kurpiers, L.A., Schulte-Herbrüggen, B., Ejotre, I., and Reeder. D.M. Bushmeat and emerging infectious diseases: lessons from africa., In: *Problematic Wildlife*, 507–551. Cham: Springer International Publishing; 2016. https://doi.org/10.1007/978-3-319-22246-2_24.

207 Megid, J., Kotait, I. Appolinário, C.M. and Carrieri. M.L. Rabies in Brazil. In: *History of Rabies in the Americas: From the Pre-Columbian to the Present, Volume II: Historical Introductions and Disease Status to Date*, 341–365. Springer; 2024. https://doi.org/10.1007/978-3-031-25405-5.

208 Vigilato, M.A.N., Clavijo, A., Knobl, T., et al. Progress towards eliminating canine rabies: policies and perspectives from Latin America and the caribbean. *Philos. Trans. R. Soc. B, Biol. Sci.* 2013; 368(1623): 20120143. https://doi.org/10.1098/rstb.2012.0143.

209 Schneider, M.C., Min, K.-D., Romijn, P.C., et al. Fifty years of the national rabies control program in brazil under the one health perspective. *Pathogens* 2023; 12(11): 1342. https://doi.org/10.3390/pathogens12111342.

210 Annand, E.J., Horsburgh, B.A., Xu, K., et al. Novel Hendra virus variant detected by sentinel surveillance of horses in Australia. *Emerg. Infect. Dis.* 2022; 28(3): 693. https://doi.org/10.3201/eid2803.211245.

211 Field, H., Crameri, G., Kung, N.Y.H., and Wang. F. Ecological aspects of Hendra virus. In: *Henipavirus: Ecology, Molecular Virology, and Pathogenesis, Current Topics in Microbiology and Immunology Vol. 359*(ed. B. Lee and P. Rota), 11–23, Berlin, Heidelberg: *Springer*;,; 2012. https://doi.org/10.1007/82_2012_214.

212 Middleton, D., Pallister, J., Klein, R., et al. Hendra virus vaccine, a one health approach to protecting horse, human, and environmental health. *Emerg. Infect. Dis.* 2014; 20(3): 372–379. https://doi.org/10.3201/eid2003.131159.

213 Yuen, K.Y., Fraser, N.S., Henning, J., et al. Hendra virus: epidemiology dynamics in relation to climate change, diagnostic tests and control measures. *One Health* 2021; 12: 100207. https://doi.org/10.1016/j.onehlt.2020.100207.

214 Melidou, A., Enkirch, T., Willgert, K.C., et al. Drivers for a pandemic due to avian influenza and options for One Health mitigation measures. *EFSA J.* 2024; 22(4): e8735, 2024. https://doi.org/10.2903/j.efsa.2024.8735.

215 Kanaujia, R. Bora, I. Ratho, R.K. et al. Avian influenza revisited: concerns and constraints. *VirusDisease* 2022; 33(4): 456–465. https://doi.org/10.1007/s13337-022-00800-z.

216 Sims, L.D. and M. Peiris. One health: the Hong Kong experience with avian influenza. In: *One Health: The Human-Animal-Environment Interfaces in Emerging Infectious Diseases. Current Topics in Microbiology and Immunology*, Springer, Berlin, Heidelberg (ed. Mackenzie, J., Jeggo, M., Daszak, P., Richt, J), 365: 281–298, 2013. https://doi.org/10.1007/82_2012_254.

217 Guyonnet, V. and Peters. A.R. Are current avian influenza vaccines a solution for smallholder poultry farmers?. *Gates Open Res.* 2020; 4: 122. https://doi.org/10.12688/gatesopenres.13171.1.

218 Wedari, N.L.P.H., Sukrama, I.D.M., Budayanti, N.N.S., et al. One health concept and role of animal reservoir in avian influenza: a literature review. *Bali Med. J.* 2021; 10(2): 515–520.

219 Ramadan, O.P.C., Berta, K. K., Wamala, J.F., et al. Analysis of the 2017-2018 rift valley fever outbreak in Yirol East County, South Sudan: a one health perspective. *Pan. Afr. Med. J.* 2022; 42(Suppl 1): 5. https://doi.org/10.11604/pamj.supp.2022.42.1.33769.

220 Mwangi, D.K. Institutional one health and animal-human health connections in Nthongoni, Eastern Kenya. *Health & Place.* 2022; 77: 102818. https://doi.org/10.1016/j.healthplace.2022.102818.

221 Lang'at, N.K. Rift Valley Fever Disease Surveillance and Control Strategies in Marigat Sub County, Baringo County, Kenya. *University of Nairobi*, 2023. http://erepository.uonbi.ac.ke/handle/11295/164911.

222 Kalyanaraman, A., Preethi, L., and Bhukya. P.L. An imminence to humans and animals: the rift valley fever virus., In: *Emerging Human Viral Diseases, Volume I: Respiratory and Haemorrhagic Fever*, 419–442. Springer; 2023. https://doi.org/10.1007/978-981-99-2820-0_17.

223 Ohimain, E.I. and Silas-Olu, D. The 2013–2016 Ebola virus disease outbreak in West Africa. *Curr. Opin. Pharmacol.*. 2021; 60: 360–365. https://doi.org/10.1016/j.coph.2021.08.002.

224 Jacob, S.T., Crozier, I., Fischer, W.A., et al. Ebola virus disease. *Nat. Rev. Dis. Primers.* 2020; 6(1): 13. https://doi.org/10.1038/s41572-020-0147-3.

225 Maudling. R. How can One health contribute to pandemic prevention? looking at Ebola through a one health lens. *CABI One Health.* 2022; (2022): ohcs20220004. https://doi.org/10.1079/cabionehealth20220004.

226 Tusabe, F., Tahir, I.M., Akpa, C.I. et al., Lessons learned from the ebola virus disease and COVID-19 preparedness to respond to the human monkeypox virus outbreak in low-and middle-income countries. *Infect. Drug Resist.* 2022; 15: 6279–6286. https://doi.org/10.2147/IDR.S384348.

227 World Health Organization. *Second Meeting of the International Health Regulations (2005) (IHR) Emergency Committee Regarding the Multi-Country Outbreak of Monkeypox.* https://www.who.int/News/Item/23-07-2022-Second-Meeting-of-the-International-Health-Regulations-(2005)-(Ihr)-Emergency-Committee-Regarding-the-Multi-Country-Outbreak-of-Monkeypox (accessed 30 August 2024).

228 Decaro, N., Martella, V., Saif, L.J., and Buonavoglia, C. COVID-19 from veterinary medicine and one health perspectives: what animal coronaviruses have taught us. *Res. J. Vet. Sci.* 2020; 131: 21–23. https://doi.org/10.1016/j.rvsc.2020.04.009.

229 Plowright, R.K., Reaser, J.K., Locke, H.S.J., et al. Land use-induced spillover: a call to action to safeguard environmental, animal, and human health. *Lancet Planet. Health* 2021; 5(4): e237–e245. https://doi.org/10.1016/S2542-5196(21)00031-0.

230 Sachs, J.D., Karim, S.S.A., Aknin, L., et al. The lancet commission on lessons for the future from the COVID-19 pandemic. *Lancet.* 2022; 400(10359): 1224–1280. https://doi.org/10.1016/S0140-6736(22)01585-9.

231 Khanna, R.C., Cicinelli, M.V., Gilbert, S.S. et al., COVID-19 pandemic: lessons learned and future directions. *Indian J. Ophthalmol.* 2020; 68(5): 703–710. https://doi.org/10.4103/ijo.IJO_843_20.

232 Harrington, W.N., Kackos, C.M., and Webby, R.J. The evolution and future of influenza pandemic preparedness. *Exp. Mol. Med.* 2021; 53(5): 737–749. https://doi.org/10.1038/s12276-021-00603-0.

233 Pervaiz, R., Aslam, H., Sarwar, T., et al. Assessment of programs to control the endemic dengue fever: a literature review. *Pak. J. Intensive Care Med.* 2022; 2022: 13. https://doi.org/10.54112/pjicm.v2022i1.13.

234 Shaheen. M.N.F. The concept of one health applied to the problem of zoonotic diseases. *Rev. Med. Virol*. 2022; 32(4): e2326. https://doi.org/10.1002/rmv.2326.

235 Caputo, B., Russo, G., Manica, M.A., et al. comparative analysis of the 2007 and 2017 Italian chikungunya outbreaks and implication for public health response. *PLoS Negl. Trop. Dis*. 2020; 14(6): e0008159. https://doi.org/10.1371/journal.pntd.0008159.

236 de Oliveira, R.C., Júnior, D.S.T., dos Santos Filho, C.R., et al. Lessons learned on health information, education and communication for Chikungunya prevention in countries with risk areas: a scoping review. *Res. Soc. Dev*. 2021; 10(14): e376101421901–e376101421901. https://doi.org/10.33448/rsd-v10i14.21901.

237 Abdul-Ghani, R., Fouque, F., Mahdy, M.A.K., et al. Multisectoral approach to address chikungunya outbreaks driven by human mobility: a systematic review and Meta-analysis. *J. Infect. Dis*. 2020; 222(Suppl 8): S709–S716. https://doi.org/10.1093/infdis/jiaa500.

238 Panigrahi, P. 2003 Severe acute respiratory syndrome (SARS) epidemic: a one health perspective. *Va. J. Public Health*. 2020; 4(3): 6. https://commons.lib.jmu.edu/vjph/vol4/iss3/6.

239 Dhama, K., Patel, S.K., Sharun, K., et al. SARS-CoV-2 jumping the species barrier: zoonotic lessons from SARS, MERS and recent advances to combat this pandemic virus. *Travel Med. Infect. Dis*. 2020; 37: 101830. https://doi.org/10.1016/j.tmaid.2020.101830.

240 Davis. I.M. SARS-CoV: lessons learned; opportunities missed for SARS-CoV-2. *Rev. Med. Virol*. 2021; 31(18): e2152-e2147. https://doi.org/10.1002/rmv.2152.

241 Yang, Y., Peng, F., Wang, R., et al. The deadly coronaviruses: the 2003 SARS pandemic and the 2020 novel coronavirus epidemic in China. *J. Autoimmun*. 2020; 109: 102434. https://doi.org/10.1016/j.jaut.2020.102434.

242 Hemida. M.G. The middle east respiratory syndrome coronavirus (MERS-CoV). *Anim.-Orig. Viral Zoonoses*. 2020; 241–254. https://doi.org/10.1007/978-981-15-2651-0_11.

243 Azhar, E.I., Velavan, T.P., Rungsung, I., et al. Middle East respiratory syndrome coronavirus—a 10-year (2012–2022) global analysis of human and camel infections, genomic sequences, lineages, and geographical origins. *J. Infect. Dis*. 2023; 131: 87–94. https://doi.org/10.1016/j.ijid.2023.03.046.

244 Te, N., Ciurkiewicz, M., van den Brand, J.M.A., et al. Middle east respiratory syndrome coronavirus infection in camelids. *Vet. Pathol*. 2022; 59(4): 546–555. https://doi.org/10.1177/03009858211069120.

245 Laurenson-Schafer, H., Sklenovská, N., Hoxha, A., et al. Description of the first global outbreak of mpox: an analysis of global surveillance data. *Lancet Glob. Health*. 2023; 11(7): e1012–e1023. https://doi.org/10.1016/S2214-109X(23)00198-5.

246 Kuehn, R., Fox, T., Guyatt, G., et al. Infection prevention and control measures to reduce the transmission of mpox: a systematic review. *PLOS Glob. Public Health*. 2024; 4(1): e0002731. https://doi.org/10.1371/journal.pgph.0002731.

247 Bunge, E.M., Hoet, B., Chen, L., et al. The changing epidemiology of human monkeypox—A potential threat? A systematic review. *PLoS Negl. Trop. Dis*. 2022; 16(2): e0010141. https://doi.org/10.1371/journal.pntd.0010141.

248 Jhaveri. R. Echoes of 2009 H1N1 influenza pandemic in the COVID pandemic. *Clin. Ther*. 2020; 42(5): 736–740. https://doi.org/10.1016/j.clinthera.2020.04.003.

249 Vargha, D. and Wilkins. I. Vaccination and pandemics. *Isis* 2023; 114(S1): S50–S70. https://doi.org/10.1086/726980

250 Keusch, G.T., Amuasi, J.H., Anderson, D.E., et al. Pandemic origins and a One Health approach to preparedness and prevention: Solutions based on SARS-CoV-2 and other RNA viruses. *Proc. Natl. Acad. Sci*. 2022; 119(42): e2202871119. https://doi.org/10.1073/pnas.2202871119.

251 Ribeiro, C.D.S., van de Burgwal, L.H.M., and Regeer. J. Overcoming challenges for designing and implementing the one health approach: a systematic review of the literature. *One Health* 2019; 7: 100085. https://doi.org/10.1016/j.onehlt.2019.100085.

252 Bhatia. R. Implementation framework for one health approach. *Indian J. Med. Res*. 2019; 149(3): 329. https://doi.org/10.4103/ijmr.IJMR_1517_18.

253 Mbugi, E.V., Kayunze, K.A., Katale, B.Z., et al. "One Health" infectious diseases surveillance in Tanzania: are we all on board the same flight? *Onderstepoort J. Vet. Res.* 2012; 79(2). https://doi.org/10.4102/ojvr.v79i2.500.

254 Valeix, S.F. One health integration: a proposed framework for a study on veterinarians and zoonotic disease management in Ghana. *Front. Vet. Sci.* 2018; 5. https://doi.org/10.3389/fvets.2018.00085.

255 Erkyihun, G.A., Gari, F.R., Edao, B.M., and Kassa. M. A review on one health approach in ethiopia. *One Health Outlook* 2022; 4(1): 8. https://doi.org/10.1186/s42522-022-00064-z.

256 Chatterjee, P. Kakkar, M. and Chaturvedi. S. Integrating one health in national health policies of developing countries: india's lost opportunities. *Infect. Dis. Poverty* 2016; 5(1): 87. https://doi.org/10.1186/s40249-016-0181-2.

257 Ferrinho, P. and Fronteira. I. Developing one health systems: a central role for the one health workforce. *Int. J. Environ. Res. Public. Health.* 2023; 20(6): 4704. https://doi.org/10.3390/ijerph20064704.

258 Machalaba, C., Raufman, J., Anyamba, A., et al. Applying a one health approach in global health and medicine: enhancing involvement of medical schools and global health centers. *Ann. Glob. Health.* 2021; 87(1): 30. https://doi.org/10.5334/aogh.2647.

259 Nana, S.D., Duboz, R., Diagbouga, P.S., et al. A participatory approach to move towards a one health surveillance system for anthrax in Burkina Faso. *PLOS One* 2024; 19(6): e0304872. https://doi.org/10.1371/journal.pone.0304872.

260 Nyatanyi, T., Wilkes, M., McDermott, H., et al. Implementing one health as an integrated approach to health in Rwanda. *BMJ Glob. Health.* 2017; 2(1): e000121. https://doi.org/10.1136/bmjgh-2016-000121.

261 Murphy, S.C., Negron, M.E., Pieracci, E.G., et al. One health collaborations for zoonotic disease control in Ethiopia. *Revue Scientifique et Technique de l'OIE.* 2019; 38(1): 51–60. https://doi.org/10.20506/rst.38.1.2940.

7

Advancing Veterinary Medicine for Biodiversity Conservation and Global Wildlife Health

Sonam Bhatt[1], Anil Kumar[1], Arzoo Nisha[1], Ashish Tripathi[1], R. S. K. Mandal[1], Rohit Jaiswal[2] and Bhavna[3]*

[1] *Department of Veterinary Medicine, Bihar Veterinary College, BASU, Patna, Bihar, India*
[2] *Department of Livestock Products Technology, Bihar Veterinary College, BASU, Patna, Bihar, India*
[3] *Department of Veterinary Gynaecology and Obstetrics, Bihar Veterinary College, BASU, Patna, Bihar, India*

*Corresponding author: sonam9363bhatt@gmail.com

TABLE OF CONTENTS

7.1 Intersection of Veterinary Medicine and Wildlife Conservation
7.1.1 Health Assessment, Disease Monitoring, Surveillance, and Control
7.1.2 Captive Propagation and Reintroduction/Wildlife Rehabilitation and Release
7.1.3 Identification of Critical Health Factors with Impact on Wildlife Population Dynamics
7.1.4 Integrated Approaches to Protect Ecosystem
7.1.5 Wildlife Management
7.1.6 Conflict Resolution
7.1.7 Legal and Ethical Considerations
7.1.8 Research and Innovation
7.1.9 Public Education and Advocacy
7.2 Addressing Health Challenges in Diverse Ecosystems
7.2.1 Veterinarians in Wildlife Conservation
7.2.2 Addressing Intensive Livestock Farming
7.2.3 Ecological Medicine
7.2.4 Integrating Ecosystem Health in Veterinary Curriculum
7.3 One Health Initiatives for Biodiversity Protection
7.3.1 Threats to Biodiversity Addressed by One Health
7.3.2 Role of Veterinarians in One Health for Biodiversity
7.3.3 Holistic One Health Strategies for Advancing Global Health
7.3.3.1 Wildlife Corridors and Transboundary Disease Control
7.3.3.2 Implementation of One Health in Education
7.3.3.3 Promoting Global Cooperation for Conservation
7.4 Conclusion
References

One Health Integration: Global Perspectives on Animal Health and Sustainable Agriculture. First Edition.
Edited by Pratik Subhash Gaikwad, Vivek Harishankar Shukla and Pintu Choudhary.

Companion Website: https://www.wiley.com/go/pratikgaikwad/onehealth

7.1 Intersection of Veterinary Medicine and Wildlife Conservation

The preservation of wildlife and biodiversity are important and intricate tasks for the field of veterinary sciences. The delicate balance between species and the interdependence of ecosystems demands a comprehensive approach to wildlife management with veterinary sciences emerging as a key component of conservation initiatives [1]. The contributions of veterinary sciences have a range of domains, including disease management, population health monitoring, animal rescue and rehabilitation, research and conservation medicine, and wildlife forensics. Scientific wildlife conservation requires understanding the link between conservation and utilization, as well as the theory of holism [2]. Modern conservation success relies on multidisciplinary approaches that address social, economic, political, and biological challenges. Veterinary medicine's role in conservation must swiftly expand to fulfill the needs of governments and nongovernmental organizations globally. Integrating veterinary medicine into conservation efforts has the potential to improve biological, social, and economic outcomes. Veterinarians can contribute to wildlife protection in numerous ways.

Wildlife health disciplines, including epidemiology, nutrition, genetics, toxicity, and reproductive research, can support conservation efforts alongside clinical and pathology services. Wildlife healthcare may involve identifying essential health factors, monitoring health status, crisis intervention, developing new technology, managing animal welfare concerns, and providing training [3]. Wildlife species are disappearing from the planet at a rate never seen before. The main reasons for the reduction in biodiversity are pollution, overexploitation, and habitat degradation. The fact that many billion wild animals have perished in recent years due to heatwaves, floods, wildfires, and other natural disasters shows how climate change intensifies these processes as a multiplier threat. Despite these obstacles, veterinarians possess special and valuable skills that allow them to support biodiversity preservation and wildlife conservation on many levels. In addition to developing links with rehabilitators to offer their services for normal wildlife rehabilitation requirements, veterinarians can plan and train to mobilize wildlife extraction, rescue, and rehabilitation units during natural catastrophes [4].

Zoological medicine also is at the forefront of veterinary research, conservation biology, and public health, offering unique ways to maintain biodiversity. Zoological medicine supports the health and well-being of individual animals and species, contributing to a better understanding of wildlife biology and motivating environmental care. Collaboration, innovation, and education are critical for ensuring the long-term health and conservation of wildlife, allowing animals to thrive in their natural habitats [5].

7.1.1 Health Assessment, Disease Monitoring, Surveillance, and Control

Wildlife health assessments help identify populations at risk of starvation, disease, and decline from anthropogenic impacts on natural habitats. The health of wildlife is also being adversely affected by several human-caused stressors that are affecting ecosystems, such as invasive species, pollution, climate change, and resource overexploitation [6]. The initial steps in obtaining an appropriate level of information of the health state of wildlife populations are surveillance and monitoring programs, and the wildlife disease surveillance is crucial due to emerging and re-emerging wildlife diseases that threaten human, animal, and ecological health, as well as possible significant economic impacts [7]. Animal disease surveillance entails the systematic collection of long-term data on disease events, risk factors, and other relevant parameters, followed by analysis with respect to temporal and spatial characteristics to reach a conclusion so that necessary preventive measures can be implemented [8].

Wildlife diseases are becoming a major global issue due to their potential impact on public health as well as the threat they pose to the welfare of domestic and wild animal populations in terms of food insecurity, economic losses, and biodiversity conservation [9]. About 72% of infectious diseases that have arisen in the last 20 years have a wildlife source, and about 60% of newly emerging infectious diseases are zoonotic. In terms of animal health, wildlife disease surveillance can help detect early signs of disease outbreaks, including those associated with emerging diseases, identify changes in patterns of disease occurrence over time, and offer useful data on the morbidity and mortality of both domestic and wild animals. It also provides valuable information for organizations to regulate and prevent diseases in wildlife populations [10].

Disease prevention is the desired method to protect the health of wildlife populations, as once a disease has been introduced into a population it can be very difficult, if not impossible, to control or eradicate [11]. The World Organization for Animal Health (WOAH) formerly called Office International des Epizooties (OIE) advises the establishment of nationwide, coordinated wildlife health surveillance (WHS) programs to better protect human and animal health by managing wildlife pathogens and informing disease management [12].

7.1.2 Captive Propagation and Reintroduction/Wildlife Rehabilitation and Release

Captive propagation, also known as captive breeding, is the only choice for species that are extinct or nearly extinct in the wild. To manage captive populations for propagation, genetic and demographic management are necessary to maintain captive populations over time, and it depends upon the basic goals of the captive program, that is, preservation of genetic diversity in captivity for return to natural environments and adapting a wild population to propagation in the captive environment. For long-term preservation of species gene pools especially toward possible reintroductions into actual environments, an attempt should be made to equalize family sizes, redress disparities in representation of founder (wild population that reproduces in captivity) alleles, avoid inbreeding and most selection, and exchange genetic material periodically with natural populations. For adaptation to captivity, managers should not regulate family sizes and thereby should permit or promote selection. Gene flow into the captive population should also be avoided. Some subdivision of the populations, optimizing number of founders, and rapid expansion of the population and stabilization at a rationally determined carrying capacity are recommended for all propagation plans [13]. Most captive breeding initiatives aim to create a self-sustaining captive population as their main objective [14].

Captive propagation projects for endangered animals aim to reintroduce them into their natural habitat. Reintroduction is a new conservation tool to restore the status of historic biodiversity in ecosystems which can help replace declining or extinct wild populations caused by natural or human-caused disasters [15]. Captive colonies are used to provide stock for reintroduction into the wild [16]. Captive populations are routinely managed to minimize inbreeding and loss of genetic variation and in order to reduce the likelihood of reintroduction failure, a series of assessments of the target species' habitat quality in reintroduction sites both before and after releases should come following successful captive propagation [15].

7.1.3 Identification of Critical Health Factors with Impact on Wildlife Population Dynamics

The health of wildlife populations is complex and includes several intrinsic parameters, including ecological (population abundance, body condition), genetic (genetic diversity), and pathological (pathogen infection) parameters. These parameters are complementary and impacted by a variety of environmental factors [16, 17]. Furthermore, ecosystems are experiencing numerous anthropogenic stressors, such as invasive species, climate change, pollution, and resource overexploitation, which all negatively affect wildlife health and increase disease [6]. Birth rate, mortality, migration, and environmental changes affect population dynamics. Analyzing these dynamics can provide insights into a species' health and ability to survive in a specific habitat [18].

7.1.4 Integrated Approaches to Protect Ecosystem

There are most diverse and rich wildlife and ecosystems in the world. When an ecosystem is destroyed or damaged, its ability to support wildlife is jeopardized, and the individuals who rely on it for survival must adapt or relocate, or they will die [19]. Ecosystem conservation is a critical practice aimed at preserving the natural environment, its biodiversity, and the intricate web of relationships among various species. Ecosystem conservation aims to preserve the health and longevity of complex systems that sustain life on the Earth. It is important for maintaining the delicate balance of nature. Ecosystem conservation includes three activities: monitoring, maintaining, and restoring damaged ecosystems [19]. Several approaches and strategies are employed to conserve ecosystems and include protected areas, sustainable resource management, habitat restoration, community engagement and enforcing policies [20].

7.1.5 Wildlife Management

Wildlife management has become increasingly important as human activities modify ecosystems, causing habitat loss, fragmentation, and species declines. The major challenges that wildlife faces, including habitat destruction and fragmentation, climate change impacts, the threat of illegal wildlife trade and poaching, the introduction and spread of invasive species, and the detrimental effects of pollution [21]. Habitat loss and fragmentation have been regarded as the most serious risks to biodiversity. Habitat refers to a location having resources and conditions suitable for an organism to live in. Food, water, cover, and any other unique elements required by a species for survival and successful reproduction are examples of these resources and conditions. Species require different combinations of abiotic and biotic components for successful reproduction and survival due to their own distinctive habitat [22]. When a large expanse of habitat breaks down into several smaller patches with a reduced overall area, separated from one another by a matrix of habitats that differs from the original, this is known as habitat fragmentation [23]. Changes in habitat structure are referred to as habitat fragmentation, and they may occur separately or in conjunction with the consequences of habitat loss, which is a decrease in habitat abundance [24].

Climate change is also a driver of habitat fragmentation. Effects of habitat fragmentation on biodiversity is huge and diverse. Habitat fragmentation is usually defined as a landscape-scale process involving both habitat loss and the breaking apart of habitat [25]. The strategies for prevention and mitigation of habitat include formation of wildlife corridors, land acquisition, conservation easements, restoration, mitigation, and Zoning and Buffer zones [26]. Wildlife management involves protecting wildlife populations and habitats to promote biodiversity, environmental stability, and the well-being of animals and humans.

Wildlife management comprises monitoring animal populations, restoring habitats, planning conservation efforts, and regulating human activities that affect wildlife. To address the ongoing concerns such as climate change, invasive species, and overexploitation, novel techniques and international cooperation, are necessary [27].

7.1.6 Conflict Resolution

The nature and intensity of human interactions with wildlife have changed over time and across place. Human–wildlife conflict varies based on habitat, geography, vegetation, and climate, and affects a varied spectrum of species. Human–wildlife conflicts occur when they share a common limited resource such as land, game animals, livestock or fish. However, the dearth of wildlife habitat caused by growing urbanization enhances human–wildlife interactions [28]. Conflicts have prompted the invention and implementation of several mitigation strategies to reduce the costs and harm caused by the conflicts. Fencing, Grassland management, habitat improvement, Conservation education and awareness of local people, and adequate compensation for human death/injuries, livestock depredation, and crop damage could be the best tools in conflict mitigation strategy [29]. To effectively address conflicts, wildlife management agencies and conservation practitioners need resources and training in outreach and public relations. They should also expand their toolkit to connect with stakeholders in diverse settings [30].

7.1.7 Legal and Ethical Considerations

Wildlife experts lack a framework and procedure for systematically and transparently incorporating ethical considerations, as well as ecological and social science, into wildlife management decision-making. It is reasonable to expect ethical considerations will play an expanded role in the future of wildlife governance. a framework and process based on three major theoretical branches developed by Western ethicists: consequentialist moral theory, which focuses on consequences and outcomes; principle- and rule-based approaches, which deal with what is considered right or wrong; and virtue ethical theory, which takes into account factors such as character, virtue, and esthetics. The framework can be used to predict the ethical repercussions of different paths of action or no action. If wildlife experts use this framework as an assessment tool to contribute input into decision-making, the outcomes will be more transparent, more understood by stakeholders, and more in line with public trust duties [31].

Ethical approaches to wild animals have five perspectives that include contractarian, utilitarian, animal rights, respect for nature and contextual (or relational) perspectives. To effectively protect nature and wildlife, global coordination is often necessary. Contractarians may support binding international agreements to protect endangered wildlife species. However, the ultimate goal is to use wildlife for human purposes. Utilitarianism is a consequentialist ethical theory that emphasizes achieving the best possible outcome for all stakeholders involved in a decision. The aim is to minimize total pain or frustration and maximize total pleasure or desire satisfaction overall. Utilitarian perspective has significant implications for wildlife management.

A wildlife policy based on animal rights would prioritize preserving wild animals' lives. Individual animals' moral value is determined by whether they promote or threaten key environmental values, according to "respect for nature" perspectives. Keystone species play a crucial role in ecosystems, while invasive species that harm native species or ecosystem health should be eliminated. A group of associated views perspectives emphasizes the ethical significance of human–animal relationships. According to this approach, humans have different moral obligations toward wild animals compared to domestic ones. Choosing one of the above approaches and rejecting the others is challenging due to the plausibility of many of the values involved. A hybrid view aims to combine some of these values. One significant hybrid viewpoint is "ecological ethics." This viewpoint advocates for the development of a comprehensive pragmatic and pluralistic ethical framework, complete with a case study database, from which research scientists and conservation managers can draw when complex moral issues arise. This ethical framework should consider various approaches to ethical theory, research ethics, and environmental and animal ethics [32].

7.1.8 Research and Innovation

Globally, nature is deteriorating at unprecedented rates, and species extinction is accelerating, with major impacts on ecosystems, climate, health, economics, and society. Protecting biodiversity is a crucial issue for the survival of our planet [33]. Digital technologies have emerged as vital instruments for understanding, monitoring, and protecting biodiversity. They provide a variety of options, ranging from remote sensing to citizen participation via science apps, delivering unprecedented amounts of data and creative tools for conservation initiatives. Despite their enormous potential, digital solutions present concerns regarding technology and data accessibility, environmental impact, and technological constraints, as well as the requirement for skilled human resources, strong cooperation networks, and effective communication methods [34].

Wildlife conservation relies heavily on technical developments to address concerns such as habitat loss, climate change, and human encroachment. Human activity has led to the rapid destruction of natural habitats, making wildlife habitat mapping and conservation crucial in ecology. Tracking and monitoring technologies have greatly advanced in recent years, providing opportunities to enhance conservation efforts. Various methodologies using drones which includes radiotracking, GPS and non-GPS transmitters, unmanned aerial vehicles or robotics aircrafts, and the artificial intelligence (AI) methods including convolutional neural network, machine learning and deep learning algorithms can be used in wildlife conservation [35].

Digital innovations like remote sensing (RS) and geographic information systems (GIS) are effective technologies for monitoring and conserving wildlife habitats. These tools enable researchers and conservationists to acquire, analyze, and interpret spatial data, thereby understanding species distribution, habitat quality, and the impact of environmental changes [36]. Furthermore, digital innovation is transforming how conservation organizations interact with local people and stakeholders. Data on wildlife observations, illegal activities, and environmental challenges is crowd sourced using mobile apps and web platforms. These technologies encourage citizens to join in conservation initiatives, fostering a sense of ownership and responsibility for the natural world. To realize the full potential of digital innovation, collaboration and cooperation among governments, NGOs, the private sector, and local communities are essential [37].

7.1.9 Public Education and Advocacy

Wildlife conservation is an educational activity in which we make purposeful and meticulous attempts to protect plant and animal species as well as their ecological niches. Wildlife conservation is critical because wildlife and wilderness play an important role in preserving ecological balance and contributing to our quality of life [38]. To involve people in biodiversity and other environmental challenges, one must provide opportunities for increased understanding, which enables individuals to make decisions and act based on sound science and credible recommendations.

Veterinarians can participate in sustainability boards at the local level to offer their knowledge and support laws that take into account wildlife conservation, biodiversity preservation, and animal health in the face of climate change. They can work in agencies whose actions impact wildlife conservation or serve on boards that advise legislators on these matters at the state or provincial level. Every state in the United States, for instance, has a department dedicated to wildlife and natural resources that creates and implements policies for environmental health and animal management. In many states, there are also agencies dedicated to sustainability and climate change [4]. To promote evidence-based policies in these areas, veterinarians can establish connections with these agencies as private individuals or as representatives of non-governmental groups. Governments should consider the knowledge of veterinarians when developing global policies aimed at minimizing the loss of biodiversity and combating climate change [39].

7.2 Addressing Health Challenges in Diverse Ecosystems

Veterinarians contribute significantly to addressing health issues in various ecosystems in several ways. One of their key roles is managing conflicts between humans and wildlife by creating and implementing conflict management programs. To identify areas of conflict and develop appropriate solutions to reduce human–animal clashes, veterinarians work closely with conservationists, wildlife managers, and local communities. These strategies may include habitat modification, deterrent methods, and the establishment of buffer zones to minimize the likelihood of conflicts. Veterinarians also promote understanding and cooperation by engaging with local populations. Through their collaboration with stakeholders such as farmers, pastoralists, and indigenous groups, they help build trust, facilitate communication, and develop consensus-driven solutions to human–wildlife conflicts. By offering valuable expertise and guidance, veterinarians play a crucial role in creating sustainable and culturally sensitive conflict resolution strategies that address the needs of both humans and animals [40].

7.2.1 Veterinarians in Wildlife Conservation

Veterinarians can use their veterinary skills and expertise to ensure the safe and ethical handling of wildlife in conflict situations. This involves logistical planning and collaboration with other stakeholders [41]. The existing and anticipated threats to wildlife species highlight an urgent and critical need for swift, large-scale intervention. Veterinarians, both as individuals and as a professional community, are uniquely equipped to contribute to the protection, conservation, and restoration of biodiversity through various means.

Table 7.1 Role of veterinarian in wildlife conservation.

S. No.	Role	Details	References
1.	Conservation medicine	• Discuss the connections between ecological, human, and animal health. • Investigating the transmission of diseases between animals and humans, including zoonotic and interspecies spread. • Identify environmental hazards that have an impact on wildlife. • Collaborating with professionals from various disciplines to support conservation efforts.	[19]
2.	Wildlife disease monitoring & surveillance	• Conducting health assessments, ongoing surveillance, and long-term monitoring of both feral and domestic animal populations within protected areas. • Identifying key health-related factors that influence the dynamics of wildlife populations. Innovating and implementing new healthcare technologies and treatment methodologies. • Delivering preventive, diagnostic, and therapeutic medical care to wildlife species.	[7]
3.	Captive Breeding and Rehabilitation	• Participating in captive breeding initiatives for wildlife conservation. • Managing the reproductive and health needs of endangered species both in the wild (in situ) and in captivity (ex situ). • Conducting disease risk assessments and developing protocols for health screening and quarantine in wildlife relocation projects.	[15]
4.	Education, Research and public advocacy	• Investigate groups that focus on sustainability, climate change, and biodiversity, and become active in their committees, research, and policies advocacy. • Encourage student research projects that combine other One Health initiatives with biodiversity conservation. • Contributing to the development of policies and guidelines at the local, national, and international levels.	[42]
5.	Disaster Response	• Training field personnel to enhance their capabilities in managing wildlife health challenges during natural or anthropogenic disasters.	[43]

Historically, wildlife veterinarians primarily focused on intervening and managing health crises in free-ranging animal populations. Outbreaks of wildlife diseases were mainly addressed when they posed a zoonotic threat such as rabies, brucellosis, or tuberculosis or had negative impacts on domestic animals or economically important game species. Meanwhile, veterinarians in zoological settings concentrated on individual animal care in captivity, ensuring welfare standards were met, and were mainly involved in conservation projects through tasks like chemical immobilization to facilitate research. The role of wildlife veterinarians has been summarized in Table 7.1.

7.2.2 Addressing Intensive Livestock Farming

The outputs of agricultural farming rely on the type of production, as various farming systems yield different products. Within animal farming, the livestock sector is the fastest-growing area of agriculture. The global trend toward intensive animal farming for higher productivity has negatively affected the environment and biodiversity, contributing to global warming. This approach has also led to pollution of soil, water, and air due to greenhouse gas emissions from animal waste. Additionally, the excessive use of antimicrobials in these systems has resulted in the rise of drug-resistant microorganisms. Thus, there is a need for a comprehensive and integrated approach that addresses the nonmarket outputs of farming to monitor these global trends [44].

Meat production is considered a major factor in the ongoing biodiversity loss crisis [45]. According to the 2019 IPBES (Intergovernmental Science-Policy Platform on Biodiversity and Ecosystem Services) Global Assessment Report on Biodiversity and Ecosystem Services, industrial agriculture is driven in large part by the meat and dairy industries and overfishing are leading causes of species extinction. The meat industry is not only one of the largest contributors to global greenhouse gas emissions, but it is also a key driver of habitat destruction and biodiversity decline. Furthermore, it is widely recognized as a primary source of water pollution in both developed and developing nations [46].

Veterinarians play a pivotal role in addressing the challenges and consequences of intensive farming by encompassing not only the health and well-being of animals but also environmental preservation, sustainable agriculture, and public health. They educate farmers on alternative disease prevention methods and proper antibiotic stewardship. Vets guide farmers on balanced feeding practices and herd management that enhance productivity while minimizing environmental impact. Veterinarians can also play a key role in promoting environmental sustainability by offering expert advice on managing animal waste. When not handled correctly, waste from farm animals can become a significant source of environmental pollution. By guiding farmers on proper waste disposal and treatment methods, veterinarians help reduce environmental risks and protect public health. Veterinarians contribute to policymaking by working with governments and organizations to shape regulations that balance production efficiency with ethical standards. They play a role in educating the public about animal welfare, sustainable food systems, and the consequences of intensive farming.

7.2.3 Ecological Medicine

The ecological medicine deals with the health of the ecosystem. The art and science of addressing how health and disease are shaped by biophysical and socioeconomic factors connected to the environment across all levels from local to global is known as EcoMedicine. Veterinarians can use their expertise to promote ecosystem health by applying an ecosystem approach to veterinary medicine. This approach can be applied at the level of individuals, populations, and ecosystems [47]. The use of EcoMedicine to promote ecosystem health closely aligns with the concept of "conservation medicine." This term has been championed by organizations like EcoHealth alliance which originated from the wildlife conservation trust founded by Gerald Durrell over three decades ago. Although the organization maintains a strong focus on wildlife, it has expanded its scope to encompass broader issues. Conservation medicine is now defined as "an emerging, interdisciplinary field that examines the connections between human and animal health and the surrounding environmental conditions."

In addressing both animal and human health issues, veterinarians acquire a range of scientific and professional skills that equip them to tackle complex environmental and socioeconomic challenges. Their assessments often include factors such as housing, nutrition, air quality, and biosecurity across various species, including exotic animals. Veterinarians are trained to consider health and disease across multiple spatial scales ranging from individual animals to entire populations and to understand the interactions between them. In recent years, some veterinarians have begun examining health and disease not only through traditional epidemiological frameworks but also within the broader context of farming systems and multilevel ecoregional dynamics [48].

Several specialized veterinary organizations focused on ecosystem health, such as the American Association of Zoo Veterinarians, the American Association of Wildlife Veterinarians, and the Alliance of Veterinarians for the Environment, are thriving. Veterinarians with expertise in fields like epidemiology, wildlife disease, toxicology, and public health are particularly well-equipped to contribute to ecosystem health initiatives [49]. For instance, veterinary epidemiologists use various tools to identify the factors influencing health, productivity, and disease skills that can be applied at the ecosystem level. Understanding wildlife populations and their diseases can provide important insights into the overall health of their habitats. Toxicologists play a critical role in safeguarding all living organisms from the harmful effects of chemical use, while public health outcomes serve as a key indicator of the well-being of ecosystems [50].

7.2.4 Integrating Ecosystem Health in Veterinary Curriculum

It has been suggested that the veterinary profession has the potential to play an important role in advancing ecosystem health. Most veterinary experience to date in delivering an ecosystem health curriculum has focused on problem-based special rotations or summer courses targeting senior students with special interest in the topic. Programs like Envirovet [51] and the ecosystem health rotations that offered by four Canadian veterinary schools [52] have fostered the veterinary application of an ecosystem health perspective by offering unique and valuable experiences. Self-selected students who are motivated to pursue brief specialized exposure to ecosystem health are the focus of these teaching opportunities. Short courses or senior student rotations can offer knowledge and experience in ecosystem health practice and research in a veterinary context. Due to the broad scope of ecosystem, the curriculum for teaching should be evidence based.

Incorporation of ecosystem health education into an existing curriculum in fields like veterinary public health, wildlife health, and agriculture medicine is logical, as these fields are actively applying ecosystem health perspectives [53]. In veterinary public health, systems perspectives are becoming more and more important for managing infectious diseases, preventing emerging diseases, and guaranteeing the safety of food from farm-to-fork. Environmental health challenges like pollution, water quality, and climate change are increasing public health concerns and are emerging "user groups" for ecosystem health concepts. Programs for food security, a crucial aspect of veterinary public health (particularly in foreign development), are developing community-based and comprehensive solutions. Concepts from ecosystem health are now seen as important components of the wildlife veterinarian's toolbox [54]. While developing policies and plans, wildlife health professionals are increasingly seeking ways to balance ecological services, conflicting social values, science, and management alternatives. There is growing interest in engaging private veterinarians to provide public services that address the requirements of the entire community, not just the animal owner, in response to emerging diseases and their effects on rural economies [55], on-farm food safety, surveillance, vector management, bio-security, disease investigation, emergency response, and community education are all examples of public-good services that are expanding to the sphere of private practice [56].

7.3 One Health Initiatives for Biodiversity Protection

One Health represents a transdisciplinary framework that emphasizes the interconnectedness of human, animal, and environmental health which is collectively known as One Health triad (Figure 7.1) at local, regional, national, and global levels [57]. The concept of One Health originated in the early 1900s when the need for collaboration between human and veterinary medicine was recognized as essential for combating the rising threat of zoonotic diseases, especially after the outbreak of diseases like the bubonic plague and rabies that highlighted the interconnectedness of human and animal health.

Over time, the scope of One Health has expanded to include public health and ecosystem health, recognizing the integrated nature of these domains [58]. The core principle of One Health is that collaborative efforts across diverse disciplines can lead to more effective and sustainable solutions to complex health challenges [59]. This approach acknowledges that the health of humans, animals, and the environment are inextricably linked and that diseases can transmit between these different populations [58]. Environmental changes, such as deforestation, urbanization, and agricultural expansion, can disrupt ecosystems and lead to increased contact between humans and wildlife, raising the risk of zoonotic disease emergence and transmission [60]. Moreover, human actions that harm biodiversity, such as overexploitation of natural resources and pollution, can have cascading effects on ecosystem services, affecting both human and animal health.

The One Health paradigm recognizes that human health is deeply intertwined with animal and environmental health, with approximately 75% of emerging infectious diseases being zoonotic, meaning they can spread between

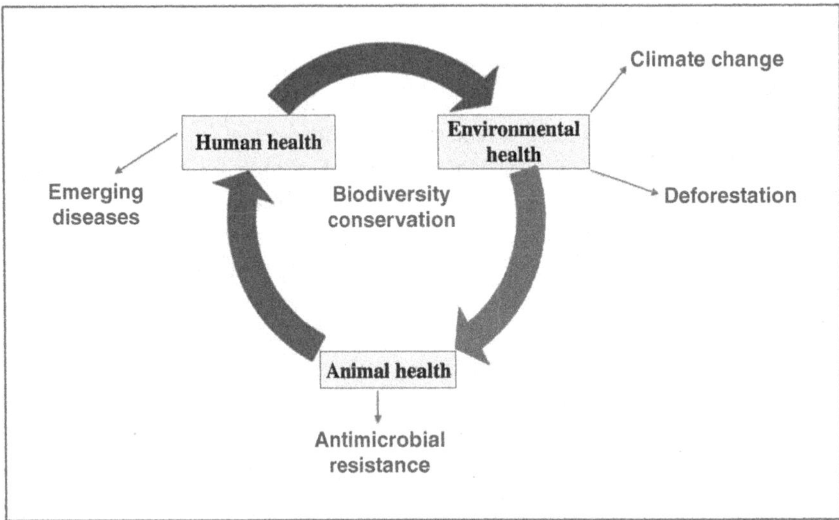

Figure 7.1 The One Health Triad and determinants affecting biodiversity.

animals and humans [61]. These diseases often emerge when ecological changes or human activities disrupt natural ecosystems, bringing humans and animals into closer contact. For instance, deforestation and agricultural expansion can lead to habitat loss for wildlife, forcing animals to seek food and shelter in human-dominated landscapes, increasing the risk of disease transmission.

7.3.1 Threats to Biodiversity Addressed by One Health

Biodiversity faces numerous threats that have significant implications for human, animal, and environmental health. Habitat loss and fragmentation, driven by deforestation, urbanization, and agricultural expansion, result in the destruction and fragmentation of natural habitats, reducing the space and resources available for wildlife [62]. This loss of habitat can lead to decreased biodiversity and increased interactions between humans and animals, heightening the risk of zoonotic disease spillovers and the emergence of new infectious diseases. Additionally, climate change can alter ecosystems, disrupt species distributions, and increase the frequency and intensity of extreme weather events, further exacerbating the threat of emerging diseases.

One health strategies provide a crucial framework for addressing these multifaceted threats through the promotion of interdisciplinary collaborations and holistic, integrated approaches as mentioned in Table 7.2. These strategies can mitigate habitat loss and fragmentation through land-use planning and conservation efforts that promote biodiversity and ecosystem services [62]. One Health approaches can also reduce the risk of zoonotic disease spillover by implementing surveillance programs that monitor wildlife populations for emerging pathogens, as well as promoting responsible agricultural practices that minimize the use of antimicrobials in food animals.

7.3.2 Role of Veterinarians in One Health for Biodiversity

Veterinarians play a crucial role in the One Health approach to biodiversity conservation and ecosystem health, and their expertise extends beyond traditional animal health practices to include wildlife conservation, disease surveillance, and ecosystem management as shown in Figure 7.2. They play a crucial role in wildlife health monitoring by actively tracking wildlife populations for signs of disease, which enables early detection of emerging zoonoses and contributes to global health security [67, 68]. They also promote ecosystem health by advocating

Table 7.2 Traditional conservation vs. One Health approach.

Aspect	Traditional conservation	One Health approach	References
Focus	Species-centric	Ecosystem and health-centric	[19]
Stakeholders	Foresters, conservation biologists	Veterinarians, ecologists, public health experts, policy makers	[63]
Disease Management	Often reactive	Emphasizes surveillance, early detection, and prevention	[7]
Community Involvement	Limited	Central – includes indigenous and local knowledge	[64]
Policy Coordination	Single sector	Multisectoral integration	[65]
Scope	Protection and preservation	Health promotion and sustainable coexistence	[66]
Data Sharing	Often siloed	Encourages cross-sectoral sharing and transparency	[63]

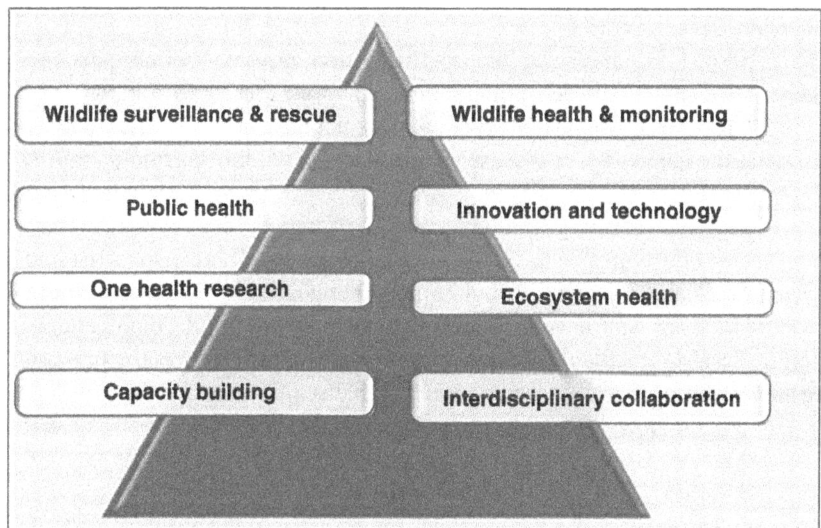

Figure 7.2 Veterinarians' roles in One Health initiatives.

for environmentally responsible agricultural practices, reducing the use of harmful chemicals, and supporting land management strategies that sustain biodiversity [69]. Through their efforts to enhance food security, animal productivity, and disease control, especially in low-income regions, veterinarians contribute to public health and poverty alleviation, thereby advancing both human health and socioeconomic development [70, 71].

Additionally, they work in interdisciplinary collaborations with professionals across medical, ecological, and policy domains, co-designing solutions to address biodiversity and ecosystem threats [72]. Veterinarians are also committed to raising public awareness and educating communities about conservation and ecosystem health through outreach initiatives [73]. They further contribute to capacity building by training future One Health professionals and supporting interdisciplinary academic programs [74]. In addition to disease surveillance, they are involved in wildlife rescue, rehabilitation, and health assessments during conservation operations [7, 75].

Veterinarians are also at the forefront of innovation and technology, contributing to the development of diagnostic tools, vaccines, and biosecurity measures that help prevent diseases across species [76, 77]. Finally, their involvement in One Health research integrates environmental science into health studies, advancing a holistic understanding of the interactions between human, animal, and environmental health [78, 79].

7.3.3 Holistic One Health Strategies for Advancing Global Health

Intersectoral coordination is essential for addressing the complex challenges posed by zoonotic diseases and other One Health issues [80]. Effective collaboration between human health, animal health, and environmental sectors can improve disease surveillance, prevention, and control efforts. In some instances, poor sectoral integration, insufficient advocacy, financial constraints, and limited research may challenge One Health implementation, which may contribute to worsening zoonotic and infectious diseases as well as environmental issues [81]. Policy frameworks that support One Health approaches are needed to ensure that relevant sectors work together effectively to address health threats. These frameworks should include clear roles and responsibilities for different sectors, as well as mechanisms for data sharing, communication, and joint decision-making. In addition to supporting collaboration, these frameworks must also ensure that the requirements of individual countries and regions are considered, as a "one size fits all" strategy to implementing One Health is unlikely to succeed [82].

7.3.3.1 Wildlife Corridors and Transboundary Disease Control

Establishing and maintaining wildlife corridors is crucial for facilitating the natural movement of animals, preserving biodiversity, and ensuring genetic exchange between populations. However, these corridors can also serve as pathways for the transmission of infectious diseases between wildlife populations and, potentially, to domestic animals and humans. Addressing the challenges of disease transmission in wildlife corridors requires a collaborative.

One Health approach that integrates ecological, veterinary, and public health expertise. To effectively manage transboundary diseases in wildlife, coordinated efforts are needed at the international level. This can involve establishing joint surveillance programs, sharing data and information, and implementing harmonized disease control measures [83]. These efforts can contribute to sustainable development by increasing economic development and restoration [84]. The flowchart of wildlife disease surveillance is shown in Figure 7.3 which depicts the practical application of One Health integrating animal, human, and environmental health disciplines for collaborative and cross-sectoral solutions.

7.3.3.2 Implementation of One Health in Education

The inclusion of One Health principles in veterinary curricula is crucial for preparing future veterinarians to address the complex challenges at the interface of human, animal, and environmental health. By equipping veterinarians with a comprehensive understanding of One Health concepts, they can effectively contribute to disease prevention, surveillance, and control efforts [85]. Integrating One Health concepts into training programs for veterinary and environmental science professionals is essential for building a workforce capable of addressing complex health challenges [86]. By incorporating One Health principles into veterinary and environmental science curricula, educational institutions can equip future professionals with the knowledge and skills necessary to address complex health challenges at the human–animal–environment interface [87].

Continuing education programs that provide professionals with the latest information and tools to address One Health challenges can improve their ability to effectively contribute to disease prevention, surveillance, and control efforts. Such programs play a vital role in bridging the gap between developed and resource-poor settings, ensuring veterinarians are well-prepared to contribute effectively, as their education in developed countries might not fully translate to the realities of resource-limited environments [88]. These initiatives might emphasize the importance of livestock in local microeconomics and food security, enabling veterinarians to recognize the crucial

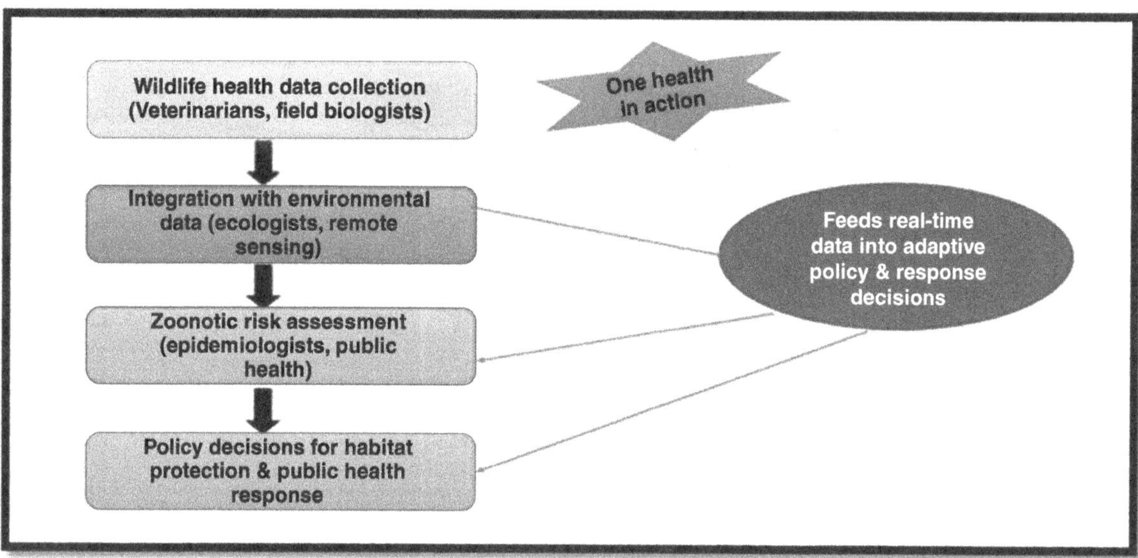

Figure 7.3 Flowchart of wildlife disease surveillance.

role of animal health within the broader community context. Veterinarians possess skills in comparative medicine, which involves drawing comparisons across different species to understand diseases, which is a unique skill that enhances their ability to address complex health issues within a One Health framework [89].

7.3.3.3 Promoting Global Cooperation for Conservation

A key barrier to implementing One Health approaches is the lack of dedicated funding and resources. Without sufficient funding, it can be difficult to establish and sustain collaborative initiatives, conduct research, and implement interventions [90]. Effective governance structures are needed to coordinate One Health activities across sectors and ensure accountability. Establishing clear roles and responsibilities, developing shared goals and objectives, and implementing monitoring and evaluation mechanisms can improve the effectiveness of One Health initiatives.

To facilitate effective collaboration and decision-making, it is crucial to establish standardized systems for data collection, analysis, and sharing across sectors [91]. Sharing data between human and animal health sectors can be challenging due to differences in data collection methods, data formats, and privacy regulations [92]. However, collaborative efforts to harmonize data and establish data-sharing agreements can improve disease surveillance and response. A robust surveillance system with the capacity of rapid reporting of newly diagnosed threats, publicizing best practices to public health workers, epidemiological disease modelling enabled interventions, simulating transmission dynamics and enhanced forecasting is crucial to mitigate upcoming emerging public health threats [92].

Global cooperation and coordination are essential for addressing health challenges that transcend national boundaries, such as transboundary animal diseases, zoonotic diseases, and antimicrobial resistance [93]. International organizations, governments, and research institutions must work together to share information, coordinate surveillance and response efforts, and develop and implement harmonized policies. The increasing demand for natural resources is simultaneously impacting the health of humans, animals, and ecosystems [93]. There is an increasingly urgent need to recognize that ecosystem health directly influences human health, and that conservation efforts must be integrated into One Health initiative to protect biodiversity, preserve ecosystem services, and prevent the emergence and spread of diseases [94].

7.4 Conclusion

To protect biodiversity and endangered species, veterinary medicine presents enormous opportunities for collaboration and innovation. By working with other stakeholders and applying their expertise, veterinarians may play a vital role in preserving biodiversity and protecting endangered animals for future generations. There are many opportunities for collaboration, ingenuity, and capacity building to overcome the difficulties a veterinarian encounters in preserving ecosystem health and biodiversity. Additionally, it is crucial for promoting innovation and interdisciplinary collaboration. By working with ecologists, conservation biologists, lawmakers, and local communities, veterinarians can develop comprehensive methods for managing biodiversity conservation. Applying One Health approach, promoting sustainable land use, and integrating veterinary knowledge into conservation planning are all necessary for global wildlife health.

References

1 Pathade, A., Jadhav, A., Bobde, K., et al. The role of veterinary sciences in wildlife conservation and biodiversity protection. *Rev. Electron. Vet.* 2024; 25(1): 225–245.
2 Zhou, X.H., Wan, X.T., Jin, Y.H., et al. Concept of scientific wildlife conservation and its dissemination. *Zool. Res.* 2016; 37(5): 270–274. https://doi.org.10.13918/j.issn.2095-8137.2016.5.270.
3 Karesh, W.B. and Cook, R.A. Applications of veterinary medicine to in situ conservation efforts. *Oryx* 1995; 29(4): 244. https://doi.org.10.1017/S0030605300021232.
4 Cerda, J.R., MPH, J.D, and Webb, T.L. Wildlife conservation and preserving biodiversity: impactful opportunities for veterinarians? *J. Am. Vet. Med. Assoc.* 2023; 261(7): 1077–1085. https://doi.org/10.2460/javma.23.02.0094.
5 Espinosa Garcia-San Roman, J., Quesada-Canales, Ó., Arbelo Hernandez, M., et al. Veterinary education and training on non-traditional companion animals, exotic, zoo, and wild animals: concepts review and challenging perspective on zoological medicine. *Vet. Sci.* 2023; 10: 357. https://doi.org/10.3390/vetsci10050357.
6 Kophamel, S., Illing, B., Ariel, E., et al. Importance of health assessments for conservation in noncaptive wildlife. *Conserv. Biol.* 2022; 36(1): 13724. https://doi.org.10.1111/cobi.13724.
7 Sleeman, J.M. Has the time come for big science in wildlife health? *EcoHealth* 2013; 10(4): 335–338.
8 Kumar, H.C., Hiremath, J., and Yogisharadhya, R. Animal disease surveillance: its importance & present status in India. *Indian J. Med. Res.* 2021; 153(3): 299–310.
9 Cupertino, M.C., Resende, M.B., Mayers, N.A., et al. Emerging and re-emerging human infectious diseases: a systematic review of the role of wild animals with a focus on public health impact. *Asian Pac. J. Trop. Med.* 2020; 13(3): 99–106. https://doi.org.10.4103/1995-7645.277535.
10 Delgado, M., Ferrari, N., Fanelli, A., et al. Wildlife health surveillance: gaps, needs and opportunities. *Sci. Tech. Rev.* 2023; 42: 161–172.
11 Wobeser, G.A. *Essentials of Disease in Wild Animals.* Ames, Iowa: Blackwell Pub; 2006.
12 Mazzamuto, M.V., Schilling, A.K., and Romeo, C. Wildlife disease monitoring: methods and perspectives. *Animals* 2022; 12(21): 3032.
13 Foose, T.J., Lande, R., Flesness, N.R., et al. Propagation plans. *Zoo Biol.* 1986; 5(2): 139–146.
14 Ralls, K. and Ballou, J. D. Captive breeding and reintroduction. *Encycl. Biodivers.* 2013; 662–667. https://doi.org.10.1016/B978-0-12-384719-5.00268-9. https://repository.si.edu/bitstream/handle/10088/21037/nzp_Captive_breeding_2013.pdf
15 Park, S.R., Yoon, J., and Kim, S.K. Captive propagation, habitat restoration, and reintroduction of oriental white storks (*Ciconia boyciana*) extirpated in South Korea. *Reintroduction* 2011; 1: 31–36.

16 Gray, R.L. Captive propagation as a tool in wildlife management. In: *Proceedings of Northern California Herpetological Society and Bay Area Amphibian and Reptile Society Conference on Captive Propagation and Husbandry of Reptiles and Amphibians*, 1–165; 1985.

17 Stephen, C. Toward a modernized definition of wildlife health. *J. Wildl. Dis.* 2014; 50(3): 427–430.

18 Duval, E., Quéméré, E., Loot, G., et al. A multifaceted index of population health to detect risk-prone populations and underlying stressors in wildlife. *Biol. Conserv.* 2022; 274: 109706.

19 Musk, H. Chronicles of biodiversity: the dynamics of wildlife ecology. *Poultry Fish. Wildl. Sci.* 2023; 11: 250.

20 Wilson, J.W. and Primack, R.B. *Conservation Biology in Sub-Saharan Africa*. Open Book Publishers; 2019. https://doi.org.10.11647/OBP.0177.

21 Kevin, E. Conservation of ecosystem and its diversity of policies, challenges. *J. Environ. Occup. Health* 2023; 13(9): 1–2.

22 Hall, L.S., Krausman, P.R., and Morrison, M.L. The habitat concept and a plea for standard terminology. *Wildl. Soc. Bull.* 1997; 25: 173–182.

23 Wilcove, D.S., McLellan, C.H., and Dobson, A.P. Habitat fragmentation in the temperate zone. *Conserv. Biol.* 1986; 237–256.

24 Fahrig, L. Effects of habitat fragmentation on biodiversity. *Annu. Rev. Ecol. Evol. Syst.* 2003; 34: 487–515.

25 Fletcher, R.J. Jr., Betts, M.G., Damschen, E.I., et al. Addressing the problem of scale that emerges with habitat fragmentation. *Global Ecology and Biogeography*. 2023; 32: 828–841. https://doi.org/10.1111/geb.13658.

26 Silvy, N.J. *The Wildlife Techniques Manual: Management*. 7th ed. Vol. 2. Baltimore: The Johns Hopkins University Press; 2012.

27 Gupta, S., Kumaresan, P. R., Saxena, A., et al. Wildlife conservation and management: Challenges and strategies. *Uttar Pradesh J. Zool.* 2023; 44(24): 280–286.

28 Tarique, M. Wildlife management: protecting and conserving nature's richness. *Int. J. Pure Appl. Zool.* 2025; 13(1): 1–2.

29 Basak, S.M., Rostovskaya, E., Birks, J., and Wierzbowska, I.A. Perceptions and attitudes to understand human-wildlife conflict in an urban landscape – a systematic review. *Ecol. Indic.* 2023; 151: 110319. https://doi.org.10.1016/j.ecolind.2023.110319.

30 Chouksey, S., Singh, S., Pandey, R., et al. Monitoring the status of human-wildlife conflict and its impact on community-based conservation in Bandhavgarh tiger reserve, Madhya Pradesh, India. *J. Appl. Nat. Sci.* 2018; 10(2): 710–715.

31 Miller, J., Linnell, J.D.C., Athreya, V., and Sen, S. Human-wildlife conflict in India: addressing the source. *Econ. Polit. Wkly.* 2017; 23–24.

32 Smith, C.A., Tantillo, J.A., Hale, B., et al. A practical framework for ethics assessment in wildlife management decision-making. *J. Wildl. Manag.* 2024; 88: e22502. https://doi.org.10.1002/jwmg.22502.

33 Gamborg, C., Palmer, C., and Sandoe, P. Ethics of wildlife management and conservation: what should we try to protect? *Nat. Educ. Knowl.* 2012; 3(10): 8.

34 Soriano-Redondo, A., Correia, R.A., Barve, V., et al. Harnessing online digital data in biodiversity monitoring. *PLoS Biology*. 2024; 22(2): e3002497. https://doi.org/10.1371/journal.pbio.3002497.

35 Freitas, H. and Gouveia, A.C. Biodiversity futures: digital approaches to knowledge and conservation of biological diversity. *Web Ecol.* 2025; 25: 29–37. https://doi.org.10.5194/we-25-29-2025.

36 Aarju, R., Bahuguna, S., Pandey, R., et al. Enabling technologies for wildlife conservation. In: *IEEE Devices for Integrated Circuit* (DevIC), 217–220; 2023. https://doi.org.10.1109/DevIC57758.2023.10134561.

37 Richardson, N. Technological innovations in wildlife conservation through remote sensing and GIS. *J. Remote Sens. GIS.* 2024; 13: 351.

38 Bhilave, M. Education and awareness programs through partnership for promoting wildlife conservation. In: *Conserving Wildlife Together*. VYD Publisher; 2023.

39 Kiran, D., Sander, W.E., and Duncan, C. Empowering veterinarians to be planetary health stewards through policy and practice. *Front. Vet. Sci.* 2022; 9: 775411. https://doi.org.10.3389/fvets.2022.775411.

40 Upreti, J. Exploring digital innovation in wildlife conservation. *Acta Sci. Vet. Sci.* 2024; 6(3): 140–141.

41 Dhungana, R., Maraseni, T., Allen, B. L., et al. (2024). Multi-stakeholder identification and prioritization of human–tiger conflict reduction measures in Chitwan National Park, Nepal. *Oryx.* 2024; 58(5): 655–663. https://doi.org/10.1017/S0030605323001734.

42 Rabinowitz, P.M. and Conti, L.A. Links among human health, animal health, and ecosystem health. *Annu. Rev. Public Health* 2010; 31: 189–204.

43 Deem, S.L., Karesh, W.B., and Weisman, W. Putting theory into practice: wildlife health in conservation. *Conserv. Biol.* 2001; 15(5): 1224–1233.

44 Fernandes, R.N. and Pinto, M.D.L.R. *Veterinarian's Role in Conservation Medicine and Animal Welfare.* IntechOpen; 2019. https://doi.org.10.5772/intechopen.84173.

45 Manzoor, S., Syed, Z., and Abubabakar, M. Global perspectives of intensive animal farming and its applications. In: *Intensive Animal Farming – A Cost-Effective Tactic.* IntechOpen; 2023.

46 Shankar, T., Praharaj, S., Sahoo, U., and Maitra, S. Intensive farming: its effect on the environment. *Int. Bi-Monthly* 2021; 12: 37480–37487.

47 Brondizio, E.S., Settele, J., Diaz, S., and Ngo, H.T. *Global Assessment Report of the Intergovernmental Science-Policy Platform on Biodiversity and Ecosystem Services.* IPBES; 2019.

48 Nielsen, N.O., Waltner-Toews, D., Nishi, J.S., and Hunter, D.B. Whither ecosystem health and ecological medicine in veterinary medicine and education. *Can. Vet. J.* 2012; 53(7): 747–753.

49 Faye, B. and Waltner-Toews, D. McDermott, J. From "ecopathology" to "agroecosystem health." *J. Epidemiol. Santé Anim.* 1997; 31: 17–21.

50 Boyce, W.M., Yuill, T., Homan, J., et al. A role for veterinarians in wildlife health and conservation biology. *J. Am. Vet. Med. Assoc.* 1992; 200: 435–437.

51 VanLeeuwen, J.A., Waltner-Toews, D., Abernathy, T., et al. Evolving models of human health toward an ecosystem context. *Ecosyst. Health* 1998; 4(4): 229–241. https://doi.org.10.1046/j.1526-0992.1998.00070.x.

52 Gilardi, K.V.K., Else, J.G., and Beasley, V.R. Envirovet summer institute: integrating veterinary medicine into ecosystem health practice. *Ecohealth* 2004; 1(1): 50–55.

53 Ribble, C.S., Hunter, B., Lariviere, N., et al. Ecosystem health as a clinical rotation for senior students in Canadian veterinary schools. Can. *Vet. J.* 1997; 38: 485–490.

54 Nielsen, N.O. Will the veterinary profession flourish in the future? *J. Vet. Med. Educ.* 2003; 30: 301–307.

55 Umali, D.L., Feder, G., and de Haan, C. Animal health services: finding the balance between public and private delivery. *World Bank Res. Observ.* 1994; 9: 71–96.

56 Ghai, R.R., Carpenter, A., Liew, A., et al. Animal reservoirs and hosts for emerging alphacoronaviruses and betacoronaviruses. *Emerg. Infect. Dis.* 2021; 27(4). https://doi.org.10.3201/eid2704.203945.

57 Linder, D.E., Cardamone, C.N., Cash, S.B., et al. Development, implementation, and evaluation of a novel multidisciplinary One Health course for university undergraduates. *One Health.* 2020; 9: 100121. https://doi.org.10.1016/j.onehlt.2019.100121.

58 Yasmeen, N., Jabbar, A., Shah, T., et al. One health paradigm to confront zoonotic health threats: a Pakistan perspective. *Front. Microbiol.* 2022; 12: 719334.

59 Lebov, J., Grieger, K., Womack, D., et al. A framework for One Health research. *One Health.* 2017; 3: 44–50.

60 Khan, I.A., Ali, M.Z., Rashid, M.H., et al. The role of veterinary professionals in the One Health approach: challenges and future directions. *Vet. Med. Sci.* 2020; 6(3): 573–581. https://doi.org.10.1002/vms3.259.

61 Tan, W.S., Law, S.H., Tan, T.L., et al. Exploring the link between animal diseases and human health: the role of veterinarians in preventing zoonotic diseases. *J. Vet. Sci. Technol.* 2021; 12(6): 530. https://doi.org.10.4172/2157-7579.1000530.

62 Bruno, A., Arnoldi, I., Barzaghi, B., et al. The one health approach in urban ecosystem rehabilitation: an evidence-based framework for designing sustainable cities. *iScience* 2024; 27: 110959. https://doi.org/10.1016/j.isci.2024.110959.

63 Beck, A. J., Martin, B. M., Konkel, M. E., & Bobe, J. R. Integrating the One Health concept in the education of future veterinarians. *Vet. Educ. J.* 2014; 34: 56–60.

64 Atlas, R.M. and Maloy, S. *One Health: People, Animals, and the Environment*. ASM Press; 2014.

65 Lebov, J., Grieger, K., Womack, D., et al. A framework for One Health research. *One Health* (2017); 3: 44–50. https://doi.org/10.1016/j.onehlt.2017.03.004

66 Mackenzie, J.S., Jeggo, M., Daszak, P., and Richt, J.A. One Health: the human-animal-environment interfaces in emerging infectious diseases. *Curr. Top. Microbiol. Immunol.* 2013; 365: 1–13. https://doi.org/10.1007/82_2012_263

67 Gibbs, E.P.J. The evolution of One Health: a decade of progress and challenges for the future. *Vet. Rec.* 2014; 174(4): 85–91. https://doi.org/10.1136/vr.g143

68 Haider, M.Z., Aslam, T., Anwar, S., et al. One Health approach: a way forward to prevent zoonotic diseases in the region. *Acta Tropica* 2018; 181: 134–141. https://doi.org.10.1016/j.actatropica.2018.01.006.

69 Chikunda, A., Maredza, M., Njokweni, D., et al. Zoonoses and veterinary public health: a review of the epidemiology, control strategies, and veterinary role in One Health. *J. Public Health Epidemiol.* 2020; 12(7): 189–198. https://doi.org.10.5897/JPHE2020.1234.

70 Clift, B. R., Thorne, E., Smith, J., & Jones, L. A review of strategies for enhancing One Health collaboration between human and veterinary professionals. *One Health.* 2021; 13: 100244. https://doi.org/10.1016/j.onehlt.2021.100244

71 García, P., Tella, J. L., Martínez, A., & Rodríguez, M. One Health: integrating environmental, animal, and human health into a unified framework. *Environ. Int.* 2020; 136: 105465. https://doi.org/10.1016/j.envint.2020.105465

72 O'Keefe, L., Thomas, A., Murphy, B., & Williams, C. A multidisciplinary One Health approach: an effective tool for addressing emerging infectious diseases. *Epidemiol. Infect.* 2019; 147: 233. https://doi.org/10.1017/S0950268819002152

73 Barros, M., Dias, M., Carvalho, L., & Silva, R. Zoonotic diseases and the role of veterinary professionals in controlling emerging pathogens. *J. Vet. Anim. Sci.* 2021; 53(3): 65–70. https://doi.org/10.1029/jvsas.2021.30456

74 Cook, J. A., Doyle, M., Smith, R., & Patel, A. Cross-sectoral collaboration for One Health: a study on addressing zoonotic diseases in high-risk environments. *Global Health Action*. 2022; 15(1): 98–107. https://doi.org/10.1080/16549716.2022.1905631

75 Cook, J. A., Doyle, M., Adams, L. E., & Patel, A. H. Cross-sectoral collaboration for One Health: a study on addressing zoonotic diseases in high-risk environments. *Global Health Action*. 2022; 15(1): 98–107. https://doi.org/10.1080/16549716.2022.1905631

76 Thomson, P., Wilson, S., Carter, R., & Evans, L. One Health: addressing the intersections of human, animal, and environmental health in disease prevention. *One Health.* 2023; 17: 100376. https://doi.org/10.1016/j.onehlt.2023.100376

77 Lee, L. Y., Chan, K., Wong, P., & Lim, J. Pathogen transmission across animal-human-environment interfaces: the case for a One Health framework. *BMC Infect. Dis.* 2020; 20(1): 217. https://doi.org/10.1186/s12879-020-05075-w

78 Bonny, P. E., Li, H., Zhang, L., & Chen, Y. The One Health approach to preventing zoonotic diseases: strategic research directions. *Vet. Res.* 2019; 50(1): 89–95. https://doi.org/10.1186/s13567-019-0699-0

79 Rossetti, A., Olsson, J., Müller, S., & Pérez, L. Evaluating One Health interventions in multi-stakeholder environments: evidence from zoonotic outbreaks. *J. Appl. Environ. Stud.* 2020; 15(4): 63–77. https://doi.org/10.1142/9789811234652_0009

80 Hsu, W., Puglisi, R., and Zhang, L. Re-thinking One Health in the context of infectious disease research. *Front. Public Health.* 2021; 9: 780. https://doi.org/10.3389/fpubh.2021.707031

81 Gibbs EP, Anderson TC. One world-One Health and the global challenge of epidemic diseases of viral aetiology. *Vet Ital.* 2009; 45(1): 35–44

82 Mastroeni, P., Rossetti, C., Giacometti, A., & Morelli, R. Innovations in One Health approaches to disease surveillance in high-risk areas. *Global Health.* 2023; 19(1): 1–7. https://doi.org/10.1186/s41256-023-00112-4

83 Smith, J. A., Thompson, L., Nguyen, T., & García, M. One Health and emerging zoonotic diseases: connecting veter inary and human health efforts. *Int. J. Zoonotic Dis.* 2024; 22(1): 25–31. https://doi.org/10.1016/j.ijzd.2023.09.011

84 Martins, A., Costa, R., Silva, L., & Pereira, M. Zoonotic transmission dynamics and control in wildlife populations. *Vet. Anim. Sci. Rev.* 2023; 9(3): 55–60. https://doi.org/10.1016/j.vetres.2023.06.014

85 Brown, E., Joris, A., Müller, T., & Silva, R. Implementing One Health initiatives in rural communities: a framework for collaboration. *One Health J.* 2022; 8(2): 120–130. https://doi.org/10.3389/oneh.2022.00567

86 Thomas, J. and Williams, T. The role of wildlife veterinarians in zoonotic disease surveillance: contributions to One Health. *J. Wildl. Manag.* 2024; 88(3): e22502. https://doi.org.10.1002/jwmg.22502.

87 Sharan, M., Vijay, D., Yadav, J. P., & Bedi, J. S. Surveillance and response strategies for zoonotic diseases: a comprehensive review. *Science in One Health.* 2023; 2: 100050. https://doi.org/10.1016/j.soh.2023.100050

88 Pant, H., Verma, J., & Richhariya, S. Wildlife Conservation and Management using GIS and Remote Sensing. In Geospatial Technology and Its Applications in Resource Management (pp. 191–202). New Delhi: AkiNik Publications. 2022. ISBN 978-93-91498-40-9.

89 Fasina, F. O., Fasanmi, O. G., Makonnen, Y. J., et al. The One Health landscape in Sub-Saharan African countries. *One Health.* 2021; 13: 100325. https://doi.org/10.1016/j.onehlt.2021.100325

90 Bouabdallah, S. 'Ethical considerations in One Health research', in Drug Discovery and One Health Approach in Combating Infectious Diseases. 2025. Elsevier, pp. 363–379.

91 Johnson, D., Carter, S., & Lee, R. Integrating One Health into global health systems: challenges and opportunities. *Global Health Action.* 2024; 17(1): 1–9. https://doi.org/10.1080/16549716.2024.1937581

92 Pettan-Brewer, C., Martins, A. F., de Abreu, D. P. B., et al. From the approach to the concept: One Health in Latin America—Experiences and perspectives in Brazil, Chile, and Colombia. *Front. Public Health.* 2020; 8: 389. https://doi.org/10.3389/fpubh.2020.00389

93 World Health Organization (WHO), Food and Agriculture Organization (FAO), and World Organization for Animal Health (WOAH). *Global Framework for the Progressive Control of Transboundary Animal Diseases (GF-TADs): Strategic Action Plan 2021–2025.* Geneva: WHO; 2021.

94 Zinsstag, J., Schelling, E., Waltner-Toews, D., et al. *One Health: The Theory and Practice of Integrated Health Approaches.* 2nd ed. Wallingford: CABI; 2020.

8

Emerging Global Technologies in Veterinary Sciences

*Benedict Terkula Iber[1,2], Pranshul Sethi[3,4], Ramandeep Saini[5], Nainci Dhiman[5], and Ayush Madan[2,6]**

[1] *Department of Fisheries and Aquaculture, Joseph Sarwuan Tarka University (Formerly, Federal University of Agriculture Makurdi), Makurdi, Benue State, Nigeria*
[2] *Institute of Tropical Aquaculture and Fisheries (AKUATROP), Universiti Malaysia Terengganu, Kuala Nerus, Terengganu, Malaysia*
[3] *College of Pharmacy, Shri Venkateshwara University, Gajraula, Uttar Pradesh, India*
[4] *Chitkara College of Pharmacy, Chitkara University, Rajpura, Punjab, India*
[5] *Chandigarh College of Technology, Chandigarh Group of Colleges, Greater Mohali, Punjab, India*
[6] *Department of Biotechnology, School of Research & Technology (SORT), People's University, Bhopal, Madhya Pradesh, India*

*Corresponding author: madanayushmadan@gmail.com

TABLE OF CONTENTS

8.1 Introduction
8.1.1 Overview of Veterinary Sciences
8.1.2 Conventional vs. Advanced Methods in Veterinary Sciences
8.1.3 Importance of Technological Advancements in Veterinary Medicine
8.2 Diagnostic Technologies
8.2.1 Imaging Techniques in Veterinary Diagnostics
8.2.1.1 Radiography (X ray)
8.2.1.2 Ultrasonography
8.2.1.3 Computed Tomography
8.2.1.4 Nuclear Scintigraphy
8.2.2 Molecular Diagnostics in Veterinary Medicine
8.2.2.1 Polymerase Chain Reaction
8.2.3 Point-of-care Testing Devices for Rapid Diagnosis
8.2.3.1 Blood Glucometer
8.2.3.2 Rapid Immunoassay
8.2.3.3 Lactate Meter
8.2.3.4 Coagulation Analyzers
8.3 Treatment and Therapeutic Technologies
8.3.1 Advanced Surgical Techniques in Veterinary Medicine
8.3.1.1 Laparoscopy
8.3.1.2 Laser Surgery
8.3.1.3 Advanced Fracture Repair
8.3.1.4 Thoracoscopy
8.3.2 Emerging Therapies in Veterinary Oncology
8.3.2.1 Immunotherapy
8.3.2.2 Radiation Therapy
8.3.2.3 Photodynamic Therapy

One Health Integration: Global Perspectives on Animal Health and Sustainable Agriculture. First Edition.
Edited by Pratik Subhash Gaikwad, Vivek Harishankar Shukla and Pintu Choudhary.

Companion Website: https://www.wiley.com/go/pratikgaikwad/onehealth

8.3.3 Rehabilitation and Physiotherapy for Animals
8.3.4 Gene Therapy and Regenerative Medicine for Animals
8.3.5 Nanotechnology Applications for Drug Delivery in Animals
8.3.6 Immunotherapy and Vaccines: Advancements in Preventative Medicine
8.4 Digital Health and Telemedicine
8.4.1 Teleconsultation Services for Remote Diagnosis
8.4.2 Wearable Health Monitoring Devices for Pets
8.4.2.1 Biosensors
8.4.3 Remote Surgery Guidance: Advancements in Teleoperation
8.4.3.1 M7 Surgical Robot System
8.4.3.2 The Zeus System
8.4.3.3 Viky Endoscopic Robot
8.4.4 Mobile Applications for Animal Healthcare
8.4.4.1 The Pet Mobile App
8.5 Impact of Technology on Animal Welfare and Management
8.5.1 Precision Livestock Farming
8.5.1.1 Monitoring Devices
8.5.1.2 Drug Tracking
8.5.1.3 Feed Follow-up System
8.5.2 Use of VR in Animal Training
8.6 Technological Innovations in Animal Nutrition
8.6.1 Precision Feeding System for Livestock
8.6.2 Nutrigenomics in Animal Nutrition Research
8.6.2.1 Nutragenomics in Pig
8.6.2.2 Nutragenomics in Poultry
8.6.3 Smart Feeders and Automated Diet Management
8.6.3.1 Data-driven Farm Decision System
8.7 Future Perspectives
8.8 Conclusion
References

8.1 Introduction

This chapter explores the transformative role of emerging technologies in veterinary sciences, with a focus on advancements in diagnostics, treatments, digital health, and animal welfare. It covers innovations such as advanced imaging techniques, molecular diagnostics, point-of-care (POC) testing, and minimally invasive surgeries, highlighting their impact on improving diagnostic accuracy and treatment outcomes. The chapter also covers the rise of telemedicine, wearable health devices, and mobile apps, which are enhancing accessibility and real-time monitoring for pet health. Additionally, it examines how technologies like precision livestock farming (PLS) and virtual reality (VR) are revolutionizing animal welfare and management, while innovations in animal nutrition, such as smart feeders and nutrigenomics, are optimizing feeding practices.

8.1.1 Overview of Veterinary Sciences

Veterinary science is a critical component of the medical and scientific field that specifically aims at treating animals. It applies to all animals, whether those that people use to keep as pets, those that people rear for food, the wild animals, and even the exotic ones. This field involves assembling information from many scientific disciplines for the efficient diagnosing, treating and eliminating diseases in animals [1, 2]. In addition, veterinary science has special significance to human health by eliminating diseases from animals, food hygiene, and preserving the nation's environment. The history of Veterinary medicine can be traced back to other ancient civilization including Egypt, Mesopotamia, and China where early societies included the welfare of animals they reared.

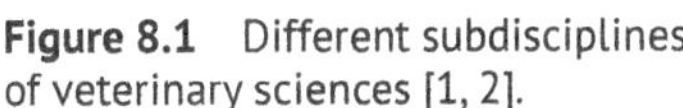

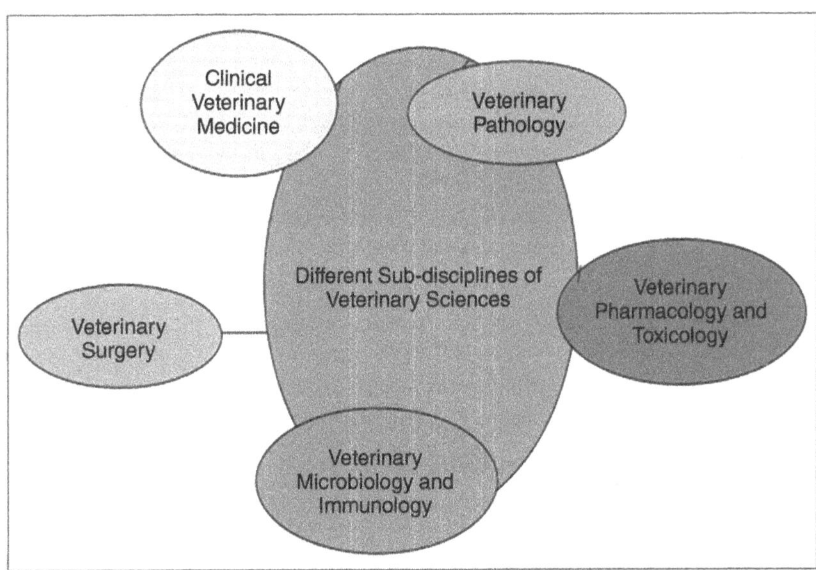

Figure 8.1 Different subdisciplines of veterinary sciences [1, 2].

Veterinary sciences have known a revolution characterized by a fast advancement in technology in the last couple of years. These advancements not only improved diagnosis and treatment of animal diseases, but also greatly expanded the veterinary practice [1]. There are many subdisciplines within veterinary sciences that focus on different aspects of animal health and care for, for example, clinical veterinary medicine, veterinary pathology, veterinary surgery (Figure 8.1). As a result of new discoveries and technical developments that increase the scope and accessibility of veterinary treatment, the field of veterinary science is continuously developing. To treat animals properly and make a positive contribution to society, a veterinarian must be skilled in clinical, scientific, and humanitarian endeavors.

This chapter explores various ways that worldwide advances in technology are changing veterinary sciences, highlighting the significant consequences on animal health, animal welfare, and the veterinary profession as an entity. In this context, technological innovation has been well-applied in the modernization of veterinary medicine [3–5]. Technology is responsible for some of the biggest breakthroughs in veterinary medicine, making care not only more precise and efficient, but also more effective. Innovations in telemedicine, wearable technology for animals, and artificial intelligence (AI) are helping to transform the way that veterinarians are diagnosing and treating animals' diseases, monitoring their health and managing their practices [2].

8.1.2 Conventional vs. Advanced Methods in Veterinary Sciences

Conventional veterinary sciences play a critical role in maintaining and preserving animal health, which is essential to public health and food safety. Veterinarians can serve as agents for the protection of humans from zoonotic diseases by preventing and managing diseases among animal populations. They also play a crucial role in maintaining food production systems and providing proper care for pets and working animals. By employing conventional methods, the branch of veterinary science has achieved remarkable strides despite obstacles including drug resistance, the emergence of infectious diseases, and raising the standard of living for animals. Preventive measures, treatment effectiveness, and diagnosis accuracy will likely be enhanced by combining new scientific discoveries and technological advancements with traditional or conventional methods (Table 8.1). Over time, the veterinary sciences sector has seen tremendous evolution, moving from traditional or conventional techniques to embracing cutting-edge technologies and methodologies. As the field continues to evolve, these conventional

Table 8.1 Overview of different emerging technologies in veterinary medicine.

Technology	Application	Benefits	References
Regenerative Medicine	Joint repair, wound healing, organ regeneration	Enhanced healing and minimal recovery time	[6–8]
Next-Gen Sequencing	Breed-specific health screening, personalized medicine	Early detection of genetic disorders	[9]
Gene Editing	Genetic disease correction	Potential eradication of genetic diseases	[6, 10, 11]
3D Printing	Orthopedic implants, surgical planning models	Improved surgical outcomes	
Wearable Devices	Early disease detection	Continuous health monitoring	[12, 13]
Telemedicine	Rural veterinary care	Increased access to veterinary care	[14]
Robotic Surgery	Minimally invasive procedures	Reduced surgical trauma	[15]
Digital Pathology	Histopathology, remote consultations	Faster diagnosis, improved accuracy	[16–18]

practices will undoubtedly adapt and integrate with innovative approaches, ensuring comprehensive and effective veterinary care for all species [3].

8.1.3 Importance of Technological Advancements in Veterinary Medicine

Technology is transforming every part of our life, and veterinary medicine is no exception. In actuality, the technology is now more important in veterinary care. The integration of cutting-edge technologies in veterinary medicine and animal care has improved animal health and welfare in all aspects, including enhanced and improved diagnostic approach, new treatment modalities, and innovative therapeutic approach. It has also been able to promote research and innovation in the field of animal care. These advancements have made a significant impact not only on biomedical research, public health, and food safety but also on animal welfare [4].

Diagnostic capacities have been meaningfully enhanced by modern technology. For instance, high-tech imaging methods such as magnetic resonance imaging (MRI), computed tomography (CT) scans, and ultrasonography enable the earlier and more precise diagnosis of numerous illnesses, allowing for timely treatment. Additionally, certain molecular diagnostics, such as next-generation sequencing (NGS) and polymerase chain reaction (PCR), have totally changed the way that infections and genetic illnesses as well as cancer indicators are detected. Advancements in technology have given rise to novel therapeutic options for, for example, regenerative medicine offers potential therapies for degenerative diseases and injuries. Modern surgical techniques, such as robotic-assisted treatments and minimally invasive surgeries (laparoscopy, endoscopy) have shortened the recovery period and increased the likelihood of favorable outcomes. According to the research, genomics and bioinformatics have revolutionized medicine and are the reason behind precision medicine as well. Tremendous improvement in veterinary technology directly affects animal well-being. Automated health and behavior monitoring enables early illness detection and the identification of stress indicators [3, 4].

8.2 Diagnostic Technologies

The field of veterinary science continues to play a pivotal role in promoting general well-being, health, and welfare of livestock, wildlife, and companion animals. Accurate and specific diagnosis forms the foundation for effective veterinary medical interventions, ensuring the sustainability of animal health and the prevention of diseases. Over the years, advancements in molecular biology, biotechnology, and a deeper understanding of animal physiology have revolutionized diagnostic methods in veterinary sciences [19–21]. These innovations have significantly improved the precision, speed, and reliability of diagnostic procedures, enabling veterinarians to provide evidence-based and targeted treatments.

Modern diagnostic techniques such as PCR, NGS, mass spectrometry, and advanced imaging modalities like CT and MRI have transformed veterinary diagnostics. For example, PCR-based diagnostics are widely used for identifying infectious agents with high specificity and sensitivity, which is crucial in controlling outbreaks in livestock populations [22]. Similarly, NGS has facilitated genomic studies to detect genetic disorders and pathogens, providing insights into the epidemiology of zoonotic diseases.

POC diagnostic tools, including portable biosensors and lateral flow assays, have further enhanced field-based diagnostic capabilities, particularly in rural and resource-limited settings. These technologies enable rapid and on-site detection of diseases, minimizing the delay between diagnosis and treatment [23]. In addition, advancements in AI and machine learning are beginning to assist in the interpretation of diagnostic data, contributing to more accurate prognostic assessments.

Despite these advancements, challenges persist, such as the need for cost-effective diagnostic solutions, especially for developing countries, and the requirement for continuous improvement in diagnostic accuracy to cater to diverse animal species [24, 25]. The development of novel diagnostic techniques and the refinement of existing methodologies remain active areas of research, holding immense potential to enhance the quality of veterinary care [5].

The field of veterinary medicine has undergone significant transformation in recent years due largely to the rapid advancement of technology. From imaging techniques and molecular diagnostics to POC testing devices and minimally invasive surgical procedures, these innovations are not only making diagnoses quicker and more accurate but are also helping to improve treatment outcomes and overall animal welfare [1, 2, 26]. By harnessing new technologies, veterinary professionals can provide higher-quality care, enabling animals to lead healthier and more comfortable lives.

8.2.1 Imaging Techniques in Veterinary Diagnostics

In veterinary diagnostics, imaging techniques aid in providing detailed insights into an animal's health. The ability to see beyond the surface through technologies like X-rays, ultrasound, CT scans, and nuclear scintigraphy has revolutionized how veterinarians approach disease diagnosis and treatment [3, 27, 28]. These imaging technologies have proven highly effective for diagnosing a wide range of conditions, from bone fractures to soft tissue abnormalities, as well as helping plan surgical interventions. The application of imaging allows for a noninvasive examination of an animal's internal or anatomic systems and helps in the identification of diseases and disorders. This technology has made it possible to detect diseases at earlier stages, determine the precise plan of actions to create a treatment plan, and monitor the results of therapies [29]. Veterinary professionals provide high-quality care because, while each imaging modality has limitations of its own, when combined with one another, they become completely inclusive. Routine diagnostics are based on conventional techniques such as radiography, ultrasound, and fluoroscopy, while advanced, detailed insights into complex disorders are provided by contemporary techniques including CT, MRI, nuclear medicine, digital radiography, and thermography. As technology develops, novel imaging modalities are going to complement and improve current conventional techniques, substantially enhancing veterinary medicine's diagnostic capabilities [6].

8.2.1.1 Radiography (X ray)

Radiographs, also known as X-rays, are among the most basic and frequently utilized imaging methods in veterinary diagnostics. They contribute to the diagnosis and treatment of a variety of ailments by offering insightful information about the interior architecture of animals. Although the methods used to create radiographs, or X-ray images, are similar to those used in human medicine, the equipment's dimensions are adjusted to suit the needs of animals [30]. Some large animal clinics use transportable equipment to treat horses and other large animals. Pets may need to be sedated prior to this surgery, even though it doesn't hurt. This helps the animal remain motionless while being positioned and allows the owner to feel more at ease. Bones, foreign objects, and vast bodily cavities can all be clearly seen with X-ray technology. Their use is frequently in the diagnosis of deformities, fractures, malignancies, and infections. The precise cause of a disease may not always be ascertained using radiography [7]. The introduction of computed radiography (CR) has brought about a significant shift in how radiographs are captured, moving away from traditional film-based systems to digital formats [31]. This transition has made it easier to store, manipulate, and share images, which is particularly helpful for mobile veterinary services that reach underserved areas [25]. CR is especially useful in diagnosing bone fractures, dental issues, and internal conditions such as pneumonia or abdominal problems. However, the upfront costs of CR equipment and the need for specialized training to use these systems properly can be barriers, especially for smaller practices or those operating in resource-limited settings. While CR has numerous advantages, it still requires careful calibration and quality control to ensure that the images obtained are both clear and accurate.

8.2.1.2 Ultrasonography

In veterinary medicine, ultrasonography, or ultrasound imaging, has become one of the most essential diagnostic tools for identifying and managing diseases. This noninvasive imaging technique utilizes high-frequency sound waves to produce cross-sectional images of internal organs, offering veterinarians a reliable and detailed view of an animal's internal structures [32]. The ability to visualize these structures in real time has significantly enhanced diagnostic accuracy and therapeutic monitoring.

Ultrasound technology has proven to be a game-changer in veterinary diagnostics due to its ability to provide real-time imaging of soft tissues. It is particularly invaluable for examining the abdominal organs, guiding biopsies, and assessing heart function [19]. One of the reasons ultrasounds have become so indispensable is their versatility. It is noninvasive, does not require sedation in many cases, and offers immediate results, which allows veterinarians to make quick decisions. Ultrasound has also seen advances in imaging techniques, such as elastography (which assesses tissue stiffness) and the use of microbubble contrast agents, which enhance the ability to detect diseases like cancer at an early stage [30]. While ultrasound is extremely effective, its application can be limited by the skill of the operator, and it may not always offer clear results in cases of obesity or thick fur, which can obstruct the view of internal organs [13]. Despite these challenges, the promise of ultrasound in veterinary care continues to expand as technology improves, showcasing its vital role in modern veterinary diagnostics, delivering precision and confidence to veterinarians in their efforts to ensure animal health and well-being [8, 9].

8.2.1.3 Computed Tomography

CT has become a cornerstone in the diagnosis of various ailments and diseases in animals due to its ability to produce high-quality, detailed images of internal body structures. CT operates by utilizing automated X-rays and relies on multiple measurements to create sectional images of the body, which can be further reconstructed into 3D models of internal organs, bones, or limbs. This advanced imaging modality has revolutionized veterinary diagnostics by offering unparalleled accuracy in visualizing complex anatomical details [19]. One of the key advantages of CT in veterinary practice is its noninvasive nature, coupled with the capability to provide high-resolution images, which significantly aids in the precise diagnosis and effective management of diseases. Its applications span a wide range, including the evaluation of tumors, fractures, and organ abnormalities. Additionally, the ability to generate 3D reconstructions enhances surgical planning and treatment outcomes [22].

CT scans provide a deeper level of detail than traditional X-rays by taking multiple cross-sectional images of the body, which can then be reconstructed into 3D models [9, 12]. This is invaluable when diagnosing complex conditions like tumors, fractures, or neurological disorders, where precise visualization of anatomical structures is essential. CT is also critical for surgical planning, especially in oncology, as it helps determine the size and boundaries of tumors, ensuring that surgeries are planned with precision. Despite its benefits, CT remains costly and is not always available in smaller veterinary clinics, especially in lower-income regions [26, 31]. The equipment itself is expensive, and proper interpretation requires skilled professionals, which can make CT inaccessible for some practices. As technology continues to evolve, there is hope that the cost will decrease, and accessibility will improve, making CT an even more vital tool in everyday veterinary care. Despite these factors, the benefits of CT, including its diagnostic precision and versatility, make it an invaluable tool in modern veterinary medicine [10].

8.2.1.4 Nuclear Scintigraphy

Nuclear scintigraphy, also known as radionuclide imaging, is a diagnostic imaging technique that utilizes radioactive materials to evaluate the health and functionality of various tissues and organs. Widely applied in both veterinary and human medicine, this method provides valuable insights into disease diagnosis and organ function assessment [33]. The process involves administering a radioactive tracer, often Technetium-99m, which emits gamma rays detectable by a gamma camera. The choice of tracer depends on the specific organ or system being examined. Following intravenous injection of the tracer, the animal is positioned in front of a gamma camera, and multiple images are captured over time to monitor the tracer's distribution and accumulation. These sequential images help visualize dynamic physiological processes within the body.

Regions of abnormal tracer uptake, whether increased or decreased, are identified during image analysis and can indicate potential pathological changes [12]. Nuclear scintigraphy, a functional imaging technique, plays a significant role in diagnosing bone disorders and assessing organ function. Unlike traditional imaging methods that focus on anatomical details, nuclear scintigraphy focuses on how well tissues and organs are functioning [34]. This is especially useful in identifying early-stage infections, tumors, and even in evaluating how well treatments are working for certain conditions. Newer imaging technologies like positron emission tomography (PET) and single-photon emission CT (SPECT) have shown promise in enhancing diagnostic accuracy, particularly in the field of oncology, where understanding tumor metabolism is crucial [1]. However, despite its promise, nuclear scintigraphy remains underused in routine practice due to the high cost of equipment and the complexity of the procedures, which often require specialized training [26]. Continued research into making these technologies more accessible and cost-effective will be essential for expanding their use in veterinary care.

8.2.2 Molecular Diagnostics in Veterinary Medicine

In veterinary medicine, molecular diagnostics is a game-changing technique that makes molecular disease detection accurate and timely. This field integrates novel techniques for pathogen, host, and environmental sample genetic molecules (DNA and RNA) identification and assessment [14]. Molecular diagnostics has given veterinarians the ability to identify the precise gene chromosomes linked to a range of disorders, allowing for early diagnosis, treatment planning, and disease control. The implementation of these effective veterinary infectious disease management tools into normal vet practice could assume a vital role in the promotion of animal well-being, the demand management of diseases, and as a result the general public health. Thus, with advancing knowledge, more novel diagnostic technologies are expected to be discovered, and the existing ones are set to be improved and optimized to provide broader potential and utilization within the sphere of veterinary medicine [15]. Molecular diagnostics provides the tools to detect pathogens, genetic mutations, and disease markers at a molecular level [5, 11]. Technologies like PCR, NGS, and fluorescence in-situ hybridization (FISH) have enabled veterinarians to diagnose diseases with unprecedented accuracy [1]. This enables more personalized treatment options and improving the overall standard of care.

8.2.2.1 Polymerase Chain Reaction

PCR has been useful for the molecular identification of a wide range of diseases. This highly efficient technique enables the rapid and accurate detection of pathogens, genetic mutations, and other molecular markers by amplifying specific DNA or RNA sequences. Its precision and sensitivity have revolutionized the diagnosis and management of infectious and genetic disorders in animals [26]. Various types of PCR are employed in veterinary medicine, each with unique advantages suited to specific applications. Conventional PCR serves as a fundamental method for amplifying target sequences, while multiplex PCR allows the simultaneous detection of multiple targets in a single reaction, increasing efficiency and reducing diagnostic time [31, 35]. Real-time PCR, or quantitative PCR (qPCR), provides real-time data on amplification, enabling both qualitative and quantitative analysis of genetic material. These advanced methodologies have significantly improved diagnostic capabilities in veterinary practice, facilitating timely and accurate interventions.

By amplifying small amounts of DNA, PCR enables veterinarians to identify infections even when they are present in low quantities, making it invaluable for diagnosing viral infections, bacterial and parasitic diseases [29]. The development of real-time PCR has further increased its utility by offering faster results and the ability to quantify pathogens with high sensitivity [1]. However, the high cost of PCR machines and reagents, along with the need for specialized skills to operate them, can be a barrier to their widespread use, particularly in resource-constrained areas [1]. Despite these challenges, PCR remains one of the most reliable tools for diagnosing infectious diseases and monitoring antimicrobial resistance in veterinary settings [16]. The various types of PCR used in veterinary medicines are as follows:

8.2.2.1.1 Next-generation Sequencing

NGS, also called high-throughput sequencing, is a set of technologies that allow for sequencing numerous DNA or RNA samples at the same time. Specifically, it has transformed the field of genetics and genomics by providing more efficient, less costly, and accurate sequencing than previously used techniques [6]. This technique is available for diagnosing in veterinary medicine and can assist in analyzing all the genetic contents. The use and advantages of histology in the diagnosis, treatment, and study of diseases in animals cannot be overstated [17, 18].

NGS has transformed the ability to explore the genetic landscape of both pathogens and the host. This technology provides in-depth insights into the genetic makeup of diseases, which can help identify mutations, track disease outbreaks, and tailor treatments based on an animal's genetic profile [3, 36]. In oncology, NGS allows for detailed tumors profiling, providing critical information for personalized cancer treatment. However, like other high tech diagnostic techniques, the widespread use of NGS in veterinary medicine is limited by its high costs and the complexity of data interpretation, which requires specialized bioinformatics knowledge [10]. As NGS technology becomes more accessible and user-friendly, it has the potential to revolutionize how veterinarians diagnose and treat a wide range of conditions, from infectious diseases to genetic disorders.

8.2.2.1.2 Fluorescence In-situ Hybridization

FISH is a molecular cytogenetic technique widely utilized in veterinary diagnostics to detect specific DNA sequences in animal tissue samples. This advanced method involves the use of fluorescent probes that bind to specific regions of chromosomes, allowing visualization of genetic material under a fluorescence microscope [15]. FISH provides veterinarians with precise insights into the genetic composition and abnormalities within tissue samples, making it a valuable tool in modern veterinary medicine. The applications of FISH are extensive, offering detailed information about specific strains of pathogens and pathological conditions affecting the tissues of various animal species. It is particularly effective in cancer screening, diagnosing infectious diseases, identifying genetic disorders, and managing infertility. By enabling targeted and accurate detection, FISH contributes significantly to the early diagnosis and treatment of complex conditions in animals [19, 20].

In addition, FISH allows for the precise localization of specific DNA or RNA sequences within tissues. This can be especially useful for identifying infections at the cellular level or monitoring gene expression in cancer [33]. This technique is invaluable for studying gene expression and understanding the molecular mechanisms behind certain diseases. However, FISH is currently a labor-intensive and time-consuming process that requires specialized equipment and expertise, which limits its use in routine clinical practice [5]. Despite these limitations, FISH remains an essential tool in research and has the potential to be adapted for more widespread use in clinical veterinary diagnostics as technology continues to improve.

8.2.2.1.3 Enzyme-linked Immunosorbent Assay

Enzyme-linked immunosorbent assay (ELISA) is a widely employed diagnostic technique in veterinary medicine, utilizing immunological principles to detect the presence of specific antigens or antibodies in biological samples such as blood, serum, or plasma [37]. This method has become indispensable in veterinary diagnostics due to its precision, sensitivity, and reliability. ELISA is particularly effective in diagnosing a range of infectious diseases in animals, such as canine parvovirus in dogs and feline leukemia virus in cats. The test functions by utilizing antibodies conjugated to an enzyme that reacts with the target substance, either antigen or an antibody. When the target is present, the enzyme catalyzes a color change, indicating a positive result. This colorimetric change provides a clear, quantifiable outcome, making ELISA a valuable tool for accurate disease detection. The high sensitivity and specificity of ELISA ensures its critical role not only in diagnosing diseases but also in monitoring disease progression and treatment efficacy. Its adaptability to various pathogens and conditions makes it a cornerstone in veterinary clinics, aiding in the early detection and management of infectious diseases, thereby improving animal health and welfare [21, 22].

8.2.3 Point-of-care Testing Devices for Rapid Diagnosis

POC diagnostics are a way of diagnosing medical conditions that involve tests carried out at the patient's bedside. It is revolutionizing the healthcare sector by giving prompt test outcomes on location, which is advantageous mainly in areas such as veterinary science because rapid identification could greatly influence the way a patient responds to therapy. POC diagnostic tools are mostly wireless and simple to handle, such that the results can be delivered without having to send samples to a central laboratory. Such devices are relevant in different domains or situations like hospitals, outdoor activities and homes [23]. These devices, which range from glucometers to lactate meters and rapid immunoassays, allow veterinarians to make quick decisions, particularly in emergency situations where time is of the essence [18].

8.2.3.1 Blood Glucometer

Among the various diagnostic tools available, blood glucometers are essential for monitoring diabetes and other conditions that influence an animal's blood glucose level. It provides instant readings, enabling veterinarians to quickly assess an animal's health status and make informed decisions regarding diagnosis and treatment plans [38]. The immediate feedback from blood glucometers is particularly valuable in managing diabetic animals, ensuring timely interventions and accurate adjustments to therapy.

By facilitating precise glucose monitoring, blood glucometers contribute significantly to the effective treatment and care of diabetic animals, ultimately improving their well-being and quality of life. Their accessibility and ease of use make them indispensable tools in veterinary practice, allowing veterinarians to confidently diagnose and monitor diseases in real time. This not only enhances the standard of care but also fosters better health outcomes for animal patients [24]. It has also been found extremely useful in managing chronic conditions like diabetes in veterinary patients [23]. The device provides rapid blood glucose measurements, which are essential for adjusting insulin treatments in real-time. Its portability and ease of use makes it ideal for both veterinary clinics and home care, providing an efficient way for pet owners to manage their animal's condition [24]. However, ensuring the accuracy of this device is critical, and regular calibration and proper training are necessary to minimize user error and obtain reliable results.

8.2.3.2 Rapid Immunoassay

Rapid immunoassays are diagnostic tests designed to detect specific antigens or antibodies in biological samples such as blood, urine, or saliva, leveraging immunological principles. These tests are particularly valuable in veterinary medicine due to their ability to deliver quick results, often within minutes, making them ideal for use in both veterinary clinics and field settings [25]. The applications of rapid immunoassays extend beyond routine diagnostics, encompassing the screening of physiological parameters and the detection of various infectious diseases. They are also instrumental in assessing the immunization status of animals, enabling veterinarians to make informed decisions about vaccination and disease prevention. The speed and ease of use of these tests significantly enhance the efficiency of veterinary practice, ensuring timely and accurate diagnosis. While these assays offer convenience and speed, their accuracy can be affected by factors such as the quality of the test kits and the operator's skill. For optimal performance, it is crucial to follow standardized protocols and provide appropriate training [39]. By providing reliable and immediate results, rapid immunoassays play a critical role in improving animal health care and supporting effective disease management strategies [25].

8.2.3.3 Lactate Meter

A lactate meter is a portable diagnostic tool widely used in veterinary medicine to measure lactate concentrations in blood samples. Lactate levels provide crucial information about an animal's oxygenation status and metabolic condition, as lactate is a byproduct of anaerobic metabolism. Elevated lactate levels often indicate inadequate tissue oxygenation or metabolic disturbances, making this tool invaluable for rapid assessment in critical situations. Lactate meters are particularly essential in emergency settings, operating theaters, sports medicine, and field conditions, where quick and accurate results can facilitate timely and appropriate treatment. It is useful in critical care settings, where they help assess tissue oxygenation and metabolic function in patients experiencing conditions like sepsis or shock [24, 25, 39]. The ability to monitor lactate levels in real-time allows veterinarians to make quick decisions that can be lifesaving. However, lactate meters require regular calibration and may not always provide a comprehensive picture of a patient's condition, necessitating further testing to confirm a diagnosis [25, 40]. Their portability and ease of use make them a reliable choice for monitoring the health of animals under various circumstances, ensuring better outcomes and improved care in veterinary practice [26].

8.2.3.4 Coagulation Analyzers

A coagulation analyzer is an essential diagnostic tool for veterinarians, enabling the evaluation of an animal's blood clotting capacity. This device plays a pivotal role in diagnosing various hemostatic disorders and monitoring patients undergoing anticoagulation therapy. It is also critical for assessing bleeding tendencies in animals scheduled for surgical procedures, ensuring their safety during and after the operation. These devices are invaluable for diagnosing conditions such as hemophilia and disseminated intravascular coagulation, where timely treatment is crucial. Although coagulation analyzers offer quick results, their effectiveness relies on proper training and understanding of the device's limitations [24]. By identifying coagulation abnormalities, these analyzers assist veterinarians in accurately diagnosing and treating coagulation disorders. They are indispensable in regulating patient safety during surgical treatments involving anticoagulant therapy, allowing for precise adjustments to minimize risks. The timely and reliable information provided by coagulation analyzers empowers veterinarians to deliver high-quality care and improve clinical outcomes for their patients [27].

8.3 Treatment and Therapeutic Technologies

Veterinary care has developed a lot in the past, accompanying development in human healthcare. The main purpose of veterinary treatment and therapeutic technologies is to guarantee the health and well-being of such animals as pets, stock, wild animals, exotic species. Such advances do not just make health care better but also improve the cause of numerous diseases. From advanced diagnostics and surgical techniques to regenerative therapies and holistic approaches, veterinarians are better equipped than ever to ensure the health and well-being of their patients. As research and innovation continue to drive progress, the future of veterinary medicine holds the promise of even more sophisticated and effective care solutions for all types of animals [28].

8.3.1 Advanced Surgical Techniques in Veterinary Medicine

With the advent of a new era of accuracy and effectiveness in surgical techniques brought about by advancements in veterinary medicine, the care given to animal patients has undergone a revolutionary change. Veterinarians today possess a wide range of technologies to treat a vast array of medical diseases with unparalleled precision, ranging from minimally invasive procedures that reduce trauma and speed recovery to advanced imaging and robotic-assisted surgeries that improve precision and outcomes. Innovative surgical treatments are used to improve animals' quality of life and well-being, and these cutting-edge techniques demonstrate the ongoing progress of veterinary research [29, 30]. Advanced surgical techniques, particularly minimally invasive procedures, have dramatically improved veterinary care. These techniques reduce recovery times, minimize complications, and improve overall surgical outcomes for animal patients [34].

8.3.1.1 Laparoscopy

Laparoscopy in veterinary medicine entails the use of a camera and other medical instruments to carry out a surgery on animals through small cuts on the body. It is used for various reasons due to its noninvasiveness compared to the traditional open surgery hence it causes less pain, the recovery time is short, and the chances of getting a complication are very rare [31]. Furthermore, this minimally invasive technique has become increasingly popular in veterinary medicine. By using small incisions and a camera, veterinarians can perform surgeries with reduced blood loss, improved visualization, and faster recovery times [41]. Procedures such as biopsies, ovariectomies, and even adrenalectomies are now routinely performed using laparoscopy [41]. However, the high cost of laparoscopy equipment and the need for specialized training remain significant barriers to its adoption, especially in smaller or rural practices.

8.3.1.2 Laser Surgery

Laser surgery is a surgical technique where light beams are being focused on performing specific medical operations to animals. The benefits over conventional procedures include Bleeding time, pain and recovery time are substantially much less compared to typical procedures. It is majorly employed for soft tissue surgery and orthopedic procedures. Laser surgery involves anesthesia, laser settings, final surgery and post-operative care prior to discharge of the animal patient [32]. This particular technique is quite popular in veterinary medicine for its precision and ability to minimize bleeding [42]. Lasers are particularly effective for soft tissue surgeries, such as tumor removal and dental procedures [27]. In addition to reducing bleeding, laser surgery accelerates the healing process and reduces postoperative pain, improving recovery times [43]. Regrettably, laser surgery is costly, and its use requires specialized training, which can be a barrier in some veterinary practices.

8.3.1.3 Advanced Fracture Repair

Modern fracture management in veterinary procedure promotes enhanced management of fractures among animals, thereby enhancing its healing process and recovery. This ability will improve steadily with technology and techniques over the years for treatment of any of the difficult to treat fractures thus improving on the quality of life for veterinary patients.

8.3.1.4 Thoracoscopy

Thoracoscopy in veterinary medicine is a relatively new procedure that allows the visualization and treatment of certain conditions located in the chest cavity (thorax) of animals. Like laparoscopy, thoracoscopy utilizes a thoracoscope, which serves as a less traumatic intervention as opposed to the classic thoracoscopic surgery or thoracotomy. Thoracoscopy, or video-assisted thoracic surgery (VATS), offers a minimally invasive approach to treating thoracic conditions such as pericardial effusion, pulmonary neoplasia, and spontaneous pneumothorax [28]. Small incisions (ports) are made between the ribs to enter the thoracoscope and surgical equipment once the animal has been sedated and positioned appropriately. The smaller incisions, less postoperative pain, and quicker recovery times associated with this technique puts it ahead of traditional open surgery. To make a working cavity and increase visibility, carbon dioxide is frequently inhaled into the pleural space. After inserting the thoracoscope, the chest cavity is inspected. Specific tools are used to carry out therapeutic treatments or biopsies. Following the procedure, the thoracoscope and equipment are taken out, the carbon dioxide is expelled, and the incisions are sealed with surgical glue or stitches [33, 34]. However, thoracoscopy requires specialized equipment and expertise, limiting its use to practices with the necessary resources [27].

8.3.2 Emerging Therapies in Veterinary Oncology

Some relatively new trends in this field are aimed at improving the therapy of cancer diseases in animals, especially dogs, and cats. The main goals of these therapies are to raise the probability of the positive outcome, decrease the side effects, and increase the quality of life of pets with cancer. These therapies include immunotherapy, radiation therapy, gene therapy, and nanotechnology applications.

8.3.2.1 Immunotherapy

Immunotherapy involves different kind of cancer vaccines, monoclonal antibodies and some kind of checkpoint inhibitors that work by modulating the immune system. Cancer vaccines work by alerting the human immune system to identify cancer cells as foreign bodies and destroys them. Some examples include the melanoma vaccine for canine, where lungs melanoma cells in dogs are targeted. Several monoclonal antibodies are artificially synthesized in the laboratory to have the ability of gearing towards antigens found on the surface of cancerous cells in order to be destroyed by the body's immune system. Monoclonal antibodies that are recognized in dog's lymphoma cells are still under development [35, 36]. Immunotherapy has shown considerable promise in veterinary applications, where it can enhance immune responses or directly target cancer cells, offering a more personalized and effective treatment strategy [6]. While immunotherapy is still in the experimental stages in veterinary medicine, its integration into clinical practice is expected to improve the outcomes of cancer treatment for animals.

8.3.2.2 Radiation Therapy

This form of treatment is especially useful in veterinary oncology as it helps to eliminate cancerous cells while the healthy cells surrounding them stay intact. It is often administered as a cure and an alleviation measure in companion animals with special reference to pets such as dogs and cats [37, 38]. Advanced forms of radiation therapy, such as intensity-modulated radiation therapy (IMRT) and helical tomotherapy, allow for the precise targeting of tumors' while minimizing damage to surrounding tissues. These therapies have been shown to improve local tumor control and reduce normal tissue toxicity. This further enhances survival and quality of life for veterinary cancer patients. When combined with immunotherapy, radiation therapy holds potential for even greater efficacy, although challenges such as overlapping toxicities and preclinical model limitations remain [31].

8.3.2.3 Photodynamic Therapy

Photodynamic therapy (PDT) is a modern; effective type of treatment launched in veterinary medicine for cancer treatment and some other diseases. It entails the administration of a chemical which on illumination by light of a particular wavelength, generates toxic products that kills cancerous cells [39, 40].

8.3.3 Rehabilitation and Physiotherapy for Animals

Animal rehabilitation and animal physiotherapy are quite unique branches of veterinary medicine that embrace the use of treatment techniques applied to enhance the levels of functional ability of animals. These practices are most helpful in taking care of animals with injuries, surgical operations, or animals with conditions like arthritis [41]. This is through techniques such as massaging, hydrotherapy, electric stimulation, and development of proper exercise regimes that will help in relieving pain and helping animal functional ability throughout their life span as a pet or working animal. These therapies are slowly finding acceptance in the mainstream approach to an animal's well-being due to increased awareness in the welfare of animals and the fact that such therapies are effective and encompassing [41, 42].

8.3.4 Gene Therapy and Regenerative Medicine for Animals

There are two fields that are quickly advancing and have application in veterinary science gene therapy and regenerative medicine. In gene therapy, which is the modification or manipulation of an animal's genetic material to cure or prevent diseases, there is potential for treatment of genetic disorders and cancers among other conditions not amenable to standard modes of therapy [44]. On the contrary, regenerative medicine seeks to repair or replace injured organs and tissues by using stem cells, growth factors, and biomaterials. These novel techniques are intended to improve the well-being of animals through new effective treatments for wounds as well as chronic diseases [43, 44].

8.3.5 Nanotechnology Applications for Drug Delivery in Animals

With the ability to treat animals precisely and effectively, nanotechnology is transforming the way that drugs are delivered in veterinary medicine. Researchers can target certain tissues, increase medication stability, improve treatment outcomes, and reduce adverse effects by modifying materials at the nanoscale. By improving drug delivery methods, this technique has the potential to treat a variety of ailments in animals, including infectious disorders and cancer. With nanotechnology's further advancements, veterinary applications stand to revolutionize animal health care by guaranteeing safer and more effective therapies [45, 46]. Nanotechnology, particularly the use of graphene oxide (GO), has emerged as a promising tool in drug delivery and cancer therapy. GO nanostructures can improve the bioavailability and pharmacokinetics of drugs, enhancing their accumulation at tumor sites and minimizing side effects [44]. While the use of GO in veterinary medicine is still in its early stages, its application in cancer treatment shows significant promise, particularly in targeted drug delivery.

8.3.6 Immunotherapy and Vaccines: Advancements in Preventative Medicine

In veterinary medicine, immunotherapy refers to a variety of procedures intended to enhance or adjust the immune system. This method is especially helpful for treating allergies, cancer, and chronic illnesses in animals. Utilizing the body's innate defense mechanisms, immunotherapy presents a viable substitute for conventional treatments, which can have severe side effects [47]. These include newly developed vaccine formulations that offer more comprehensive and long-lasting immunity, such as DNA, vector, and recombinant vaccines. As the idea of One Health suggests, vaccinations are constantly evolving to prevent the transmission of infectious diseases among animal populations and protect human and animal health at the same time [47, 48].

8.4 Digital Health and Telemedicine

Digital health technologies, such as remote monitoring systems, are being adapted from human healthcare to veterinary applications. These systems facilitate the continuous assessment of health parameters, enabling timely interventions. Digital health and telemedicine in veterinary medicine are rapidly evolving fields, leveraging technology to enhance animal healthcare [17, 18]. These innovations include teleconsultation services, wearable health monitoring devices, biosensors, and advancements in remote surgery guidance. Each of these components plays a crucial role in improving the accessibility and quality of veterinary care.

These technologies provide affordable and continuous monitoring solutions for various diseases such as diabetes, heart diseases, and Alzheimer's disease. These systems integrate multiple sensors to monitor physiological parameters, enabling real-time data collection and storage in the cloud for continuous health assessment by healthcare professionals [45]. While wearable devices offer economical and effective solutions for health monitoring, there are technical limitations in the current devices, particularly in the integration of multiple parameters for consistent measurements. There is a need for improved integration techniques to enhance the functionality and performance of wearable systems.

8.4.1 Teleconsultation Services for Remote Diagnosis

A remote pathology interpretation service is called telepathology, or teleconsulting [49]. Though not particularly new, the phenomena have gained significance as technology advances. During the COVID-19 epidemic, teleconsulting became more popular as veterinary clinics searched for substitutes for in-person consultations [50]. Even though the word "telepathology" was coined in 1986, the field's first known use was in 1969, when live, black-and-white images of blood smears and histology slides were transmitted using microwave-based telecommunication [51]. After half a century, there have been notable developments in the fields of telecommunications and information technology; consequently, telepathology has grown in sophistication, accessibility, and usage in both human and veterinary medicine [52]. Acquiring cytologic, hematologic, histologic, or macroscopic pictures for transmission over telecommunication channels for diagnosis, consulting, teaching, and research is known as telepathology [53–57]. The importance that telepathology played in providing much-needed pathology expertise to rural areas was highlighted when it was initially reported in the literature on human pathology. Teleconsulting is especially useful because many rural veterinary offices in North America are located far from the laboratory and veterinary specialists. All animal species are served by these clinics, and prompt test results are essential for happy clients and well-timed treatment decisions [58].

Furthermore, quick answers are essential in animal production operations were figuring out the reason of an illness is critical for the general well-being of the herd as well as for identifying any newly emerging, zoonotic, or foreign animal diseases, ensuring food safety, and protecting public health [59]. In a recent study, development, implementation, and evaluation of myHealthE (MHE), a digital innovation designed for Child and Adolescent Mental Health Services (CAMHS) to automate the remote collection and reporting of patient-reported outcome measures (PROMs) into the National Health Services (NHS) electronic healthcare records was achieved [38]. Such studies can be modified for application in veterinary medicine as it highlights the feasibility and acceptability of the system within clinical services, demonstrating its potential to enhance the efficiency of data collection and integration into existing NHS infrastructure. The application of teleconsultation services enables veterinarians to diagnose and treat animals remotely, reducing the need for in-person visits. This is especially useful for routine check-ups and minor ailments. These services rely on digital platforms to collect and transmit data, ensuring that veterinarians have access to the necessary information to make informed decisions [38].

8.4.2 Wearable Health Monitoring Devices for Pets

Animal health is a major concern in the modern world. We must wait for veterinary specialists to evaluate and diagnose an animal before we can keep an eye on its health. This ultimately results in delayed therapy and a decline in the health of the animals. Thus, designing a system that monitors an animal's health to facilitate primary health diagnosis by the animal owner is crucial. In this direction, sensors including blood pressure, heart rate, respiration rate, temperature, and ECG module can be applied [16]. This can be done by creating a system that has sensors that can be attached to an animal's body to measure physiological data including blood pressure, temperature, heart rate, respiration rate, and ECG. For farmed animals, it can mean the difference between life and death if biomarkers or certain substances cannot be promptly, precisely, and consistently detected. Microelectronics and biotechnology have made it feasible to create transistors smaller than 100 nm and combine hundreds of them into a usable circuit on a tiny chip. New enabling technologies have also been made possible by the rapid advancements in nanofabrication [60].

Wearable devices integrate multiple sensors to monitor physiological parameters, enabling real-time data collection and storage in the cloud for continuous health assessment by healthcare professionals. While wearable devices offer economical and effective solutions for health monitoring, there are technical limitations in the current devices, particularly in the integration of multiple parameters for consistent measurements. Need for improved integration techniques to enhance the functionality and performance of wearable systems. Addressing these integration challenges could lead to earlier symptom identification and better disease management [45]. Furthermore, integration of the Internet of Things (IoT) in healthcare, emphasizing its transformative impact on health monitoring. The ability of IoT devices to monitor vital health indicators such as pulse rate, body temperature, blood pressure, and blood oxygen saturation. These devices also track bodily movements to detect risks like falls and injuries, highlighting their potential in everyday health monitoring due to their portability, lightweight design, and ease of use. The system's construction involves data collection, sensor reading preprocessing, and the use of a cloud platform for feature extraction, recognition algorithms, and emergency callouts. However, the peculiar challenges with this system include data privacy concerns, the need for robust data security measures, or the integration of these systems with existing healthcare infrastructure. Additionally, there is a lack of discussion on the long-term reliability and accuracy of these IoT devices in diverse real-world settings, which are critical for widespread adoption [37].

8.4.2.1 Biosensors

Biosensors are the most widely used technique to prevent health risks, a range of techniques are employed to measure the amount of antibiotics in the body. The biosensors' operation and design are highly straightforward and comprehensible, enabling prompt and precise identification of antibiotics. A transducing device and a recognition element enable biosensors to function. The method of affinity-pairing, such as enzyme/substrate and antibody/antigen receptors, is worked on by the recognition element [61]. Biosensors integrated into wearable devices can detect specific health markers, offering real-time insights into an animal's health status. The data collected can be stored and analyzed to identify trends and potential health issues early on [45].

8.4.3 Remote Surgery Guidance: Advancements in Teleoperation

Remote surgery guidance involves using teleoperation technologies to assist veterinarians in performing surgeries from a distance. This can be particularly useful in complex cases where specialist input is required. Systems like the M7 surgical robot, Zeus system, and Viky endoscopic robot are examples of advanced technologies that facilitate remote surgical procedures, enhancing precision and outcomes [38]. Robots have gradually moved outside of industry to help people more directly over the past few decades. Service robots are currently employed in a variety of industries today [58]. Surgeons are using robots more and more to help them with a variety of procedures, most notably minimally invasive surgery (MIS). Robotically assisted surgical systems (RASS) enable MIS by utilizing extremely skilled equipment to create a smaller, less painful incision into the patient's body [62]. This facilitates quicker healing, which lowers hospital stays and, consequently, patient expenses. Surgical assistants are relieved of their manual holding duties when robot arms are used to position and hold surgical instruments, and surgeons get mental comfort as a result of their increased confidence in the accuracy of the instruments' placement and operation [63]. Below are a few instances of RASS:

8.4.3.1 M7 Surgical Robot System

The M7 robotic system was developed in 1998 by the Stanford Research Institute. M7 has two robotic arms that resemble humans and have seven degrees of freedom that reflect force. Stereo vision allows surgeons to teleoperate. There are 4.5 kg in each arm. Suturing corneal lacerations have been demonstrated using microsurgical technology. During the ninth NEEMO experiment in April 2006, real-time abdominal surgery was conducted on a patient simulator using the M7 system [64].

8.4.3.2 The Zeus System

In 1995, Computer Motion created the Zeus system, which was approved by the FDA in 2001. This system combined an Aesop robot developed by Computer Motion with two robotic arms that could grasp instruments. Zeus has a robotic arm that he controls with a computer-assisted remote-control device. In 2001, a group of French surgeons in New York performed the first "Lindbergh surgery operation" on a patient in Strasbourg, France, with the help of the Zeus system [65].

8.4.3.3 Viky Endoscopic Robot

Endo control Medical makes a lightweight endoscopic robot called Viky.31 Its job is to provide stable images and move the endoscope precisely as directed by the surgeon to maximize the exposure of the operative site. It is commonly utilized for gynecological, urological, and digestive laparoscopic procedures. Without the assistance of a helper, the surgeon can directly check the position of the robot. Many other robotic systems were made to help with remote surgeries which have helped a lot in the veterinary sciences [66].

8.4.4 Mobile Applications for Animal Healthcare

The rapid advancement of technology has made mobile terminals an essential everyday requirement for humans. They have a developed application foundation already, both in private and public enterprise. Businesses are becoming more competitive as a result of the economic shift. Our lives are becoming more and more dependent on the use of terminals [14, 17]. Animal health monitoring and epidemic prevention are currently dealing with a transformation issue due to the quick advancement of medical treatment. As more sophisticated and comprehensive systems continue to evolve, the transition from traditional manual statistics to electronic terminal statistics offers a more practical and effective method of working for the prevention of animal epidemics and health supervision. For real-time statistics, data updating, and data prediction, it offers efficient data assurance and accuracy [67].

Mobile applications have become a significant tool in veterinary medicine, offering innovative solutions for animal healthcare. These applications leverage the capabilities of smartphones to provide a range of services, from monitoring animal health to facilitating communication between pet owners and veterinarians. The integration of mobile technology in veterinary medicine is part of a broader trend in healthcare, where mobile health (m-health) applications are increasingly used to enhance healthcare delivery [18]. Mobile applications provide pet owners with easy access to veterinary services and information. They allow for remote monitoring and management of animal health, which is particularly beneficial in rural or underserved areas where veterinary services may be limited. Also highlighted are SMS medicine's potential to enhance healthcare delivery through cost-effectiveness, scalability, and improved communication, especially in low-resource settings, while identifying challenges such as data privacy, technological limitations, and integration with existing systems as areas needing further attention [46].

These applications can track vital signs and other health parameters in real-time, enabling early detection of health issues. This is crucial for timely interventions and can significantly improve health outcomes for animals. The potential of machine learning algorithms in transforming animal healthcare by enabling early disease detection, handling large datasets, providing error-free results, and supporting real-time applications has already been explored [9]. In addition, Mobile applications can reduce the cost of veterinary care by minimizing the need for in-person visits and enabling efficient management of chronic conditions. This is particularly important in low-resource settings where cost can be a barrier to accessing veterinary services [46].

8.4.4.1 The Pet Mobile App

Our lives are significantly impacted by mobile technologies, and as these technologies improve, users can enable new kinds of healthcare systems with the use of rule-based expert systems. In particular, the availability of affordable smartphones running the Android OS with a more user-friendly interface opens new possibilities for the ongoing monitoring of the health of pets, including healthy dogs and cats as well as those that have ingested harmful substances. It is possible to stop illness outbreaks in pets by using the pet smartphone app. Mobile applications can reduce the cost of veterinary care by minimizing the need for in-person visits and enabling efficient management of chronic conditions. This is particularly important in low-resource settings where cost can be a barrier to accessing veterinary services [46]. Using this app, you may locate the closest animal hospital in your neighborhood [68]. Applications facilitate better communication between pet owners and veterinarians, allowing for more effective management of animal health. Features such as appointment scheduling, medication reminders, and direct messaging can improve adherence to treatment plans and overall care quality. These applications are particularly beneficial in areas like chronic disease management, lifestyle interventions, and behavioral therapy, offering functionalities such as drug guides, medical calculators, and remote monitoring. Help in reducing the frequency of hospital visits by enabling self-management of conditions like diabetes, where they assist in monitoring glucose levels, diet, and physical activity. In cardiology, apps are used for heart monitoring and blood pressure tracking, aiding in the self-management of cardiovascular diseases.

Nevertheless, some of the challenges in diabetes management apps often involve lack of educational content, which is crucial for effective self-management. Similarly, weight management apps fail to incorporate behavioral strategies that could enhance their effectiveness. In the realm of mental health, apps for conditions like bipolar disorder often do not adhere to clinical guidelines or provide comprehensive tools for symptom monitoring and patient education [17]. Additionally, there is a lack of integration with personal health records, which could improve the usability and effectiveness of these apps. Future Directions: To address these gaps, there is a need for a medical apps accreditation program to ensure quality and adherence to clinical guidelines. This would involve regular assessment and certification of apps to keep up with rapid technological advancements [14]. Moreover, leveraging social networks could create support groups for individuals with similar health concerns, enhancing the effectiveness of health management practices. Understanding the context that influences health activities is also crucial for developing effective chronic disease management strategies [9, 46].

8.5 Impact of Technology on Animal Welfare and Management

The environment that animals raised in farms must learn to interact with has become more complex due to the introduction of new husbandry practices and management technologies. For instance, laying hens must learn the temporal and spatial design elements of new free range and aviary systems, and cattle may need to learn how to interact with virtual fences and automated milking systems. Variations in learning capacities among farmed animals may affect how new technologies or AI (Figure 8.2) affect specific individuals, which could have an impact on welfare when new livestock management techniques are introduced [69]. In addition, platform variability, which complicates the standardization of technological applications across different devices, and concerns about security and privacy, which are paramount given the sensitive nature of medical data. Additionally, issues such as cost-effectiveness, energy consumption, user interface design, and the quality of medical data collected by different technological applications are highlighted as areas requiring further research and development [14].

8.5.1 Precision Livestock Farming

A lot of exciting new and developing technologies have the potential to completely transform the livestock farming industry, and one of the most significant ones is probably PLF. When properly applied, PLF or Smart Farming has

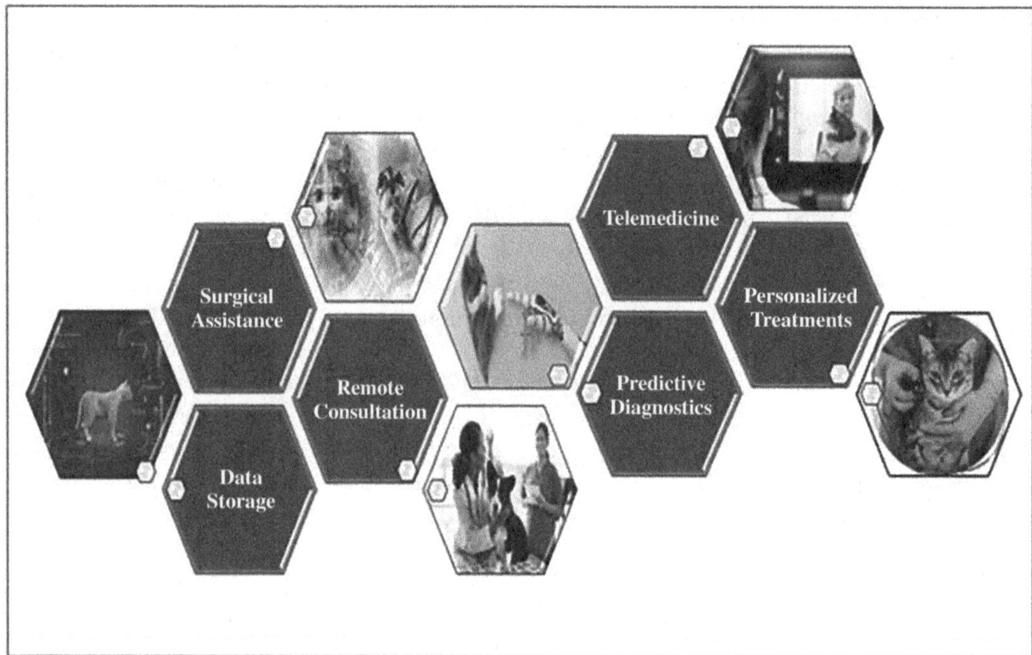

Figure 8.2 Role of artificial intelligence in different areas of veterinary medicine.

the potential to enhance or at least objectively record farm animal welfare; lower greenhouse gas emissions and enhance farm environmental performance; enable better livestock product marketing and product segmentation; lessen the illicit trade in livestock products; and enhance the economic stability of rural areas [70]. The definition of PLF is "the application of principles and techniques of process engineering to livestock farming to automatically monitor, model, and manage animal production." It involves translating bio responses into pertinent data that can be readily applied to various management aspects that prioritize the environment and the animal [71]. Automated measurement techniques are increasingly being used to track animal behavior, and several models that can discern fairly accurate features of daily physiological routines have been developed. The core framework of PLF has been established by various behavioral monitoring studies conducted on activity, eating and milking. PLF is a management system that combines a range of data from many hardware sources for monitoring using highly intelligent software and processes. With sophisticated monitoring techniques like tele-surveillance, this data-driven system minimizes unfavorable environmental effects while promoting better health, welfare, and productivity [72].

PLF technologies have the potential to improve animal welfare by detecting health issues early and ensuring optimal environmental conditions, but their current ability to promote positive welfare states is limited. Technology is effective in reducing negative experiences like diseases and injuries, but promoting positive affective states remains a challenge due to early development stages and lack of evidence for positive welfare indicators. PLF technologies can monitor various parameters such as feeding behavior, environmental conditions, and health indicators, which can help in making informed management decisions to improve welfare. There are concerns about the impact of PLF on human–animal relationships (HAR), as reduced human interaction could affect farmers' empathy and concern for animal welfare. The adoption of PLF technologies is slow due to innovation uncertainty and the need for validation to ensure reliability and trust among farmers. Technology is mostly available for cattle, with fewer options for smaller animals like poultry and fish, which are often monitored at the group level rather than individually. There is a need for further research to validate PLF technologies and develop reliable positive welfare indicators, as well as to encourage collaboration between industry, researchers, and farmers. The potential for PLF to improve welfare depends on how the data is used to adapt management practices and address root causes of welfare issues rather than just treating symptoms [15].

These technologies, such as camera systems and accelerometers, have been developed primarily to boost production efficiency but also contribute to welfare improvements by enabling early detection of health issues and optimizing feeding systems, thus reducing hunger and discomfort. Environmental monitoring and automatic milking systems further enhance animal comfort and improve human–animal interactions. However, a significant gap remains as current PLF systems do not provide a comprehensive, multidimensional assessment of animal welfare. The integration of PLF sensor data into automated welfare assessment systems is a potential solution, but further research is needed to define and validate this approach, ensuring a holistic evaluation of animal welfare [47].

Furthermore, the application of PLF in grazing land management has shown promise in improving livestock production efficiency and animal welfare by automating data collection and enhancing decision-making processes. Machine learning, remote sensing, and precision agriculture are significantly enhancing the efficiency of data collection and monitoring in grazing land management. These advancements support better decision-making on farms, which is crucial for improving livestock production efficiency while maintaining animal welfare, environmental sustainability, and profitability. One major issue is the lack of reliable reference data and the low variability in datasets used for model calibration, which can hinder the effectiveness of these technologies. Additionally, there is a need for stronger relationships between farmers and researchers, clearer communication of the benefits of PLF, and increased cooperation among professionals from various fields. The development of user-friendly software and applications is also necessary to make these technologies more accessible and widely implemented in real-world conditions [12].

8.5.1.1 Monitoring Devices

Many technologies were used to monitor the many aspects of the animals, such as image and sound analysis using cameras, sensors, or other devices like water/feed consumption, scales, etc. In image analysis, no additional stress is caused by the devices' requirement not to be placed on the animal; however, in the prediction stage, it is challenging to maintain good precision because the developed software for target tracking and animal foreground extraction depends on several intricate image factors. Images are analyzed to estimate body condition and weight, measure water and feed intake, evaluate gait and lameness, and identify marked animals in estrus behavior [73]. Variability in mobile phone platforms and technological limitations can affect the performance and reliability of these applications.

Additionally, disparities in access to smartphones and internet connectivity can limit their reach [16]. Many mobile applications are developed without proper validation by veterinary authorities, which can lead to issues with accuracy and reliability. Establishing standards and regulations for these applications is necessary to ensure their safety and effectiveness. There is growing prevalence of healthcare-related mobile applications aimed at patients, emphasizing the need to understand their limitations, safety concerns, and challenges related to legalization. While these applications are increasingly used, the benefits they claim are not always supported by evidence. A significant concern is that many of these applications are developed by nonexperts and lack validation from healthcare authorities, which poses potential risks to patient safety. More research is needed to assess the long-term effects of these applications on healthcare systems and individual psychosocial well-being. Also, existing research often lacks a universal perspective and may be biased by financial interests promoting the use of these applications [17]. Another recent study identified lack of comprehensive evaluation of healthcare Apps, which should consider both clinical and technological aspects due to the nascent evidence of their clinical effectiveness and associated risks. In Chile, while the use of mobile technology and Apps is on the rise, there is a notable absence of regulations governing their use. The paper points out that few national institutions are dedicated to the development of healthcare Apps, with the Digital Transformation Committee and the National Center for Health Information Systems being notable exceptions [18].

Monitoring devices, such as accelerometers and GPS, are used to track animal behavior and health, allowing for early detection of diseases and stressors. These devices can improve animal welfare by enabling timely interventions and optimizing environmental conditions. Precision livestock management (PLM) is a developing field that uses technology like GPS and accelerometers to monitor animal welfare on rangelands, aiming to improve sustainable meat production and animal welfare by providing real-time data to livestock managers. The "Five Freedoms" framework is used to evaluate animal welfare, focusing on aspects like freedom from thirst, hunger, discomfort, pain, and the ability to express normal behavior. PLM can help address these freedoms by providing data to detect issues like water scarcity, heat stress, and disease early on. GPS and accelerometers can track livestock movements and behaviors, helping to identify welfare concerns such as lameness, parturition, and heat stress. These technologies can alert managers to intervene promptly, potentially improving animal health and productivity. The use of multiple sensors, including remote sensing imagery, can enhance the detection of changes in animal behavior, although challenges remain in terms of cost, data processing, and the physical impact of sensors on animals. There is a need for more research on the use of sensors to detect cold and heat stress, and the integration of these technologies into commercial operations due to cost and expertise barriers [13]. In poultry farming, PLF systems have been developed to provide a continuous picture of welfare states, facilitating fast interventions that benefit the flock. However, the commercial adoption of these systems remains limited. While PLF systems have the potential to enhance animal welfare by providing real-time monitoring and enabling swift interventions, their primary focus has been somewhat ambiguous between improving welfare and increasing production efficiency. The development of PLF has predominantly concentrated on broiler farming, followed by laying hens, utilizing technologies such as environmental and wearable sensors and cameras. Notably, more publications have prioritized animal health and welfare over production, suggesting a current trend towards welfare improvement. However, a significant gap remains in the commercial application of these technologies, which is crucial for realizing their full potential in enhancing bird welfare [48].

8.5.1.2 Drug Tracking

Misuse of veterinary antimicrobial drugs on a global scale has resulted in a concerning rise in bacterial resistance, which has caused clinical treatment failure in both humans and animals. Risk depends on the optimization of pharmacokinetics by measurement and characterization of interindividual variability of drug intake to obtain the optimal dosing regimen of antibiotics for prevention and treatment of diseases along with minimizing resistance. Therefore, these novel systems allow not only for early disease detection and early medication interventions, but also for transparent/traceability, follow-up on recovering patients, and refined phenotypes, as well as the assessment of feed and water intake to calculate the precise amount of drug and associate with certain health effects [74]. The integration of PLF technologies can indirectly support drug management by providing data on animal health and behavior, which can inform treatment decisions and reduce the need for antibiotics and growth hormones. It offers transformative solutions to longstanding ethical concerns in traditional livestock farming, such as overcrowding, antibiotic use, and environmental harm. There is need for the development of standardized ethical guidelines, global adoption, and cross-sector collaboration to ensure ethical treatment of animals in the PLF era [32].

8.5.1.3 Feed Follow-up System

Measuring the amount of grain that cattle consume is thought to be a great way to estimate their overall health. Because they are not hungry, sick cattle will spend less time eating. Initially, research concentrated mostly on pressure sensors attached to the jaw using a halter to identify patterns of rumination [75]. Next, using a computer collection system, Burfeind [76] collected the data and transformed it into a monitoring system that can analyze the data to distinguish between eating and rumination. These days, it is feasible to forecast feed intake, health, and environmental effects using rumination activity patterns. As a result, it is possible to distinguish between physiologically sound and pathological states, such as metabolic abnormalities and stress-related situations [77].

8.5.2 Use of VR in Animal Training

The use of animals in scientific research and training has long been a topic of ethical debate. With hundreds of experiments involving animal models conducted each month, concerns are frequently raised about the welfare of animals and the ethical implications of their use. Animal rights and welfare organizations advocate for the recognition of animals as sentient beings capable of experiencing pain and emotions, urging for their humane treatment. This has led to widespread support for the "3Rs" principle in scientific practices: Replacement, Reduction, and Refinement, which aim to minimize the use and suffering of animals in research and training [9, 46].

VR emerges as a transformative tool in addressing these ethical challenges, particularly in animal training and veterinary education. VR technology offers immersive, interactive environments that can simulate real-world scenarios without the need to involve live animals. For example, VR-based training programs are being developed to help veterinary students acquire surgical skills [37]. These programs use stereoscopic viewing and minimally interactive virtual environments to provide a realistic and detailed understanding of surgical procedures. Students can practice techniques in a controlled, risk-free environment, improving their proficiency and confidence before performing surgeries on live animals. The benefits of VR in animal training and veterinary education extend beyond ethical considerations. It allows repeated practice, which is critical for mastering complex skills, without causing harm to animals [38]. Additionally, VR can simulate rare or high-risk scenarios that may not frequently occur in real life, ensuring that trainees are well-prepared to handle a wide range of challenges. By integrating VR into training programs, institutions can significantly reduce the reliance on animal models, aligning with the ethical goals of the 3Rs. Beyond veterinary education, VR has potential applications in the behavioral training of animals. For instance, VR environments can be designed to simulate different scenarios, aiding in desensitization training for animals with anxiety or fear-related behaviors. This innovative approach not only enhances animal welfare but also opens new possibilities for humane training techniques [78, 79].

8.6 Technological Innovations in Animal Nutrition

Technological innovations in animal nutrition have significantly advanced the field, particularly through precision feeding systems, nutrigenomics, and smart feeders. These innovations aim to optimize livestock production by enhancing feed efficiency, reducing environmental impact, and improving animal health and welfare. Precision feeding systems, nutrigenomics in pigs and poultry, and smart feeders are at the forefront of these advancements, each contributing uniquely to the field.

8.6.1 Precision Feeding System for Livestock

Precision livestock feeding represents a transformative approach in animal agriculture, aiming to align the nutritional supply with the specific nutrient requirements of individual animals in real-time. By utilizing advanced sensor technology and data-driven strategies, this method ensures that each animal receives the optimal amount of nutrients at the right time, significantly improving the efficiency and sustainability of livestock management [15, 47]. This approach is supported by advanced technologies such as sensors and automation, which enable real-time monitoring and data collection. The method enhances feed efficiency, reduces environmental impacts such as greenhouse gas emissions, and improves animal welfare by allowing for real-time health monitoring [49].

The foundation of precision livestock feeding lies in real-time sensor data, which provides continuous and accurate information about the environment, the animals, and the composition of feed. Sensors monitor various parameters, such as the animals' health, metabolic status, and feed intake, enabling the accurate assessment of each animal's unique nutritional needs. This data is then used by automated systems or smart machines to deliver precise quantities of feed to individual animals, ensuring their specific dietary requirements are met [12]. The benefits of precision livestock feeding extend across multiple dimensions. Economically, it optimizes feed utilization, reducing waste and maximizing returns by ensuring no excess feed is supplied. Environmentally, it minimizes nutrient runoff and greenhouse gas emissions, contributing to reduced environmental pollution and supporting sustainable farming practices. Socially, it promotes animal welfare by ensuring animals are neither underfed nor overfed, aligning with the ethical standards of responsible livestock management [12, 47].

To achieve these outcomes, the integration of advanced technologies with animal models is crucial. The continuous development of smart machines, such as automated feeders and robotic systems, is necessary to handle the complexities of individualized feeding. These systems rely on sophisticated algorithms to interpret sensor data and make real-time adjustments, delivering the right feed composition to the right animal at the right moment [12]. The implementation of precision livestock feeding not only enhances economic efficiency and environmental sustainability but also reinforces the social responsibility pillar of agricultural sustainability. By reducing resource waste, lowering the ecological footprint, and promoting ethical treatment of animals, this approach aligns with global efforts to create a more sustainable and responsible agricultural sector [13, 48].

As technology continues to evolve, precision livestock feeding is poised to become a cornerstone of modern livestock management, fostering a balance between productivity, environmental stewardship, and animal welfare [80, 81]. However, the need for real-time monitoring solutions, cost-effective large-scale implementation, and a deeper understanding of the long-term effects on animal health and welfare. Addressing these challenges is crucial for optimizing resource efficiency and developing personalized nutritional strategies that contribute to a more sustainable and ethically sound agricultural landscape [49]. In pig production, precision feeding has been shown to reduce lysine intake by over 25%, decrease feeding costs by more than 8%, and lower nitrogen and phosphorus excretion by nearly 40%, thus minimizing the environmental footprint. These improvements are achieved by tailoring diets daily to the individual nutritional requirements of pigs, which not only optimizes nutrient efficiency but also minimizes environmental impacts. Nevertheless, there is a need for a better understanding of the technology and its implementation to fully realize its benefits in real-world settings. Additionally, while increasing the number of feeding phases can prevent nutrient oversupply, it complicates feed management and raises production costs, indicating a need for more efficient strategies to balance these factors [50].

In broilers production, precision nutrition strategies that adjust diets daily can enhance production efficiency and sustainability by reducing nutrient oversupply and undersupply throughout the production cycle. This approach uses modern technologies to blend feed components daily, ensuring nutrients are neither under nor oversupplied, which is a common issue with traditional multiphase feeding systems [32]. While some farms may already have the necessary technology to implement precision nutrition, the initial investment and logistical challenges of integrating these systems into existing operations are concerns. The adoption of precision nutrition and feeding technologies could represent a paradigm shift in poultry feed formulation, helping the industry meet the rising global demand for animal protein more sustainably and efficiently [51].

8.6.2 Nutrigenomics in Animal Nutrition Research

Nutrigenomics, one of the most rapidly advancing fields in animal nutrition research, focuses on understanding how nutrition influences gene expression patterns and epigenetic modifications such as DNA methylation and histone alterations [52]. This field bridges the gap between nutrition and genomics, providing insights into how dietary components can impact on the genetic makeup and overall health of animals. In addition, it can also improve animal performance, health, and welfare by tailoring diets to the genetic makeup of livestock [51]. In livestock, the understanding of imprinted genes whose expression depends on their parental origin is relatively limited compared to humans and mice. However, these genes hold immense potential in shaping economically important traits. For instance, the maternally imprinted *Insulin-like Growth Factor 2* (*IGF2*) gene in pigs have been shown to play a pivotal role in muscle development and fat deposition, traits crucial for meat quality and yield

[53–57]. Nutrigenomics research is gradually unraveling the potential of such genes, enabling targeted nutritional interventions to optimize desirable traits in livestock.

Although most of the experimental work in nutrigenomics has been conducted on mouse models, this research has laid a strong foundation for expanding studies to livestock. Studies in mice and rats have explored the effects of nutrition during specific life stages, such as pregnancy, and have conducted multigenerational experiments to assess the long-term impacts of dietary interventions. For example, maternal diet during pregnancy has been shown to influence offspring's gene expression and metabolic health through epigenetic modifications. These findings provide valuable insights that can be translated to livestock systems, enabling researchers to understand how targeted nutritional strategies during critical periods can influence animal health and productivity. Nutrigenomics holds transformative potential in animal nutrition research by paving the way for precision feeding strategies that align with genetic predispositions. This approach not only optimizes growth, reproduction, and health outcomes in animals but also contributes to sustainable livestock production by reducing resource wastage and improving feed efficiency. As research in this field expands, it promises to revolutionize how we approach animal nutrition, integrating genomic knowledge with tailored dietary strategies to maximize both economic and biological gains [63, 82].

The field of nutrigenomics is supported by related disciplines such as nutrigenetics, transcriptomics, proteomics, and metabolomics, which collectively contribute to understanding the dietary effects on genes responsible for phenotypic traits in livestock. Despite its potential, the application of nutrigenomics in tropical regions remains underexplored due to several challenges. These include the fragmented nature of research efforts, insufficient funding for comprehensive studies, technical complexities associated with multi-omics research, and ethical considerations. There should be a renewed focus on integrating nutrigenomics into nutrition and genetics research to improve the nutritional efficiency of livestock, suggesting that overcoming these barriers could unlock significant advancements in the field [53–57]. In pigs, nutrigenomics can help identify key molecular players involved in physiological adaptations to dietary changes, offering insights into optimizing feed formulations for better growth and health outcomes. Nutrigenomics studies the impact of nutrients on gene functioning, focusing on gene expression and epigenetic changes like DNA methylation and histone modifications. This field is rapidly growing, especially in livestock, where it can influence production traits and animal health. In livestock, dietary changes have been explored to improve meat quality, such as enhancing fatty acid profiles in beef and milk composition in dairy cattle. Despite advancements, there are significant gaps in understanding the proteome level in livestock, which is crucial for a comprehensive view of how diets affect animals. More studies are needed to explore the effects of nutrition on epigenetic mechanisms, such as DNA methylation and noncoding RNA interactions. Cutting-edge technologies like whole-genome bisulfite sequencing and RNA-sequencing are underutilized in livestock studies compared to human and rodent research. These tools could provide deeper insights into the genetic and epigenetic impacts of nutrition [52].

8.6.2.1 Nutragenomics in Pig

One of the main suppliers of meat is the pig farming sector. The majority of swine nutrigenomic research has focused on the genes that control the operation of the gut, liver, adipose, and muscular tissues [83]. In a study conducted, a hybrid Duroc Large White Landrace pig line was fed a low-protein diet containing three distinct types of fat: palm kernel oil, soybean oil, and palm oil. They investigated the expression and activity of SCD, a crucial lipogenic gene, in subcutaneous adipose and muscular tissues. Additionally, they measured the protein concentrations of FAS and ACACA, two important enzymes in the production of new fatty acids [84].

8.6.2.2 Nutragenomics in Poultry

The farm animal with the greatest number of breeding herds and individuals worldwide is poultry, which is primarily made up of chickens. Additionally, chicken meat is the most consumed meat. The correct growth and health status of chickens and hens are the main goals of the various food treatment methods used. Adding phytonutrients to chicken feed is thought to be an all-natural way to ward against illnesses. In one study, the transcriptome of intestinal intraepithelial lymphocytes was examined using a microarray technique, supplementing with carvacrol, cinnamaldehyde, and capsicum oleoresin from day 7 after hatching [85, 86].

8.6.3 Smart Feeders and Automated Diet Management

The relationship that exists between people and their pets goes beyond simple friendship and develops into a deep tie that makes our furry friend essential parts of our households. Their happiness and health become vital to us, and their well-being becomes entwined with our own. Nonetheless, given the hectic pace of contemporary life, making sure our cherished dogs receive the best care, and nourishment may frequently turn into a difficult balancing act [51]. Nutrition is one of the most important but also the most difficult areas of pet care. It can be challenging to maintain regular feeding regimens that are customized to each pet's needs, especially for pet owners who lead busy lives. Traditional automatic feeders may seem convenient, but they frequently lack the intelligence and adaptability needed to satisfy the specific needs of every pet. This may lead to problems including overfeeding, erratic behavior patterns, and eventually weakened pet health [87, 88]. Smart feeders and automated diet management systems are integral to PLF, allowing for the efficient delivery of tailored diets. These systems use electronic animal identification and computer-aided technologies to monitor and adjust feeding regimens based on individual animal needs. Automated systems can improve labor efficiency and reduce costs by streamlining routine workflows and ensuring precise nutrient delivery, which is crucial for maintaining animal health and optimizing production. However, implementation of precision feeding and nutrigenomics requires substantial investment in technology and infrastructure, which may be prohibitive for small-scale farmers. Additionally, the complexity of integrating these systems into existing farming practices can pose practical difficulties [30, 50].

8.6.3.1 Data-driven Farm Decision System

With the latest technological advancements, smart farm management can be implemented to reduce agricultural decision-making, which previously required hiring skilled individuals at a reasonable cost. Data recording devices with sensors and robotics-based automation tools that are linked to data-driven farm decision systems facilitate smart farm management. A vast amount of data can be produced by continuously recording real-time data logging of individual animals thanks to the development and affordability of a variety of sensors that can be used to monitor location, movement, sound, physiological parameters, product quality, etc. These sensors can be integrated with the creation of animal-friendly wearable technologies. Combining all these technologies to achieve precision animal farming is known as smart animal management [89].

8.7 Future Perspectives

Advancements in technology have revolutionized veterinary medicine, enabling rapid and accurate diagnosis of animal illnesses through robotics, imaging technology, and molecular procedures. These innovations allow veterinarians to examine and diagnose animals in a short amount of time, facilitating early disease detection and faster recovery. Speedy diagnostic tools not only help identify illnesses promptly but also play a crucial role in improving animal health and welfare. In therapeutics, gene-based treatments have been transformative, allowing veterinarians to target and eliminate disease-causing genes, potentially leading to healthier, disease-free generations. Additionally, the integration of nanotechnology into veterinary medicine has enhanced drug delivery systems. By utilizing nanoscale particles, medications can be precisely delivered to the affected areas without impacting other body systems, significantly reducing adverse side effects.

Moreover, remote diagnostic devices have further advanced veterinary care by enabling the detection of diseases and monitoring of health parameters from a distance. These tools provide veterinarians with real-time insights into an animal's condition, streamlining the diagnostic process and enabling timely interventions. Together, these technological advancements have elevated the standard of veterinary diagnostics and therapeutics, ensuring improved care and outcomes for animals.

8.8 Conclusion

It is also noteworthy that due to the application of the newest international technologies in the field of veterinary sciences, there is a qualitative change in the fight against diseases and the increase in capabilities for their detection, treatment and prevention. Telemedicine expands people's options for seeking treatment, whereas genetics and precision medicine are already providing more targeted treatments. Besides, vaccine development in cases of zoonotic diseases is crucial, and AI and machine learning enhance disease detection and treatment. Besides changing the portfolios of veterinary practice, these innovations in technology are also improving sustainability and health in the international context. Thus, there is evidence of optimism in the future of animal health.

References

1. Chauhan, R.S., Malik, Y.S., Saminathan, M., and Tripathi, B.N. Molecular biology techniques of pivotal importance in veterinary diagnostics. In: *Essentials of Veterinary Immunology and Immunopathology*, 623–645. Singapore: Springer; 2024. https://doi.org/10.1007/978-981-99-2718-0_22.
2. Gazalle, P.F., Lima, D.D., Martins, K.R., and Cunha, R.C. PCR and other genomic techniques applied to veterinary medicine. *Foco* 2023; 16(3): e1226–e1226. https://doi.org/10.54751/REVISTAFOCO.V16N3-010.
3. Middleton, J.R., Getchell, R.G., Flesner, B.K., et al. Considerations related to the use of molecular diagnostic tests in veterinary clinical and regulatory practice. *J. Am. Vet. Med. Assoc.* 2021; 259(6): 590–595. https://doi.org/10.2460/JAVMA.259.6.590.
4. Sériot, P., Dunié-Mérigot, A., Tréhiou, C.B., et al. Treatment and outcome of spontaneous pneumothorax secondary to suspected migrating vegetal foreign body in 37 dogs. *Vet. Rec.* 2021; 189(4): e22. https://doi.org/10.1002/VETR.22.
5. Ossiboff, R.J. Molecular diagnostic techniques. *Schalm's Vet. Hematol.* 2022; 1331–1336. https://doi.org/10.1002/9781119500537.CH145.
6. Gupta, K., Sharma, V., and Siddiqui, T. Transforming medicine: advances in gene therapy, immunotherapy, and targeted cures. *Curr. Protein Pept. Sci.* 2025; 26(6): 436–450. https://doi.org/10.2174/011389203733613725010210 4842.
7. Thakur, S., Bi, A., Mahmood, S., et al. Graphene oxide as an emerging sole adsorbent and photocatalyst: chemistry of synthesis and tailoring properties for removal of emerging contaminants. *Chemosphere* 2024; 352: 141483. https://doi.org/10.1016/J.CHEMOSPHERE.2024.141483.
8. Lu, Q. Bioresponsive and multifunctional cyclodextrin-based non-viral nanocomplexes in cancer therapy: building foundations for gene and drug delivery, immunotherapy and bioimaging. *Environ. Res.* 2023; 234: 116507. https://doi.org/10.1016/J.ENVRES.2023.116507.
9. Das, S., Roy, R.K., and Bezboruah, T. Machine learning in animal healthcare: a comprehensive review. *IJRES* 2024; 11(3): 89–93. https://doi.org/10.14445/23497157/IJRES-V11I3P109.
10. Domrazek, K. and Jurka, P. Application of next-generation sequencing (NGS) techniques for selected companion animals. *Animals* 2024; 14(11): 1578. https://doi.org/10.3390/ANI14111578.
11. Sue, M.J., Yeap, S.K., Omar, A.R., and Tan, S.W. Application of PCR-ELISA in molecular diagnosis. *Biomed. Res. Int.* 2014; 2014: 653014. https://doi.org/10.1155/2014/653014.

12 Bretas, I.L., Dubeux, Jr, J.C., Cruz P.J., et al. Precision livestock farming applied to grazing land monitoring and management – a review. *Agron. J.* 2023; 116(3): 1164–1186. https://doi.org/10.1002/AGJ2.21346.

13 Tobin, C.T., Bailey, D.W., Stephenson, M.B., et al. Opportunities to monitor animal welfare using the five freedoms with precision livestock management on rangelands. *Front. Anim. Sci.* 2022; 3: 928514. https://doi.org/10.3389/FANIM.2022.928514.

14 Talmale, R. and Sonwane, S. Mobile healthcare applications and platforms. *Proceedings - 2024 International Conference on Healthcare Innovations, Software and Engineering Technologies, HISET 2024*, 293–295; 2024. https://doi.org/10.1109/HISET61796.2024.00091.

15 Schillings, J., Bennett, R., and Rose, D.C. Exploring the potential of precision livestock farming technologies to help address farm animal welfare. *Front. Anim. Sci.* 2021; 2: 639678. https://doi.org/10.3389/FANIM.2021.639678.

16 Huang, W., Li, J., and Alem, L. Towards preventative healthcare: a review of wearable and mobile applications. *Stud. Health Technol. Inform.* 2018; 251: 11–14. https://doi.org/10.3233/978-1-61499-880-8-11.

17 Karia, J., Mohamed, R., and Petrushkin, H. Patient-targeted mobile applications in healthcare. *Br. J. Hosp. Med.* 2023; 84(8): 1–5. https://doi.org/10.12968/HMED.2023.0158.

18 Tala, Á., Vásquez, E., Rojas, E., and Marín, R. An appraisal of healthcare mobile applications. *Rev. Med. Chile.* 2022; 150(2): 206–215. https://doi.org/10.4067/S0034-98872022000200206.

19 Shen, Q., Li, Z., Meyer, M.D., et al. 50-nm gas-filled protein nanostructures to enable the access of lymphatic cells by ultrasound technologies. *Adv. Mater.* 2024; 36(28): 2307123. https://doi.org/10.1002/ADMA.202307123.

20 Navarro-Becerra, J. A., Castillo, J.I., and Borden, M.A. Effect of poly (ethylene glycol) configuration on microbubble pharmacokinetics. *ACS Biomater. Sci. Eng.* 2024; 10(5): 3331–3342. https://doi.org/10.1021/ACSBIOMATERIALS.3C01764.

21 Gupta, J., Ahmed, A.T., Tayyib, N.A., et al. A state-of-art of underlying molecular mechanisms and pharmacological interventions/nanotherapeutics for cisplatin resistance in gastric cancer. *Biomed. Pharmacother.* 2023; 166. 115337 https://doi.org/10.1016/J.BIOPHA.2023.115337.

22 Paramasivam, G., Palem, V.V., Meenakshy, S., et al. Advances on carbon nanomaterials and their applications in medical diagnosis and drug delivery. *Colloids Surf B Biointerfaces.* 2024; 241, 114032. https://doi.org/10.1016/J.COLSURFB.2024.114032.

23 Morgan, T.J. and Anstey, C.M. Expanding the boundaries of point of care testing. *J. Clin. Monit. Comput.* 2020; 34(3): 397–399. https://doi.org/10.1007/S10877-019-00344-6.

24 Stern, J.K. and Camus, M.S. Point-of-care instruments. *Vet. Clin. North Am. Small Anim. Pract.* 2022; 53(1): 17–28. https://doi.org/10.1016/J.CVSM.2022.08.001.

25 Alkhabiry, S.S.H., Alonizan, A.F.M., Almalki, Z.S.S., et al. Point-of-care testing: the use of portable and rapid diagnostic tests for immediate patient care. *J. Surv. Fish. Sci.* 2022; 9(4). 169–171. https://doi.org/10.53555/SFS.V9I4.2589.

26 Moreira, L.M. and Lyon, J.P. Photodynamic therapy in veterinary medicine: applications in dogs and cats. *Pubvet* 2022; 16(6): 1–4. https://doi.org/10.31533/PUBVET.V16N06A1129.1-4.

27 Barbur, L.A., Rawlings, C.A., and Radlinsky, M.A.G. Epicardial exposure provided by a novel thoracoscopic pericardectomy technique compared to standard pericardial window. *Vet. Surg.* 2018; 47(1): 146–152. https://doi.org/10.1111/VSU.12739.

28 Kanai, H., Furuya, M., Hagiwara, K., et al. Efficacy of bloc thoracic duct ligation in combination with pericardiectomy by video-assisted thoracoscopic surgery for canine idiopathic chylothorax. *Vet. Surg.* 2020; 49(S1): O102–O111. https://doi.org/10.1111/VSU.13370.

29 Arya, N. and Kaur, A. A review paper on application of PCR-ELISA in the molecular diagnosis. *IJIREM* 2022; 9(1): 341–344. https://doi.org/10.55524/IJIREM.2022.9.1.69.

30 Ahmad, H.I. and Hamid, M. (eds.) Recent trends in livestock innovative technologies. In: *Recent Advances in Biotechnology (Vol. 4)*. Bentham Science Publishers; 2023. https://doi.org/10.2174/9789815165074123070l.

31 Bhalla, N., Brooker, R., and Brada, M. Combining immunotherapy and radiotherapy in lung cancer. *J. Thorac. Dis.* 2018; 10: S1447–S1460. https://doi.org/10.21037/JTD.2018.05.107.

32 Egon, K., KARL, L., and Eugene, R. *Animal Welfare and Ethical Considerations in Precision Livestock Farming (PLF)*; 2023. https://doi.org/10.31219/OSF.IO/DH984.

33 Guimarães T.G., Cardoso, K.M., Marto, C.M., et al. Oncological applications of photodynamic therapy in dogs and cats. *Appl. Sci. (Switzerland).* 2022; 12(23): 12276. https://doi.org/10.3390/APP122312276.

34 Case, J.B. Advances in video-assisted thoracic surgery, thoracoscopy. *Vet. Clin. North Am. Small Anim. Pract.* 2016; 46(1): 147–169. https://doi.org/10.1016/j.cvsm.2015.07.005.

35 Sharon, E., Polley, M.Y., Bernstein, M.B., and Ahmed, M. Immunotherapy and radiation therapy: considerations for successfully combining radiation into the paradigm of immuno-oncology drug development. *Radiat. Res.* 2014; 182(2): 252–257. https://doi.org/10.1667/RR13707.1.

36 Hikmawati, F., Susilowati, A., and Setyaningsih, R. Colony morphology and molecular identification of *Vibrio* spp. on green mussels (*Perna viridis*) in Yogyakarta, Indonesia tourism beach areas. *Biodiversitas* 2019; 20(10): 2891–2899. https://doi.org/10.13057/BIODIV/D201015.

37 Elango, S., Manjunath, L., Prasad, D., et al. Super artificial intelligence medical healthcare services and smart wearable system based on IoT for remote health monitoring. *Proceedings - 5th International Conference on Smart Systems and Inventive Technology, ICSSIT 2023*, 1180–1186; 2023. https://doi.org/10.1109/ICSSIT55814.2023.10060928.

38 Morris A.C., Ibrahim, Z., Moghraby, O.S., et al. Moving from development to implementation of digital innovations within the NHS: myHealthE, a remote monitoring system for tracking patient outcomes in child and adolescent mental health services. *Digit Health* 2023; 9. 1–14. https://doi.org/10.1177/20552076231211551.

39 Still, V., Petley, L., and McDowell, G. Point-of-care testing. *Biomed. Sci. Pract.* 2022. 441. https://doi.org/10.1093/HESC/9780198831228.003.0016.

40 Makic, M.B.F. and Barton, A.J. Point of care testing: ensuring accuracy. *Clin Nurse Spec.* 2015; 29(6): 306–307. https://doi.org/10.1097/NUR.0000000000000165.

41 Saha, M. Laparoscopy minimally invasive surgery for pet animals. *IJRAPS.* 2023; 7(6): 6–13. https://doi.org/10.47070/IJRAPS.V7I6.135.

42 Guedes, R.L., Höglund, O.V., Brum, J.S., et al. Resorbable self-locking implant for lung lobectomy through video-assisted thoracoscopic surgery: first live animal application. *Surg. Innov.* 2018; 25(2): 158–164. https://doi.org/10.1177/1553350617751293.

43 Chaves, L.K.M., De Oliveira, M.D., Da Silva, I.C.C.C., et al. Inovações em técnicas minimamente invasivas em cirurgias de animais. *Int. Seven Multidiscip. J.* 2024; 3(5): 1397–1402. https://doi.org/10.56238/ISEVMJV3N5-004.

44 Sadeghi, M.S., Sangrizeh, F.H., Jahani, N. et al. Graphene oxide nanoarchitectures in cancer therapy: drug and gene delivery, phototherapy, immunotherapy, and vaccine development. *Environ. Res.* 2023; 237: 117027. https://doi.org/10.1016/J.ENVRES.2023.117027.

45 Devi, M.P., Sathya, T., and Raja, G.B. Remote human's health and activities monitoring using wearable sensor-based system—a review. In: *Internet of Things*, 203–228. Cham: Springer Nature Link; 2021. https://doi.org/10.1007/978-3-030-66633-0_9.

46 Rahman, M.Z. and Bhuiyan, M.S.A. SMS medicine: revolutionizing healthcare delivery through mobile technology. *Ann. Innov. Med.* 2024; 2(4): 22–30. https://doi.org/10.59652/AIM.V2I4.368.

47 Van Erp-Van der Kooij, E. and Rutter, S.M. Using precision farming to improve animal welfare. *CABI Rev.* 2020; 15(51). https://doi.org/10.1079/PAVSNNR202015051.

48 Rowe, E., Dawkins, M.S., and Gebhardt-Henrich, S.G. A systematic review of precision livestock farming in the poultry sector: is technology focussed on improving bird welfare? *Animal* 2019; 9(9): 614. https://doi.org/10.3390/ANI9090614.

49 Sonea, C., Gheorghe-Irimia, R.A., Tapaloaga, D. et al. Optimizing animal nutrition and sustainability through precision feeding: a mini review of emerging strategies and technologies. *Ann. Valahia Univ. Targ. – Agric.* 2023; 15(2): 7–11. https://doi.org/10.2478/AGR-2023-0011.

50 Pomar, C. and Remus, A. Precision pig feeding: a breakthrough toward sustainability. *Anim. Front.* 2019; 9(2): 52–59. https://doi.org/10.1093/AF/VFZ006.

51 Moss, A.F., Chrystal, P.V., Cadogan, D.J. et al. Precision feeding and precision nutrition: a paradigm shifts in broiler feed formulation? *Anim. Biosci.* 2021; 34(3): 354–362. https://doi.org/10.5713/AB.21.0034.

52 Nowacka-Woszuk, J. Nutrigenomics in livestock-recent advances. *J. Appl. Genet.* 2020; 61(1): 93–103. https://doi.org/10.1007/S13353-019-00522-X.

53 Okani-Onyejiaka, M.C., Etuk, E.B., and Ogundu, U.E. Nutrigenomics in livestock research and production: principles, applications and challenges. *Niger. J. Anim. Prod.* 2024; 155–158. https://doi.org/10.51791/NJAP.VI.4328.

54 Mark, J.J. A brief history of veterinary medicine. *Anc. Hist. Encycl.* 2020. https://www.worldhistory.org/article/1549/a-brief-history-of-veterinary-medicine/.

55 Ogilvie, T., and Kastelic, J. Technology is rapidly changing our world, including veterinary medicine. *Can. Vet. J.* 2022; 63(12): 1177.

56 Chmurzynska, A., Mlodzik, M.A., Radziejewska, A. et al. Caloric restriction can affect one-carbon metabolism during pregnancy in the rat: a transgenerational model. *Biochimie.* 2018; 152: 181–187.

57 El Idrissi, A.H., Larfaoui, F., Dhingra, M. et al. Digital technologies and implications for veterinary services. *Rev. Sci. Tech.* 2021; 40(2): 455–468.

58 El-Husseiny, H.M., Mady, E.A., Helal, M.A.Y., and Tanaka, R. The pivotal role of stem cells in veterinary regenerative medicine and tissue engineering. *Vet. Sci.* 2022; 9(11): 648.

59 Yitbarek, D. and Dagnaw, G.G. Application of advanced imaging modalities in veterinary medicine: a review. *Vet. Med.Res. Rep.* 2022; 13: 117–130.

60 Meomartino, L., Greco, A., Di Giancamillo, M. et al. Imaging techniques in veterinary medicine. Part I: radiography and ultrasonography. *Eur. J. Radiol. Open.* 2021; 8: 100382.

61 Samir, H., Swelum, A.A., and Kandiel, M.M.M. Exploring roles of diagnostic ultrasonography in veterinary medicine. *Front. Vet. Sci.* 2022; 9: 1084676.

62 Anglart, D., Hallén-Sandgren, C., Emanuelson, U., and Rönnegård, L. Comparison of methods for predicting cow composite somatic cell counts. *J. Dairy Sci.* 2020; 103(9): 8433–8442.

63 Rogers, L., Galezowski, A., Ganshorn, H., et al. The use of telepathology in veterinary medicine: a scoping review. *J. Vet. Diagn. Invest.* 2024; 36(4): 490–497. https://doi.org/10.1177/10406387241241270.

64 Daniel, G.B. and Neelis, D.A. Thyroid scintigraphy in veterinary medicine. *Semin. Nucl. Med.* 2014; 44(1): 24–34.

65 Greco, A., Meomartino, L., Gnudi, G., et al. Imaging techniques in veterinary medicine. Part II: computed tomography, magnetic resonance imaging, nuclear medicine. *Eur. J. Radiol. Open.* 2023; 10: 100467.

66 Debnath, M., Prasad, G.B.K.S., and Bisen, P.S. *Molecular Diagnostics: Promises and Possibilities.* Springer Science & Business Media; 2010.

67 Dahlhausen, B. Future veterinary diagnostics. *J. Exot. Pet. Med.* 2010; 19(2): 117–132.

68 Pestana, E., Belak, S., Diallo, A. et al. *Early, Rapid and Sensitive Veterinary Molecular Diagnostics-Real Time PCR Applications.* Springer Science & Business Media; 2010.

69 Dunisławska, A., Łachmańska, J., Sławińska, A., and Siwek, M. Next generation sequencing in animal science—a review. *Anim. Sci. Pap. Rep.* 2017; 35(3): 205–224.

70 Kubacki, J., Fraefel, C., and Bachofen, C. Implementation of next-generation sequencing for virus identification in veterinary diagnostic laboratories. *J. Vet. Diagn. Invest.* 2021; 33(2): 235–247.

71 Moter, A. and Göbel, U.B. Fluorescence in situ hybridization (FISH) for direct visualization of microorganisms. *J. Microbiol. Methods.* 2000; 41(2): 85–112.

72 Khatate, P., Savkar, A., and Patil, C.Y. Wearable smart health monitoring system for animals. *2018 2nd International Conference on Trends in Electronics and Informatics, ICOEI*, 162–164. IEEE; 2018.

73 El-Sayed, A. and Kamel, M. Advanced applications of nanotechnology in veterinary medicine. *Environ. Sci. Pollut. Res. Int.* 2020; 27: 19073–19086.

74 Pezzuto, F., Scarano, A., Marini, C. et al. Assessing the reliability of commercially available point of care in various clinical fields. *Open Public Health J.* 2019; 12(1): 342–368.

75 Troccaz, J., Dagnino, G., and Yang, G.Z. Frontiers of medical robotics: from concept to systems to clinical translation. *Annu. Rev. Biomed. Eng.* 2019; 21: 193–218.

76 Cepolina, F. and Razzoli, R.P. An introductory review of robotically assisted surgical systems. *Int. J. Med. Robot. Comput. Assist. Surg.* 2022; 18(4): e2409.

77 Bhadesiya, C.M., Patel, V.A., Anikar, M.J., and Gajjar, P.J. A disquisition on telehealth and teleguidance for veterinary healthcare professionals. *Pharma Innov.* 2021; 10: 154–160.

78 Brodie, A. and Vasdev, N. The future of robotic surgery. *Ann. R. Coll. Surg. Engl.* 2018; 100(Suppl 7): 4–13.

79 Almekkawy, M., Chen, J., Ellis, M.D., et al. Therapeutic systems and technologies: state-of-the-art applications, opportunities, and challenges. *IEEE Rev. Biomed. Eng.* 2019; 13: 325–339.

80 Naniwadekar, R.G. Innovative surgical techniques in veterinary medicine: enhancing animal health and welfare. *REDVET.* 2024; 25(1): 440–451.

81 Fossum, T.W. *Small Animal Surgery-Inkling Enhanced E-Book: Small Animal Surgery E-Book.* Elsevier Health Sciences; 2018.

82 Bordoni, L. and Gabbianelli, R. Primers on nutrigenetics and nutri (epi) genomics: origins and development of precision nutrition. *Biochimie* 2019; 160: 156–171.

83 Macdonald, A., Hawkes, L.A., and Corrigan, D.K. Recent advances in biomedical, biosensor and clinical measurement devices for use in humans and the potential application of these technologies for the study of physiology and disease in wild animals. *Philos. Trans. R Soc. Lond B Biol. Sci.* 2021; 376(1831): 20200228.

84 Tullo, E., Finzi, A., and Guarino, M. Environmental impact of livestock farming and precision livestock farming as a mitigation strategy. *Sci. Total Environ.* 2019; 650: 2751–2760.

85 Han, Q. Application of intelligent mobile terminal in animal epidemic prevention and animal health supervision. *Rev. Cient. Facult. Cienc. Vet.* 2019; 29(1): 32–43.

86 Lee, C., Colditz, I.G., and Campbell, D.L.M. A framework to assess the impact of new animal management technologies on welfare: a case study of virtual fencing. *Front. Vet. Sci.* 2018; 5: 187.

87 Luo, W., Chen, D., Wu, M., et al. Pharmacokinetics/pharmacodynamics models of veterinary antimicrobial agents. *J. Vet. Sci.* 2019; 20(5).

88 Norton, T., Chen, C., Larsen, M.L.V., and Berckmans, D. Precision livestock farming: building 'digital representations' to bring the animals closer to the farmer. *Animal* 2019; 13(12): 3009–3017.

89 Tekin, K., Yurdakök, B., Kanca, H., and Guatteo, R. Precision livestock farming technologies: novel direction of information flow. *Ankara Univ. Vet. Fak. Derg.* 2021; 68(2): 193–212.

9

Global Policy Frameworks and Future Directions for Veterinary Sciences

*Bernabé Vidal[1], Lorenzo Verger[2,3], Linda Ternova[4], and Gustavo J. Nagy[5]**

[1] *Graduate Programme in Environmental Sciences, Faculty of Sciences, University of the Republic (FC-UdelaR), Montevideo, Uruguay*
[2] *Department of Public Health, Faculty of Veterinary Medicine, University of the Republic (FVET-UdelaR), Montevideo, Uruguay*
[3] *Zoonosis Division, Ministry of Public Health (MSP), Montevideo, Uruguay*
[4] *Faculty of Medicine Carl Gustav Carus, TUD Dresden University of Technology, Fetscherstraße 74, 01037, Dresden, Germany*
[5] *Graduate Programme in Environmental Sciences and Institute of Ecology and Environmental Sciences (IECA), Faculty of Sciences, University of the Republic (FC-UdelaR), Montevideo, Uruguay*

*Corresponding author: gnagy@fcien.edu.uy

TABLE OF CONTENTS

9.1 Introduction
9.2 International Policies Shaping Veterinary Sciences
9.2.1 Origins and Early Drivers of International Collaboration for Animal Disease Control
9.2.2 Incorporation of Veterinary Sciences into the Global Public Health Sphere
9.2.3 New Fields of Action, New Policies: Animal Welfare and Wildlife Health
9.2.3.1 Animal Welfare in the International Sphere
9.2.3.2 Wildlife Health in the International Policy
9.2.4 Development of Holistic Health Concepts
9.2.5 Current International Policies on OH and Planetary Health
9.3 Collaborative Frameworks for Global Health Initiatives
9.3.1 Introduction to Collaborative Frameworks: Origins and Core Concepts
9.3.2 Global Health Stakeholders, Evolving Relationships, and Interdisciplinarity
9.3.3 Key Principles, Strategies, and Successful Initiatives for Effective Development
9.3.4 Current Situation, Barriers, and Problems
9.4 Anticipated Future Trends and Policy Considerations
9.4.1 Veterinary Sciences, Policies, and Public Health Challenges and Trends
9.4.2 Climate Change, Environmental Shifts, Increased Endemic Areas, and the Emergence of Zoonotic Vector-borne Diseases
9.4.3 Science and Policy in Action: Future Trends and Challenges in Decision-making in Animal Health and Epidemiology
9.4.4 The United Nations SDGs Framework for Addressing Future Global Challenges in Veterinary Science and Policies
9.4.4.1 Veterinary Science and Sustainability
9.4.4.2 Animal Welfare and SDGs
9.4.4.3 Environmental Sustainability in Animal Health
9.4.4.4 Human–Animal Connection
9.4.5 Planetary Health: A Bibliometric Review of Current and Expected Trends and Policy Implications
9.4.5.1 Documents by the Year of Publication
9.4.5.2 Documents by Affiliation

One Health Integration: Global Perspectives on Animal Health and Sustainable Agriculture. First Edition.
Edited by Pratik Subhash Gaikwad, Vivek Harishankar Shukla and Pintu Choudhary.

Companion Website: https://www.wiley.com/go/pratikgaikwad/onehealth

9.4.5.3 Documents by Country
9.4.5.4 Documents by Type
9.4.5.5 Co-authorship Analysis
9.4.5.6 Co-occurrence Analysis
9.4.5.7 Citation Analysis
9.5 Summary of Chapter
9.5.1 International Policies Shaping Veterinary Sciences
9.5.2 Collaborative Frameworks for Global Health Initiatives (GHIs)
9.5.3 Future Trends and Policy Considerations
9.5.4 Bibliometric Research Findings (2017–2024)
9.6 Conclusion
References

9.1 Introduction

In today's interconnected world, veterinary sciences play a pivotal role that transcends traditional animal health boundaries. This chapter explores the global policy frameworks shaping the future of the field, examining their influence on animal health, public health, environmental sustainability, and wildlife welfare. It traces the historical evolution of international cooperation in animal disease control and highlights the broadening of veterinary priorities to include animal welfare and wildlife health.

A key focus is placed on the emerging, interrelated approaches of One Medicine, One Health (OH), Global Health, EcoHealth, and Planetary Health, which emphasize the intricate interdependencies between human, animal, and environmental well-being. Readers will gain insight into the international policies and collaborative frameworks that guide veterinary practice across borders, along with the anticipated global trends influencing the profession, such as climate change, the increasing prevalence of zoonotic diseases, and the drive toward sustainable development.

After reading this chapter, readers should be able to understand the evolving concepts of these holistic health approaches and examine how global health partnerships and policy mechanisms are shaping the future of veterinary sciences. The chapter also highlights the relevance of the United Nations Sustainable Development Goals (SDGs) as a guiding framework to address future challenges and to promote a more integrated, resilient, and sustainable approach to global veterinary practice.

9.2 International Policies Shaping Veterinary Sciences

In today's hyperconnected world, controlling animal diseases requires considering their global implications. Recent examples such as the H5N1 Influenza and African Swine Fever pandemic underscore the urgent need for international cooperation to share epidemiological information and prepare the national veterinary services to prevent, detect, and control emerging animal diseases [1, 2]. This section explores, from a historical perspective, the processes that led to the creation of prominent international organizations safeguarding animal and human health.

9.2.1 Origins and Early Drivers of International Collaboration for Animal Disease Control

At the beginning of the twentieth century, the veterinary profession was predominantly concerned with preventing, diagnosing, and controlling diseases in livestock and poultry, equine medicine, and certain zoonotic diseases such as brucellosis and tuberculosis.

As international trade expanded alongside new modes of transport and the widespread movement of people and animals, it became increasingly evident that controlling animal diseases could not be managed on a national scale alone. In 1920, rinderpest, a highly contagious and deadly viral cattle disease, was reintroduced into Europe through cattle in transit from India to Brazil, the only documented outbreak of rinderpest on the American continent. Coupled with the increase in diseases spurred by World War I, this situation hastened the decades-old push for international collaboration in controlling animal diseases. It led to the International Conference for the Study of Epizootics in Paris in 1921, which established the foundations for the creation of the Office International des Epizooties (OIE), or World Organization for Animal Health (WOAH) in English, in 1924 [3, 4].

The establishment of the OIE/WOAH initiated a new era of international cooperation in animal health policy, which would continue to develop over the following decades. The countries of the League of Nations, founded in 1920, recognized the importance of international dialogue to address issues related to agriculture, food shortages, and their connection to nutrition and public health. Consequently, collaborating with the International Institute of Agriculture, they began collecting agricultural statistics from various countries, organizing meetings, and producing publications. These efforts laid the groundwork for founding the Food and Agriculture Organization (FAO) in 1945 as an agency of the newly formed United Nations (UN) [5, 6].

Soon after its founding, the FAO established a specialized unit called the Animal Health Service. This unit collaborated with the OIE and the World Health Organization (WHO) to develop the first FAO/WHO/OIE Animal Health Yearbook in 1956. This document compiled information on over 100 animal diseases reported by member countries, which were considered significant in public health, socio-economic impact, and international trade. The yearbook also included data on livestock populations and veterinary resources in these countries, laying the foundation for modern animal health surveillance systems [7].

9.2.2 Incorporation of Veterinary Sciences into the Global Public Health Sphere

What we now know as Veterinary Public Health (VPH), the concept of applying veterinary science and resources to protect and promote human health has been integral to the profession since its inception. Throughout the nineteenth century, numerous texts explored the relationship between animals and human health. During this time, veterinary professionals became members or advisors of central national and regional hygiene and public health institutions [8, 9]. Shortly after the establishment of the WHO in 1948, member countries requested that it, along with other agencies like FAO and OIE, take actions to develop areas such as zoonosis control, food hygiene, and advice on developing national VPH services. The first international efforts to control zoonoses focused on five specific diseases identified at a seminar sponsored by the WHO and the FAO in Vienna in 1952: rabies, Q fever, bovine tuberculosis, brucellosis, and hydatidosis [10].

A particularly successful example of the inclusion of VPH in international health organizations is the program developed in the Americas by the PAHO (Pan American Health Organization). PAHO, one of the oldest international health organizations in the world, was founded in 1902 and became the regional office for the Americas of the WHO in 1948. The need for a VPH program within the organization became evident in 1945 and 1946, following outbreaks of anthrax, equine encephalitis, and foot-and-mouth disease in Haiti, Panama, and Mexico, respectively. Thanks in part to the guidance and technical resources provided by PAHO, these outbreaks, which caused significant economic and human losses, were controlled. This situation and constant requests from member countries for advice on animal disease control led to the establishment of the VPH Unit in 1949. Under the technical guidance of the VPH unit, the Pan American Foot and Mouth Disease Center (PANAFTOSA) was established in 1951 and headquartered in Rio de Janeiro. PANAFTOSA led and coordinated international efforts to control and eradicate Foot and Mouth Disease (FMD). In 1956, the Pan American Zoonoses Center was created in Azul, Buenos Aires Province. This center later evolved into the Pan American Institute for Food Protection and Zoonoses and ultimately merged with PANAFTOSA in 2005. The resulting center serves the countries in the region by controlling FMD, combating zoonotic diseases, and ensuring food safety. This center is arguably the world's most extensive VPH program. It has been instrumental in the significant advances made in the region regarding the control and eradication of FMD, urban rabies, and numerous zoonotic diseases [11, 12].

One of the primary areas of focus for VPH is the sanitary control of animal-derived foods and preventing diseases transmitted to humans through food [13]. A significant international achievement in this field was establishing a regulatory body to unify the various and often contradictory food standards, terminologies, and guidelines across different countries. To address this issue, the FAO and WHO brought together health professionals, scientists, and civil servants from member countries, creating a commission that had its first meeting in 1963. Initially composed of 120 members from 30 countries and 16 international organizations, this commission was named the Codex Alimentarius Commission (CAC). The CAC implemented the Joint FAO/WHO Food Standards Programme. The CAC drafted and approved guidelines and food standards in a series of documents known as the Recommended Standards (CAC/RS series), later compiled into a comprehensive compendium called the *Codex Alimentarius*. The *Codex* standards are voluntary and require ratification by national regulations for effective implementation [14, 15].

9.2.3 New Fields of Action, New Policies: Animal Welfare and Wildlife Health

At the turn of the twenty-first century, international organizations officially addressed two topics of growing interest in the veterinary community: animal welfare and wildlife health. Initially developed out of concern for the suffering of farm animals, animal welfare has become a full-fledged scientific discipline with important international implications [16]. Moreover, the second half of the twentieth century saw a dramatic increase in biodiversity loss driven by habitat destruction, pollution, overexploitation and anthropogenic disasters, generating opportunities for the application of veterinary sciences to address this reality [17]. This section describes the processes of international organizations to incorporate these new concerns into their range of action.

9.2.3.1 Animal Welfare in the International Sphere

Over the last four decades, animal welfare has gained international recognition because it can be assessed and measured scientifically. This broader understanding includes the absence of disease and animals' behavioral and emotional well-being as they adapt to their environments [16].

Although no dedicated international organization has advised animal welfare policies, the OIE/WOAH was well-suited for this role. In 2001, its International Committee established a new department focused on animal welfare in response to increasing public interest. By 2002, member countries had endorsed specific recommendations to develop a comprehensive vision and strategy. A permanent working group coordinates these efforts, prioritizing issues such as the use of animals in food production, transportation, and humane slaughter. Since then, the OIE (WOAH) has provided global leadership on animal welfare issues. Other vital international players include the World Society for the Protection of Animals, industry organizations like the International Meat Secretariat, and veterinary organizations like the World Veterinary Association [18].

9.2.3.2 Wildlife Health in the International Policy

In the late 1990s, emerging zoonotic diseases were well established. Outbreaks of Ebola, Nipah, Hendra, and others had made it clear that there were common underlying factors. These factors primarily included pathogens originating from a wildlife reservoir, human or domestic animal exposure due to environmental changes or interaction with wildlife, and the exacerbation of the phenomenon through global trade and human travel. Recognizing this reality, the OIE established its Wildlife Working Group in 1994. This group encouraged the creation of specialized collaborating centers focused on wildlife, developed a network of national focal points on this topic, and included reporting wildlife diseases in the World Animal Health Information System (WAHIS) under a section called WAHIS-Wild. Additionally, it outlined the Wildlife Health Framework intending to "protect wildlife health worldwide to achieve OH," supported by two objectives [18]:

1. "Improve the ability of OIE/WOAH members to manage the risk of pathogen emergence in wildlife and transmission at the human–animal–ecosystem interface whilst considering wildlife protection."

2 "Support OIE/WOAH members to improve surveillance systems, early detection, notification, and management of wildlife diseases."

The OIE/WOAH collaborates on this issue with the Convention on International Trade in Endangered Species of Wild Fauna and Flora (CITES) to address the problem of pathogens transmitted through the wildlife trade and with the Wildlife Health Specialist Group of the International Union for Conservation of Nature (IUCN). Established in 1984, this group comprises approximately 350 experts in wildlife diseases. Several NGOs, such as the Wildlife Disease Association and the Wildlife Conservation Society, have extensive experience studying wildlife diseases [19, 20].

9.2.4 Development of Holistic Health Concepts

Understanding the development of the holistic concepts of One Medicine, OH, Global Health, EcoHealth, the Planetary vision for OH, and Planetary Health can help us appreciate their evolution and significance. Table 9.1 summarizes these concepts.

9.2.5 Current International Policies on OH and Planetary Health

One of the most important documents defining the international framework for applying the OH concept is the OH Joint Plan (OH-JPA) of Action, written first by the Tripartite and recently by the Quadripartite (OIE/FAO/WHO/UNEP). In its 2022–2026 program, this document proposes six action areas to help achieve sustainable health and food systems, reduce global health threats, and improve ecosystem management [33].

1. Enhancing OH's capacities to strengthen health systems.
2. Reducing some of the risks posed by emerging and re-emerging zoonotic epidemics and pandemics.
3. Controlling and, whenever possible, eliminating endemic zoonotic, neglected tropical and vector-borne diseases (VBDs).
4. Hardening the assessment, communication and management of food safety risks.
5. Controlling the increasing antimicrobial resistance (AMR).
6. Integrating the environment into OH.

The Quadripartite also developed guidelines for implementing the OH-JPA at a national level through five steps [38, 39]:

1. Situation analysis.
2. Setting up/strengthening OH governance and coordination.
3. Planning the implementation.
4. Implementing national OH action plans.
5. Reviewing, sharing, and Incorporating lessons learned.

Unlike the OH concept, international agencies have yet to widely incorporate other approaches like Planetary Health into their guidelines. Planetary Health involves monitoring and evaluating the drivers of emerging zoonotic diseases, such as land use change, urbanization, and climate change, including extreme weather events. However, the WHO has published a series of reports on climate change and health since 1990, highlighting the risks that extreme weather events and global temperature increases pose to human health. Additionally, since 2000, the WHO has been working with the World Meteorological Organization and UNEP, mainly focused on the climate-related impacts in vulnerable regions [39]. The Sixth Assessment Report (AR-6) of the Intergovernmental Panel on Climate Change (IPCC) shared the evidence on the increasing influence of climate change, variability and extreme events on human health and well-being and animal health [40].

Table 9.1 Resume of developing holistic concepts One Medicine, One Health, Global Health, EcoHealth, and Planetary Health.

Approaches	Comments	References
One Medicine (OM)	• Rudolf Virchow introduced the term "zoonosis" in the nineteenth century	[21–24]
	• He proclaimed that there should be no dividing line between human and animal medicine. His Canadian disciple, Sir William Osler, continued his concepts in the 1870s	
	• The US Communicable Diseases Center (CDC) founded the Veterinary Public Health division in 1947 to integrate human and veterinary public health professionals to address zoonotic disease concerns	
	• OM underscores the interconnectedness of human and animal health	[25]
	• The inter-related health of humans, animals, and the environment is complex and a relationship we all share	[26, 27]
	• OM calls to action to work together for a sustainable future based on the understanding that diseases can seamlessly cross species barriers: Zoonotic transmission	[26, 27]
	• OM recognizes this interconnectedness and collaborates between human and animal healthcare to ensure equal and sustainable medical progress for humans and animals without compromising animal welfare	[26, 27]
	• OM aims to improve global health and address emerging challenges as a transformative approach	[26, 27]
	• Veterinary and human Medicine practitioners and researchers ensure sustainable medical progress without compromising an animal's life	[27]
	• OM underscores the vital role of veterinarians in monitoring, preventing, and controlling zoonotic diseases, focusing on early animal detection as a crucial early warning system for potential human outbreaks	[27]
One Health and EcoHealth	• One Medicine evolved into One Health (OH), emphasizing promotion rather than treating diseases	[26, 28]
	• The 2007 One World, One HealthTM document about managing avian influenza introduced the OH, which focused on safeguarding the health of vertebrates, including humans	[29, 30]
	• Given the global health thinking in recent decades, primarily focused on the health of populations worldwide, ecosystem approaches to health have emerged aimed at optimal health outcomes	[31, 32]
	• OH encompasses the health of people, animals, and ecosystems, emphasizing interdependence	[31, 33, 34]
	• By considering the health of all living beings and their shared environment, we can more effectively address emerging diseases, antimicrobial resistance, food safety, and other health threats	[31, 33, 34]
	• OH has a significant global impact, and its implementation could benefit the international community by at least US$37 billion annually	[33]
	• The WHO formed an OH Initiative, "One Health Quadripartite," working with the UN FAO, UNEP, and the WOAH to integrate work on human, animal, and environmental health across the Organization	[34]
	• OH integrates and unifies health to balance and optimize people's, animals, and environmental health	[33, 34]
	• OH involves diverse sectors, disciplines, and communities at varying levels of society working together to foster health and well-being by addressing the need for safe water, nutritious food, energy, and air and contributing to sustainable development goals, including climate action	[33, 34]
	• The EcoHealth approach emphasizes biodiversity and ecosystems, aiming to understand and address health issues within the context of ecosystems and their interactions	[31]

Approaches	Comments	References
Global Health (GH) and	• GH aims to improve health outcomes worldwide through understanding how local health is a shared and intertwined common good	[32]
Planetary Health (PH)	• PH focuses on the broad perspective on health and the state of natural systems, recognizing that human well-being is intimately associated with the planet's health.	[31, 35, 36]
	• The Planetary Health Alliance understands PH as a solutions-oriented, transdisciplinary field that analyses and addresses the anthropogenic transformations of Earth's natural systems regarding human health and all life on Earth	[36–38]
	• The "planetary" vision for OH encompasses essential aspects of the OH and PH frameworks, which facilitate going from "local to global" to address the health, well-being, and sustainability of humans, animals, and the environment	[37]

9.3 Collaborative Frameworks for Global Health Initiatives

Collaborative frameworks have emerged as essential tools to address these challenges, bringing together stakeholders who developed comprehensive and sustainable solutions [41–43]. In this chapter, we analyze the foundations, actors, strategies, and current challenges of collaborative frameworks in Global Health, focusing on their intersection with veterinary medicine, human health, and environmental sustainability.

9.3.1 Introduction to Collaborative Frameworks: Origins and Core Concepts

Global Health intersectoral collaboration began in 1946 when the WHO was founded and evolved through contemporary OH initiatives [42]. This integrative approach tackles complex challenges, from pandemics to climate change, by fostering cross-sector synergies. This section traces the origins of these collaborative frameworks, examines their core concepts, and highlights their pivotal role in addressing global health crises.

Global Health (GH) aims to achieve better health outcomes for populations worldwide by transcending national borders and working to eliminate disparities in low-resource settings through research, education, and collaborative intervention. Global Health focuses on multidisciplinary challenges and considers specific factors for each case [41]. Although the conceptual foundations are hundreds of years old, the origins of collaborative frameworks in GH can be traced back to the WHO formation in 1946. The WHO focuses on physical, mental, and social well-being, necessitating collaboration across various sectors and disciplines [42]. GH has a holistic nature, encompassing multilayered concepts from molecular levels to complex assemblages, addressing matters such as climate change, stratospheric ozone depletion, pandemics, and biological crises on a global scale [43]. Inter-sectorial collaborations are now recognized as crucial for health systems, even though their application in the OH domain remains complex, and the concept has evolved [44].

Inter-sectorial collaboration provides different perspectives, skills and knowledge exchange among countries and stakeholders, fostering a more integrated approach to solving health problems [42]. However, Global Health Initiatives (GHIs) have experienced rapid growth, raising concerns about coherence and synergy among activities. Improving health in the era of SDGs requires leadership from all stakeholders to ensure that GHIs promote coherence and synergy among their activities [45]. GH financing has dramatically increased in recent years, creating policy environments that often overlap or contradict each other, raising concerns about equity [46]. Achieving objectives requires innovations that align with new political and economic realities within a multilevel, multiparty, and multipurpose partnership framework of global health governance. The frameworks should be inclusive, equitable, flexible, democratic, and sustainable. The resources available to GHIs have increased the number of

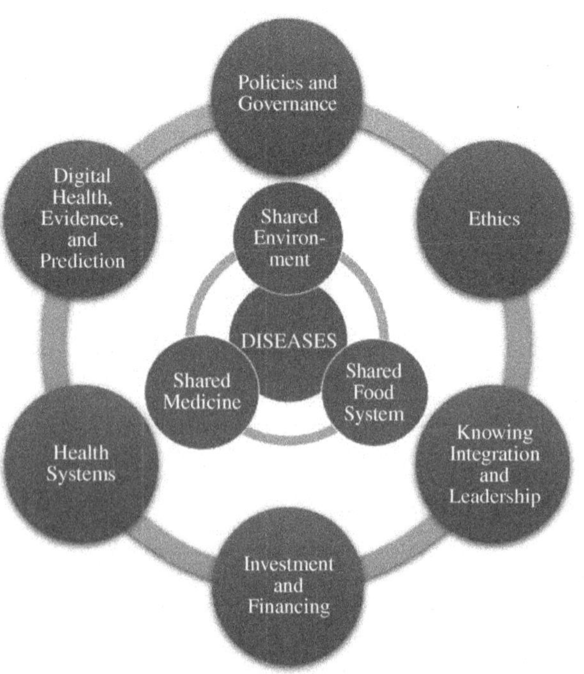

Figure 9.1 Disease dynamics between shared human–animal systems and the external factors. *Source*: Adapted from [49].

related institutions, including bilateral donors, United Nations agencies, and global and regional funds. This rapid growth has sometimes shown a need for coordination [47].

While veterinary medicine is increasingly essential in GH and food security (Figure 9.1), animal health services and the livestock sector have been marginalized and underfunded for decades, even though the sector is continuously growing (and is expected to expand further). Few small livestock farmers in the developing world receive veterinary care, which is problematic considering the strong correlation found in studies between poverty, livestock keeping, and endemic zoonoses, with zoonoses responsible for most human cases of infectious diseases. In 2014, 56 zoonotic diseases caused about 2.5 billion cases and 2.7 million human deaths each year, affecting animal health and production, food security, and various economic sectors. Many zoonoses remain uncontrolled due to insufficient veterinary professionals to face outbreaks [48].

9.3.2 Global Health Stakeholders, Evolving Relationships, and Interdisciplinarity

GH stakeholders range from international organizations to NGOs and community-based entities. Addressing the multiple, complex, and emerging global and public health challenges requires stakeholders' interactions to foster interdisciplinary relationships and collaborative networks [47, 50, 51]. This sub-section examines the evolution of these relationships and presents examples of successful initiatives that have transformed the Global Health landscape.

Many actors are involved in GHIs, ranging from traditional international organizations, such as the WHO, to regional, community-level, and NGO that provide distinct perspectives and capacities. Such diversity creates a collaborative environment where innovative solutions emerge [47]. The existing networks, partnerships, and initiatives to address complex health challenges and assist countries are evidence of the evolution of interdisciplinary collaboration in Global Health. Notable examples include the International Ministerial Conference on Avian and Pandemic Influenza (2007), the World Medical Association Resolution (2008), the First One Health Congress (2011), the World Medical and Veterinary Association on One Health Collaboration (2012), and the One Health Global Conference (2015) (Table 9.2).

Table 9.2 Chronology of various collaborative frameworks for GHIs relevant to veterinary sciences.

Collaborative Framework	Year	References
FAO/WHO/OIE Joint Expert Committee on Zoonoses (JEZ)	1958	[58]
Emergency Prevention System for Animal Health (EMPRES-AH)	1994	[59]
The Global Rinderpest Eradication Programme	1994	[59]
The International Livestock Research Institute (ILRI)	1994	[60]
The Global Framework for the Progressive Control of Transboundary Animal Diseases	2004	[61]
The International Health Regulations (IHR)	2005	[62]
Global Early Warning System (GLEWS)	2006	[63]
World Bank's Global Program for Avian Influenza Control and Human Pandemic Preparedness and Response	2006	[64]
International Ministerial Conference: Avian and Pandemic Influenza	2007	[50]
The Global Alliance for Rabies Control (GARC)	2007	[65]
The World Medical Association Resolution	2008	[50]
The Predict Project	2009	[66]
Tripartite agreement among three international organizations (FAO, WOAH, WHO)	2010	[50]
The First One Health Congress	2011	[50]
The World Medical and Veterinary Association on One Health Collaboration	2012	[50, 67]
The Global Health Security Agenda (GHSA)	2014	[68]
The One Health Global Conference	2015	[50]
Cooperation between FAO, WOAH, WHO, United Nations International Children Emergency Fund (UNICEF), World Bank and UNESCO	2017	[50]
Operational Framework of One Health for strengthening animal, human and environmental health systems	2018	[50]
The World Bank's One Health Operational Framework	2018	[67]
Quadripartite understanding of the One Health collaboration	2022	[50]
Central Asia One Health project	2023	[51]
Global Framework. Integrating Well-being into Public Health Promotion Approach	2023	[56]
Collaboration Framework Arrangement Among the Department of Health and Human Services of the United States of America, the Pan American Health Organization, and the WHO European Regional Office	2023	[57]

The key players in this landscape are the WHO, the FAO, and the OIE/WOAH [51]. These organizations play pivotal roles in advancing global health agendas, with WHO leading efforts to promote health equity and universal health coverage (connecting and facilitating partnerships between governments, civil society, the private sector and individuals, with over 800 institutions in more than 80 countries as support), FAO leading the OH approach in agrifood system transformation (with a spectrum of work and actors that involve agriculture, animal, plant, forest and aquaculture health), and animal health and welfare, which are the WOAH's expertise [52–55].

GH initiatives such as the Central Asia OH project, supported by the World Bank, exemplify coordinated and integrated efforts to align strategies and resources across organizational boundaries. A key conclusion from these initiatives was the need for a systems-wide approach rather than isolating zoonoses, leveraging existing monitoring tools [51]. Furthermore, adopting frameworks like the "Global Framework for Integrating Well-being into Public Health Utilizing a Health Promotion Approach" underscores the importance of holistic, collaborative approaches to addressing health challenges [56].

After the challenges posed by the Pandemic since 2020, the future of global health governance will likely include continued efforts and international collaborative initiatives to strengthen interdisciplinary collaboration, increase inclusivity and integrative approaches, and foster synergies among diverse stakeholders. By harnessing diverse actors' collective expertise and resources, the global health community is better equipped to tackle complex health challenges and promote Health and well-being for all [57].

9.3.3 Key Principles, Strategies, and Successful Initiatives for Effective Development

Effective governance in GH requires clear principles and strategies to build resilient and integrated systems [51, 69, 70]. This sub-section explores the foundational principles guiding intersectoral collaboration, from revising the International Health Regulations (IHR) to implementing frameworks like OH [62, 69]. Empirical evidence of inter-institutional and interdisciplinary collaboration demonstrates the profound impact of strategic cooperation at both global and local levels, inspiring us with the potential of our collective efforts.

Human and veterinary medicine stakeholders should act cohesively and efficiently, synergizing with other relevant services to address emerging ZIDs. Health governance emerged as a pivotal concern, prompting the WHO Assembly in 1995 to advocate for revising the IHR. Global health governance and enforcement principles help address transnational health threats. Clear targets and strategies and robust health information systems capable of monitoring progress are imperative [51, 62].

A paramount principle for developing a common strategic framework is establishing resilient public and animal health systems grounded in good governance and aligned with the IHR (2005) and OIE/WOAH intergovernmental standards to contribute to a sustainable, horizontal approach to strengthening public health systems [51, 62]. The WHO developed the IHR Monitoring and Evaluation Framework to aid countries in monitoring and enhancing their capacities and compliance with the IHR (2005) and the OH approach [69]. For instance, the COVID-19 pandemic and climate crisis underscored the necessity of evidence-based decision-making to shape the success of health interventions worldwide. Effective policymaking requires consideration of specific contextual factors for each country. Experience, expertise, political context, values judgments, resources, policy narratives, pressure groups, and cultural traditions should inform policy formulation [69, 70].

Examples include rabies, salmonellosis, Q Fever or Bovine Amyloidotic Spongiform Encephalopathy. Future collaborations will require operational interventions and improved collaboration between medical and veterinary services [70, 71]. For key stakeholders such as WHO, OIE and FAO, coordination mechanisms include establishing frameworks with specific stakeholder roles, communication systems, capacity building, and developing local, national, regional, and international strategies [50].

A review of OH operations highlighted 12 crucial individual, organizational, and network factors contributing to successful collaboration during significant health events. Individual factors like prior education and training are critical for quick mobilization during health events. Organizational factors, including adaptive policies and protocols, benefit from being flexible and monitored. Networks must be in place before health events, and a supportive political environment is crucial for their development. Critical aspects of network functioning include leadership, monitoring, evaluation, and successful communication [67].

In global health research, relational and operational aspects are crucial across all partnerships. Seven core concepts are considered equally important: focus, values, equity, benefit, leadership, communication, and resolution. Large, complex partnerships progress well when the involved participants reach a minimum program and have adequate resources allocated. While attributes may vary, these core concepts remain essential for successful research partnerships in global Health [72].

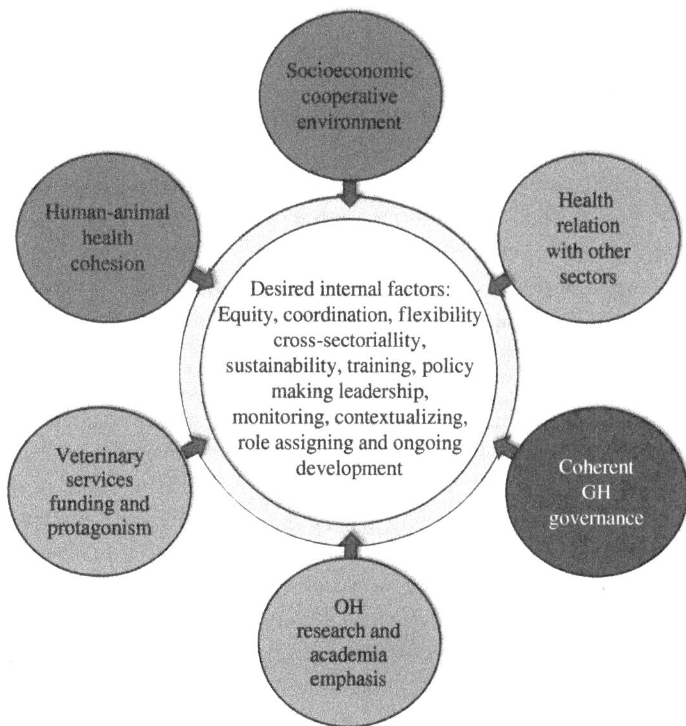

Figure 9.2 Desired external and internal framework factors.

9.3.4 Current Situation, Barriers, and Problems

Despite advances in GH collaboration, significant persisting barriers hinder its full potential. Challenges include gaps in coordination, misallocated resources, and psychological and professional resistance between sectors [50, 73–76]. This sub-section explores obstacles to implementing collaborative frameworks and proposes solutions to overcome these issues, emphasizing the need for integrated and sustainable approaches.

The Pandemic in 2020–2021 highlighted many challenges and some opportunities, underscoring the importance of strong GHI and local health systems to protect nations and economies, emphasizing prevention and equitable access to healthcare [73]. However, significant challenges hinder effective collaboration. According to FAO and WOAH, the increasing demand for animal protein (plus 70% of additional animal protein in 2050), coupled with human encroachment on wildlife habitats (human actions severely alter 75% of the terrestrial environments), are a significant threat to human and animal health. Moreover, vulnerable rural communities facing poverty and inadequate resources are particularly susceptible to these health risks. Besides, diseases can also be passed from humans to animals and generate significant impacts [73, 74]. This reality underscores the validity of the OH approach in a scenario of changes that require innovation, technology and resources to address the objectives (Figure 9.2).

Despite the pressing need for collaboration, psychological and professional barriers persist among healthcare professionals while it is perceived as something that exceeds their operation and is not sufficiently meaningful. Overcoming these barriers requires reevaluating professional identities and fostering a shared sense of purpose (even fewer than 25% of the individuals read a journal related to another sector) [75]. The authors also mentioned that resource allocation and wrong assignations hinder effective control measures for zoonotic diseases [50].

Institutionalizing the OH approach within government institutions remains challenging since deficiencies in coordination and integration and weak legislation persist [50]. Furthermore, system-level barriers impede the uptake and implementation of WHO technical guidelines worldwide [76]. In addressing these challenges, comprehensive, multi-level integrated activities are essential. Encouraging higher education institutions to incorporate

OH principles into curricula, expanding laboratory capacities, and fostering government leadership are critical steps [50]. Local initiatives, such as OH Clinics in the USA, demonstrate promising potential and could evolve into more developed centers [44].

Efforts to collaborate under the OH approach worldwide can be categorized into level-based, solution-based, and third party-based collaborations. For example, in a country like India (the most populated one), solution-based collaborations often need more ownership from other ministries and suffer from policy uncertainties. Level-based collaborations in research need more explicit guidelines and advocacy, while solution-based collaborations focus only on specific diseases during pandemics, needing more sustainable guidelines; third party-based collaborations frequently need evaluation plans. Differing approaches, the absence of a standard evaluation framework and adequate monitoring complicate the effectiveness of these collaborations [44]. Moreover, despite the increased interest in OH and similar concepts, few studies analyze the factors supporting effective practices and collaborations, limiting the ability to learn from past experiences [67] and leading to impossibilities in the speculation of which functions better, even though there is not a worldwide fitted health system. Therefore, incorporating localities and stakeholders is needed to implement practical OH initiatives [44]. The ongoing interest in health system strengthening presents an opportunity to enhance inter-sectoral OH collaboration. However, several authors specified that many challenges exist, such as more transparency [44].

The WOAH promotes Veterinary Services to improve legal frameworks and resources, recognizing their critical role in global health security; however, veterinary services must often be better organized [77]. Addressing this requires raising awareness among competent authorities about the essential role of veterinary services in protecting animal and human Health [62]. Financial sustainability will depend on appropriate resource allocation and efficient management strategies [77].

9.4 Anticipated Future Trends and Policy Considerations

Several global health stakeholders and authors anticipate or project future trends, including changes and new scientific and policy challenges in veterinary practice and public health [78–80]. The most common expected worldwide trends are climate change, population increases and globalization, technological advancement, increased spread of infectious zoonotic diseases and their transmission, broad incorporation of animal welfare concepts, and antimicrobial resistance (AMR), all of which will demand enhanced stakeholders collaboration, as explained in Sections 9.2 and 9.3. We underscore the pressing need for a new professional, teaching, research, practice and policy landscape that integrates and unifies OH and Planetary concepts [79, 81].

9.4.1 Veterinary Sciences, Policies, and Public Health Challenges and Trends

Because veterinary public health safeguards animal and human health, concerted actions of all veterinary practice and policymaking stakeholders are needed. The OH approach is advocated in veterinary sciences, practice and policymaking, demanding updated information on anticipated dynamic trends shaping the field. Therefore, progress will depend on collaboration, innovation, and a holistic approach. Each professional in their respective field has a crucial role in advancing veterinary sciences and OH. Three key areas are population increase, new technologies, and climate change [78–81]. Table 9.3 presumes some anticipated trends.

Decision-making in animal health and epidemiology faces several challenges, especially as we strive to improve resource allocation, disease control, and research efforts. Decision-making in animal health and epidemiology requires a multidisciplinary approach, innovative methods, and a holistic view of the impact on animals and humans. Some key aspects are disease prioritization methods [88], monetary value [89] and emerging challenges in epidemiology [90]. Some methods used for disease prioritization, aid decision-making related to disease control strategies, organizational planning, risk assessment, surveillance, and research priority setting are as follows [88]:

Table 9.3 Resume of anticipated future trends in veterinary sciences and One Health.

Future trends in veterinary sciences and OH	Examples	References
Population Increases and Globalization:	• Veterinarians have to face new professional duties due to our changing world. For instance, the • Globalization of animal trade and its products • Impact of disease spread and control • Rapid movement of pathogens across borders	[81]
Advancements in Technology	• New technologies, such as telemedicine, wearable devices, genomics, data analytics, and digital health records, are transforming veterinary practice • Telehealth platforms will enable remote consultations, while genomics will transform disease diagnostics and personalized treatments. Data-driven approaches will strengthen disease surveillance and management • Artificial intelligence (AI) can aid veterinarians' practice and research	[82–84]
Extreme Weather and Climate	• Environmental changes and habitat shift: The spread and redistribution of VBDs are leading to new public health worries	[80]
Antimicrobial Stewardship	• Veterinarians must use antibiotics responsibly and prudently, as it is essential to combat antimicrobial resistance	[80]
Education and Training	• Veterinarians must stay updated on emerging trends and maintain their expertise. Education programs focusing on interdisciplinary skills and global health challenges motivate professionals to remain committed to their learning and growth • Training programs focus on interdisciplinary skills and global health challenges. Veterinarian curricula and continuing education programs must address climate change and Planetary Health and its effects on animal health • Veterinarians should advocate for climate action and promote environmental sustainability within clinical practices to protect animal health and contribute to public health	[80, 85]
Workforce Challenges and Veterinary Burnout in the United States.	• Burnout is a real challenge: Practice owners must support and retain their teams, recognize the consequences of expecting them to do more with less, and protect them as best as possible in conflicts with pet owners	[86, 87]
Product Shortages and Online Pet Pharmacies	• Several significant products have been placed on long-term backorders, affecting practice protocols and revenues • Streamlining the process for approving new products and nurturing vendor relationships can reduce the impact • Practices may consider partnering with online pharmacies to capture at least some revenue	

- Economic impact assessment of diseases to allocate resources effectively.
- Multicriteria evaluation of severity, cost, and feasibility to rank diseases.
- Assessment of the likelihood and consequences of disease occurrence.
- Prioritization of diseases based on straightforward criteria.
- Identification of high-risk areas or populations.
- Mathematical modeling to predict disease dynamics.

Beyond the monetary value of zoonotic diseases, we must recognize the broader impact of animal health to make informed decisions that benefit humans and animals [90]. Some emerging challenges in epidemiology in the twenty-first century include addressing novel threats across diverse content areas, leveraging advanced analytical techniques, and effectively handling large datasets [89].

9.4.2 Climate Change, Environmental Shifts, Increased Endemic Areas, and the Emergence of Zoonotic Vector-borne Diseases

Environmental changes induce veterinarians to adapt their practices and animal and public health policies [85]. Changing temperatures and habitats may affect the range of disease vectors, reservoir hosts (such as wildlife), and disease pattern shifts. Increased zoonotic diseases and pandemics will likely demand urgent action to safeguard global health [90–92]. Veterinarians, policymakers, and researchers' collaboration will facilitate the development of effective climate adaptation strategies. Some examples are the following [93–95]. Table 9.4 illustrates the impact of climate change on animal health and zoonotic vector-borne diseases in new environments.

Environmental shifts due to climate change will impact animal health. As ecosystems change, new diseases may appear; veterinarians must monitor and respond to these emerging animal (and human health) threats [95, 96].

Table 9.4 Summary of some climate change impacts on animal health and zoonotic vector-borne diseases (ZVBDs) in new environments.

Future trends in veterinary sciences	Impacts	References
Heat stress	• Global warming and heat waves can be catastrophic for livestock. The severity and duration of heat stress can disrupt their metabolism, induce oxidative stress, and weaken their immune system, rendering them more vulnerable to diseases and even death	[96, 97]
Increased Endemic Areas and Spillover Risk	• Under a medium climate change scenario, the endemic ZVBD regions will increase by about 10% on average across all 101 specific ZVBDs and pathogens worldwide	[94]
Emergence/ re-emergence of ZVBDS	• Climate change is likely increasing ZVBDs worldwide. Therefore, enhanced cooperation in veterinary and public health services is needed to reduce this climate-related health risk • Altered climatic and ecological determinants can influence the distribution and prevalence of VBDs. As climatic conditions shift, the range of disease vectors may expand, affecting animal health • Some diseases may become more prevalent due to altered environmental conditions, affecting wild and domestic animals • Climatic shifts (e.g., rainfall and temperature) can induce the emergence of pathogens and ZVBDs in new environments, underscoring the urgent need for public health agencies to foster their capacity to detect, respond to, and manage ZVBDs in these new areas • The climate-modeled suitability of environments for both hosts and vectors of 165 ZVBDs until 2080 project the risk of human exposure to different ZVBDs, underscoring the connection between human disease risk and global environmental change	[94, 96]
Extreme Weather Events	• Extreme weather events can disrupt animal habitats, health, food sources, and breeding patterns. These events can lead to animal stress and injuries, malnutrition, and disease outbreaks • Altered climatic and vegetation patterns affect livestock access to food and water, animal health, and productivity	[96, 98]
Agriculture and Food Security	• Climate-related shifts such as temperature and precipitation changes and pests affect animal health, water availability, food systems, crop growth, and livestock feed quality • The global community must invest in research and technologies to enhance the sustainability of food systems worldwide. Veterinarians are critical in ensuring resilient food production systems	[100]

However, veterinarians have the power to face these challenges head-on by implementing effective adaptation strategies and preventive measures, such as heat stress management plans for livestock, community participation, and efficient veterinary services to reduce these effects and protect the health of our animal populations. By understanding these challenges and implementing these strategies, we can work towards safeguarding both animal and human well-being in a changing climate [97–99].

9.4.3 Science and Policy in Action: Future Trends and Challenges in Decision-making in Animal Health and Epidemiology

Public policy decisions underlie the societal response to animal health, public health, food safety and the sustainability of animal breeding. Although animal health policy often emerges at the science-politics interface, scientists tend to disdain politics, which limits their involvement in policy formulation. On the other hand, epidemiologists are qualified to bring scientific knowledge to complex policy issues through analytical, macro-epidemiological approaches considering policy issues' economic, legal, and cultural contexts and bio-medical concepts. Risk analysis is a systematic approach that helps evaluate animal health and compare policy options. Capturing these opportunities for applied epidemiology requires understanding the policymaking process, the basic principles of epidemiology, communication skill-building, and experiential learning opportunities in a team environment [78, 86, 101].

9.4.4 The United Nations SDGs Framework for Addressing Future Global Challenges in Veterinary Science and Policies

The UN SDGs help address global veterinary science and animal welfare challenges. There is a positive relationship between the SDGs and animal welfare [102, 103]. Aligning animal welfare policies and practices with the SDGs helps achieve sustainability and commiseration regarding animals [104–106]. Some examples are as follows:

9.4.4.1 Veterinary Science and Sustainability

Science is crucial in achieving sustainability goals. It guides policy decision-making by integrating knowledge into designing sectoral policies that balance societal needs with environmental limitations. As part of this broader scientific effort, veterinary science can contribute to sustainable practices in animal health, food production, and ecosystem management [107, 108].

9.4.4.2 Animal Welfare and SDGs

Animal welfare is a multifaceted, growing concern encompassing scientific, ethical, economic, cultural, legal, social, religious, and political aspects and a key driver of sustainability [109, 110]. The SDGs aim to create a future without poverty, hunger, and the worst effects of climate change and biodiversity loss [105]. Two SDGs, # 12: responsible production and consumption and # 14: life below water, have mutual solid reinforcement with animal welfare. Improved animal welfare practices are necessary to address current and future global challenges. Animal health, welfare, human health, and sustainable socio-economic and ecological systems are closely interlinked [109, 110]. A workshop conducted with agricultural and veterinary scientists analyzed the compatibility between achieving the SDGs and improving animal welfare. They found that working toward the SDGs aligns with improving animal welfare [102] and benefits farming systems and society [110].

9.4.4.3 Environmental Sustainability in Animal Health

The SDGs emphasize ecological sustainability, which includes aspects relevant to animal health. For example, SDG 15 (Life on Land) focuses on biodiversity conservation and sustainable land use, indirectly impacting animal habitats and health [103].

9.4.4.4 Human–Animal Connection

Improving animal welfare can positively affect human health and well-being. Recognizing this connection is essential for achieving the SDGs [106, 110]. Better animal health contributes to better animal welfare. In particular, controlling terrestrial and aquatic animal diseases reduces pain and distress, reducing the need to cull to prevent the spread of diseases that can have a high economic impact or pose a risk to public health [110].

9.4.5 Planetary Health: A Bibliometric Review of Current and Expected Trends and Policy Implications

Planetary health (PH) is a novel interdisciplinary and transdisciplinary approach to understanding environmental change's consequences on human health and the institutions that influence those effects [111]. PH relies on the health of human civilization and the quality of the natural systems on which it depends [35]. PH aims to comprehensively analyze global environmental transformations' complex and interrelated connections, their impact on natural systems, and how their alterations influence human health and well-being [112]. SDGs emphasize global leadership and collaboration across sectors and precise evaluation of the benefits and trade-offs concerning health, the environment, and sustainable development. PH is a cohesive topic within this framework that fosters integrated action towards the SDGs by states, the United Nations system, and other stakeholders [113].

We examined the relationship between PH, SDGs, and international policies through bibliometric analysis. We used the Scopus database and applied the search string, summarized in Table 9.5. Then, we exported the results (as of November 18, 2024) to a CSV file, converted them into an Excel file, and checked for duplicate records. We identified one hundred thirty-three documents after applying the exclusion criteria. We did not impose any publishing period restrictions; the articles are from 2017 to 2024. We used the VOSviewer software for additional analysis.

9.4.5.1 Documents by the Year of Publication

The scientific literature published between 2017 and 2024 (until November 18) increased since 2019 (Figure 9.3).

9.4.5.2 Documents by Affiliation

Five universities share five publications, followed by other organizations (Figure 9.4).

9.4.5.3 Documents by Country

The countries with the greatest number of publications are the United States ($n = 28$), followed by China ($n = 23$), Australia ($n = 22$), the United Kingdom ($n = 21$), Italy and South Africa ($n = 12$, each), Canada ($n = 9$), and Germany and Peru ($n = 8$, each).

Table 9.5 Scopus search strategy.

Search string/identified documents	Exclusion criteria	Duplicate records	Bibliometric analysis documents
ALL ("Planetary health") AND (ALL ("sustainable development goals") OR ALL (sdg*)) AND ALL ("future trends") AND (ALL (international) OR ALL (global)) AND (ALL (policy) OR ALL (policies)) ($n = 143$)	Non-English documents ($n = 2$) Not yet in the final stage of publication ($n = 8$)	$n = 0$	$n = 133$

Source: The authors.

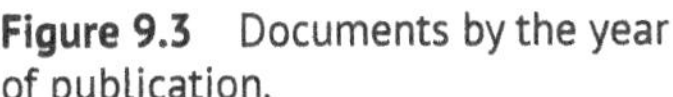

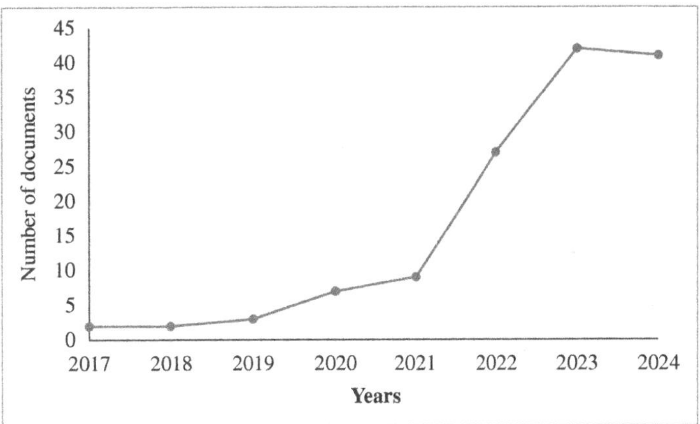

Figure 9.3 Documents by the year of publication.

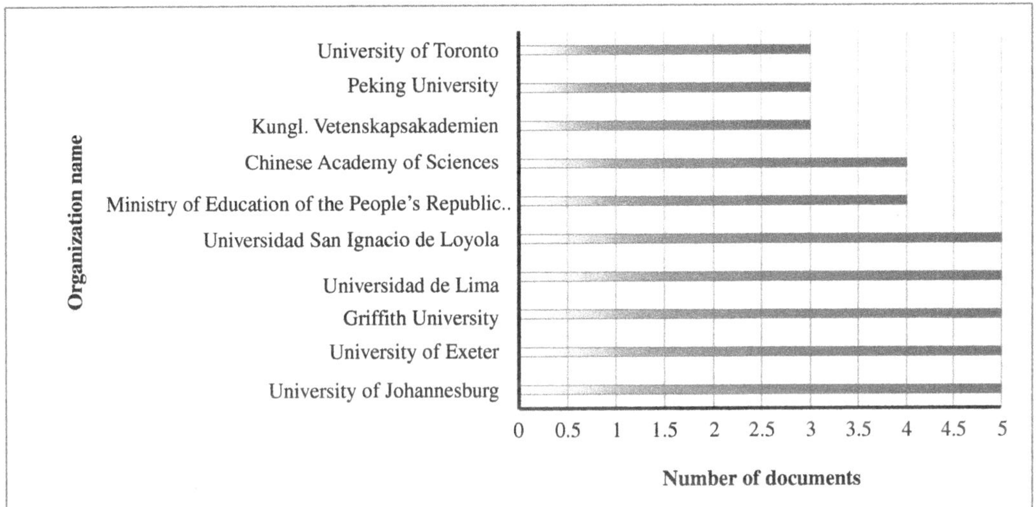

Figure 9.4 Documents by affiliation.

9.4.5.4 Documents by Type

The "Articles" category, with 59 publications (44%), accounted for the most significant percentage of the literature, followed by "Reviews" with 41 publications (31%), "Book" with 17 publications (13%), and "Book chapter" with 13 publications (10%).

9.4.5.5 Co-authorship Analysis

For the co-authorship analysis, we chose "countries" as the unit of study, determining the minimum number of documents and citations required for each country to be five, respectively. Only 23 out of the 73 nations meet the criteria, led by the United States (28 documents and 887 citations) and followed by China (23 documents and 299 citations.) With 600 citations, Australia ranked third ($n = 22$), the United Kingdom fourth (823 citations and 21 publications), and South Africa and Italy fifth with equal publications ($n = 12$) and 627 and 538 citations, respectively.

Using the VOSviewer, five clusters were visible (Figure 9.5): (Brazil, Malaysia, Denmark, Sweden, the Netherlands, Spain, and the United Kingdom); (France, Germany, India, Peru, Switzerland, and the

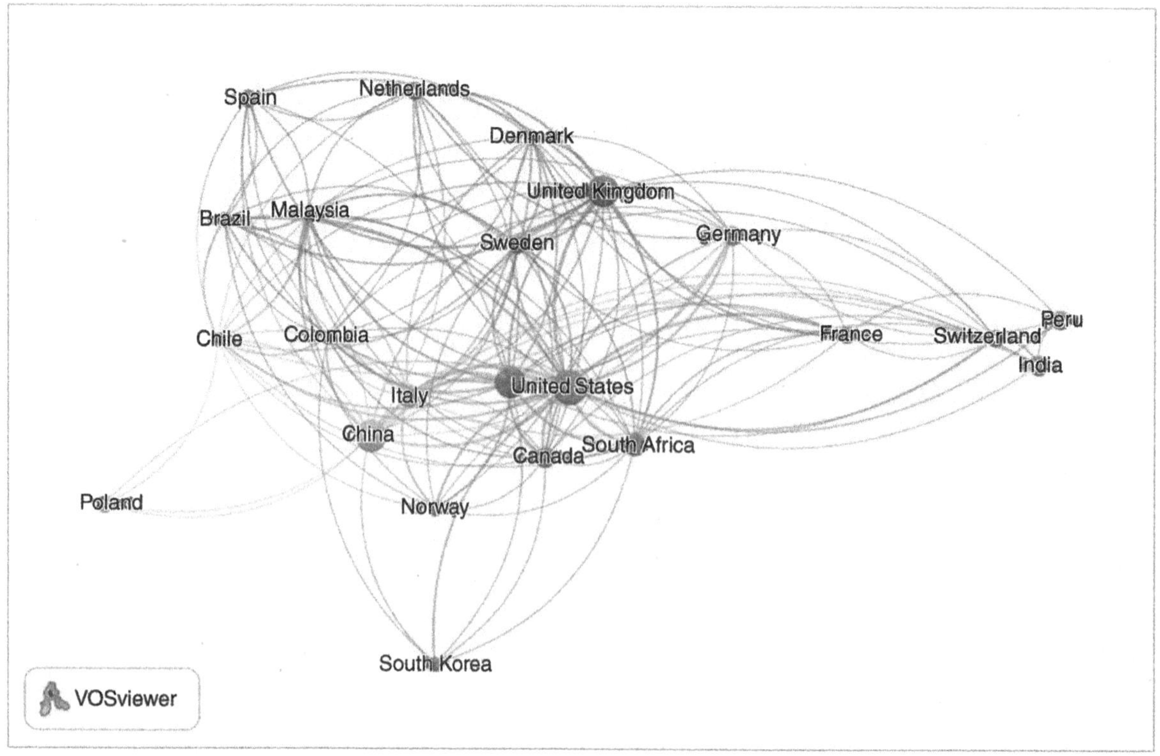

Figure 9.5 Co-authorship analysis by countries.

United States); (Australia, Canada, Colombia, South Africa, and South Korea); (Chile, China, Italy, and Poland); and (Norway). The most published documents came from the United States (28 documents), consistent with the results obtained in 9.4.5.3. "Documents by Country," where the United States had the highest number of published documents. The same can be affirmed if referring to the large node visualized on the VOSviewer map. Besides, the proximity of the nodes indicates strong cooperation between the United States and Australia.

9.4.5.6 Co-occurrence Analysis

In the co-occurrence analysis, we used the "author keywords" as the unit of analysis, setting a minimum threshold of five keyword occurrences. Based on this criterion, only 6 out of 528 keywords met the threshold. The keywords "Sustainability," "climate change," "sustainable development," and "sustainable development goals" showed the highest total link strength. VOSviewer visualization revealed two clusters (not shown): one cluster comprised sustainability, entrepreneurship, and SDGs, while the other included climate change, sustainable development, and bibliometric analysis.

9.4.5.7 Citation Analysis

We conducted citation analysis using the "documents" counting method, determining that ten citations are the minimal amount for a given document. Consequently, 42 out of 133 sources met the requirement. With 360 citations, Landrigan et al. [114] received the most citations. Perez-Escamilla et al. [115] and Ayeleru et al. [116] received 161 and 143 citations each.

9.5 Summary of Chapter

This chapter reviews the Global Policy Frameworks and Future Directions for Veterinary Sciences, focusing on evolving concepts, international policies, collaborative frameworks, and anticipated future trends.

Key findings are summarized as follows:

9.5.1 International Policies Shaping Veterinary Sciences

- In today's interconnected world, managing animal diseases requires a global perspective. International cooperation is vital for sharing epidemiological data and strengthening national veterinary systems.
- Veterinary Public Health plays a critical role in safeguarding human health, marking its longstanding importance in the profession.
- The early twenty-first century saw international veterinary bodies address emerging concerns like animal welfare and wildlife health.
- Key global frameworks by OIE, FAO, WHO, and UNEP illustrate the growing importance of the OH approach in tackling health challenges.

9.5.2 Collaborative Frameworks for Global Health Initiatives (GHIs)

- Since the WHO's inception in 1946, collaborative frameworks (as illustrated in Table 9.2) have become central to addressing global health issues.
- Organizations like WHO, FAO, and OIE/WOAH collaborate through integrated models and international regulations (e.g., IHR).
- The COVID-19 pandemic has emphasized the need for early zoonotic disease detection and response, likely reshaping future global health governance.
- Despite collaborative efforts, ongoing barriers such as conflicting priorities, limited resources, and disciplinary silos hinder effective OH implementation.

9.5.3 Future Trends and Policy Considerations

- Future challenges include climate change, globalization, the rise of zoonoses, antimicrobial resistance, and animal welfare, requiring adaptive policies and intersectoral coordination.
- Climate shifts demand strong veterinary services and community engagement in early warning and health preparedness.
- Veterinarians must be equipped to address environmental challenges, calling for a unified teaching, research, and policy framework based on OH and PH principles.
- The UN SDGs indirectly support veterinary-related themes such as animal welfare, sustainable food systems, and ecosystem management.

9.5.4 Bibliometric Research Findings (2017–2024)

- A marked increase in literature on planetary health and sustainability was observed post-2019, particularly from 2021 to 2023.
- Leading publishing countries include the USA, China, Australia, and the UK.
- Frequent keywords include "Sustainability," "climate change," and "sustainable development goals."

9.6 Conclusion

In this chapter, we explored the global policy frameworks shaping the future of veterinary sciences. The evolution from animal disease control to a broader public health agenda highlights the need for collaborative efforts in addressing complex health challenges. The integration of animal welfare and wildlife health into international discourse reflects the recognition of interdependencies among human, animal, and environmental health. Holistic health concepts, particularly through OH and PH, emphasize the interconnectedness of global health systems.

The challenges of climate change, environmental shifts, and zoonotic diseases underscore the urgency for adaptive policy measures. While key principles and strategies from successful collaborations have been identified, barriers remain. Ongoing dialogue among global health stakeholders is essential to address the complexities of veterinary sciences and public health effectively.

Looking forward, aligning veterinary sciences with the United Nations SDGs is crucial for confronting future global challenges. The future of veterinary sciences is linked to robust, inclusive, and forward-thinking policies, necessitating commitment to international collaboration and interdisciplinary approaches for a healthier tomorrow.

References

1 Gilbert, W.D., Adamson, D., Donachie, K., et al. A cost–benefit analysis of preparing national veterinary services for transboundary animal disease emergencies. *Transbound. Emerg. Dis.* 2023; 1: 1765243. https://doi.org/10.1155/2023/1765243.

2 Sharan, M., Vijay, D., Yadav, J.P., et al. Surveillance and response strategies for zoonotic diseases: a comprehensive review. *Sci. One Health* 2023; 2: 100050. https://doi.org/10.1016/j.soh.2023.100050.

3 Brückner, G. and Teissier, M. A brief historical overview of the World Organization for Animal Health (OIE) and its historical relationship with countries in southern Africa. *Proceedings of the 44th International Congress of the World Association for the History of Veterinary Medicine. Praetoria, South Africa*. 2023. https://repository.up.ac.za/bitstream/handle/2263/74482/2020_WAHVM_BrucknerGideon.pdf?sequence=1.

4 Barrett, T. and Rossiter, P.B. Rinderpest: the disease and its impact on humans and animals. *Adv. Virus Res.* 1999; 53: 89–110. https://doi.org/10.1016/s0065-3527(08)60344-9.

5 Biswas, M. FAO: its history and achievements during the first four decades, 1945–1985. Doctoral dissertation. University of Oxford. 2008. https://ora.ox.ac.uk/objects/uuid:0b79db50-0d09-422e-8a11-d0ef8e9d47c3/download_file?file_format=application/pdf&safe_filename=602448518.pdf&type_of_work=Thesis.

6 Mayne, J.B. FAO-the history. *Rev. Mark. Agric. Econ.* 1947; 15(11), 418–426. https://doi.org/10.22004/ag.econ.8403.

7 Kouba, V. History of animal health service of the food and agriculture organization of the United Nations. In *XXXIII International Congress of the World Association for the History of Veterinary Medicine, Wittenberg, Germany*, 21–24; 2002. https://doi.org/10.13140/RG.2.2.28739.91683.

8 Steele, J.H. The history of public health and veterinary public service. *J. Am. Vet. Med. Assoc.* 2000; 217(12): 1813–1821.

9 Hardy, A. Professional advantage and public health: British veterinarians and state veterinary services, 1865–1939. *Twent. Century Br. Hist.* 2003; 14(1): 1–23. https://doi.org/10.1093/tcbh/14.1.1.

10 Kaplan, M.M. The concept of veterinary public health and its application in the World Health Organization. *Chron. World Health Organ.* 1953; 225–267. https://iris.who.int/handle/10665/250667.

11 Arambulo III, P. International programs and veterinary public health in the Americas—success, challenges, and possibilities. *Prev. Vet. Med.* 2008; 86(3–4): 208–215. https://doi.org/10.1016/j.prevetmed.2008.02.008.

12 Belotto, A., Held, J.R., Fernández, D., and Alvarez, E. Veterinary public health activities in the Pan American Health Organization over the past 58 years: 1949–2007. *Vet. Ital.* 2007; 43(4): 789–798. https://doi.org/10.1016/j.virusres.2005.03.006.

13 Pappaioanou, M. Veterinarians in global public health. *J. Vet. Med. Educ.* 2003; 30(2): 105–109. https://doi.org/10.3138/jvme.30.2.105.

14 Ramsingh, B. The Codex in historical perspective: food safety standards and the Codex Alimentarius Commission (1962–1973). *Mcis Briefings* 2010; 98. https://tspace.library.utoronto.ca/bitstream/1807/42553/3/Ramsingh_Brigit_LN_201111_PhD_thesis.pdf

15 Vojir, F., Schübl, E., and Elmadfa, I. The origins of a global standard for food quality and safety: codex Alimentarius Austriacus and FAO/WHO Codex Alimentarius. *Int. J. Vitam. Nutr. Res.* 2012; 82(3): 223. https://doi.org/10.1024/0300-9831/a000115.

16 Broom, D.M. A history of animal welfare science. *Acta Biotheor.* 2011; 59: 121–137. https://doi.org/10.1007/s10441-011-9123-3.

17 Veit, W. and Browning, H. Perspectival pluralism for animal welfare. *Eur. J. Philos. Sci.* 2021; 11: 1–14. https://doi.org/10.1007/s13194-020-00322-9.

18 Cunningham, A.A., Daszak, P., and Wood, J.L. One Health, emerging infectious diseases and wildlife: two decades of progress. *Philos. Trans. R. Soc. B, Biol. Sci.* 2017; 372(1725): 20160167. https://doi.org/10.1098/rstb.2016.0167.

19 Cerda, J.R. and Webb, T.L. Wildlife conservation and preserving biodiversity: impactful opportunities for veterinarians? *JAVMA* 2023; 261(7): 1077–1085. https://doi.org/10.2460/javma.23.02.0094.

20 OIE. *Wildlife Health Framework*. 2021. https://www.woah.org/fileadmin/Home/eng/Internationa_Standard_Setting/docs/pdf/WGWildlife/A_Wildlifehealth_conceptnote.pdf.

21 Mörner, T. Fischer, J., and Bengis, R. The value of increasing the role of private individuals and organisations in One Health. *Sci. Tech. Rev.* 2014; 33(3): 605–613. https://doi.org/10.20506/rst.33.2.2308.

22 Schultz, M. Rudolf virchow. *Emerg. Infect. Dis.* 2008; 14: 1480–1481. https://doi.org/10.3201/eid1409.086672.

23 Roland, C.G. *OSLER, Sir WILLIAM, in Dictionary of Canadian Biography, vol. 14*, University of Toronto/Université Laval; 2003. http://www.biographi.ca/en/bio/osler_william_14E.html.Dictionary of Canadian Biography. Available from: http://www.biographi.ca/en/bio/osler_william_14E.html.

24 Gyles, C. One Medicine, One Health, One World. *Can. Vet. J.* 2016; 57(4): 345–6.

25 CDC. History. timeline: people and events in one health. Centers for Disease Control and Prevention. *History of One Health*. 2022. https://www.cdc.gov/onehealth/basics/history/index.html?CDC_AA_refVal=https%3A%2F%2Fwww.cdc.gov%2Fonehealth%2Fp eople-events.html.

26 Philpott, J. One medicine: bridging the gap between human and animal health. News Medical. *Life Sciences*. 2023. https://www.news-medical.net/health/One-Medicine-Bridging-the-Gap-Between-Human-and-Animal-Health.aspx#:~:text=One%20Medicine%3A%20Bridging%20the%20Gap%20Between%20Human%20and%20Animal%20Health.

27 Humanimal Trust. *One Medicine for Humans and Animals*. 2018. https://www.humanimaltrust.org.uk/one-medicine.

28 Schneider, M.C., Munoz-Zanzi, C., Kyung-duk Min. K-D., and Aldighieri, S. *One Health From Concept to Application in the Global World*. Oxford Research Encyclopedia of Global Public Health; 2019. https://doi.org/10.1093/acrefore/9780190632366.013.29.

29 Zinsstag, J., Schelling, E., Waltner-Toews, D., and Tanner, M. From "one medicine" to "one health" and systemic approaches to health and well-being. *Prev. Vet. Med.* 2010; 101(3–4): 148–156. https://doi.org/10.1016/j.prevetmed.2010.07.003. PMID: 20832879.

30 Brown, H.L., Pursley, I.G., Horton, D.L., and La Ragione, R.M. One Health: a structured review and commentary on trends and themes. *One Health Outlook* 2024; 6(1): 17. https://doi.org/10.1186/s42522-024-00111-x.

31 Lerner, H. and Berg, C.A, Comparison of three holistic approaches to Health: One Health, EcoHealth, and planetary health. *Front. Vet. Sci.* 2016; 4: 163. https://doi.org/10.3389/fvets.2017.00163.

32 Parsons, J. Global and planetary health. In: *Good Health and Well-Being. Encyclopedia of the UN Sustainable Development Goals* (eds. W. Leal Filho, T. Wall, A.M. Azul, L. Brandli, and P.G. Özuyar), Cham: Springer; 2020. https://doi.org/10.1007/978-3-319-95681-7_5.

33 WHO. *One Health. World Health Organization.* 2023. https://www.who.int/news-room/fact-sheets/detail/one-health.

34 FAO, UNEP, WHO, and WOAH. *One Health Joint Plan of Action (2022–2026). Working Together for the Health of Humans, Animals, Plants and the Environment. Rome.* 2022. https://doi.org/10.4060/cc2289en.

35 Whitmee, S., Haines, A., Beyrer, C., et al. Safeguarding human health in the Anthropocene epoch: report of the Rockefeller Foundation—Lancet Commission on Planetary Health. *Lancet* 2015; 386(10007): 1973–2028. https://doi.org/10.1016/S0140-6736(15)60901-1.

36 Ruiz de Castañeda, R., Villers, J., Faerron Guzmán, C.A., et al. One Health and planetary health research: leveraging differences to grow together. Comment. *Lancet Planet Health* 2023; 7: e111. https://doi.org/10.1016/S2542-5196(23)00002-5.

37 Rabinowitz, P.M., Pappaioanou, M., Bardosh, K.L., and Conti. L.A planetary vision for one health. *BMJ. Glob. Health* 2018; 3: e001137. https://doi.org/10.1136/bmjgh-2018-001137.

38 Deem, S.L., Lane-deGraaf, K.E., and Rayhel, E.A. *Introduction to One Health: An Interdisciplinary Approach to Planetary Health.* Wiley-Blackwell; 2018.

39 FAO, UNEP, WHO, and WOAH. *A Guide to Implementing the One Health Joint Plan of Action at National Level.* Geneva; 2023. https://www.who.int/publications/i/item/9789240082069.

40 Cissé, G., McLeman, R., Adams, H., et al. Health, well-being, and the changing structure of communities. In: *Climate Change 2022: Impacts, Adaptation and Vulnerability. Contribution of Working Group II to the Sixth Assessment Report of the Intergovernmental Panel on Climate Change* (eds. H.-O. Pörtner, D.C Roberts, M. Tignor, and E.S. Poloczanska), 1041–1170. Cambridge, UK and New York, NY, USA: Cambridge University Press; 2022. https://doi.org/10.1017/9781009325844.009.

41 Duke Global Health Institute. *What Is Global Health*? n.d. https://globalhealth.duke.edu/what-global-health

42 Rutgers Global Health Institute. *What Is Global Health*? n.d. https://globalhealth.rutgers.edu/what-we-do/what-is-global-health/

43 Bozorgmehr, K. Rethinking the 'global' in global health: a dialectic approach. *Glob. Health* 2010; 6(19). https://doi.org/10.1186/1744-8603-6-19.

44 Yasobant, S., Bruchhausen, W., Saxena, D., and Falkenberg, T. One Health collaboration for a resilient health system in India: learnings from global initiatives. *One Health* 2019; 8: 100096. https://doi.org/10.1016/j.onehlt.2019.100096.

45 Zicker, F., Faid, M., Reeder, J., and Aslanyan, G. Building coherence and synergy among global health initiatives. *Health Res. Policy Syst.* 2015; 13(75). https://doi.org/10.1186/s12961-015-0062-3.

46 Labonté, R. and Gagnon, M.L. Framing health and foreign policy: lessons for global health diplomacy. *Glob. Health* 2010; 6(14). https://doi.org/10.1186/1744-8603-6-14.

47 Sridhar, D., Khagram, S., and Pang, T. Are existing governance structures equipped to deal with today's global health challenges – towards systematic coherence in scaling up. *Glob. Health Gov.* 2009; 2(2). https://www.ghgj.org/Sridhar%20Khagram%20and%20Pang_Are%20Existing%20Governance.pdf.

48 Kelly, A.M., Ferguson, J.D., Galligan, D., et al. *J. Am. Vet. Med. Assoc.* 2013; 242(6): 739–743. https://doi.org/10.2460/javma.242.6.739.

49 Veterinary Schools Council UK. *One Health.* n.d. https://www.vetschoolscouncil.ac.uk/policy/one-health-agenda/.

50 Adane-Erkyihun, G. and Bekele-Alemayehu, M. One Health approach for the control of zoonotic diseases. *Zoonoses* 2022; 2(37). https://doi.org/10.15212/ZOONOSES-2022-0037.

51 OIE, WHO. *WHO-OIE Operational Framework*. 2014. https://cdn.who.int/media/docs/default-source/documents/publications/who-oie-framework-for-good-governance-human-animal-interface.pdf?sfvrsn=f9f92e6b_2&download=true.

52 The Global Fund. *Strategic Framework for Collaboration between the Global Fund to Fight AIDS, Tuberculosis and Malaria and the World Health Organization*. 2018. https://www.theglobalfund.org/media/7849/other_strategicframeworkcollaborationglobalfundwho_framework_en.pdf.

53 WHO. *Collaborating Centres Fact Sheet*. 2018. https://www.who.int/docs/default-source/documents/aboutus/factsheetwhocc2018.pdf?sfvrsn7166ee_2#:~:text=Over%20800%20institutions%20in%20over%2080%20countries%20supporting,support%20of%20the%20Organization%27s%20programme%20at%20all%20levels.

54 FAO. *One Health*. n.d. https://www.fao.org/one-health/en/.

55 WOAH. *Improving Veterinary Services*. n.d. https://www.woah.org/en/what-we-offer/improving-veterinary-services/.

56 WHO. *76th World Health Assembly Adopts the Global Framework for Integrating Well-Being into Public Health Utilising a Health Promotion Approach*. 2023. https://www.who.int/news/item/29-05-2023-76th-world-health-assembly-adopts-the-global-framework-for-integrating-well-being-into-public-health-utilizing-a-health-promotion-approach.

57 WHO. *Collaboration Framework Arrangement Among the Department of Health and Human Services of the United States of America, the Pan American Health Organization, and the European Regional Office of the World Health Organization*. 2023. https://cdn.who.int/media/docs/librariesprovider2/regional-committee-meeting-reports/paho-euro-hhs-collaboration-framework-arrangement-final.pdf?sfvrsn=a83af4a6_1&download=true.

58 WHO. Joint WHO/FAO Expert Committee on Zoonoses [meeting held in Stockholm from 11 to August 16 1958]: second report. n.d. https://iris.who.int/handle/10665/40435.

59 FAO. *Emergency Prevention System for Animal Health (EMPRES-AH)*. n.d. https://www.fao.org/animal-health/our-programmes/emergency-prevention-system-for-animal-health-(empres-ah)/en.

60 International Livestock Research Institute. *Better Lives Through Livestock*. n.d. https://www.ilri.org/

61 WHO. *International Health Regulations*. 2005. https://www.who.int/health-topics/international-health-regulations#tab=tab_1.

62 WOAH. *The "Global Framework – Transboundary Animal Diseases"*. n.d. https://rr-americas.woah.org/en/projects/gf-tads/

63 WOAH. *Launch of Global Early Warning System for Animal Diseases Transmissible to Humans*. 2006. https://www.woah.org/en/launch-of-global-early-warning-system-for-animal-diseases-transmissible-to-humans/#:~:text=The%20Global%20Early%20Warning%20and%20Response%20System%20%28GLEWS%29,and%20alert%20mechanisms%20of%20OIE%2C%20FAO%20and%20WHO.

64 World Bank. *Global Program for Avian Influenza and Human Pandemic Preparedness and Response: GPAI program framework document (English)*. n.d. https://documents.worldbank.org/en/publication/documents-reports/documentdetail/908811468140057837/global-program-for-avian-influenza-and-human-pandemic-preparedness-and-response-gpai-program-framework-document.

65 Global Alliance for Rabies Control. *Our Story*. n.d. https://rabiesalliance.org/about/our-story.

66 UC DAVIS. *Predict*. n.d. https://ohi.vetmed.ucdavis.edu/programs-projects/predict-project.

67 Myhre-Erracaborde, K., Wuebbolt-Macy, K., Pekol, A., et al. Factors that enable effective One Health collaborations – a scoping review of the literature. *PLoS One* 2019; 14(12). https://doi.org/10.1371/journal.pone.0224660.

68 Global Health Security Agenda. *A Partnership Against Global Health Threats*. n.d. https://globalhealthsecurityagenda.org/.

69 De La Rocque, S., Caya, F., El Idrissi, A., et al. One Health operations: a critical component in the international health regulations monitoring and evaluation framework. *Rev. Sci. Tech. (International Office of Epizootics)* 2019; 38(1). https://doi.org/10.20506/rst.38.1.2962.

70 GHPP. *Partnership to Drive One Health Policy with Evidence*. 2023. https://www.openagrar.de/servlets/MCRFileNodeServlet/openagrar_derivate_00059624/GHPP-20231127.pdf.

71 De Giusti, M., Barbato, D., Lia, L., et al. Collaboration between human and veterinary medicine as a tool to solve public health problems. *Planet. Health* 2019; 3. https://www.thelancet.com/pdfs/journals/lanplh/PIIS2542-5196%2818%2930250-X.pdf.

72 Larkan, F., Uduma, O., Akinmayowa-Lawal, S., and Van Bavel, B. Developing a framework for successful research partnerships in global health. *Global. Health* 2016; 12(17). https://doi.org/10.1186/s12992-016-0152-1.

73 Department of Health & Social Care. *Global Health Framework: Working Together Towards a Healthier World, May 2023*. 2023. https://www.gov.uk/government/publications/global-health-framework-working-together-towards-a-healthier-world/global-health-framework-working-together-towards-a-healthier-world-may-2023.

74 WOAH. *One Health*. n.d. https://www.woah.org/en/what-we-do/global-initiatives/one-health/.

75 Eussen, B.G.M., Schaveling, J., Dragt, M.J., and Blomme, R.J. Stimulating collaboration between human and veterinary health care professionals. *BMC Vet. Res.* 2017; 13(174). https://doi.org/10.1186/s12917-017-1072-x.

76 Thiessen, M., Heiss, L., McGee, T., and Bawden, G. *The Future Is Participatory: Collaborative Communication Design for Global Health Initiatives*. University of Cincinnati Press; 2023. https://muse.jhu.edu/pub/330/article/893660/summary.

77 Romero, J. *Sustainability of Veterinary Services: Experiences and Challenges*. OIE Regional Commission. 2018. https://doi.org/10.20506/TT.2933.

78 Kaba, T., Zerihun, T., Abera, B., and Kassa, T. A review on the role of veterinary public health and its current challenges. *Arch. Vet. Sci.* 2017; VST-114. https://doi.org/10.29011/AVST-114/100014.

79 Rooke, F., Burford, J., and Freeman, S. Quality Improvement: origins, purpose and the future for veterinary practice. In: *Veterinary Evidence Vol. 6(2)*. 2021. https://www.ivis.org/library/veterinary-evidence/veterinary-evidence-vol-6-n%C2%B02-jun-2021/quality-improvement-origins-purpose-and-future-for-veterinary-practice.

80 Rillera-Marzo, R., Kisa, A., Adhikari, A., and Padhi, B. *One Health Approach in Global Abstract Submission Deadline May 31 2024*. 2024. https://www.mdpi.com/topics/One_Health#:~:

81 WHO. Future trends in veterinary public health. World Health Organization. *WHO Technical Report Series 907*. 2002.

82 Akinsulie, O.C., Idris, I., Aliyu, V.A., and Shahzad, S., et al. Application of artificial intelligence in veterinary clinical practice and biomedical research. *Front. Vet. Sci.* 2024; 11: 1347550. https://doi.org/10.3389/fvets.2024.1347550.

83 FutureDoctor. AI. *AI in Veterinary Medicine: Revolutionizing Pet Healthcare*. 2024. https://futuredoctor.ai/ai-in-veterinary-medicine/.

84 Hamadani, A., Ahmad-Ganai, N., Hamadani, H., et al. (eds.) Applications and impact of artificial intelligence in veterinary sciences. In: *A Biologist's Guide to Artificial Intelligence: Building the Foundations of Artificial Intelligence and Machine Learning for Achieving Advancements in Life Sciences*, 139–150. 2024. https://doi.org/10.1016/C2023-0-01341-3.

85 Kramer, C.G., McCaw, A.K., Zarestky, J., and Duncan. C.G. Veterinarians in a changing global climate: educational disconnect and a path forward. *Front. Vet. Sci.* 2020; 7: 613620. https://doi.org/10.3389/fvets.2020.613620.

86 AVMA. JAVMA News. *Report Looks to Future of Veterinary Profession*. 2020. https://www.avma.org/javma-news/2020-04-01/report-looks-future-veterinary-profession.

87 Whittall, D. Trending issues in veterinary medicine for 2023 and beyond. *Practice LIFE*. 2022. https://www.practicelife.com/en/latest/trending-issues-in-veterinary-medicine-for-2023-and-beyond/.

88 Amenu, K., McIntyre, K.M., Moje, N., et al. Approaches for disease prioritisation and decision-making in animal health, 2000–2021: a structured scoping review. *Front. Vet. Sci.* 2023; 10: 1231711. https://doi.org/10.3389/fvets.2023.1231711.

89 Lau, B., Duggal. P., Ehrhardt, S., et al. Perspectives on the future of epidemiology: a framework for training. *Am. J. Epidemiol.* 2020; 189(7): 634–639. https://doi.org/10.1093/aje/kwaa013.

90 Liz Paola, N.Z., Torgerson, P.R., and Hartnack, S. Alternative paradigms in animal health decisions: a framework for treating animals not only as commodities. *Animals* 2022; 12, 1845. https://doi.org/10.3390/ani12141845.

91 European Commission. *Veterinary Services in a Changing World: Climate Change and Other External Factors. KNOWLEDGE FOR POLICY. Supporting Policy with Scientific Evidence.* 2021. https://knowledge4policy.ec.europa.eu/publication/veterinary-services-changing-world-climate-change-other-external-factors_en.

92 Kiran, D., Sander, W.E., and Duncan, C. Empowering veterinarians to be planetary health stewards through policy and practice. *Front. Vet. Sci.* 2022; 9: 775411. https://doi.org/10.3389/fvets.2022.775411.

93 Michigan State University. *Climate Change and Veterinary Medicine.* College of Veterinary Medicine, Michigan State University. 2019. https://cvm.msu.edu/vetschool-tails/climate-change-and-veterinary-medicine.

94 Parsons, D. *Forecasting Zoonotic Disease Risks in a Changing Climate.* BMC BugBitten Blog Network. 2024. https://blogs.biomedcentral.com/bugbitten/2024/04/19/forecasting-zoonotic-.disease-risks-in-a-changing-climate/.

95 WWF. *How the Climate Crisis Could Impact Our Future.* 2023. https://www.worldwildlife.org/stories/how-the-climate-crisis-could-impact-our-future.

96 Magiri, R., Muzandu, K., Gitau, G., et al. Impact of climate change on animal health, emerging and re-emerging diseases in Africa. In: *African Handbook of Climate Change Adaptation Oguge* (eds. N. Oguge, D. Ayal, L. Adeleke, and I. da Silva), Cham: Springer; 2021. https://doi.org/10.1007/978-3-030-45106-6_19.

97 Lacetera, N. Impact of climate change on animal health and welfare. *Anim. Front.* 2019; 9(1): 26–31. https://doi.org/10.1093/af/vfy030.

98 Hiko, A. and Malicha, G. *Climate Change and Animal Health Risk, Climate Change and the 2030 Corporate Agenda for Sustainable Development (Advances in Sustainability and Environmental Justice, Vol. 19)*, Leeds: Emerald Group Publishing Limited; 2016. https://doi.org/10.1108/S2051-503020160000019004.

99 Renae Charalambous, J.J., Pahuja, H., Fox, D., et al. Impacts of climate change on animal welfare. *CABI Rev.* 2023. https://doi.org/10.1079/cabireviews.2023.0020.

100 UNDESA. Food security and nutrition and sustainable agriculture. SDG #2. *End Hunger, Achieve Food Security and Improved Nutrition and Promote Sustainable Agriculture.* N.d. https://sdgs.un.org/topics/food-security-and-nutrition-and-sustainable-agriculture.

101 CEDEFOD. The external factors influencing VET. Cedefop project 'Changing nature and role of vocational education and training in Europe' – Working Paper 3. European Centre for the Devclopment of Vocational Training. 2017. https://www.cedefop.europa.eu/files/wp3_external_factors_influencing_vet.pdf.

102 Keeling, L., Tunón, H., Olmos-Antillón, G., et al. Animal welfare and the United Nations sustainable development goals. *Front. Vet. Sci.* 2019; 6: 336. https://doi.org/10.3389/fvets.2019.00336.

103 Keeling, L.J., Marier, E.A., Olmos-Antillón, G., et al. A global study to identify a potential basis for policy options when integrating animal welfare into the UN sustainable development goals. *Front. Anim. Sci.* 2022; 3: 974687. https://doi.org/10.3389/fanim.2022.974687.

104 MSD. *Public Policy Statement Environmental Sustainability in Animal Health.* MSD Animal Health. 2023. https://www.msd-animal-health.com/wp-content/uploads/sites/2/2023/01/Updated-Sustainability-Public-Policy-Statement-MSD.pdf.

105 Herdoiza, N., Worrell, E., and Van den Berg, F. Including animal welfare targets in the SDGs: the case of animal farming. *Agric. Hum. Values* 2024; 41: 815–830. https://doi.org/10.1007/s10460-023-10521-8.

106 United Nations. *Transforming Our World: The 2030 Agenda for Sustainable Development.* n.d. https://sdgs.un.org/sites/default/files/publications/21252030%20Agenda%20for%20Sustainable%20Development%20web.pdf.

107 Tricarico, J.M., Kebreab, E., and Wattiaux, M.A. MILK symposium review: sustainability of dairy production and consumption in low-income countries with emphasis on productivity and environmental impact. *J. Dairy Sci.* 2020; 103: 9791–9802. https://doi.org/10.3168/jds.2020-18269.

108 UNESCO. *How Science Can Help to Create a Sustainable World*. UNESCO News. 2016. https://www.unesco.org/en/articles/how-science-can-help-create-sustainable-world.

109 WOAH. *Animal Welfare. Global Strategy on Animal Welfare*. 2017. https://www.woah.org/app/uploads/2021/03/en-oie-aw-strategy.pdf.

110 WOAH. *Animal Welfare: A Vital Asset for a More Sustainable World*. Vision paper. 2024. https://www.woah.org/app/uploads/2024/01/en-woah-visionpaper-animalwelfare.pdf.

111 The Lancet Planetary Health. Welcome to the Lancet Planetary Health. *Lancet Planet. Health* 2017; 1: e1. https://doi.org/10.1016/S2542-5196(17)30013-X.

112 Issue Brief – Planetary Health [WWW Document]. 2017. https://www.undp.org/publications/issue-brief-planetary-health.

113 Pongsiri, M.J., Bickersteth, S., Colón, C., et al. Planetary health: from concept to decisive action. *Lancet Planet. Health* 2019; 3: e402–e404. https://doi.org/10.1016/S2542-5196(19)30190-1.

114 Landrigan P.J., Stegeman, J.J., Fleming, L.E., et al. Human health and ocean pollution. *Ann. Glob. Health* 2020; 86(1): 151. https://doi.org/10.5334/aogh.2831.

115 Perez-Escamilla, R., Bermudez, O., Buccini, G.S., et al. Nutrition disparities and the global burden of malnutrition. *BMJ* (Clin. Res. Ed.) 2018; 361: k2252. https://doi.org/10.1136/bmj.k2252.

116 Ayeleru, O.O., Dlova, S., Akinribide, O.J., et al. Challenges of plastic waste generation and management in sub-Saharan Africa: a review. *Waste Manage.* 2020; 110: 24–42. https://doi.org/10.1016/j.wasman.2020.04.017.

10

Challenges, Opportunities, and Future Directions in One Health Collaboration

Ahmed Abdulkadir Hassan-Kadle[1], *Zainab Ali Abbas Magar*[2], *Aamir Muse Osman*[1,3] *and Pratik Subhash Gaikwad*[2*]

[1] *Somali One Health Centre, Abrar University, Mogadishu, Somalia*
[2] *School of Biotechnology and Bioinformatics, D Y Patil Deemed to be University, Navi Mumbai, Maharashtra, India*
[3] *Ministry of Livestock, Forestry, and Range, Federal Government of Somalia, Mogadishu, Somalia*

*Corresponding author: pratik.gaikwad@dypatil.edu

TABLE OF CONTENTS

10.1 Introduction
10.2 Current Landscape of One Health Collaboration
10.3 Challenges in One Health Collaboration
10.3.1 Lack of Integrated One Health Approach
10.3.2 Sectionalism and Fragmented Governance
10.3.3 Resource Constraints
10.3.4 Communication Barriers
10.3.5 Conflicting Agendas
10.3.6 Leadership and Continuity Challenges
10.3.7 Cultural and Behavioral Differences
10.3.8 Knowledge and Data Sharing Obstacles
10.4 Opportunities in One Health Collaboration
10.4.1 Strengthening Surveillance and Response
10.4.2 Ensuring Sustainable Food Systems
10.4.3 Promoting Environmental Sustainability
10.4.4 Facilitating Research and Development
10.4.5 Building Public Trust and Advocacy
10.5 Future Directions in One Health Collaboration
10.5.1 One Health Governance
10.5.2 Multisectoral Communication and Coordination
10.5.3 Building Sustainable One Health Systems
10.5.4 Interdisciplinary Research
10.5.5 Public–Private Partnerships in One Health
10.5.6 Investing in One Health Education
10.5.7 Ethical Considerations in Implementing One Health Practices
10.5.8 Leveraging New Technologies and Tools
10.5.9 Untapped Opportunities for Global Collaborations
10.5.10 Envisioning a Sustainable and Healthier Future
10.6 Conclusion
References

One Health Integration: Global Perspectives on Animal Health and Sustainable Agriculture. First Edition.
Edited by Pratik Subhash Gaikwad, Vivek Harishankar Shukla and Pintu Choudhary.

Companion Website: https://www.wiley.com/go/pratikgaikwad/onehealth

10.1 Introduction

The One Health concept is a collaborative, interdisciplinary framework that recognizes the interconnectedness of human, animal, and environmental health. This chapter explores an in-depth examination of the challenges and opportunities within One Health collaboration, focusing on its potential to address global health issues such as zoonotic diseases, environmental degradation, and antimicrobial resistance (AMR).

The current status of One Health initiatives is provided, emphasizing the progress achieved and the obstacles that hinder effective cross-sector collaboration. Key challenges such as fragmented governance, resource limitations, communication gaps, and conflicting priorities are discussed. Despite these challenges, One Health presents valuable opportunities in areas such as enhancing disease surveillance, promoting sustainable food systems, safeguarding environmental health, and encouraging international cooperation.

The chapter also outlines prospective directions for advancing One Health practices, highlighting the need for improved governance structures, enhanced communication and coordination, interdisciplinary research, and greater investments in education and public–private collaborations. These aspects contribute to providing a roadmap to strengthen One Health integration, contributing to a healthier and more sustainable future for humans, animals, and ecosystems.

10.2 Current Landscape of One Health Collaboration

The One Health collaboration is evolving rapidly, with significant progress in integrating human, animal, plant, and environmental health [1]. This evolution is driven by global challenges like the COVID-19 pandemic, AMR, and climate change [2]. Key developments include data-driven approaches, heightened public awareness, and the growing recognition of One Health's role in addressing complex health challenges [1, 2].

International organizations, such as WHO, FAO, WOAH, and UNEP, are promoting One Health through joint initiatives [3]. Academic institutions are increasingly adopting interdisciplinary research and education programs that foster collaboration across medical, veterinary, agricultural, and environmental sciences [1, 4]. Regions with high zoonotic disease risks are also implementing robust One Health frameworks to enhance surveillance and response systems [1, 5]. Table 10.1 provides an overview of major organizations, programs, and initiatives actively promoting One Health collaboration, highlighting their goals, geographical scope, and key activities.

Despite this progress, significant challenges remain, including institutional barriers, data sharing concerns, and the need for standardized guidelines that hinder comprehensive implementation at local, national, regional, and global levels [2]. Although One Health platforms and grassroots initiatives are emerging to address these barriers, greater coordination, public awareness, and sustained political commitment are essential to fully realize the potential of One Health in preventing and managing health threats at the human–animal–plant–environment interface [14]. As the world continues to face health threats, strengthening One Health collaboration will be crucial to achieving sustainable health outcomes. Figure 10.1 presents a conceptual framework illustrating the interconnectedness between human, animal, and environmental health sectors within the One Health approach.

10.3 Challenges in One Health Collaboration

The major barriers hindering effective One Health collaboration persist despite its strong potential to improve health outcomes by integrating human, animal, and environmental health efforts. Differences in priorities, perspectives, and terminology among sectors often lead to miscommunication and a lack of shared goals. Limited resources, funding constraints, and the absence of dedicated support mechanisms further restrict interdisciplinary efforts. Cultural resistance and varying levels of stakeholder commitment also hinder integration. Additionally,

Table 10.1 Overview of existing collaborative efforts in One Health.

Organization/program	Goals	Geographical scope	Key activities	References
World Health Organization (WHO)	To promote health, keep the world safe, and serve vulnerable populations	Global	Coordinating international health responses, providing guidelines on health policies	[6]
Food and Agriculture Organization (FAO)	To achieve food security and better nutrition, promote sustainable agriculture	Global	Implementing food safety measures, enhancing agricultural practices, and improving animal health	[7]
World Organisation for Animal Health (OIE)	To improve animal health and welfare globally, ensuring safe trade of animals and animal products	Global	Setting international standards for animal health, conducting capacity-building programs	[8]
Global Health Security Agenda (GHSA)	To accelerate progress toward a world safe and secure from infectious disease threats	Global	Strengthening national capacities for detection and response to infectious diseases	[9]
EcoHealth Alliance	To promote conservation of ecosystems and improve health outcomes through an integrated approach	Global	Conducting research on the links between health and ecosystems, promoting community engagement	[10]
One Health Commission	To advance the One Health approach to solve complex health issues	Global	Facilitating collaboration among professionals across human, animal, and environmental health sectors	[11]
International Livestock Research Institute (ILRI)	To improve food security and reduce poverty in developing countries through livestock research	Africa and South Asia	Conducting research on animal health and productivity, enhancing livestock systems	[12]
Centers for Disease Control and Prevention (CDC)	To protect public health and safety through the control and prevention of disease	United States and Global	Conducting disease surveillance, outbreak response, and public health research	[13]

short-term funding cycles disrupt the long-term collaboration needed to address complex issues such as zoonotic diseases and environmental degradation. Overcoming these barriers is crucial to strengthening effective One Health partnerships.

10.3.1 Lack of Integrated One Health Approach

Challenges in adopting an integrated One Health approach are multifaceted, with a significant barrier being the lack of interdisciplinary collaboration among key stakeholders. This fragmentation prevents the effective integration of human, animal, plant, and environmental health perspectives, resulting in strategies that fail to account for the interconnectedness of these sectors, ultimately leading to suboptimal outcomes in disease prevention and environmental conservation. Although the One Health concept is increasingly recognized, its practical implementation often remains limited due to siloed operations within the health, agriculture, and environmental sectors, where efforts are frequently rebranded without genuine integration [15].

Resistance to adopting the One Health framework can also stem from cultural differences and the reluctance to abandon traditional disciplines, especially difficulty in engaging medical doctors who often see the concept as

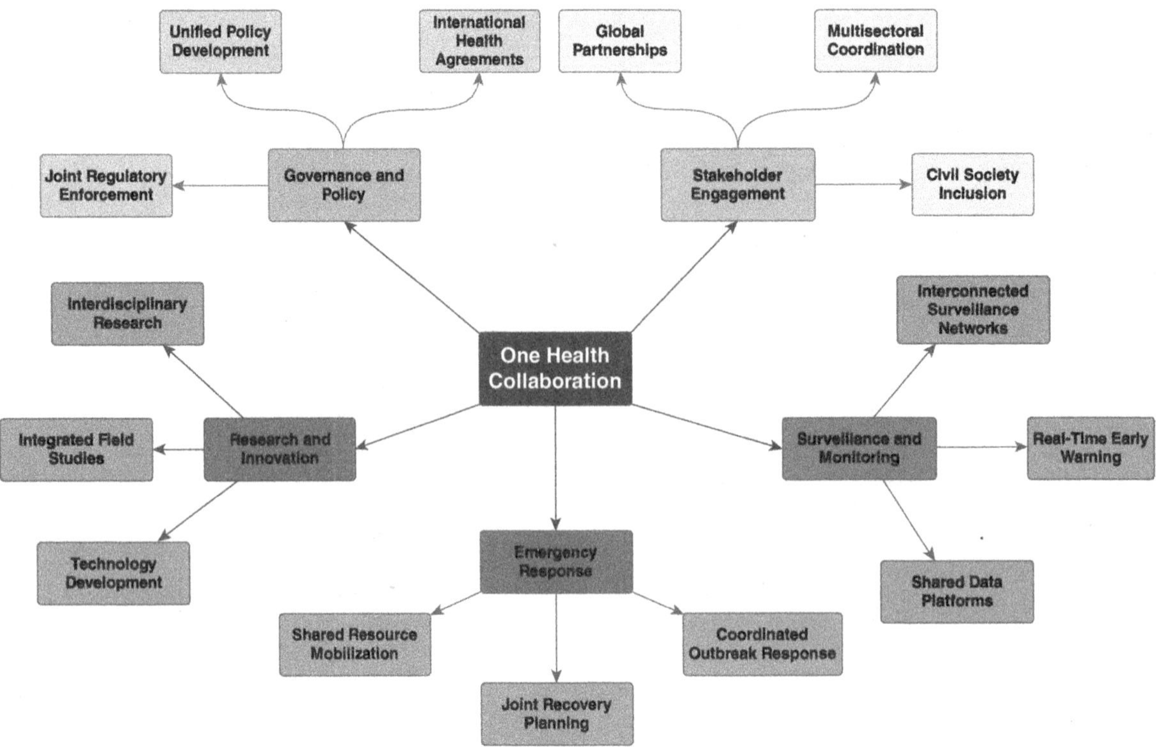

Figure 10.1 Conceptual framework of One Health collaboration.

an encroachment of other disciplines into medicine [16]. A clear example of this challenge was evident during the 2014–2016 West African Ebola outbreak, where inadequate coordination between human and animal health sectors delayed the identification of the zoonotic source, thereby hindering control efforts [17].

Overcoming these challenges requires high-level institutional support, including the integration of One Health principles into educational curricula, capacity building, and political commitment to establish clear budgets and agendas that foster collaboration [18]. Additionally, experts advocate for enhanced One Health education, continuous workforce training, and strong advocacy from national and regional leaders to promote the widespread adoption of the One Health framework.

10.3.2 Sectionalism and Fragmented Governance

Sectionalism and fragmented governance pose significant challenges to the effectiveness of the One Health approach, which depends on the integration of human, animal, plant, and environmental health disciplines to address complex global health issues. Sectionalism arises when different sectors such as health, agriculture, and environmental agencies operate independently, each focusing on their own priorities with insufficient coordination with other sectors. This siloed approach leads to fragmented governance, where policies and actions are developed in isolation, resulting in disjointed and often ineffective responses to health threats [18, 19].

Fragmentation in health governance is a longstanding issue observed in various contexts, often compounded by sectionalism. For example, the global health landscape is marked by a proliferation of actors with divergent interests, creating accountability issues and power imbalances that undermine the effectiveness of health programs and jeopardize the achievement of health-related Sustainable Development Goals (SDGs) [20]. The COVID-19 pandemic has starkly highlighted the detrimental effects of sectionalism and fragmented governance on public health. Countries with fragmented health systems struggled to effectively manage the crisis, underscoring the urgent need for integrated investments in global health security and universal health coverage to build more resilient and equitable health systems [21].

Sectionalism and fragmented governance significantly weaken health systems by creating institutional silos, where sectors like public health, environmental agencies, and veterinary services operate in isolation, hindering coordinated responses [22]. Complex and overlapping regulations further cause confusion and slow actions, especially in managing cross-border zoonotic diseases [23]. Additionally, global health governance is often dominated by wealthier nations, leaving the needs of low-income countries overlooked and worsening existing health disparities. Resource allocation tends to focus on immediate crises rather than on long-term prevention and preparedness, leaving systems vulnerable to future emergencies [24]. Addressing these challenges calls for stronger cross-sector collaboration, simplified regulatory frameworks, empowerment of vulnerable nations, and sustained investments in resilient health infrastructure [25].

To overcome these challenges, it is crucial to foster cross-sectoral collaboration, develop unified regulatory frameworks, address power imbalances to ensure equitable participation, and shift funding priorities from reactive crisis management to proactive prevention and capacity building. By addressing sectionalism and fragmented governance, stakeholders can enhance the operationalization of the One Health approach, ultimately leading to better health outcomes for humans, animals, and the environment.

10.3.3 Resource Constraints

Resource constraints significantly undermine the effectiveness of One Health initiatives in addressing potential pandemic threats by limiting their capacity to implement holistic and preventive measures, particularly in low- and middle-income countries (LMICs). Limited funding, inadequate infrastructure, and a shortage of skilled personnel lead to gaps in surveillance, response, and interdisciplinary collaboration, all of which are critical for the success of One Health [18, 26]. For instance, limited financial resources often result in fragmented efforts where human, animal, and environmental health sectors cannot effectively integrate their operations. Additionally, the shortage of trained personnel in critical areas such as epidemiology and veterinary sciences exacerbates the problem, as it hampers the ability to detect and respond to zoonotic diseases promptly [18]. These limitations not only reduce the ability to prevent outbreaks but also impair the capacity to manage them efficiently when they do occur, ultimately increasing the risk of pandemics.

In sub-Saharan Africa, a study by Cleaveland et al. [27] highlighted that the lack of laboratory infrastructure severely limits effective zoonotic disease surveillance. In resource-constrained countries, integrating public health and animal health priorities often faces significant policy challenges. For instance, in Zambia, efforts to prepare for avian and pandemic influenza revealed the difficulties of aligning disease control interventions with trade and development realities. The focus on mitigating disease risks often sidelines broader public health concerns, thereby limiting the effectiveness of pandemic preparedness [26]. This scenario is likely applicable to other resource-constrained countries, suggesting that effective disease governance requires a holistic approach that incorporates trade and development sectors alongside veterinary and public health sectors.

10.3.4 Communication Barriers

Effective communication is essential for the success of One Health collaboration, yet it is often hampered by language differences, technical jargon, and varying levels of expertise among stakeholders. Key communication barriers that impede effective One Health responses during global health crises include disciplinary silos, where professionals from different sectors – such as human health, animal health, plant health, and environmental health – tend to work in isolation without sufficient cross-disciplinary dialogue [28]. This lack of communication across disciplines leads to fragmented responses and missed opportunities for collaborative problem-solving.

For example, veterinarians and physicians may have differing approaches to disease management, which can result in misaligned interventions and reduced effectiveness [29].

These communication gaps not only cause inefficiencies but also lead to duplication of efforts. Additionally, differences in language, terminology, and organizational culture between sectors further exacerbate misunderstandings and hinder the development of cohesive, unified strategies. Bureaucratic challenges, such as hierarchical structures and rigid protocols, also slow down the communication process, delaying critical decisions. Furthermore, inconsistent messaging and a lack of trust among stakeholders, including the public, contribute to the spread of misinformation and diminish the effectiveness of health interventions during crises [30].

Bridging these communication gaps requires the development of clear and inclusive communication strategies that facilitate understanding and collaboration across diverse disciplines and cultures.

10.3.5 Conflicting Agendas

One Health initiative often involves a diverse range of stakeholders with differing priorities and agendas, which can create conflicts and hinder effective collaboration. Conflicts frequently arise between economic development, environmental conservation, and public health objectives, making it challenging to achieve a unified approach. For example, agricultural intensification may prioritize productivity and economic gains, but this can compromise environmental sustainability and increase the risk of zoonotic disease emergence [31]. Additionally, One Health initiatives often struggle to foster meaningful and equitable participation across various disciplines and sectors, leading to ineffective collaborations. These challenges are exacerbated by difficulties in monitoring and evaluating the success of such initiatives, which are essential for their long-term effectiveness [32].

The recent increase in political and financial focus on One Health has further intensified power struggles among key stakeholders, particularly in the human and animal health sectors. This has led to a siloed, disease-specific approach that undermines the broader goals of the One Health movement [33]. Operational challenges related to global health governance, such as institutional proliferation, competition for resources, and the absence of a central authority, also diminish the effectiveness of One Health initiatives. Balancing these competing interests requires careful negotiation, compromise, and a strong commitment to finding common ground that supports the overarching objectives of One Health.

10.3.6 Leadership and Continuity Challenges

One Health initiative that requires continuity of care faces several leadership challenges, particularly due to the complex, interdisciplinary nature of these efforts. A significant challenge is managing collaboration across different sectors and disciplines, which often have varying priorities and operational practices, and due to changes in political administrations. These changes can disrupt ongoing projects, reduce continuity, and undermine long-term commitments to One Health goals. Leaders must foster meaningful participation from all stakeholders, ensuring that diverse professional and cultural perspectives are integrated effectively. This is crucial to maintaining continuity of care, as disjointed efforts can lead to gaps in service and reduced effectiveness [32]. Additionally, maintaining sustained commitment over time is crucial, as One Health issues often require long-term strategies rather than short-term solutions. Leadership must also manage complex governance frameworks that involve multiple agencies and jurisdictions, which can complicate decision-making and resource allocation. Moreover, aligning diverse interests and ensuring that all parties remain engaged and motivated over extended periods poses a significant challenge [34]. Another challenge is ensuring effective communication and coordination across various levels of care. In integrated care settings, leadership must facilitate smooth transitions and information sharing between different care providers to maintain continuity, which is often complicated by structural and cultural barriers within healthcare systems [35].

Sustaining engagement and accountability within teams over the long term is also critical. Leaders must ensure that all members remain committed to shared goals and that strategies are continuously evaluated and adapted to meet evolving needs [36]. Moreover, the complexity of managing integrated services heightens the need for sustained collaboration and adaptability, especially in response to global health challenges.

The COVID-19 pandemic has underscored the urgency of these challenges. Leaders are now tasked with managing care, making critical decisions, and ensuring employee well-being while preparing for unexpected situations [34, 37]. Effective time management and accountability are essential, as leaders must prioritize tasks and transparently acknowledge their responsibilities to maintain quality care [34]. These factors make leadership in One Health initiatives particularly demanding, requiring vision, adaptability, and the ability to build and maintain trust among diverse stakeholders.

10.3.7 Cultural and Behavioral Differences

Cultural and behavioral differences play a crucial role in shaping the effectiveness of One Health initiatives in global health. These differences often lead to varying perceptions of disease risk, health-seeking behaviors, and attitudes toward animals and the environment. For example, traditional practices and local beliefs can influence how communities perceive zoonotic diseases, sometimes resulting in resistance or hesitation to adopt preventive measures recommended by global health authorities [38, 39]. In some cultures, practices such as traditional hunting and the consumption of bushmeat are deeply rooted but carry risks for zoonotic disease transmission [40].

The importance of community involvement and the decolonization of health governance further underscores the need to consider local contexts and adopt participatory approaches in program implementation. The decolonization agenda emphasizes correcting power imbalances between high-income and low-income countries, advocating for diverse representation and the inclusion of local knowledge in health governance [41].

Addressing these cultural and behavioral differences requires cultural competence, sensitivity, and the ability to build trust and mutual respect among diverse participants. For One Health interventions to be effective, they must be tailored to fit the cultural contexts in which they are implemented, ensuring both their acceptability and sustainability.

10.3.8 Knowledge and Data Sharing Obstacles

The success of One Health relies on the effective sharing of knowledge and data across sectors. However, obstacles such as data privacy concerns, intellectual property rights, and a lack of standardized data-sharing protocols often impede this process. Disparities in data quality and accessibility between high-income and low-income regions further exacerbate these challenges, leading to inequities that limit the effectiveness of One Health interventions. As a result, data often becomes fragmented, making it difficult to consolidate and analyze effectively.

Ethical and legal constraints also complicate data sharing. Human health data are typically subject to stricter regulations than environmental data, creating discrepancies that can lead to reluctance in sharing due to privacy concerns and fears of losing control over information [42]. Additionally, motivational and institutional barriers arise when there is a lack of perceived benefits for sharing data, combined with institutional inertia and a lack of trust between sectors.

The absence of robust, integrated digital platforms exacerbates these issues. Existing systems often fail to integrate data from diverse sources, limiting the potential for comprehensive surveillance and response strategies in One Health initiatives [43]. These combined obstacles significantly impede the ability of One Health initiatives to effectively utilize shared knowledge and data, which is crucial for addressing complex global health challenges.

The operationalization of One Health through digital technologies, such as artificial intelligence (AI) and big data, offers potential solutions but also introduces new challenges. A proposed global framework for One Digital Health aims to promote fair and equitable data sharing across various health domains, addressing issues related to data control and accessibility [44]. The COVID-19 pandemic has underscored the importance of international collaborations and global data sharing. However, legal obstacles continue to prevent data sharing for nonpandemic-related research, potentially hindering public health efforts [45]. Additionally, the adoption of health information technology faces resistance due to organizational, technical, and financial barriers, which must be addressed to create a cohesive knowledge ecosystem [46]. Addressing these barriers requires efforts to develop standardized data systems, harmonize ethical and legal frameworks, incentivize data sharing, and create robust digital infrastructure.

Table 10.2 provides a consolidated view of the major challenges faced in One Health collaboration, including their descriptions, potential impacts, and relevant examples from real-world experiences. Figure 10.2 provides a visual summary of the interconnected challenges impeding effective One Health collaboration.

10.4 Opportunities in One Health Collaboration

One Health approach highlights the interconnectedness of human, animal, and environmental health. With growing global challenges, cross-disciplinary collaboration is more crucial than ever. This section explores how partnerships among healthcare workers, veterinarians, environmental scientists, and policymakers can create

Table 10.2 Challenges faced in One Health collaboration.

Challenge	Description	Potential impacts	Examples	References
Resource Constraints	Limited funding and human resources hinder the implementation of One Health initiatives	Inadequate research, insufficient training, and reduced program effectiveness can result from resource limitations	Many local health departments struggle to allocate sufficient funds for cross-sectoral initiatives	[47, 48]
Communication Barriers	Differences in terminology, language, and communication styles among stakeholders can lead to misunderstandings	Misalignment of goals and objectives among sectors can impede collaboration and reduce effectiveness	Miscommunication between agricultural and healthcare sectors regarding disease reporting protocols	[49, 50]
Cultural Differences	Diverse cultural perspectives and values can affect stakeholder engagement and collaboration efforts	Resistance to collaborative approaches and diminished trust can arise from cultural misunderstandings	Variations in attitudes toward animal health practices in different communities can create friction	[51, 52]
Regulatory Challenges	Inconsistent regulations across regions can complicate collaborative efforts and hinder data sharing	Delays in response to health threats and increased vulnerability to zoonotic diseases may occur	Differences in veterinary and public health regulations between countries can obstruct coordinated responses	[53, 54]
Data Sharing Issues	Concerns over data privacy and ownership can limit the sharing of critical information among sectors	Incomplete data can lead to ineffective responses to health threats and missed opportunities for prevention	Hesitance to share surveillance data between public health and animal health agencies	[53, 55, 56]
Lack of Training	Insufficient training in One Health principles among professionals can reduce collaboration effectiveness	Professionals may not fully understand the interconnectedness of health sectors, leading to siloed approaches	Limited educational programs integrating One Health concepts in veterinary and medical schools	[53, 14, 57]

innovative solutions to complex health problems. One Health not only addresses health crises but also supports sustainable development, food security, and biodiversity conservation. By aligning efforts across sectors, it enables better resource use and policymaking, leading to improved outcomes for all. This section emphasizes the need for strong partnerships to strengthen public health, enhance resilience, and safeguard ecosystems in an increasingly complex world.

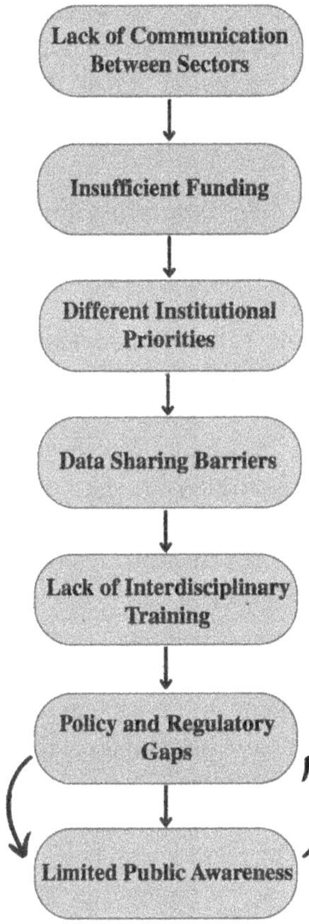

10.4.1 Strengthening Surveillance and Response

One Health collaboration offers significant opportunities to strengthen surveillance systems and enhance response capabilities to health threats. By integrating surveillance strategies across sectors, the One Health framework addresses the interconnected nature of zoonotic diseases, improving the ability to anticipate and mitigate outbreaks before they escalate into larger public health crises. This integrated approach enhances the early detection of emerging diseases, recognizing the critical role of cross-sectoral data sharing and coordination. Given that approximately 75% of emerging infectious diseases are zoonotic, it is essential to implement strategies that leverage these collaborative efforts to bolster early detection and intervention [58].

This holistic approach is especially vital in regions where zoonotic diseases are prevalent and where traditional, siloed methods have proven inadequate. In resource-constrained settings, where the burden of neglected tropical diseases (NTDs) is high, effective surveillance and response systems are crucial for disease elimination. Innovative approaches tailored to local contexts, such as dynamic mapping of transmission, geographic information systems (GIS), AI, and mobile health technologies, can enhance the monitoring and understanding of disease transmission pathways, thereby informing more targeted control measures [59, 60].

Moreover, the successful implementation and sustainability of One Health surveillance systems depend on the active engagement of stakeholders through participatory processes [61]. By fostering multisectoral partnerships and prioritizing joint outbreak responses, the One Health approach can significantly strengthen global health security against zoonotic diseases.

Figure 10.2 Challenges to effective One Health collaboration.

10.4.2 Ensuring Sustainable Food Systems

Integrating One Health principles into agricultural practices provides a promising framework for addressing the multifaceted challenges posed by current food systems. Sustainable food systems are essential for achieving the SDGs and ensuring global health and well-being. These systems aim to reduce the environmental impact of agriculture, improve food security, and enhance the nutritional quality of food. However, existing food system practices have exposed populations to various health issues, including malnutrition, infectious diseases, AMR, and noncommunicable diseases [62].

The One Health approach emphasizes the importance of interdisciplinary collaboration to create resilient and sustainable food systems that can meet the growing demands of the global population while preserving environmental and natural resources [63]. This approach is particularly relevant in the context of global crises such as the COVID-19 pandemic and climate change, which have highlighted the vulnerabilities and interdependencies within our food systems [64].

To ensure sustainable food systems, it is crucial to integrate health, equity, sustainability, and resilience into food production and consumption practices. Achieving this requires a paradigm shift in agriculture and diet, supported by policy reforms, research, and advocacy [62]. Innovations in crop management, pest control, and food waste reduction, along with the promotion of diversified agroecological systems, can play a significant role in meeting these goals [64]. Additionally, promoting animal welfare and reducing antibiotic use in livestock production can mitigate the risk of AMR, thereby contributing to safer food systems.

10.4.3 Promoting Environmental Sustainability

Integrated approaches to environmental sustainability and One Health collaboration can significantly enhance the resilience of both ecosystems and human health by acknowledging the interdependence of humans, animals, and their shared environment. These approaches are grounded in social-ecological systems thinking, which recognizes the complex and adaptive nature of human-environment interactions [65]. One Health collaboration can promote efforts to protect and restore natural habitats, reduce pollution, and mitigate the impacts of climate change. By fostering partnerships between environmental and health sectors, One Health contributes to biodiversity conservation and the sustainable use of natural resources, ultimately supporting long-term ecological health [66]. However, the environmental aspect of One Health is often underrepresented, despite its profound impact on human and animal health.

Addressing the root causes of environmental degradation and disease emergence through these integrated approaches promotes ecosystem balance and reduces the risk of zoonotic diseases. Additionally, these efforts support the sustainable use of natural resources, contribute to climate change mitigation, and enhance the adaptive capacity of human communities and ecosystems in the face of environmental changes. Collaboration across sectors such as public health, veterinary sciences, and environmental management enables the development of comprehensive strategies that are more effective in preventing and responding to health and environmental challenges, thereby strengthening the overall resilience of both ecosystems and human populations [65, 67].

The relationship between public health and the environment is crucial, as climate change and environmental degradation pose significant risks to health. Integrated actions and holistic thinking, especially in the settings where people live, are essential for promoting health, equity, and sustainability. A settings-based approach to health promotion, which considers the interconnected nature of these issues, is key to addressing them effectively [68].

10.4.4 Facilitating Research and Development

One Health collaboration offers a valuable platform for interdisciplinary Research and Development (R&D) to tackle complex health challenges at the intersection of humans, animals, and the environment. By recognizing the interconnectedness of health threats such as zoonotic diseases, AMR, and ecosystem degradation One Health promotes integrated, multidisciplinary approaches. Bringing together experts from medicine, veterinary science, environmental science, and public health, these collaborations foster comprehensive research that yields more impactful results.

The pooling of resources, expertise, and data through One Health collaborations accelerates the discovery of innovative solutions, including new treatments, vaccines, and technologies that improve health outcomes across multiple sectors. The rapid development of COVID-19 vaccines demonstrates the potential of global cooperation in speeding up R&D efforts [69]. For example, integrating environmental surveillance with clinical data allows for the early detection of emerging zoonotic diseases, facilitating rapid response and containment measures. Additionally, R&D within the One Health framework is well-suited to address complex challenges such as AMR by promoting responsible antibiotic use across both human and animal sectors [70]. These collaborations also open opportunities for implementing novel environmental monitoring tools to predict and mitigate health risks. The inclusion of diverse scientific perspectives in R&D not only strengthens the reliability of findings but also ensures that interventions are sustainable and relevant on a global scale [71].

Table 10.3 Opportunities for enhancing One Health collaboration.

Opportunity	Specific areas for improvement	Potential benefits	Stakeholders involved	References
Strengthening Surveillance	Implementing integrated disease surveillance systems	Early detection of zoonotic diseases, improved public health	Public health agencies, veterinary services, NGOs	[73, 74]
Promoting Environmental Sustainability	Enhancing sustainable agricultural practices	Reduced environmental impact, improved ecosystem health	Farmers, environmental organizations, government	[52, 74]
Fostering Interdisciplinary Research	Encouraging collaboration among various disciplines	Innovative solutions to health challenges, shared knowledge	Academic institutions, research organizations	[75–77]
Improving Communication	Developing effective communication channels	Enhanced collaboration, better public awareness	Media, community organizations, health authorities	[48, 78]
Capacity Building	Training programs for professionals in One Health	Increased expertise, better preparedness for health crises	Educational institutions, professional bodies	[79, 80]
Engaging Local Communities	Involving communities in health initiatives	Increased community ownership, tailored health solutions	Local governments, community leaders, NGOs	[79]
Leveraging Technology	Utilizing digital tools for data sharing	Improved data access, real-time monitoring	Tech companies, researchers, health agencies	[47]
Policy Advocacy	Promoting supportive policies for One Health	Better funding, enhanced collaboration	Policymakers, advocacy groups, international bodies	[77, 80]

10.4.5 Building Public Trust and Advocacy

To effectively promote One Health collaboration and its benefits, advocacy strategies must be tailored to foster public trust by emphasizing the interconnectedness of human, animal, and environmental health. These strategies should involve transparency, accountability, and a commitment to the well-being of communities that highlight the tangible benefits of One Health, such as preventing pandemics and ensuring food security [72]. Engaging diverse stakeholders, including communities, policymakers, and scientific experts, is crucial for building a shared understanding and commitment to One Health principles. Trust can be further strengthened by demonstrating successful One Health initiatives and ensuring that communication is culturally sensitive and locally relevant [72]. Public trust can be built through consistent, clear messaging that underscores the mutual benefits of collaborative action, ultimately leading to greater acceptance and support of One Health initiatives.

Table 10.3 outlines the key opportunities for enhancing One Health collaboration, detailing specific focus areas such as strengthening surveillance, promoting environmental sustainability, and building public trust, along with potential benefits and key stakeholders involved.

10.5 Future Directions in One Health Collaboration

One Health concept has emerged in recent years as a comprehensive approach to addressing health issues that span across different sectors. This framework emphasizes the importance of collaboration among various sectors, including healthcare, veterinary science, environmental management, and public policy. Looking ahead, it is

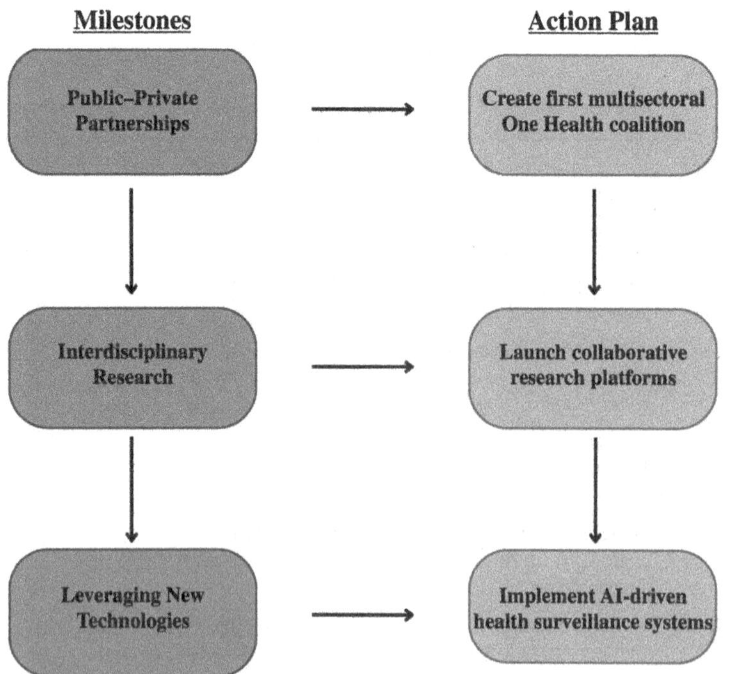

Figure 10.3 Future directions in One Health collaboration.

crucial to develop a clear and actionable strategic plan that identifies essential milestones and steps to enhance global One Health efforts.

Figure 10.3 illustrates this strategic roadmap, highlighting the critical phases and milestones necessary for advancing One Health collaboration. The roadmap serves as a guide for stakeholders to align their efforts, ensuring that all sectors work synergistically toward common goals.

10.5.1 One Health Governance

One Health governance is increasingly recognized as a crucial framework for addressing the intricate connections between human, animal, plant, and environmental health. This governance model underscores the importance of integrated policies, cross-sectoral collaboration, and a multidisciplinary approach to managing and mitigating health risks that span across species and ecosystems [81]. As the global health landscape becomes increasingly interconnected, the demand for robust One Health governance structures has intensified, driving the development of frameworks that not only promote synergy among health sectors but also ensure equitable resource distribution, effective communication, and coordinated response strategies [82].

To enhance One Health governance, integrating knowledge through multicriteria analyses and systems thinking is essential. These strategies enable policymakers to create a shared vision and direction, facilitating evidence-based decision-making and transforming observations into actionable insights. Additionally, adopting transdisciplinary approaches can strengthen the effectiveness of existing systems and foster the creation of new networks for collective action [83].

Leadership and partnership competencies are also critical for the success of One Health initiatives. Effective leadership can champion collaborations, build trust, and ensure that initiatives are adequately resourced and supported [82]. Moreover, meaningful community engagement and the identification of "win–win" strategies can enhance the legitimacy and credibility of collaborative efforts, thereby strengthening intersectoral partnerships [84]. This governance approach is not just a response to current health challenges but a proactive strategy for future preparedness. By fostering cooperation across diverse sectors, One Health governance is positioned as a future-oriented direction for health collaboration, crucial for achieving global health security and sustainable development goals.

10.5.2 Multisectoral Communication and Coordination

In the evolving landscape of One Health collaboration, effective multisectoral communication and coordination have become essential for addressing the complex challenges at the intersection of human, animal, and environmental health. The increasing threats posed by zoonotic diseases, climate change, and AMR highlight the critical need for strong communication channels and coordinated efforts across these sectors [85, 86].

Multisectoral communication fosters mutual understanding and data sharing among stakeholders from different sectors, enhancing the ability to respond quickly and efficiently to public health crises. Meanwhile, coordination, on the other hand, ensures that actions taken by various sectors are aligned, synergistic, and avoid duplication of efforts. The integration of these two components communication and coordination into One Health initiatives is vital for building resilience against emerging health threats [86].

Looking ahead, it is imperative to develop platforms and tools that enable seamless communication across disciplines, sectors, and geographic regions. For example, the One Health Systems Mapping and Analysis Resource Toolkit (OH-SMART) serves as an integrative tool designed to systematically enhance coordination and collaboration across sectors. This toolkit aids in revising emergency response frameworks, improving national action plans for AMR, and creating multiagency infectious disease collaboration protocols, thereby addressing complex health issues through a structured, stepwise approach [87].

10.5.3 Building Sustainable One Health Systems

Building sustainable One Health systems requires a multisectoral approach that integrates the expertise, resources, and efforts of various sectors, including human, animal, plant, and environmental health. This approach is essential for addressing the complex and interconnected challenges of emerging infectious diseases, AMR, and other health threats. Recent studies have highlighted the need to expand the One Health approach to incorporate additional dimensions such as food systems and resilience. For instance, the Food Systems, One Health, and Resilience (FOR) approach advocates for a more comprehensive framework that includes food security and resilience as critical components. This expanded model aims to foster collaborative, multisectoral, and transdisciplinary efforts to ensure sustainable and resilient health outcomes for all [63].

Digital transformation is another crucial aspect of modernizing One Health systems. The One Digital Health framework proposes integrating digital health technologies with One Health principles to create a unified health ecosystem. This approach emphasizes the importance of citizen engagement, education, and the use of advanced technologies to manage health data and improve health outcomes at both individual and population levels [88].

Future directions in One Health collaboration should focus on strengthening institutional frameworks, enhancing cross-sectoral communication, and fostering partnerships that promote shared goals and responsibilities. By aligning policies, strategies, and interventions across sectors, it is possible to create resilient health systems that can effectively prevent, detect, and respond to health crises [89]. This holistic approach not only enhances public health outcomes but also supports sustainable development by ensuring that the health of people, animals, and ecosystems are maintained in harmony [90].

10.5.4 Interdisciplinary Research

Interdisciplinary research stands as a crucial future direction in One Health collaboration, highlighting the need to integrate diverse fields to address the intricate relationships between human, animal, plant, and environmental health. The interconnectedness of these domains requires a collaborative approach that draws on the strengths of various disciplines, including veterinary science, medicine, environmental science, social sciences, and public health [91]. This collaborative effort is vital for comprehensively understanding and mitigating emerging health threats such as zoonotic diseases, AMR, and ecosystem degradation challenges that no single discipline can tackle alone.

The drive for interdisciplinary research in healthcare stems from the complexity of health problems, which demand insights from fields such as medicine, epidemiology, social sciences, engineering, and digital health technologies. For example, the integration of mathematics, physics, and engineering into medical research has shown significant potential for enhancing clinical training and care delivery [92]. Similarly, collaborations between biological sciences, epidemiology, and social sciences are essential for shaping public health policies, particularly in the context of One Health and zoonotic diseases [93].

The importance of interdisciplinary research in achieving global health objectives, such as the SDGs, cannot be overstated. The interconnected nature of these goals requires a multiperspective approach to health issues, leveraging the strengths of various disciplines to develop innovative and effective interventions [94]. As global health challenges grow more complex and intertwined, interdisciplinary research within the One Health framework will play an essential role in advancing our collective capacity to safeguard public health, protect biodiversity, and promote sustainable development.

10.5.5 Public–Private Partnerships in One Health

Public–private partnerships (PPPs) hold immense potential for shaping the future of One Health systems, offering a collaborative approach that harnesses the strengths of both sectors to address complex health challenges at the animal, human, plant, and environmental interface. These partnerships can provide the financial investment, technical expertise, and infrastructure needed to support surveillance, diagnostic, and response systems crucial for tackling complex issues that cannot be solved by single entities alone [2, 95, 96].

In the health domain, PPPs have shown promise in areas such as developing new drugs and vaccines for neglected diseases, enhancing community health services, and improving primary health care delivery. For example, product development PPPs (PD PPPs) have successfully attracted investments from multinational drug companies to combat neglected diseases, reducing the suffering of over one billion people worldwide [97]. These partnerships are pivotal in driving innovation and advancing public health by facilitating the discovery and development of essential medicines.

To advance global health security, future collaborations should focus on creating sustainable models that incentivize private sector engagement in developing health technologies, research innovations, and capacity building. Effective PPPs must emphasize shared responsibility, mutual benefits, transparent governance, equitable resource allocation, and a commitment to capacity building in low-resource settings, where the need for enhanced health systems is most critical [2].

10.5.6 Investing in One Health Education

Investing in One Health education is a critical component for the advancement of One Health systems and the enhancement of future collaborations across various sectors. As the interconnectedness between human, animal, plant, and environmental health becomes increasingly evident, there is a growing need for a well-trained workforce that comprehensively understands these relationships. Educational programs that emphasize interdisciplinary learning are essential in bridging the existing gaps between different sectors, ensuring that professionals whether they are in medicine, veterinary science, environmental studies, or public health are equipped with the knowledge and skills to collaborate effectively [1, 98]. This includes integrating One Health concepts into existing curricula in medical, veterinary, environmental, and agricultural schools, as well as offering specialized training programs for professionals already in the field. Additionally, public education campaigns can raise awareness of the One Health approach among broader audiences, fostering a culture of collaboration and shared responsibility for health. Education serves as the foundation for equipping future professionals with the necessary skills and knowledge to operate within integrated health systems. By promoting a curriculum that emphasizes the interconnectedness of human, animal, and environmental health, educational institutions can cultivate a workforce adept at anticipating, identifying, and mitigating health risks that cross these domains. This forward-looking investment not only strengthens One Health systems but also ensures the sustainability of collaborative efforts in tackling emerging and re-emerging health threats globally [99].

Moreover, such education fosters a culture of cooperation and mutual understanding, which is vital for the development of cohesive strategies to tackle complex global health challenges, including zoonotic diseases, AMR, and climate change impacts [98]. By prioritizing and investing in One Health education, we not only build a workforce capable of responding to current health issues but also create a foundation for sustainable, integrated health systems [98]. These systems will be better prepared to anticipate and mitigate future health threats, thereby promoting resilience and adaptability in the face of emerging global challenges.

10.5.7 Ethical Considerations in Implementing One Health Practices

Ethical considerations in implementing One Health practices are pivotal as they influence every stage of its implementation from research and policymaking to practical applications. The integration of human, animal, and environmental health sectors raises complex ethical challenges that must be addressed to ensure equitable and effective outcomes. These include concerns about animal welfare, the fair distribution of resources, and the rights of communities affected by One Health interventions. For instance, the prioritization of human health over animal and environmental health can lead to ethical dilemmas, especially in resource-constrained settings [100, 101]. This requires a nuanced understanding of the interdependencies and interconnections among these domains, as well as a commitment to ethical principles that guide decision-making processes [102].

Additionally, the involvement of various stakeholders from different sectors requires transparent decision-making processes that respect cultural values and ethical norms. Ethical frameworks that guide the allocation of resources, the conduct of research, and the implementation of interventions are crucial to maintaining trust and fostering cooperation among all parties involved [100, 101].

Moreover, the governance of One Health initiatives must address ethical issues related to data sharing, transparency, accountability, and trust. Effective surveillance systems, for instance, must be designed with ethical considerations in mind to ensure responsible self-governance and community empowerment. This involves creating frameworks that facilitate collective deliberation and expert evaluation, thereby promoting a more inclusive and democratic approach to health governance [101, 103].

The future of One Health collaboration hinges on the integration of ethical considerations into every aspect of its implementation. By fostering a multispecies understanding of health and promoting ethical debate and guidelines, we can build a robust framework that supports sustainable and equitable health outcomes for humans, animals, plant, and the environment [101, 104].

10.5.8 Leveraging New Technologies and Tools

The rapid advancement of technology presents transformative opportunities for enhancing collaboration within the One Health framework, which integrates human, animal, plant, and environmental health [105]. Innovations in digital health, big data analytics, and AI are pivotal in facilitating real-time surveillance and response to health threats [60]. For example, AI algorithms can analyze vast datasets to predict disease outbreaks and identify potential zoonotic threats, enabling timely interventions [74, 60].

Mobile health applications play a crucial role in improving communication among veterinarians, farmers, and public health officials, fostering a more interconnected approach to disease management [60, 106]. These applications empower communities by providing real-time information on health risks and preventive measures, thus enhancing public engagement in One Health initiatives [76].

Moreover, remote sensing technologies and GIS are instrumental in monitoring environmental changes and their impacts on health outcomes [107–109]. Drones equipped with sensors can assess livestock health and environmental conditions, offering timely data that informs interventions [110]. Additionally, genomic technologies such as metagenomics and next-generation sequencing enable rapid pathogen identification and tracking of AMR genes, contributing to a deeper understanding of microbial ecosystems [111].

Blockchain technology is emerging to enhance transparency and traceability in food supply chains, addressing food safety and security issues [111]. The Internet of Things (IoT) introduces smart sensors and wearable devices in livestock management, continuously monitoring vital parameters like temperature and activity, which provides early alerts for illnesses and reduces antibiotic dependency through precision farming [112].

Overall, the integration of these new technologies and tools can significantly strengthen the One Health framework, promoting a more proactive and sustainable approach to health management. However, achieving equitable access and responsible usage of these technologies requires international cooperation, sufficient funding, and capacity building, particularly in LMICs.

10.5.9 Untapped Opportunities for Global Collaborations

Despite the advancements in One Health initiatives, there remain significant untapped opportunities for global collaborations that could enhance the effectiveness of health interventions. One key opportunity is fostering partnerships between LMICs and high-income nations to build capacity within health systems. Collaborative efforts can focus on sharing best practices, resources, and expertise to strengthen surveillance and response capabilities in LMICs, which often bear the brunt of zoonotic diseases [113, 114].

International organizations can play a pivotal role in facilitating multi-sectorial collaborations that address the root causes of health threats [115, 116]. For instance, joint initiatives that integrate agriculture, environmental management, and public health can promote sustainable development while enhancing resilience against emerging health risks [117]. Additionally, collaborative research efforts are essential for the development of novel vaccines and treatments targeting zoonotic diseases, which are increasingly prevalent due to heightened human–animal interactions [118].

The establishment of international networks for knowledge sharing and resource allocation can facilitate a more coordinated response to global health threats. Existing frameworks, such as the One Health Global Network, can be leveraged alongside new models of collaboration that utilize shared resources and expertise [119]. By fostering a culture of collaboration, stakeholders can collectively address challenges such as AMR and food security, ultimately leading to improved health outcomes worldwide [120, 121].

Addressing global health challenges, including pandemics, climate change, and food insecurity, necessitates transdisciplinary and cross-border collaborations that extend beyond traditional boundaries [122]. Capacity-building initiatives targeting LMICs are critical, as these regions often face the highest burden of zoonotic diseases while possessing limited institutional capacities [123]. Establishing regional centers of excellence, promoting south–south cooperation, and supporting localized research initiatives can help bridge these gaps and facilitate inclusive knowledge sharing [121].

Moreover, the rise of citizen science and community-led surveillance systems offers valuable insights and early warning signals [124]. Engaging local communities in data collection, wildlife monitoring, and health education not only empowers citizens but also fosters culturally relevant and sustainable solutions [125, 126]. By capitalizing on these untapped opportunities, stakeholders can create a more robust global network that effectively addresses the interconnected challenges of health, agriculture, and environmental sustainability [127, 128].

10.5.10 Envisioning a Sustainable and Healthier Future

The vision for a sustainable and healthier future through the One Health paradigm necessitates a holistic approach that recognizes the interconnectedness of human, animal, and environmental health [129]. Achieving this vision requires a commitment to sustainability, equity, and inclusivity, ensuring that all stakeholders have a voice in shaping health policies and practices [130, 131].

To realize this future, it is essential to integrate One Health principles into educational curricula and training programs, fostering a new generation of professionals equipped to tackle health challenges from a multidisciplinary perspective [129, 131]. Empowering local communities with knowledge about the One Health approach can stimulate grassroots movements that advocate for health and environmental stewardship [130, 131]. Furthermore, promoting community engagement and participatory governance can empower populations to take an active role in health initiatives, leading to sustainable and culturally relevant solutions [116, 132].

A strategic shift toward integrative and forward-thinking methodologies is fundamental. This includes embedding One Health principles into national development policies, climate action strategies, and agricultural reform agendas [130]. Policymakers must acknowledge the interdependence of human health, animal welfare, and environmental integrity, addressing these aspects concurrently [130, 133, 134].

Additionally, integrating sustainability metrics into health policies can guide decision-makers in prioritizing actions that benefit both health and the environment [130]. A collective commitment to envisioning resilient, equitable, and sustainable health systems is essential for ensuring that both current and future generations can thrive in harmony with the planet [130, 133, 135]. Investing in education and youth engagement is crucial for nurturing the next generation of One Health professionals, through the development of interdisciplinary curricula and promoting One Health fellowships [133, 135, 136].

By embracing this vision and working collectively, stakeholders can pave the way for a healthier planet, safeguarding health and well-being while preserving ecosystems and ensuring the equitable distribution of resources for generations to come [130, 137, 138].

10.6 Conclusion

The integration of One Health principles into sustainable agriculture is both essential and complex, highlighting the interconnectedness of human, animal, plant, and environmental health. This chapter has elucidated the current landscape of One Health collaboration, revealing significant progress alongside persistent challenges such as fragmented governance, communication barriers, resource constraints, and conflicting agendas. Addressing these challenges is crucial for dismantling silos and fostering trust among sectors, thereby enabling a cohesive and interdisciplinary approach.

Numerous opportunities exist to advance One Health initiatives, including the strengthening of disease surveillance systems, promotion of sustainable food production models, and enhancement of environmental stewardship. Additionally, interdisciplinary research and PPPs can drive transformative change, building public trust and advocacy for collaborative health initiatives.

Looking forward, the future of One Health collaboration demands visionary leadership and inclusive governance structures that prioritize multi-sectoral coordination and investment in education and capacity building. Ethical considerations must be embedded in all stages of planning and implementation to ensure that One Health initiatives are effective, equitable, and socially responsible. Embracing technological innovations will further enhance our ability to proactively address health threats and safeguard ecosystems.

Global collaboration, particularly through PPPs and international cooperation, presents a significant opportunity for cultivating resilient agricultural systems capable of adapting to evolving challenges such as climate change and environmental degradation. The One Health approach serves as a powerful framework for reimagining sustainable agriculture, urging stakeholders across disciplines to unite in cultivating a healthier, more equitable world. This collective action is not only desirable but imperative for the well-being of current and future generations.

References

1 Mwatondo, A., Rahman-Shepherd, A., Hollmann, L., et al. A global analysis of One Health networks and the proliferation of One Health collaborations. *Lancet (London, England)* 2023; 401: 605–616. https://doi.org/10.1016/S0140-6736(22)01596-3.

2 Abbas, S.S., Shorten, T., and Rushton, J. Meanings and mechanisms of One Health partnerships: insights from a critical review of literature on cross-government collaborations. *Health Policy Plan* 2022; 37: 385–399. https://doi.org/10.1093/heapol/czab134.

3 Mettenleiter, T.C., Markotter, W., Charron, D.F., et al. The One Health High-Level Expert Panel (OHHLEP). *One Health Outlook* 2023; 5: 18. https://doi.org/10.1186/s42522-023-00085-2.

4 Hassan-Kadle, A.A., Osman, A.M., Ibrahim, A.M., et al. One Health in Somalia: present status, opportunities, and challenges. *One Health* 2023; 18: 100666. https://doi.org/10.1016/j.onehlt.2023.100666.

5 Thapa, D., Canales Gómez, A.C., and Kangethe, E.K. One Health regional initiative for Eastern and Southern Africa. In: *Presented at the COHESA Workshop on Building the Capacity of Higher Educational Institutions to Educate, Train, and Empower the Next Generation Workforce to Tackle One Health Issues, Gaborone*, 22–24. Washington, DC: World Bank; 2022.

6 World Health Organization (WHO), United Nations Environment Programme, and World Organisation for Animal Health. *One Health Joint Plan of Action (2022–2026): Working Together for the Health of Humans, Animals, Plants and the Environment*. Geneva: WHO; 2022.

7 Food and Agriculture Organization (FAO) of the United Nations. *The FAO Action Plan on Antimicrobial Resistance 2021–2025: Supporting Innovation and Resilience in Food and Agriculture Sectors*. Rome: FAO; 2021.

8 World Organisation for Animal Health (OIE). *The OIE Strategy on Antimicrobial Resistance and the Prudent Use of Antimicrobials*. Paris: OIE; 2016.

9 Balajee, S.A., Arthur, R., and Mounts, A.W. Global health security: building capacities for early event detection, epidemiologic workforce, and laboratory response. *Health Secur.* 2016; 14(6): 424–432. https://doi.org/10.1089/hs.2015.0062.

10 Caceres, S.B. Global health security in an era of global health threats. *Emerg Infect. Dis.* 2011; 17: 1962. https://doi.org/10.3201/eid1710.101656.

11 Adeyemi, O.A., Agbabiaka, T.O., and Sujon, H. Global One Health post-graduate programmes: a review. *One Health Outlook* 2024; 6: 7. https://doi.org/10.1186/s42522-024-00097-6.

12 Roda, B., Bònoli, A., Sambri, V., and Careri, M. Advancements and challenges in One Health. *Class Phys. Sci.* 2024; 79: 79–98.

13 Danasekaran, R. One Health: a holistic approach to tackling global health issues. *Indian J. Community Med.* 2024; 49: 260–263. https://doi.org/10.4103/ijcm.ijcm_521_23.

14 Yopa, D.S., Massom, D.M., Kiki, G.M., et al. Barriers and enablers to the implementation of One Health strategies in developing countries: a systematic review. *Front. Public Health* 2023; 11: 1252428. https://doi.org/10.3389/fpubh.2023.1252428.

15 Prata, J.C., Ribeiro, A.I., and Rocha-Santos, T. (eds.) *One Health: Integrated Approach to 21st Century Challenges to Health*. Cambridge, MA: Academic Press; 2022.

16 Mi, E., Mi, E., and Jeggo, M. Where to now for One Health and EcoHealth? *EcoHealth* 2016; 13: 12–17. https://doi.org/10.1007/s10393-016-1112-1.

17 Marí Saéz, A., Weiss, S., Nowak, K., et al. Investigating the zoonotic origin of the West African Ebola epidemic. *EMBO Mol. Med.* 2015; 7: 17–23. https://doi.org/10.15252/emmm.201404792.

18 Lee, K. and Brumme, Z.L. Operationalizing the One Health approach: the global governance challenges. *Health Policy Plan.* 2013; 28: 778–785. https://doi.org/10.1093/heapol/czs127.

19 Queenan, K., Garnier, J., Nielsen, L.R., et al. Roadmap to a One Health agenda 2030. *CABI Rev.* 2017; 2017: 1–17. https://doi.org/10.1079/PAVSNNR201712014.

20 Spicer, N., Agyepong, I., Ottersen, T., et al. 'It's far too complicated': why fragmentation persists in global health. *Glob. Health* 2020; 16: 60. https://doi.org/10.1186/s12992-020-00592-1.

21 Lal, A., Erondu, N.A., Heymann, D.L., et al. Fragmented health systems in COVID-19: rectifying the misalignment between global health security and universal health coverage. *Lancet* 2021; 397: 61–67. https://doi.org/10.1016/S0140-6736(20)32228-5.

22 Barr, A., Garrett, L., Marten, R., and Kadandale, S. Health sector fragmentation: three examples from Sierra Leone. *Glob. Health* 2019; 15: 1–8. https://doi.org/10.1186/s12992-018-0447-5.

23 Opitz, S. Regulating epidemic space: the *nomos* of global circulation. *J. Int. Relat. Dev.* 2016; 19: 263–284. https://doi.org/10.1057/jird.2014.30.

24 Gostin, L.O., Friedman, E.A., and Finch, A. The global health architecture: governance and international institutions to advance population health worldwide. *Milbank Q.* 2023; 101(Suppl 1): 734–769. https://doi.org/10.1111/1468-0009.12627.

25 Elnaiem, A., Mohamed-Ahmed, O., Zumla, A., et al. Global and regional governance of One Health and implications for global health security. *Lancet* 2023; 401: 688–704. https://doi.org/10.1016/S0140-6736(22)01597-5.

26 Mwacalimba, K.K. and Green, J. 'One health' and development priorities in resource-constrained countries: policy lessons from avian and pandemic influenza preparedness in Zambia. *Health Policy Plan.* 2015; 30: 215–222. https://doi.org/10.1093/heapol/czu001.

27 Cleaveland, S., Sharp, J., Abela-Ridder, B., et al. One Health contributions towards more effective and equitable approaches to health in low- and middle-income countries. *Philos. Trans. R. Soc. Lond. B Biol. Sci.* 2017; 372: 20160168. https://doi.org/10.1098/rstb.2016.0168.

28 Denis-Robichaud, J., Hindmarch, S., Nswal, N.N., et al. One Health communication channels: a qualitative case study of swine influenza in Canada in 2020. *BMC Public Health* 2024; 24: 964. https://doi.org/10.1186/s12889-024-18460-7.

29 Valeix, S., Stein, C., and Bardosh, K. Knowledge flows in one health: the evolution of scientific collaboration networks. In: *One Health*, 38–57. London: Routledge; 2016.

30 Bauder, L., Giangobbe, K., and Asgary, R. Barriers and gaps in effective health communication at both public health and healthcare delivery levels during epidemics and pandemics; systematic review. *Disaster Med. Public. Health Prep.* 2023; 17: e395. https://doi.org/10.1017/dmp.2023.61.

31 Gilbert, W., Thomas, L.F., Coyne, L., and Rushton, J. Review: mitigating the risks posed by intensification in livestock production: the examples of antimicrobial resistance and zoonoses. *Animal* 2021; 15(2): 100123. https://doi.org/10.1016/j.animal.2020.100123.

32 Ribeiro, C., Burgwal, L., and Regeer, B. Overcoming challenges for designing and implementing the One Health approach: a systematic review of the literature. *One Health* 2019; 7: 100085. https://doi.org/10.1016/j.onehlt.2019.100085.

33 Spencer, J., McRobie, E., Dar, O., et al. Is the current surge in political and financial attention to One Health solidifying or splintering the movement? *BMJ Glob. Health* 2019; 4: e001102.

34 Abuhammad, S. Preparing for future pandemics: challenges for healthcare leadership. *J. Healthc. Leadersh.* 2022; 14: 131–136. https://doi.org/10.2147/JHL.S363650#d1e123.

35 Amelung, V., Chase, D., and Reichert, A. Leadership in integrated care. In: *Handbook of Integrated Care* (ed. V. Amelung, V. Stein, N. Goodwin, R. Balicer, E. Nolte, and E. Suter), 221–236. Cham: Springer International Publishing AG; 2017. https://doi.org/10.1007/978-3-319-56103-5_14.

36 Klinga, C., Hansson, J., Hasson, H., and Sachs, M. Co-Leadership – a management solution for integrated health and social care. *Int. J. Integr. Care* 2016; 16: 2236. https://doi.org/10.5334/ijic.2236.

37 Zorn, C.K., Pascual, J.M., Bosch, W., et al. Addressing the challenge of COVID-19: One Health care site's leadership response to the pandemic. *Mayo Clin. Proc. Innov. Qual. Outcomes* 2021; 5(1): 151–160. https://doi.org/10.1016/j.mayocpiqo.2020.11.001.

38 Zinsstag, J., Schelling, E., Crump, L., et al. (eds.) *One Health: The Theory and Practice of Integrated Health Approaches*. Wallingford, UK: CABI; 2021. https://doi.org/10.1079/9781789242577.0000.

39 O'Brien, M.K., Wuebbolt Macy, K., Pelican, K., et al. Transforming the One Health workforce: lessons learned from initiatives in Africa, Asia and Latin America. *Rev. Sci. Tech.* 2019; 38(1): 239–250. https://doi.org/10.20506/rst.38.1.2956.

40 Subramanian, M. Zoonotic disease risk and the bushmeat trade: assessing awareness among hunters and traders in Sierra Leone. *Ecohealth* 2012; 9(4): 471–482. https://doi.org/10.1007/s10393-012-0807-1.

41 McCoy, D., Kapilashrami, A., Kumar, R., et al. Developing an agenda for the decolonization of global health. *Bull. World Health Organ.* 2024; 102(2): 130–136. https://doi.org/10.2471/BLT.23.289949.

42 Ribeiro, C.D.S., van Roode, M.Y., Haringhuizen, G.B., et al. How ownership rights over microorganisms affect infectious disease control and innovation: a root-cause analysis of barriers to data sharing as experienced by key stakeholders. *PLoS One* 2018; 13(5): e0195885. https://doi.org/10.1371/journal.pone.0195885.

43 Redman-White, C.J., Loosli, K., Qarkaxhija, V., et al. A digital One Health framework to integrate data for public health decision-making. *IJID One Health* 2023; 1: 100012. https://doi.org/10.1016/j.ijidoh.2023.100012.

44 Ho, C. Operationalizing "One Health" as "One Digital Health" through a global framework that emphasizes fair and equitable sharing of benefits from the use of artificial intelligence and related digital technologies. *Front. Public Health* 2022; 10: 768977. https://doi.org/10.3389/fpubh.2022.768977.

45 Bentzen, H., Castro, R., Fears, R., et al. Remove obstacles to sharing health data with researchers outside of the European Union. *Nat. Med.* 2021; 27: 1329–1333. https://doi.org/10.1038/s41591-021-01460-0.

46 Alrahbi, D., Khan, M., Gupta, S., et al. Challenges for developing health-care knowledge in the digital age. *J. Knowl. Manag.* 2020; 26: 824–853. https://doi.org/10.1108/JKM-03-2020-0224.

47 Mahajan, S., Khan, Z., Giri, P.P., et al. Operationalising 'One Health' through primary healthcare approach. *Prev. Med. Res. Rev.* 2024; 1(4): 199–206. https://doi.org/10.4103/PMRR.PMRR_8_24.

48 Buregyeya, E., Atusingwize, E., Nsamba, P., et al. Operationalizing the One Health approach in Uganda: challenges and opportunities. *J. Epidemiol. Glob. Health* 2020; 10(4): 250–257. https://doi.org/10.2991/jegh.k.200825.001.

49 Rubin, C., Dunham, B., and Sleeman, J. Making One Health a reality—crossing bureaucratic boundaries. In: *One Health: People, Animals, and the Environment*, 269–283. 2014. https://doi.org/10.1128/9781555818432.ch18.

50 Conrad, P.A., Meek, L.A., and Dumit, J. Operationalizing a One Health approach to global health challenges. *Comp. Immunol. Microbiol. Infect. Dis.* 2013; 36(3): 211–216. https://doi.org/10.1016/j.cimid.2013.03.006.

51 Gruel, G., Diouf, M.B., Abadie, C., et al. Critical evaluation of cross-sectoral collaborations to inform the implementation of the "One Health" approach in Guadeloupe. *Front. Public Health* 2021; 9: 652079. https://doi.org/10.3389/fpubh.2021.652079.

52 Gray, G.C. and Mazet, J.A. To succeed, one health must win animal agriculture's stronger collaboration. *Clin. Infect. Dis.* 2020; 70(3): 535–537. https://doi.org/10.1093/cid/ciz729.

53 Johnson, I., Hansen, A., Bi, P., et al. The challenges of implementing an integrated One Health surveillance system in Australia. *Zoonoses Public Health* 2018; 65(1): 229–236. https://doi.org/10.1111/zph.12433.

54 Suryawanshi, S.J., Jain, S., Sharma, R.K., et al. Current veterinary regulations and way ahead. *Res. Vet. Sci.* 2024; 166: 105101. https://doi.org/10.1016/j.rvsc.2023.105101.

55 Ghai, S. and Hemachudha, T. Continued failure of rabies elimination—consideration of challenges in applying the one health approach. *Front. Vet. Sci.* 2022; 9: 847659. https://doi.org/10.3389/fvets.2022.847659.

56 Nienaber McKay, A.G., Brand, D., Botes, M., et al. The regulation of health data sharing in Africa: a comparative study. *J. Law. Biosci.* 2024; 11(1): lsad035. https://doi.org/10.1093/jlb/lsad035.

57 Uchtmann, N., Herrmann, J.A., Hahn, E.C., et al. Barriers to, efforts in, and optimization of integrated One Health surveillance: a review and synthesis. *EcoHealth* 2015; 12: 368–384. https://doi.org/10.1007/s10393-015-1022-7.

58 Sharan, M., Vijay, D., Yadav, J.P., et al. Surveillance and response strategies for zoonotic diseases: a comprehensive review. *Sci. One Health* 2023; 2: 100050. https://doi.org/10.1016/j.soh.2023.100050.

59 Zhou, X., Bergquist, R., and Tanner, M. Elimination of tropical disease through surveillance and response. *Infect. Dis. Poverty* 2013; 2: 1. https://doi.org/10.1186/2049-9957-2-1.

60 Singh, S., Sharma, P., Pal, N., et al. Holistic One Health surveillance framework: synergizing environmental, animal, and human determinants for enhanced infectious disease management. *ACS Infect. Dis.* 2024; 10(3): 808–826. https://doi.org/10.1021/acsinfecdis.3c00625.

61 Bordier, M., Goutard, F., Antoine-Moussiaux, N., et al. Engaging stakeholders in the design of One Health surveillance systems: a participatory approach. *Front. Vet. Sci.* 2021; 8. https://doi.org/10.3389/fvets.2021.646458.

62 Pradyumna, A., Egal, F., and Utzinger, J. Sustainable food systems, health and infectious diseases: concerns and opportunities. *Acta Tropica* 2019; 191: 172–177. https://doi.org/10.1016/j.actatropica.2018.12.042.

63 Nitzan, D., Andreuzza, B., and Chattopadhyay, D. The food systems, One Health, and resilience (FOR) approach-led by the FOR-runners. *Sustainability* 2023; 15(18): 13889. https://doi.org/10.3390/su151813889.

64 Frison, E. and Clément, C. The potential of diversified agroecological systems to deliver healthy outcomes: making the link between agriculture, food systems & health. *Food Policy* 2020; 96: 101851. https://doi.org/10.1016/j.foodpol.2020.101851.

65 Berkes, F. Making Connections: Leopold's land health, indigenous ways of knowing, social-ecological resilience, and One Health. *CABI One Health* 2023; ohcs20230008. https://doi.org/10.1079/cabionehealth.2023.0008.

66 Keesing, F. and Ostfeld, R.S. Impacts of biodiversity and biodiversity loss on zoonotic diseases. *Proc. Natl. Acad. Sci. U. S. A.* 2021; 118(17): e2023540118. https://doi.org/10.1073/pnas.2023540118.

67 Berniak-Woźny, J. and Rataj, M. Towards green and sustainable healthcare: a literature review and research Agenda for green leadership in the healthcare sector. *Int. J. Environ. Res. Public Health* 2023; 20(2): 908. https://doi.org/10.3390/ijerph20020908.

68 Poland, B. and Dooris, M. A green and healthy future: the settings approach to building health, equity and sustainability. *Crit. Public Health* 2010; 20: 281–298. https://doi.org/10.1080/09581596.2010.502931.

69 Krammer, F. SARS-CoV-2 vaccines in development. *Nature* 2020; 586(7830): 516–527. https://doi.org/10.1038/s41586-020-2798-3.

70 McEwen, S.A. and Collignon, P.J. Antimicrobial resistance: a One Health perspective. *Microbiol. Spectr.* 2018; 6(2). https://doi.org/10.1128/microbiolspec.ARBA-0009-2017.

71 Destoumieux-Garzón, D., Mavingui, P., Boetsch, G., et al. The One Health concept: 10 years old and a long road ahead. *Front. Vet. Sci.* 2018; 5: 14. https://doi.org/10.3389/fvets.2018.00014.

72 Singh, S. and Jha, S.K. One Health: a long road ahead. *Int. J. Community Med. Public Health* 2023; 10: 2657–2660.

73 Pelletier, J., Guillot, C., Rocheleau, J.P., et al. The added value of One Health surveillance: data from questing ticks can provide an early signal for anaplasmosis outbreaks in animals and humans. *Can J. Public Health* 2023; 114(2): 317–324. https://doi.org/10.17269/s41997-022-00723-8.

74 Panel, O.H.H.L.E., Hayman, D.T., Adisasmito, W.B., et al. Developing One Health surveillance systems. *One Health* 2023; 17: 100617. https://doi.org/10.1016/j.onehlt.2023.100617.

75 Shaheen, M.N. The concept of One Health applied to the problem of zoonotic diseases. *Rev. Med. Virol.* 2022; 32(4): e2326. https://doi.org/10.1002/rmv.2326.

76 Ghai, R.R., Wallace, R.M., Kile, J.C., et al. A generalizable One Health framework for the control of zoonotic diseases. *Sci. Rep.* 2022; 12(1): 8588. https://doi.org/10.1038/s41598-022-12619-1.

77 Atlas, R.M. and Maloy, S. The future of One Health. *Microbiol. Spectr.* 2014; 2(1): 10–1128. https://doi.org/10.1128/microbiolspec.oh-0018-2012.

78 Humboldt-Dachroeden, S. Lessons learned from One Health practices in Sweden and Italy. *Eur. J. Public Health* 2021; 31(3): ckab165. https://doi.org/10.1093/eurpub/ckab165.

79 Berrian, A.M., Wilkes, M., Gilardi, K., et al. Developing a global One Health workforce: the "Rx One Health Summer Institute" approach. *EcoHealth* 2020; 17: 222–232. https://doi.org/10.1007/s10393-020-01481-0.

80 Robbiati, C., Milano, A., Declich, S., et al. Building a European One Health workforce for prevention and preparedness to health threats. *Eur. J. Public Health* 2023; 33(2): ckad160-213. https://doi.org/10.1093/eurpub/ckad160.213.

81 Ruckert, A., Harris, F., Aenishaenslin, C., et al. One Health governance principles for AMR surveillance: a scoping review and conceptual framework. *Res. Dir. One Health* 2024; 2: e4. https://doi.org/10.1017/one.2023.13.

82 Stephen, C. and Stemshorn, B. Leadership, governance and partnerships are essential One Health competencies. *One Health* 2016; 2: 161–163. https://doi.org/10.1016/j.onehlt.2016.10.002.

83 Hitziger, M., Esposito, R., Canali, M., et al. Knowledge integration in One Health policy formulation, implementation, and evaluation. *Bull. World Health Organ.* 2018; 96: 211–218. https://doi.org/10.2471/BLT.17.202705.

84 Such, E., Smith, K., Woods, H., et al. Governance of intersectoral collaborations for population health and to reduce health inequalities in high-income countries: a complexity-informed systematic review. *Int. J. Health Policy Manag.* 2022; 11: 2780–2792. https://doi.org/10.34172/ijhpm.2022.6550.

85 Taaffe, J., Sharma, R., Parthiban, A.B.R., et al. One Health activities to reinforce intersectoral coordination at local levels in India. *Front. Public Health* 2023; 11: 1041447. https://doi.org/10.3389/fpubh.2023.1041447.

86 Alimi, Y. and Wabacha, J. Strengthening coordination and collaboration of One Health approach for zoonotic diseases in Africa. *One Health Outlook* 2023; 5(1): 10. https://doi.org/10.1186/s42522-023-00082-5.

87 Vesterinen, H., Dutcher, T., Errecaborde, K., et al. Strengthening multi-sectoral collaboration on critical health issues: One Health systems mapping and analysis resource toolkit (OH-SMART) for operationalizing One Health. *PLoS ONE* 2019; 14. https://doi.org/10.1371/journal.pone.0219197.

88 Benis, A., Tamburis, O., Chronaki, C. and Moen, A. One digital health: a unified framework for future health ecosystems. *J. Med. Internet Res.* 2021; 23. https://doi.org/10.2196/22189.

89 Andoh, K., Hidano, A., Sakamoto, Y., et al. Current research and future directions for realizing the ideal One-Health approach: a summary of key-informant interviews in Japan and a literature review. *One Health* 2023; 16: 100468. https://doi.org/10.1016/j.onehlt.2022.100468.

90 Johnson, M.S. and Adams, V.H. Integrating "One Health" concepts in the design of sustainable systems for environmental use. *Toxics* 2023; 11(3): 280. https://doi.org/10.3390/toxics11030280.

91 Humboldt-Dachroeden, S., Rubin, O., and Sylvester Frid-Nielsen, S. The state of One Health research across disciplines and sectors – a bibliometric analysis. *One Health* 2020; 10: 100146. https://doi.org/10.1016/j.onehlt.2020.100146.

92 Smye, S. and Frangi, A. Interdisciplinary research: shaping the healthcare of the future. *Future Healthc. J.* 2021; 8: e218–e223. https://doi.org/10.7861/fhj.2021-0025.

93 Barnett, T., Pfeiffer, D., Hoque, M., et al. Practising co-production and interdisciplinarity: challenges and implications for One Health research. *Prev. Vet. Med.* 2020; 177. https://doi.org/10.1016/j.prevetmed.2020.104949.

94 Wees, S., Målqvist, M., and Irwin, R. Achieving the SDGs through interdisciplinary research in global health. *Scand J. Public Health* 2018; 47: 793–795. https://doi.org/10.1177/1403494818812637.

95 Dokter, C., Nassiri, R., and Trosko, J. One Health. In: *University Partnerships for International Development. Innovations in Higher Education Teaching and Learning* vol. 8, 207–227; 2018. https://doi.org/10.1108/S2055-364120160000008027.

96 Maurrasse, D. *Strategic Public-Private Partnerships: Innovation and Development.* Edward Elgar Publishing; 2013.

97 Campos, K., Norman, C., and Jadad, A. Product development public-private partnerships for public health: a systematic review using qualitative data. *Soc. Sci. Med.* 2011; 73(7): 986–94. https://doi.org/10.1016/j.socscimed.2011.06.059.

98 Hobusch, U., Scheuch, M., Heuckmann, B., et al. One Health education nexus: enhancing synergy among science-, school-, and teacher education beyond academic silos. *Front. Public Health* 2024; 11: 1337748. https://doi.org/10.3389/fpubh.2023.1337748.

99 Wilkes, M.S., Conrad, P.A., and Winer, J.N. One Health-one education: medical and veterinary inter-professional training. *J. Vet. Med. Educ.* 2019; 46(1): 14–20. https://doi.org/10.3138/jvme.1116-171r.

100 Beever, J. and Morar, N. The epistemic and ethical onus of 'One Health'. *Wiley-Blackwell: Bioethics;* 2018. https://doi.org/10.1111/bioe.12522.

101 LeBlanc, A., Williams-Jones, B., and Aenishaenslin, C. Bio-ethics and One Health: a case study approach to building reflexive governance. *Front. Public Health* 2022; 10. https://doi.org/10.3389/fpubh.2022.648593.

102 Lindenmayer, J., Kaufman, G., Baker, L., et al. One Health ethics: "What Then Must We Do?" *CABI One Health* 2022. https://doi.org/10.1079/cabionehealth.2022.0011.

103 Lukas, S., Crowe, S.J., Law, M., et al. An ethics-based approach to global health research Part 2: strategies for overcoming logistic and implementation challenges. *Res. Social Adm. Pharm.* 2020; 16(11): 1580–1587. https://doi.org/10.1016/j.sapharm.2020.07.010.

104 Rock, M. and Degeling, C. Public health ethics and more-than-human solidarity. *Soc. Sci. Med.* 2015; 129: 61–67. https://doi.org/10.1016/j.socscimed.2014.05.050.

105 Bordier, M., Delavenne, C., Nguyen, D.T.T., et al. One Health surveillance: a matrix to evaluate multisectoral collaboration. *Front. Vet. Sci.* 2019; 6: 109. https://doi.org/10.3389/fvets.2019.00109.

106 Bartlett, M.L. and Uhart, M. Leveraging One Health as a sentinel approach for pandemic resilience. *Virol. J.* 2024; 21(1): 269. https://doi.org/10.1186/s12985-024-02545-1.

107 Colpaert, A. Satellite and UAV platforms, remote sensing for geographic information systems. *Sensors (Basel, Switzerland)* 2022; 22(12): 4564. https://doi.org/10.3390/s22124564.

108 Faruque, F.S. Remote sensing and geospatial technologies in public health. *ISPRS Int. J. Geo-Inf.* 2018; 7(8): 303. https://doi.org/10.3390/ijgi7080303.

109 Cingoli, G. and Rinaldi, L. Geographical information systems in buffalo health applications. *Ital. J. Anim. Sci.* 2007; 6(2): 217–222. https://doi.org/10.4081/ijas.2007.s2.217.

110 Alanezi, M.A., Shahriar, M.S., Hasan, M.B., et al. Livestock management with unmanned aerial vehicles: a review. *IEEE Access* 2022; 10: 45001–45028. https://doi.org/10.1109/ACCESS.2022.3168295.

111 Urban, L., Perlas, A., Francino, O., et al. Real-time genomics for One Health. *Mol. Syst. Biol.* 2023; 19(8): e11686. https://doi.org/10.15252/msb.202311686.

112 Džermeikaitė, K., Bačėninaitė, D., and Antanaitis, R. Innovations in cattle farming: application of innovative technologies and sensors in the diagnosis of diseases. *Animals* 2023; 13(5): 780. https://doi.org/10.3390/ani13050780.

113 Sankoh, O. Global health estimates: stronger collaboration needed with low-and middle-income countries. *PLoS Med.* 2010; 7(11): e1001005. https://doi.org/10.1371/journal.pmed.1001005.

114 Rasanathan, K., Bennett, S., Atkins, V., et al. Governing multisectoral action for health in low-and middle-income countries. *PLoS Med.* 2017; 14(4): e1002285. https://doi.org/10.1371/journal.pmed.1002285.

115 Machalaba, C.C., Salerno, R.H., Barton Behravesh, C., et al. Institutionalizing One Health: from assessment to action. *Health Secur.* 2018; 16(S1): S–37. https://doi.org/10.1089/hs.2018.0064.

116 Henley, P., Igihozo, G., and Wotton, L. One Health approaches require community engagement, education, and international collaborations—a lesson from Rwanda. *Nat. Med.* 2021; 27(6): 947–948. https://doi.org/10.1038/s41591-021-01350-5.

117 de la Rocque, S., Errecaborde, K.M.M., Belot, G., et al. One health systems strengthening in countries: tripartite tools and approaches at the human-animal-environment interface. *BMJ Glob. Health* 2023; 8(1): e011236.

118 Jesudason, T. A One Health priority research agenda for AMR. *Lancet Microbe* 2023; 4(10): e769.

119 Fanning, J.P., Murthy, S., Obonyo, N.G., et al. Global infectious disease research collaborations in crises: building capacity and inclusivity through cooperation. *Glob. Health* 2021; 17: 1–6. https://doi.org/10.1186/s12992-021-00731-2.

120 Zhang, X.X., Lederman, Z., Han, L.F., et al. Towards an actionable One Health approach. *Infect Dis. Poverty* 2024; 13(1): 28. https://doi.org/10.1186/s40249-024-01198-0.

121 Mumford, E.L., Martinez, D.J., Tyance-Hassell, K., et al. Evolution and expansion of the One Health approach to promote sustainable and resilient health and well-being: a call to action. *Front. Public Health* 2023; 10: 1056459. https://doi.org/10.3389/fpubh.2022.1056459.

122 Atkins, S., Marsden, S., Diwan, V., et al. North–South collaboration and capacity development in global health research in low-and middle-income countries–the ARCADE projects. *Glob. Health Action* 2016; 9(1): 30524. https://doi.org/10.3402/gha.v9.30524.

123 Cash-Gibson, L., Guerra, G., and Salgado-de-Snyder, V.N. SDH-NET: a South–North-South collaboration to build sustainable research capacities on social determinants of health in low-and middle-income countries. *Health Res. Policy Syst.* 2015; 13: 1–9. https://doi.org/10.1186/s12961-015-0048-1.

124 McNeil, C., Verlander, S., Divi, N., and Smolinski, M. The landscape of participatory surveillance systems across the One Health spectrum: systematic review. *JMIR Public Health Surveill.* 2022; 8(8): e38551. https://doi.org/10.2196/38551.

125 Castello, L. Filling global gaps in monitoring data with local knowledge. *Aquatic Conserv.* 2023; 33(5). https://doi.org/10.5334/cstp.665.

126 Jansen, M., Beukes, M., Weiland, C., et al. Engaging citizen scientists in biodiversity monitoring: insights from the WildLIVE! project. *Citizen Sci. Theory Prac.* 2024; 9(1). https://doi.org/10.5334/cstp.665.

127 El Bizri, H.R., Fa, J.E., Lemos, L.P., et al. Involving local communities for effective citizen science: determining game species' reproductive status to assess hunting effects in tropical forests. *J. Appl. Ecol.* 2021; 58(2): 224–235.

128 Chandler, M., Bebber, D.P., Castro, S., et al. International citizen science: making the local global. *Front. Ecol. Environ.* 2012; 10(6): 328–331. https://doi.org/10.1111/1365-2664.13633.

129 Dykstra, M.P. and Baitchman, E.J. A call for one health in medical education: how the COVID-19 pandemic underscores the need to integrate human, animal, and environmental health. *Acad. Med.* 2021; 96(7): 951–953. https://doi.org/10.1097/ACM.0000000000004072.

130 Capua, I. and Cattoli, G. One Health (r) evolution: learning from the past to build a new future. *Viruses* 2018; 10(12): 725. https://doi.org/10.3390/v10120725.

131 Adisasmito, W.B., Almuhairi, S., Behravesh, C.B., et al. One Health: a new definition for a sustainable and healthy future. *PLoS Pathog.* 2022; 18(6): e1010537. https://doi.org/10.1371/journal.ppat.1010537.

132 Faijue, D.D., Segui, A.O., Shringarpure, K., et al. Constructing a One Health governance architecture: a systematic review and analysis of governance mechanisms for One Health. *Eur. J. Public Health* 2024; 34(6): 1086–1094. https://doi.org/10.1093/eurpub/ckae124.

133 Bertram, M.G., Costi, M.P., Thoré, E.S., et al. One Health. *Curr. Biol. Mag.* 2024: 34(11): R517–R519.

134 Pepin, K.M., Carlisle, K., Anderson, D., et al. Steps towards operationalizing One Health approaches. *One Health* 2024; 18: 100740. https://doi.org/10.1016/j.onehlt.2024.100740.

135 Redford, K.H., da Fonseca, G.A., Gascon, C., et al. Healthy planet healthy people. *Conserv. Lett.* 2022; 15(3): e12864. https://doi.org/10.1111/conl.12864.

136 Barrett, M.A., Bouley, T.A., Stoertz, A.H., and Stoertz, R.W. Integrating a One Health approach in education to address global health and sustainability challenges. *Front. Ecol. Environ.* 2011; 9(4): 239–245. https://doi.org/10.1890/090159.

137 Rabinowitz, P.M., Pappaioanou, M., Bardosh, K.L., and Conti, L. A planetary vision for One Health. *BMJ Global Health* 2018; 3(5): e001137.

138 Mi, E., Mi, E., and Jeggo, M. Where to now for One Health and EcoHealth? *EcoHealth* 2016; 13(1): 12–17. https://doi.org/10.1007/s10393-016-1112-1.

11

Interactive Learning and Practical Applications of One Health

Vivek Harishankar Shukla[1,2*], *Pintu Choudhary*[3] *and Pratik Subhash Gaikwad*[4*]

[1] *Department of Livestock Products Technology, Mumbai Veterinary College, Parel, Mumbai, Maharashtra, India*
[2] *Maharashtra Animal and Fishery Sciences University, Nagpur, Maharashtra, India*
[3] *Department of Food Technology, College of Agricultural Engineering and Technology, Dr Rajendra Prasad Central Agricultural University, Samastipur, Bihar, India*
[4] *School of Biotechnology and Bioinformatics, D Y Patil Deemed to Be University, Navi Mumbai, Maharashtra, India*

*Corresponding authors: vivekshukla@mafsu.ac.in; pratik.gaikwad@dypatil.edu

TABLE OF CONTENTS

11.1 Introduction
11.2 One Health: A Holistic Approach to Learning and Interconnectivity
11.2.1 Importance of Interdisciplinary Education
11.3 Innovative Teaching Methodologies
11.3.1 Problem-based Learning
11.3.2 Simulations
11.3.3 Field-based Experiences
11.4 Case Studies in One Health
11.4.1 Real-world Applications
11.4.2 Success Stories and Lessons Learned
11.4.2.1 Investigating Salmonella and Wild Songbirds
11.4.2.2 Antimicrobial Resistance in Animals and Humans
11.4.2.3 Poisoning and Death in Sea Otters
11.4.2.4 Reduction in Cases of Rocky Mountain Spotted Fever
11.4.2.5 Namibia's Battle Against Rabies
11.4.2.6 Control of Crimean Congo Hemorrhagic Fever in Kazakhstan
11.4.2.7 Control of Rift Valley Virus Fever in East Africa
11.5 Challenges in One Health Education
11.5.1 Curriculum Integration
11.5.2 Resource Limitations
11.5.3 Interdisciplinary Collaboration
11.6 Opportunities for Enhancing One Health Learning
11.7 Conclusion
References

One Health Integration: Global Perspectives on Animal Health and Sustainable Agriculture. First Edition.
Edited by Pratik Subhash Gaikwad, Vivek Harishankar Shukla and Pintu Choudhary.

Companion Website: https://www.wiley.com/go/pratikgaikwad/onehealth

11.1 Introduction

In our increasingly interconnected world, the well-being of humans, animals, and ecosystems is interdependent, necessitating a unified and comprehensive educational strategy. The One Health framework promotes collaborative efforts across various disciplines to tackle pressing global challenges such as zoonotic diseases, antibiotic resistance, and environmental decline.

This chapter examines the pivotal role that experiential and interdisciplinary education plays in promoting the One Health initiative. Innovative methods like problem-based learning (PBL), simulations, and fieldwork foster critical thinking, engagement, and practical application of knowledge. Through diverse case studies, the chapter demonstrates how these engaging methods not only improve learners' competencies but also exemplify the effective application of One Health principles in real-world situations.

Additionally, the chapter highlights significant obstacles to integrating One Health concepts into educational programs, such as limited resources and the necessity for enhanced interdisciplinary collaboration. By pinpointing areas for enhancement, it aims to create a more inclusive and efficient framework that prepares professionals to tackle the dynamic health challenges of the twenty-first century.

11.2 One Health: A Holistic Approach to Learning and Interconnectivity

As per US Centers for Disease Control and Prevention, One Health is a collaborative, multispectral, and transdisciplinary approach working at the local, regional, national, and global levels with the goal of achieving optimal health outcomes recognizing the interconnection between people, animals, plants, and their shared environment [1]. The concept emphasizes on close connection of human health with animal health and shared environment. This is important as the interactions between the three components have changed significantly during the recent past and they have come closer to each other due to many factors. Health, environmental, and agricultural practices are conflicting one another, producing ever growing new challenges that have never been seen [2].

The idea of connections between humans and animals is not new but it has been identified since ancient times [3] and is a well-known concept from Greek era to modern time [4–6]. Hippocrates mentioned that changes in the environment, that is, air, water, and place affect the bodily changes, which could be responsible for epidemics [7], thus strengthening the believe that One Health in not a new concept but our ancestors had good knowledge One Health. Further, Edward Jenner in 1796 showed that cowpox infection in humans could protect them from smallpox, thus establishing the similarity between the human and animal medicine. Further, investigations during 1830s suggested that diseases such as glanders, rabies, and anthrax are similar in animals and humans, suggesting that concept of One Health has been followed since ancient times. During 1821–1902, Dr. Rudolf Virchow found linkages between human and veterinary medicine while studying a roundworm, *Trichinella spiralis*, in swine. Further, he coined the term "Zoonosis" to indicate the infections which can pass between humans and animals [1].

However, the transboundary separation and interactions of humans and animals has become meagre due to development of advance transportation facilities, facilitating the movement of humans and goods [8]. Similarly, the population explosion has compelled the human population to live in close connection with wild animals frequently coming in close contact with each other which makes them prone to transmit the diseases to one another [9]. The international trade and travel have facilitated the easy transmission of causative agents, thus quickly spreading the diseases from one place to other remote places [10]. All these circumstances have led to the frequent transmission of endemic diseases as well as new and emerging diseases. The occurrence of COVID-19 in the recent past has further sensitized the scientific fraternity to focus on such interactions and tackle them through One Health approach.

The major advancement in the One Health approach is possible through advancement and modifications in the One Health education. The advancement in the field of One Health Education requires novel innovative methods and interdisciplinary learning to equip the students to tackle the complex health challenges [11]. Teaching methods such as PBL, team-based learning, and workshops involving interdisciplinary and multidisciplinary approach could be an important approach in understanding and inculcating the concept of One Health. An integrated health approach is important in the era of globalization, where the movement of people and goods have facilitated the transmission of deadly zoonotic diseases. The important policy decisions could be taken based on effective understanding of these complex interconnections. Therefore, it is important to develop interactive learning about One Health approach to develop a concrete framework about such future challenges.

11.2.1 Importance of Interdisciplinary Education

The interdisciplinary education comprising different areas of the One Health is important to bring an effective outcome for fighting against the challenges arising under one health concept. As shown in Figure 11.1, the diagram illustrates the interconnectedness of disciplines like human health, veterinary science, and environmental studies, which is crucial to providing a holistic approach to One Health education.

The interdisciplinary education related to different facets of One Health shall inculcate the multidisciplinary knowledge not covered in a single discipline. As One Health deals with the uncertainty and complexity of issues that intersect the human–animal–environmental interface, incorporating data, knowledge, and skills from a range of disciplines, it is important to have the interdisciplinary approach to tackle the issues related with One Health approach. Interdisciplinary education could be used to control challenges other than one's own disciplines related to One Health principles. The importance of One Health is well recognized by international organizations such as World Health Organization [12–14], World Organisation for Animal Health (OIE) [15], Food and Agriculture Organization [16], World Bank [17, 18], and United Nations Biodiversity Convention [19] and all of them recommend for multidisciplinary collaboration to work under the One Health approach to prevent and control the conditions under One Health umbrella. The OIE was the pioneer organization which advocated the incorporation of interdisciplinary education with veterinary education [20]. The effective implementation of One Health approach and practice should have a blend and close collaboration of veterinarians, medical professionals, and environmental activists.

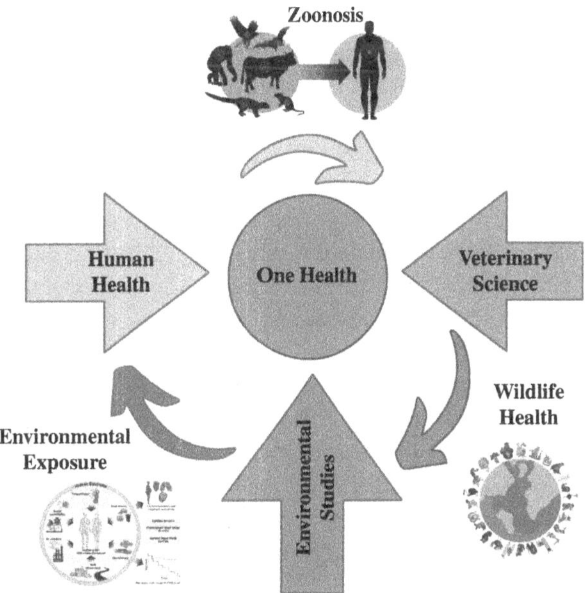

Figure 11.1 The interdisciplinary nature of One Health education.

One Health practice cannot contain a narrow spectrum of health-related medical problems; rather its purview can be elongated to local and global socio-ecological changes which affect the human health and difficult to predict [21]. Thus, there is a requirement of interdisciplinary collaboration which can provide practical solutions to the One health relevant problems such as environmental changes, demographic changes, migration, etc. At this juncture, there should be close connection between academicians with other important stakeholders such social activist, environmental activist, veterinarians, etc. to provide the practical solutions. Interdisciplinary education should be at the core of One Health practices for the improved health of humans, animals, and the environment. For effective execution of policies in these areas, medical practitioners and veterinarians must have a thorough knowledge of the humans, animals, and environmental ecosystem in which they live as well as the social, political, legal, and cultural environments in which they work [22, 23]. Even social science is one of the important aspects to control One Health problems, as various health challenges such as zoonotic infectious diseases, environmental pollution, development of antimicrobial resistance, food system challenges, malnutrition, etc. arise from interwoven spheres of humans, animals, and their ecosystem [24]. Such complex problems require interdisciplinary approach, which is the basic concept of One Health.

The interdisciplinary education shall bring the stakeholders from different disciplines to a common platform, which will enhance the interconnectedness of human, animal, and environmental health [25]. It will also open the avenues for diverse networking opportunities which shall be helpful in tackling the relevant One Health problems.

11.3 Innovative Teaching Methodologies

Innovative teaching is that teaching where teaching methods differ from the conventional patterns of knowledge-transfer teaching and teacher-centered teaching rather than solving problems in novel ways using new technologies and while guiding learners to participate in learning process and improve their creativity [26]. The innovative teaching methodologies are different from standard chalk and talk methods. They utilize creative and efficient behavior and performance that teachers use in selecting teaching materials, techniques, and evaluation methods for enhancing and developing learner creativity. The innovative teaching includes different components such as innovative teaching ideation, innovative teaching action, and innovative teaching outcome [27]. The teacher plays the most important role in teaching–learning situations, such as encouraging, supporting, and facilitating learners in discovering their talents, realizing their physical and intellectual potential, and developing characters and desirable social and human values, and functions and this becomes more easier with innovative teaching methods. The innovative teaching may include incorporation of new techniques, new concepts, and new methods of assessment [28].

The integration of technology and novel strategies in education incorporates the use of digital tools to broaden the learning areas, improved instructional design and guidance by the teachers, and creative problem-solving using digital methods [29, 30]. This integration enhances teaching and learning both within and outside the classroom. Figure 11.2 illustrates the framework of various innovative teaching methodologies employed in One Health education, showcasing their relationships and applications.

Additionally, innovative tools are associated with self-driven teaching and learning strategies and have the potential to transform educational practices [29, 31]. Since, One Health approach strives for optimal health based on the relations between the environment, people, and animals, and involves multisector and transdisciplinary collaborations [32]. Many studies have stated that the use of systems thinking approaches is important for One Health practice [33–36]. There is a growing need to inculcate One Health across different disciplines, and the use of innovative teaching methods could provide educators with tools to meet the needs of students. Few innovative teaching methods which are important in effective execution of One Health education are summarized in Table 11.1.

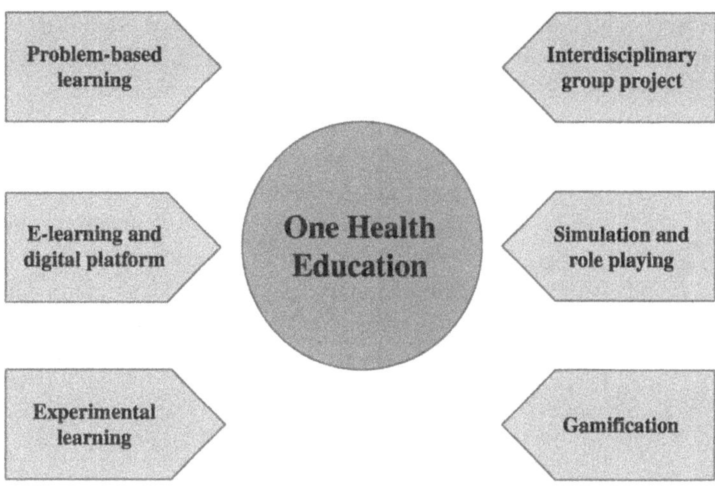

Figure 11.2 Innovative teaching methodologies framework.

Table 11.1 Innovative teaching methodologies in One Health.

Teaching methods	Description	Benefit	Examples	References
Problem-Based Learning	• Student centered • Active engagement of the students • Solving real-word problems • Directed self-collaborative learning • Case studies	• Prepare learners to address real-world challenges • Interdisciplinary projects foster collaboration and problem-solving skills • Fieldwork helps to understand real One Health situations	• Zoonotic disease such as rabies, cysticercosis, etc. • Antimicrobial resistance • Health and climate change • Food safety • Disease transmission	[37]
Simulation-Based Learning	• Solving real-world problems through simulations • Offers a real-time environment for learning	• Repeated simulation-based learning helps to develop confidence in tackling real-world challenges • More cost effective and economical than the traditional way of learning	• Simulation of disease diagnosis and treatment • Simulation of surgical procedures • Simulation of environmental hazards to their impact on humans, animals, and environment	[38]
Field-Based Experiences	• It provides opportunities that associates theoretical knowledge with real-world applications	• Detailed understanding of the problems • Provides real-world experiences • Improved collaborations	• Field trips • Community services • Case learning	[39]

11.3.1 Problem-based Learning

PBL is a student-centric approach in which learners learn about a subject by working in groups to elucidate an open-ended problem. The problem drives the motivation and the learning. The PBL provides opportunity to learn various skills such as teamwork, development of leadership qualities, critical thinking, and analyses. It also develops independent and critical thinking and inculcates self-directed learning. As per the US educator, Edgar Dale, who proposed the "Cone of Experience or Cone of Dale," about the effectiveness of the learning methods, stated that at the apex of the cone lies the methods which have the least effect on learning (verbal of written descriptions) and at base lies the methods with maximum possible effects (e.g. direct experience) of what we do by ourselves [40].

In this method of learning, rather than teaching relevant material and subsequently having students apply the knowledge to solve problems, the problem is presented first. It is a group-oriented and prepare the students to have collaborative learning setting aside the classroom teaching. During this, learning students must define the problem and then they should determine what they need to learn to solve that particular problem [41]. It is a method in which the learning starts from a problematic situation which enables students to develop a hypothesis and learning requirements to understand the problem and learning requirements [42]. In this method, students are encouraged to engage with peers and apply acquired knowledge to clinical problems, a component of One Health under the guidance of a facilitator [43].

11.3.2 Simulations

Simulation-based education is the pedagogical approach of providing students with the opportunity to practice learned skills in real-life situations. This type of learning tests knowledge and skill levels of the learners by keeping them in conditions where they must actively solve problems. The instructor defines the parameters to create a safe environment for hands-on learning experiences. While participating in a scenario, learner must quickly evaluate the situation, decide on the best course of action, and perform the correct procedural steps. Teacher can then assess whether the students understand the material and are translating their learned knowledge into skills. The biggest advantage of the simulation-based learning is that one can turn knowledge into practice and simulations help to have the hands on practice as many times as one wants and will help them feel much more comfortable when real situation arises [44].

The simulations have been used in other disciplines to present the real-time situation and could be used in the One Health approach for better understanding of the subject and the scenario. During simulation, the students can prioritize their actions and compare the different interventions and propose solution to One Health problems. A series of experiments conducted showed that simulation-based teaching activities are an effective tool for teaching One Health topics and their perception is better when compared to traditional methods such as watching videos and lectures [45]. It has also been evidenced that simulation-based teaching train the students with complex decision-making, an important perspective of One Health [46]. Further, simulations train the students for effective decision-making without any fear of adverse outcomes. There are proofs that simulation-based learning could inculcate the habit of teamwork, social, and emotional skills, which is crucial for One Health practice.

11.3.3 Field-based Experiences

In field-based learning, teaching is extended to a site outside of the classroom or laboratory, exposing students to a real-world setting. Students learn through direct interaction with an environment that reflects taught concepts rather than learning through indirect presentations such as textbooks or lectures. It provides an opportunity to present materials, objects, or phenomena that are not accessible to students in a way that enables direct contact and interaction; provides students with an opportunity to practice skills or techniques that cannot be carried out elsewhere; and stimulates higher understanding and reinforcement of previously learned classroom material [47].

Field-based experiences provide the students with opportunities to observe interaction between plant, animal, and human communities, making them an ideal tool for teaching One Health concepts [48]. Field-based experiences promote consolidation of classroom learning, real-time conceptual development, appreciation for collective actions, and environmental consciousness, which is the basic concept of One Health [49].

11.4 Case Studies in One Health

Case studies are important as they provide an idea about practical applications of One Health approach, and they define the relation between different components of One Health, that is, human, animal, and environmental health. Case studies also inform us that how modifications in one sector can influence the other sectors. Further, it also helps the policymakers to formulate suitable policies based on experiences gained through the case studies. Case studies help in formulation of suitable trainings and capacity-building program as well as development of suitable linkages and collaborations. Case studies help in controlling, preventing, and formulating suitable strategies for various diseases under the purview of One Health [50–55] Few important case studies are summarized in Table 11.2.

11.4.1 Real-world Applications

The One Health approach has been instigated in many countries for the prevention and control of zoonotic disease [63], with an increasing application in recent years in response to a surge in outbreaks. Avian influenza, rabies, anthrax, and brucellosis are the priority zoonoses across multiple countries [64] and are good instances to focus on the relevance of the One Health approach [65]. Evidence of success from One Health approaches from around the globe and the increasing trend in emerging infectious disease outbreaks will enhance the utilization of One Health in the future. There is a growing consensus on the mutually reinforcing relationship between the One Health concept and Sustainable Development Goals (SDGs) of the United Nations; many of which are directly related to the One Health approach, as it facilitates the meeting of SDGs [64].

The concept of the One Health approach has been found applicable in many areas such as antimicrobial resistance, food safety, and ecotoxicology [65]. A Memorandum of Understanding (MoU) among the FAO, WHO, WOAH, and the United Nations Environment Programme (UNEP) establishes a legal and formal framework for tackling challenges at the intersection of human, animal, and ecosystem health through an integrated and coordinated approach [66]. One Health approach has been used to prevent and control various zoonotic diseases across the world [67–70]. Another real-world application of the One Health approach was the control and prevention of avian influenza and rabies in Cambodia using the One Help approach by providing training to different stakeholders: veterinary students, human and animal lab technicians, and wildlife experts who were provided with theoretical knowledge and hands-on training for commonly occurring zoonotic diseases. The training under the One Health approach significantly helped in reduction of avian influenza and rabies by bridging the gaps in coordination, communication, and collaboration [1]. A coordinated approach based on the One Health approach between medical and veterinary professionals in China jointly executed by China CDC and US CDC reduced the occurrence of rabies [1]. Various zoonotic diseases can be controlled and prevented by propagating the concept of One Health through collaborations and training. Figure 11.3 depicts key real-world applications of the One Health approach, demonstrating its role in zoonotic disease control, environmental health, and cross-sector collaborations.

11.4.2 Success Stories and Lessons Learned

The application of the One Health concept has resolved various intermingled cases which were difficulty to crack. Few success stories which have been resolved through the One Health approach are discussed below:

Table 11.2 Real-world implementations of the One Health approach.

Studies	Key stakeholders	Major outcomes	Lessons learned	References
Investigating *Salmonella* and Wild Songbirds	• Wildlife Departments • Local Health Departments • Wildlife Laboratories	First reporting of *Salmonella* from the wild	• Collaboration among different institutions and agencies is required to control One Health hazards	[56]
Antimicrobial resistance in animals and humans	• Humans • Public Health Veterinarians • Pet owners	A lack of professional veterinary practice could lead to antibiotic resistance in humans	• Regular training for public health veterinarians • Judicious use of antibiotics • Adherence to ethical veterinary practices	[57]
Poisoning and Death in Sea Otters	• Veterinarians • Department of Fish and Wildlife • Department of Public Health • State Water Control Board • Local authorities	Changes in one part of the ecosystem can affect distant ecosystems	• The entire ecosystem is interconnected and should be preserved as a single entity	[58]
Reduction in Rocky Mountain Spotted Fever	• Humans • Local Health Veterinarians • Pet Owners	The reduction of ticks in dogs has decreased the occurrence of Rocky Mountain Spotted Fever	• The health of companion animals is important for protecting human health	[59]
Reduction of Rabies Cases	• Humans • Public Health Veterinarians • WOAH • Government Ministries	A reduction in human rabies cases has been achieved through the vaccination of dogs	• Animal vaccination can control several human diseases • Incentives in any form can enhance the success rate of any program, especially among the undereducated population.	[60]
Control of Crimean Congo Hemorrhagic Fever (CCHF)	• CDC • Government Ministries • Department of Veterinary Control and Surveillance • Entomologist	Training and awareness programs	• Training and awareness programs are among the important pillars of the One Health approach	[61]
Control of Rift Valley Fever Virus	• CDC • Public Health Professionals • Animal Health Professionals • NASA	Awareness, animal vaccination, and weather forecasting	• Collaboration among different stakeholders is an important tool for the effective execution of the One Health approach	[62]

11.4.2.1 Investigating Salmonella and Wild Songbirds

During 2020, epidemiologists in Oregon, United States, contacted CDC about a peculiar finding that a strain of *Salmonella* causing human illnesses matched a strain of *Salmonella* isolated from a wild songbird, specifically a pine siskin. Additionally, in late 2020, the Wildlife Health Laboratory in California, United States, received an increased number of reports from the public and other agencies about *Salmonella* in wild songbirds. This gave investigators a clue that the two events may be related.

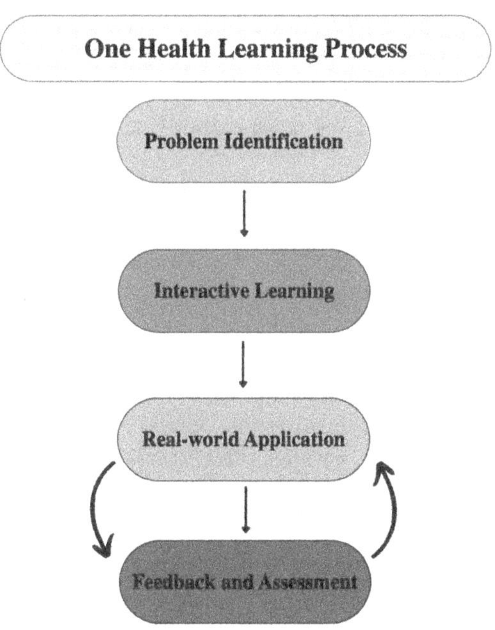

Figure 11.3 Flowchart of the One Health learning process.

To further discover the relation, CDC worked with state and local health departments, wildlife departments, and wildlife research laboratory networks to identify *Salmonella* isolates. Public health departments interviewed people infected with *Salmonella* Typhimurium to see if they had contact with wild birds before their illness started. Further, various advisories were given in order to control the disease spread. The advice, given using a One Health approach, was shared by partners to help prevent further illnesses among people, pets, and wildlife and to reduce environmental contamination. The first time *Salmonella* was recorded from the wild, and different agencies working together resolved the problem [1].

11.4.2.2 Antimicrobial Resistance in Animals and Humans

In 2016, CDC, USA, came across an outbreak of multidrug-resistant *Salmonella* linked to dairy calves, highlighting the need for farm-level tools to prevent the development of antimicrobial resistance in humans. In order to trace the origin of multidrug-resistant *Salmonella*, surveys were done at various points in the production of calves. The results revealed the indiscriminate use of antimicrobials by veterinarians who had been out of training for a long duration and used to prescribe the unwanted antibiotics, sometimes even on the pressure of clients. Another similar outbreak of drug-resistant *Campylobacter* in humans was linked to the puppies in breeding kennels. It was found that the indiscriminate use of antibiotics in kennels, mostly in breeding operations and control of diarrhea in puppies, was the major cause for the development of drug resistance.

Thereafter, steps were taken to develop a decision-making tool to encourage the calf producers to use veterinarian-developed treatment protocols. Informed training and decision-making tool for the calf producers may also help reduce the inappropriate antimicrobial use and development of resistant bacteria and outbreaks. Further, veterinarians were encouraged and trained to streamline the use of antibiotics and avoid unnecessary use. Further, the approach to improve the standardized infection control practices was encouraged to be followed in kennels to develop drug resistance [1].

11.4.2.3 Poisoning and Death in Sea Otters

The poisoning of sea otters in California, USA, was linked to microcystin secreted by cyanobacteria, which was linked to the growth of cyanobacteria in a freshwater lake called Pinto Lake, which further drains into a river and then the sea. The growth of cyanobacteria in the freshwater lake concentrated the microcystin in the sea, which accumulated in the sea otters. The real cause was traced after multiple authorities from different backgrounds, including veterinarians, the Department of Fish and Wildlife, the Department of Public Health, the State Water Control Board and Local authorities, etc. came to join hands together, providing an excellent application of One Health [1].

11.4.2.4 Reduction in Cases of Rocky Mountain Spotted Fever

In the southwestern United States and Mexico, the use of tick collars in dogs reduced the occurrence of Rocky Mountain Spotted Fever within a short span of four months' duration, which is an excellent application of the One Health approach [1].

11.4.2.5 Namibia's Battle Against Rabies

Veterinarians leading the charge, supported by the Federal Ministry of Economic Co-operation and Development, with technical support provided by the World Organization of Animal Health did remarkable work by reducing the occurrence of human rabies cases by vaccinating the dogs. A unique initiative was taken where vaccination for rabies was integrated with FMD and CBPP, which helped to enhance the vaccination status of dogs [1].

11.4.2.6 Control of Crimean Congo Hemorrhagic Fever in Kazakhstan

Crimean Congo Hemorrhagic Fever (CCHF) was a major problem in Kazakhstan, with special concentration in Zhambyl region. When studies were done using the One Health approach, it was found that the people with seroprevalence of CCHF were involved with high-risk work associated with animals such as slaughter, shearing, milking, etc., and did not use any protective equipment. Moreover, people were unaware of the preventive measures and the role of animals in the transmission of diseases. Thus, by identifying the gaps, measures were taken to curb the CCHF [1].

11.4.2.7 Control of Rift Valley Virus Fever in East Africa

Rift Valley fever was a major problem in East Africa, and during 1997 more than 90 000 cases were reported. It was also found the cases were at their peak during the years of heavy rainfall, and animals with heavy viral loads were the source of transmission of infection to humans. Thus, by application of the One Health approach in terms of predicting the years of heavy rainfall and vaccinating the animals reduced the cases of Rift Valley Virus Fever [1].

11.5 Challenges in One Health Education

The integration of One Health principles into education is a vital step toward addressing the complex and interconnected health issues facing our world today. However, the implementation of effective One Health education comes with its own set of challenges. These challenges are multifaceted and can hinder the seamless incorporation of interdisciplinary approaches into academic curricula and professional training. Issues such as curriculum integration, resource limitations, and fostering effective interdisciplinary collaboration are key obstacles that educators and institutions must navigate. This section explores these challenges in detail, offering insights into the difficulties faced by educational systems in promoting a comprehensive and unified understanding of human, animal, and environmental health. By examining these barriers, we can better understand the complexities involved in equipping future professionals with the skills needed to tackle global health challenges through the One Health approach.

11.5.1 Curriculum Integration

Curriculum integration is one of the most important challenges to One Health education, as it involves knowledge and input from multiple disciplines [23]. The incorporation of the One Health curriculum in other streams shall strengthen curricula and provide students an inherent understanding of the interconnections among human, animal, and environmental health. The curriculum integration could be in the form of core courses, optional courses, internship trainings, and collaborative programs. Students from different streams such as ecology, medicine, veterinary medicine, and public health could be offered integrative courses for the inculcation of the One Health concept. However, the curriculum integration involves the approval at different levels, which could be a difficult job for policymakers to overcome. There is need of stringent action in order to have curriculum integration and inculcation of the One Health approach in different disciplines related to One Health.

11.5.2 Resource Limitations

Resource limitation is one of the major reasons for the lack of emphasis on One Health education, especially in middle- and low-income countries. Resources in terms of money, trained manpower, knowledge about One Health are few of the important resource limitations for the execution of the One Health approach. Most of the One Health initiatives are based on interdisciplinary (ID) collaborations, which require the integration of different domains and cooperation between diverse experts, creating possibilities for knowledge co-creation. However, the inclusion of diverse stakeholders under the One Health approach can lead to conflicts due to their manifold interests and priorities.

11.5.3 Interdisciplinary Collaboration

Since One Health is associated with multiple disciplines, interdisciplinary collaboration is inevitable for its success. Doctors, veterinarians, politicians, public health workers, and all other stakeholders must join their hands together for undertaking the challenges pertaining to One Health. It requires overcoming disciplinary boundaries, establishing effective communication channels, and creating a supportive institutional framework [71]. Thus, to advance the concept of One Health, future initiatives should focus on fostering collaboration, promoting knowledge exchange, and developing interdisciplinary training programs to enhance the capacity for holistic research and action. Table 11.3 provides an overview of the challenges and opportunities in One Health education, illustrating the key points discussed in this section.

Table 11.3 Challenges and opportunities in One Health education.

Challenges in One Health education	Methods for addressing the challenges	References
Curriculum Integration	Curriculum integration may be achieved through the incorporation of core courses, internship training, collaborative programs, field training, and the introduction of special courses on One Health	[72–74]
Resource Limitations	Special provisions should be made to upgrade resource availability with respect to One Health facilities. Institutions such as WHO, FAO, the World Bank, etc., should come forward to provide support	[75–78]
Interdisciplinary Collaboration	Stakeholders from different disciplines, such as public health workers, veterinarians, environmental activists, etc., should join together to tackle challenges related to One Health.	[74, 79–81]

11.6 Opportunities for Enhancing One Health Learning

For enhancing the opportunities in One Health learning, multiple efforts must be taken to execute and make it effective. One Health learning may be enhanced by keeping books and reading material in the school and college libraries. To make the learning compulsory, the One Health content may be included in the syllabus and posted on school websites. Various platforms such as Massive Open Online Courses (MOOCs) may be used to promote information to public. Further, communication channels may be established for information sharing outside of ones' immediate sphere to ensure knowledge reaches the global level. Joint degrees, interdisciplinary events, research, and practical exchanges may be executed. Mobilization of multidisciplinary training, research, and practice initiatives should be done to assess and serve needs for improved health status at various levels. Empowerment of health professionals may be done to identify and communicate urgent threats to public health and the importance of a One Health approach to various stakeholders. Another way to enhance One Health awareness is to incorporate it in the curriculum and training of potential participants of the approach [82].

11.7 Conclusion

This chapter highlights the transformative potential of interactive learning and practical applications within the One Health framework. By promoting interdisciplinary education and collaborative strategies, it underscores the importance of integrating diverse perspectives to address the interconnected health of humans–animals–ecosystems. Innovative methods like PBL, simulations, and field experiences are key to understanding complex health issues and enhancing interdisciplinary collaboration.

Real-world case studies demonstrate the practical benefits of implementing One Health principles, yet challenges like curriculum integration, resource limitations, and the need for effective intersectoral collaboration persist. Overcoming these challenges requires cooperation across sectors, including healthcare workers, veterinarians, environmentalists, and ecologists. Curriculum integration, though critical, remains a difficult task for policymakers, while resource constraints and the shortage of trained personnel further complicate progress.

To advance One Health, it is essential to embrace new educational initiatives, such as degree courses, MOOCs, and incorporating One Health into primary education. These measures, along with enhanced interdisciplinary collaboration, will equip future professionals to tackle global health challenges effectively. By continuing to innovate and prioritize comprehensive One Health education, we can foster a more interconnected, healthier world.

References

1 Centers for Disease Control and Prevention. *One Health*. 2024. https://www.cdc.gov/one-health/about/index.html.

2 Oura, C., Conlon, K.C., Smith, W., et al. Academic and institutional 'One Health' research capacity building. In: *One Health: People, Animals and the Environment* (ed. R. Atlas and S. Maloy), 368–381. CABI; 2021. https://doi.org/10.1079/9781789242577.0368.

3 Gordon, A. and Schwabe, C. *The Quick and the Dead*. Leiden, The Netherlands: Brill; 2004. https://doi.org/10.1163/9789047404163.

4 Conti, A.A. Historical evolution of the concept of health in Western medicine. *Acta Biomed*. 2018; 89(3): 352–354. https://doi.org/10.23750/abm.v89i3.6739.

5 Evans, B.R. and Leighton, F.A. A history of One Health. *Rev. Sci. Tech*. 2014; 33(2): 413–420. https://doi.org/10.20506/rst.33.2.2298.

6 Leonardi, F. The definition of health: towards new perspectives. *Int. J. Health Serv.* 2018; 48(4): 735–748. https://doi.org/10.1177/0020731418782653.
7 Nutton, V. *Ancient Medicine.* 1st ed. London: Routledge; 2004. https://doi.org/10.4324/9780203490914.
8 Koplan, J.P., Bond, T.C., Merson, M.H., et al. Towards a common definition of global health. *Lancet* 2009; 373(9679): 1993–1995. https://doi.org/10.1016/S0140-6736(09)60332-9.
9 Esposito, M.M., Turku, S., Lehrfield, L., and Shoman, A. The impact of human activities on zoonotic infection transmissions. *Animals (Basel)* 2023; 13(10): 1646. https://doi.org/10.3390/ani13101646.
10 Tajudeen, Y.A., Oladunjoye, I.O., Bajinka, O., and Oladipo, H.J. Zoonotic spillover in an era of rapid deforestation of tropical areas and unprecedented wildlife trafficking: into the wild. *Challenges* 2022; 13(2): 41. https://doi.org/10.3390/challe13020041.
11 Cai, C., Jung, Y.S., Pereira, R.V.V., et al. Advancing one health education: integrative pedagogical approaches and their impacts on interdisciplinary learning. *Sci. One Health* 2024; 3: 100079. https://doi.org/10.1016/j.soh.2024.100079.
12 World Health Organization (WHO). *One Health.* 2017. https://www.who.int/features/qa/one-health/
13 World Health Organization (WHO). *Multisectoral and Intersectoral Action for Improved Health and Well-Being for all: Mapping of the WHO.* 2018. https://www.euro.who.int/__data/assets/pdf_file/0005/371435/multisectoralreport-h1720-eng.pdf
14 World Health Organization (WHO), Food and Agriculture Organization of the United Nations (FAO), World Organization for Animal Health (OIE). *Taking a Multisectoral, One Health Approach: A Tripartite Guide to Addressing Zoonotic Diseases in Countries.* 2019. https://www.oie.int/fileadmin/Home/eng/Media_Center/docs/EN_TripartiteZoonosesGuide_webversion.pdf
15 World Organization for Animal Health (OIE). *One Health.* 2019. https://www.oie.int/en/for-the-media/onehealth.
16 Food and Agriculture Organization of the United Nations (FAO). *One Health: Food and Agriculture Organization of the United Nations Strategic Action Plan.* 2011. http://www.fao.org/3/al868e/al868e00.pdf
17 The World Bank. *People, Pathogens, and our Planet: Towards a One Health Approach for Controlling Zoonotic Diseases.* 2010. http://documents.worldbank.org/curated/
18 Berthe, F.C.J., Bouley, T., Karesh, W.B., et al. *One Health: Operational Framework for Strengthening Human, Animal, and Environmental Public Health Systems at Their Interface.* 2018. http://documents.worldbank.org/curated/en/961101524657708673/
19 Secretariat of the Convention on Biological Diversity (COP). *Biodiversity and Human Health. COP 12 Decision XII/21.* 2014. https://www.cbd.int/decision/cop/
20 World Organization for Animal Health (OIE). *4th OIE Global Conference on Veterinary Education: Final Recommendations.* 2016. https://www.oie.int/eng/
21 Zinsstag, J., Schelling, E., Waltner-Toews, D., and Tanner, M. From 'One Medicine' to 'One Health' and systemic approaches to health and well-being. *Prev. Vet. Med.* 2011; 101 (3–4): 148–156. https://doi.org/10.1016/j.prevetmed.2010.07.003.
22 Frankson, R., Hueston, W., Christian, K., et al. One Health core competency domains. *Front. Public Health* 2016; 4: 192. https://doi.org/10.3389/fpubh.2016.00192.
23 Mor, S.M., Robbins, A.H., Jarvin, L., et al. Curriculum asset mapping for One Health education. *J. Vet. Med. Educ.* 2013; 40: 363–369. https://doi.org/10.3138/jvme.0313-0525R.
24 Rüegg, S.R., Nielsen, L.R., Buttigieg, S.C., et al. A systems approach to evaluate One Health initiatives. *Front. Vet. Sci.* 2018; 5: 23. https://doi.org/10.3389/fvets.2018.00023.
25 Errecaborde, K.M., Macy, K.W., Pekol, A., et al. Factors that enable effective One Health collaborations – a scoping review of the literature. *PLoS One* 2019; 14: e0224660. https://doi.org/10.1371/journal.pone.0224660.
26 Tan, X., Chen, P., and Yu, H. Potential conditions for linking teachers' online informal learning with innovative teaching. *Think. Skills. Creat.* 2022; 45: 101022. https://doi.org/10.1016/j.tsc.2022.101022.

27 Yu, H., Liu, P., Huang, X., and Cao, Y. Teacher online informal learning as a means to innovative teaching during home quarantine in the COVID-19 pandemic. *Front. Psychol.* 2021; 12: 596582. https://doi.org/10.3389/fpsyg.2021.596582.

28 Kayode, O.O., Ogundokun, R.O., Mohammed, R.E., and Olorundare, A.S. Review of innovative teaching strategies in senior secondary schools sciences. *i-Manager's J. Educ. Technol.* 2020; 17: 56–65. https://eric.ed.gov/?id=EJ1269287.

29 Adelabu, F.M., Ngwabe, A., and Alex, J. Self-directed learning through computer-aided mathematics instruction: first-year teacher education experience. *Int. J. High. Educ.* 2022; 11: 79–89. https://doi.org/10.5430/ijhe.v11n3p79.

30 Callaghan, M.N., Long, J.J., van Es, E.A., et al. How teachers integrate a math computer game: professional development use, teaching practices, and student achievement. *J. Comput. Assist. Learn.* 2019; 34: 10–19. https://doi.org/10.1111/jcal.12209.

31 Viberg, O., Grönlund, Å., and Andersson, A. Integrating digital technology in mathematics education: a Swedish case study. *Interact. Learn. Environ.* 2020; 31: 232–243. https://doi.org/10.1080/10494820.2020.1770801.

32 Centers for Disease Control and Prevention (CDC). *One Health.* 2023. https://www.cdc.gov/one-health/about/index.html.

33 Duboz, R., Echaubard, P., Promburom, P., et al. Systems thinking in practice: participatory modeling as a foundation for integrated approaches to health. *Front. Vet. Sci.* 2018; 5: 303. https://doi.org/10.3389/fvets.2018.00303.

34 Rocheleau, J.P., Aenishaenslin, C., Boisjoly, H., et al. Clarifying core competencies in One Health doctoral education: the central contribution of systems thinking. *One Earth* 2022; 5: 311–315. https://doi.org/10.1016/j.oneear.2022.03.005.

35 Kesselring, J. Zinsstag, J., Schelling, E., et al. One Health. The theory and practice of integrated health approaches. *Swiss Arch. Neurol. Psychiat. Psychother.* 2021. https://doi.org/10.4414/sanp.2021.03194.

36 Hitziger, M., Berezowski, J., Dürr, S., et al. System thinking and citizen participation is still missing in One Health initiatives – lessons from fifteen evaluations. *Front. Public Health* 2021; 9: 653398. https://doi.org/10.3389/fpubh.2021.653398.

37 Matsuda, Y., Falcon, A., Porter, A., et al. Implementation of problem-based learning modules in an introduction to public health course. *Front. Public Health* 2024; 12: 1405227.

38 Mustaffa-Kamal, F., Shafie, I.N.F., Zakariah, S.Z., et al. Effectiveness of field simulation approach for problem-based learning that incorporates the One Health concept. *J. Vet. Med. Educ.* 2023; 51: 405–411.

39 Shehu, N., Luka, P., Bente, D., et al. Using One Health training for interprofessional team building: implications for research, policy, and practice in Nigeria. *Front. Public Health* 2024; 12: 1375424.

40 Dale, E. Methods for analyzing the content of motion pictures. *J. Educ. Sociol.* 1932; 6: 244–250.

41 Nilson, L.B. *Teaching at Its Best: A Research-Based Resource for College Instructors*, 2nd ed. San Francisco, CA: Jossey-Bass; 2010.

42 Bodagh, N., Bloomfield, J., Birch, P., and Ricketts, W. Problem-based learning: a review. *Br. J. Hosp. Med.* 2017; 78: C167–C170. https://doi.org/10.12968/hmed.2017.78.11.C167.

43 Trullàs, J.C., Blay, C., Sarri, E., and Pujol, R. Effectiveness of problem-based learning methodology in undergraduate medical education: a scoping review. *BMC Med. Educ.* 2022; 22: 104. https://doi.org/10.1186/s12909-022-03154-8.

44 Kim, J., Park, J.H., and Shin, S. Effectiveness of simulation-based nursing education depending on fidelity: a meta-analysis. *BMC Med. Educ.* 2022; 16: 152. https://doi.org/10.1186/s12909-016-0672-7.

45 Acosta, D., Stark, H., and Hack, G. The importance of incorporating systems thinking and One Health in global health classrooms: findings from a One Health simulation activity. *Front. Public Health* 2024; 12: 1299116. https://doi.org/10.3389/fpubh.2024.1299116.

46 Vlachopoulos, D. and Makri, A. The effect of games and simulations on higher education: a systematic literature review. *Int. J. Educ. Technol. High. Educ.* 2017; 14: 22. https://doi.org/10.1186/s41239-017-0062-1.

47 Lonergan, N. and Andresen, L.W. Field-based education: some theoretical considerations. *High. Educ. Res. Dev.* 1988; 7(1): 63–77.

48 Mor, S.M., Norris, J.M., Bosward, K.L., et al. One health in our backyard: design and evaluation of an experiential learning experience for veterinary medical students. *One Health* 2018; 5: 57–64. https://doi.org/10.1016/j.onehlt.2018.05.001.

49 Lei, S.A. Field trips in college biology and ecology courses: revisiting benefits and drawbacks. *J. Instr. Psychol.* 2010; 37: 42–48.

50 Keita, I.M., Diouf, M., Ndiop, M., et al. Added value of multisectoral collaboration (One Health) for proactive vector-borne disease control in a context of climate change: the case of a joint system evaluation of malaria sentinel surveillance with its climatic factors in Senegal. *One Health Cases* 2025; 0005. https://doi.org/10.1079/onehealthcases.2025.0005.

51 Hassan-Kadle, A.A., Ibrahim, A.M., Osman, A.M., and Vieira, R.F. One Health in Somalia: bridging gaps through education, research, and outreach. *One Health Cases* 2025; 0009. https://doi.org/10.1079/onehealthcases.2025.0009.

52 Sripa, B. and Tangkawattana, S. The Lawa model: an integrated liver fluke control program using the EcoHealth/One Health approach. *One Health Cases* 2025; ohcs20250004. https://doi.org/10.1079/onehealthcases.2025.0004.

53 Manes, C., Herren, R., Cooper, E., et al. Disease, environment, and pollution: understanding drivers behind tumour outbreaks in Sea turtles. *One Health Cases* 2025; ohcs20250001. https://doi.org/10.1079/onehealthcases.2025.0001.

54 Durrance-Bagale, A., Basnet, H., Rudge, J.W., et al. Engaging community members to pinpoint priorities around zoonotic disease in Nepal. *One Health Cases* 2024; ohcs20240028. https://doi.org/10.1079/onehealthcases.2024.0028.

55 Azuba, R., Charles, W., and Khaitsa, M.L. The Coordinating Office for Control of Trypanosomiasis in Uganda (COCTU): a One Health best practice case. *One Health Cases* 2024; ohcs20240035. https://doi.org/10.1079/onehealthcases.2024.0035.

56 Patel, K., Stapleton, G.S., Trevejo, R.T., et al. Human salmonellosis outbreak linked to *Salmonella Typhimurium* epidemic in wild songbirds, United States, 2020–2021. *Emerg. Infect. Dis.* 2023; 29(11): 2298.

57 Pandey, S., Doo, H., Keum, G.B., et al. Antibiotic resistance in livestock, environment and humans: One Health perspective. *J. Anim. Sci. Technol.* 2024; 66(2): 266.

58 Miller, M.A., Moriarty, M.E., Henkel, L., et al. Predators, disease, and environmental change in the nearshore ecosystem: mortality in southern sea otters (*Enhydra lutris nereis*) from 1998–2012. *Front. Mar. Sci.* 2020; 7: 582.

59 Foley, J., López-Pérez, A., Rubino, F., et al. Roaming dogs, intense brown dog tick infestation, and emerging rocky mountain spotted fever in Tijuana, México. *Am. J. Trop. Med. Hyg.* 2024; 110(4): 779–794.

60 Freuling, C.M., van der Westhuizen, J., Khaiseb, S., et al. From field tests to molecular tools—evaluating diagnostic tests to improve rabies surveillance in Namibia. *Viruses* 2023; 15(2): 371.

61 Gabdullina, M., Gazezova, S., Ayapova, G., et al. Outbreak of Crimean-Congo hemorrhagic fever in Kyzylorda region, Kazakhstan, March–July 2022. *Open Forum Infect. Dis.* 2023; 10(Suppl 2): ofad500-140.

62 Hussein, H.E., Hassanain, S., Okwarah, P., et al. Achievement of One Health multi-sectoral collaboration in containment of Rift Valley Fever outbreak, Sudan, Red Sea State 2019. *Eur. J. Public Health* 2025; 35(Suppl 1): i66–i72.

63 Nadal, D., Beeching, S., Cleaveland, S., et al. Rabies and the pandemic: lessons for One Health. *Trans. R. Soc. Trop. Med. Hyg.* 2022; 116(3): 197–200. https://doi.org/10.1093/trstmh/trab123.

64 Rai, B.D., Tessema, G.A., Fritschi, L., and Pereira, G. The application of the One Health approach in the management of five major zoonotic diseases using the World Bank domains: a scoping review. *One Health (Amsterdam, Netherlands)* 2024; 18: 100695. https://doi.org/10.1016/j.onehlt.2024.100695.

65 Dwyer, D.E. and Kirkland, P.D. One Health in action. *NSW Public Health Bull.* 2011; 22: 123–126.

66 Dongyu, Q.U., Andersen, I., Ghebreyesus, T.A., and Eloit, M. Quadripartite call to action for One Health for a safer world. *Indian J. Health Well-Being* 2023; 14(4): 511–519.

67 Acharya, K.P., Subedi, D., and Wilson, R.T. Rabies control in South Asia requires a One Health approach. *One Health* 2021; 12: 100215. https://doi.org/10.1016/j.onehlt.2021.100215.

68 Fitzpatrick, M.C., Shah, H.A., Pandey, A., et al. One Health approach to cost-effective rabies control in India. *Proc. Natl. Acad. Sci.* 2016; 113(51): 14574–14581. https://doi.org/10.1073/pnas.1604975113.

69 Freire-Paspuel, B., Vega-Mariño, P., Velez, A., et al. "One Health" inspired SARS-CoV-2 surveillance: the Galapagos Islands experience [One Health 11 (2020) 100185]. *One Health* 2021; 13: 100345. https://doi.org/10.1016/j.onehlt.2021.100345.

70 Acharya, K.P., Acharya, N., Phuyal, S., et al. One-Health approach: a best possible way to control rabies. *One Health* 2020; 10: 100161. https://doi.org/10.1016/j.onehlt.2020.100161.

71 Andrawes, L., Johnson, T., and Coleman, M. Complexity in health: can design help support interdisciplinary solutions? *Global Health Sci. Pract.* 2021; 9(Suppl 2): S217–S225. https://doi.org/10.9745/GHSP-D-21-00222.

72 Hobusch, U., Scheuch, M., Heuckmann, B., et al. One Health education Nexus: enhancing synergy among science-, school-, and teacher education beyond academic silos. *Front. Public Health* 2024; 11: 1337748.

73 Angelos, J., Arens, A., Johnson, H., et al. One Health in food safety and security education: a curricular framework. *Compar. Immunol. Microbiol. Infect. Dis.* 2016; 44: 29–33.

74 Buregyeya, E., Atusingwize, E., Nsamba, P., et al. Operationalizing the One Health approach in Uganda: challenges and opportunities. *J. Epidemiol. Glob. Health* 2020; 10(4): 250–257.

75 Berrian, A.M., Wilkes, M., Gilardi, K., et al. Developing a global One Health workforce: the "Rx One Health Summer Institute" approach. *EcoHealth* 2020; 17: 222–232.

76 Mahajan, S., Khan, Z., Giri, P.P., et al. Operationalising 'One Health' through primary healthcare approach. *Prevent. Med. Res. Rev.* 2024; 1(4): 199–206.

77 Hassan-Kadle, A.A., Osman, A.M., Ibrahim, A.M., et al. One Health in Somalia: present status, opportunities, and challenges. *One Health* 2024; 18: 100666.

78 Viegas, S. One Health approach for the SDGs achievement. *Eur. J. Public Health* 2022; 32(Suppl 3): ckac129-017.

79 Barrett, M.A. and Bouley, T.A. Need for enhanced environmental representation in the implementation of One Health. *EcoHealth* 2015; 12: 212–219.

80 Courtenay, M., Sweeney, J., Zielinska, P., et al. One Health: an opportunity for an interprofessional approach to healthcare. *J. Interprof. Care* 2015; 29(6): 641–642.

81 Conrad, P.A., Meek, L.A., and Dumit, J. Operationalizing a One Health approach to global health challenges. *Comp. Immunol. Microbiol. Infect. Dis.* 2013; 36(3): 211–216.

82 Haider, M., Ahmed, S., and Choudhary, A. *One Health: Implementation Challenges and Need.* IntechOpen; 2023. https://doi.org/10.5772/intechopen.111933.

Multiple-choice Questions (MCQs) on One Health

Vivek Harishankar Shukla[1,2] *and Pratik Subhash Gaikwad*[3]

[1] *Department of Livestock Products Technology, Mumbai Veterinary College, Parel, Mumbai, Maharashtra, India*
[2] *Maharashtra Animal and Fishery Sciences University, Nagpur, Maharashtra, India*
[3] *School of Biotechnology and Bioinformatics, D Y Patil Deemed to Be University, Navi Mumbai, Maharashtra, India*

Introduction

The One Health concept represents a progressive, collaborative approach that highlights the complex interconnections between human, animal, and environmental health. In an age characterized by emerging infectious diseases, climate change, urban expansion, and antimicrobial resistance, the One Health framework provides a cohesive strategy to address these multifaceted challenges through cross-sector coordination and interdisciplinary insight.

This resource, structured as a comprehensive set of Multiple Choice Questions (MCQs), serves as a practical learning tool for veterinary professionals, public health practitioners, scholars, and students. By engaging with these MCQs, readers will not only strengthen their foundational and advanced knowledge but also develop critical thinking skills and readiness for academic and professional challenges.

Divided into five thematic sections, this compilation facilitates a structured exploration of key domains:

- **Section I: One Health Approach** – Covers the foundational principles, historical background, and collaborative frameworks that define One Health in both theory and practice.
- **Section II: Zoonotic Diseases** – Explores diseases transmissible between animals and humans, focusing on surveillance, control measures, and the importance of early detection and prevention.
- **Section III: Public Health** – Examines the integration of One Health into public health systems, including aspects of disease prevention, food safety, and antimicrobial resistance.
- **Section IV: Epidemiology** – Provides an overview of disease patterns and determinants, offering analytical tools for evidence-based decision-making in both animal and human health.
- **Section V: Climate Change, Environmental Health, and Urbanization** – Investigates how environmental shifts and urban development influence disease transmission and public health, reinforcing the need for a One Health perspective in global health strategies.

This resource aims to empower individuals by strengthening core knowledge, fostering critical thinking, and preparing them for practical applications in One Health research, policy, and practice. Ultimately, enabling contributions to global health initiatives and cross-sector collaboration in addressing current and future health challenges.

One Health Integration: Global Perspectives on Animal Health and Sustainable Agriculture. First Edition.
Edited by Pratik Subhash Gaikwad, Vivek Harishankar Shukla and Pintu Choudhary.

Companion Website: https://www.wiley.com/go/pratikgaikwad/onehealth

Index

a

Agricultural practices 8, 18
African Swine Fever (ASF) 162, 192, 258
AIDS 171
Animal diseases 5, 120–122
Animal health 5, 64, 72–73, 74, 94, 120, 121, 132–146
Animal rehabilitation 238
Animal welfare 5, 146–147, 213, 215, 243–244, 260, 261, 271, 272
Antibiotic 69–77, 138–139
Antimicrobial resistance (AMR) 5, 11, 12, 17, 19, 40–45, 63, 64, 69–77, 130–133, 138, 139, 176, 192, 218, 246, 261, 269, 271, 284, 291, 292, 295–298, 310–315
Aquaculture 7, 9
Artificial intelligence (AI) 5, 20, 48, 52, 140–141, 163, 244, 291, 297
Avian influenza 37, 38, 49, 162, 167, 168, 170, 171, 172, 186, 188, 189, 191

b

Biodiversity 140, 144, 210, 212, 218, 222, 260, 291, 292, 296
Biodiversity conservation 10, 140, 144, 210, 212, 218, 222, 291, 292, 296
Bioinformatics 230
Biosecurity 4, 5, 6, 7, 8, 11, 12, 135–137, 189, 216, 220, 259, 266
Biosensors 240–241
Biotechnology 5, 125–126
Blockchain technology 298
Bovine tuberculosis 184
Breeding programs 163
Brucellosis 6, 259

c

Cancer therapy 238
Centers for Disease Control and Prevention (CDC) 80, 192
Chikungunya Virus Disease (CHIKVD) 168, 170, 172, 173, 190
Cholera 143
Codex Alimentarius 260
Computed tomography (CT) Scans 232–233
COVID-19 5, 11, 17, 41, 42, 43, 52, 137, 167, 168, 172, 174, 175, 176, 180–182, 184, 185–190, 266, 267
Crimean–Congo Hemorrhagic Fever 174, 314, 316
Cultured meat 5, 164

d

Dengue 69–77, 140, 168, 172, 173, 189, 239
Diarrheal diseases 143
Disease surveillance 125–126, 134, 163, 210–211

e

EcoHealth 262–263, 268–269
Ecological medicine 216

One Health Integration: Global Perspectives on Animal Health and Sustainable Agriculture. First Edition.
Edited by Pratik Subhash Gaikwad, Vivek Harishankar Shukla and Pintu Choudhary.

Companion Website: https://www.wiley.com/go/pratikgaikwad/onehealth

Ecosystem health 8, 9, 15, 22
Ebola 47, 51, 137, 168, 170–172, 176, 183, 188, 189, 191
Environmental health 177–185
Environmental sustainability 8, 288, 292–293, 298
Epidemiology 41, 45, 47, 50, 134, 269, 271, 287, 296

f

Food and Agriculture Organization (FAO) 5, 15, 16, 17, 18, 19, 21, 35, 36, 38, 39, 43, 45, 50, 64, 69, 80, 192, 258–259, 265–266, 313, 317
Foodborne illnesses 142
Foodborne pathogens 173–174, 178
Food safety 120–121, 259–260, 272, 311, 313
Food security 5, 120–121, 164
Foot-and-mouth disease 162

g

Gene therapy 238–239
Genetic management 211–212
Genomic 5, 163
Genomic sequencing 50, 51, 52
GIS and remote sensing 213, 226
Global food security 5, 120–121, 164
Global Health 53, 133, 263–266, 285, 287, 291, 295, 296, 316, 318
Greenhouse 142, 151–152, 270

h

Habitat 140, 260, 270
Hendra Virus 188
Holistic approach 68–69
Hydatidosis 259
Human Health 63–80, 79, 82, 94, 106, 132–144
Human Metapneumovirus (hMPV) 174

i

Imaging techniques 231–233
Immunotherapy 238–239
Infectious diseases 11, 43, 63, 76, 82, 137
Integrated Disease Surveillance and Response (IDSR) 134
Integrated pest management 164
Interdisciplinary 284–296, 308–311, 316–318
Internet of Things (IoT) 140–141, 241
International Union for Conservation of Nature (IUCN) 261

l

Lactate meter 236
Laparoscopy 237
Laser surgery 237–238
Leishmaniasis 40, 47, 49
Livestock 5, 7, 8, 12, 132–133, 140–143, 148–149, 215, 216
Livestock farming 164, 243–246
Livestock management 243–246
Livestock systems 285, 292, 298
Livestock trade 258–259

m

Magnetic resonance imaging (MRI) 230
Machine learning 140–141, 243–246
Malaria 140, 173
Mastitis 136
Middle East Respiratory Syndrome (MERS) 189
Mitigation measures 148, 151–152
Monkeypox (Mpox) 167, 168, 172, 173, 189
MOOCs and online learning 318

n

Nanotechnology 239
National health systems 49
Neglected tropical diseases (NTDs) 47, 49
Neurodevelopmental disorders 144
Next-generation sequencing (NGS) 234, 298
Nipah Virus 174
Nontyphoidal Salmonella (NTSs) 174
Nuclear scintigraphy 233

o

Office International des Epizooties (OIE) 5, 13, 16–18, 192
One Health approach 63–80, 69, 176–193, 261–263, 266–269
One Health 2, 5, 13, 34, 41, 43, 45–48, 51, 122, 128–130, 162, 164, 217–221, 239, 247, 284–297, 308–318
One Health concept 43, 63
One Health Integration 47, 63
One Health Joint Plan of Action (OH-JPA) 261
One Health paradigm 64, 65, 67
One Health perspective 63–80
One Medicine concept 262
Oncology 238

p

Pathogen proliferation 143
Photodynamic therapy 238
Polymerase Chain Reaction (PCR) 233, 234
Precision agriculture 5, 140–141
Problem-based learning (PBL) 308, 311, 312
Public Health 2, 3, 35, 39, 43, 46, 47, 49, 50, 54, 63, 77–79, 82, 95, 128–130, 210, 218, 259, 268–271, 285, 287–292, 295, 296, 298
Poultry 12

r

Rabies 35–37, 168, 170, 180, 188, 259, 314, 316
Radiography (X-ray) 231–232
Remote sensing 140–141, 213–214, 226
Respiratory diseases 144
Rift Valley Fever (RVF) 168, 172, 188, 314, 316
Rinderpest 258
Rocky Mountain Spotted Fever 314, 316

s

Salmonella 142, 314
Salmonellosis 173–174
Schistosomiasis 47, 49
Severe Acute Respiratory Syndrome (SARS) 137, 168, 170, 172, 186, 189, 190, 266, 267
Simulations 308, 311, 312, 318
Smart feeders 247
Stem cell 238–239
Stewardship 71–72
Surgical robots 241–242
Surveillance 125, 163, 291, 293
Sustainability 5, 132, 148, 151, 261, 271–273
Sustainable agriculture 5, 120, 157–158
Swine Flu 172, 190

t

Teleconsultation 239–240
Telemedicine 239–242
Thoracoscopy 237–238
Toxicologic disease 76, 82
Transboundary disease 220–221, 258, 265

u

United Nations Environment Program (UNEP) 192
UNESCO 192
UNICEF 80, 19

v

Vector-borne diseases (VBDs) 140, 261, 270
Veterinary education 214–217, 220
Veterinary medicine 2, 210, 214–215, 217–221, 229
Veterinary Public Health (VPH) 259, 262, 275–269
Veterinary science 2, 3, 6, 15, 228–229, 287, 292, 293, 296, 309
Virtual reality (VR) 243

w

Wearable devices 240–241
West Nile Virus (WNV) 174, 185
Wildlife 3, 4, 9, 10, 13, 15, 20–22, 34, 39, 41, 44, 47, 49, 50, 52, 65–69, 83, 87, 95, 96, 103, 105, 108–111, 114, 116, 137, 185–190, 210–212, 219, 221, 258–261, 267, 270, 275, 276, 298, 309, 313–316

World Health Organization (WHO) 5, 15, 19, 21, 35, 36, 38, 41, 43, 45, 49, 52, 54, 55, 64, 69, 79, 80, 133, 176, 192, 313, 317
World Organisation for Animal Health (WOAH) 6, 12, 16, 17, 35, 36, 39, 42, 43, 45, 49, 54, 64, 69, 133, 192, 259–262, 265–268, 275, 313, 314

Z

Zoonoses 134, 258–260, 268–271
Zoonotic diseases 5, 39, 46, 63, 68–69, 137, 162–163, 184, 210–211, 218–221, 284, 285, 287, 289–293, 295, 297, 298, 308, 309, 313